CANCER AND CANCER CARE

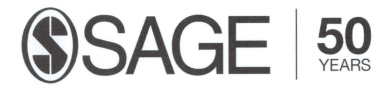

SAGE was founded in 1965 by Sara Miller McCune to support the dissemination of usable knowledge by publishing innovative and high-quality research and teaching content. Today, we publish more than 750 journals, including those of more than 300 learned societies, more than 800 new books per year, and a growing range of library products including archives, data, case studies, reports, conference highlights, and video. SAGE remains majority-owned by our founder, and after Sara's lifetime will become owned by a charitable trust that secures our continued independence.

Los Angeles | London | Washington DC | New Delhi | Singapore

CANCER AND CANCER CARE

EDITED BY
DEBBIE WYATT
NICHOLAS HULBERT-WILLIAMS

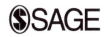

Los Angeles | London | New Delhi
Singapore | Washington DC

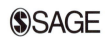

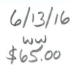

6/13/16
ww
$65.00

Los Angeles | London | New Delhi
Singapore | Washington DC

SAGE Publications Ltd
1 Oliver's Yard
55 City Road
London EC1Y 1SP

SAGE Publications Inc.
2455 Teller Road
Thousand Oaks, California 91320

SAGE Publications India Pvt Ltd
B 1/I 1 Mohan Cooperative Industrial Area
Mathura Road
New Delhi 110 044

SAGE Publications Asia-Pacific Pte Ltd
3 Church Street
#10-04 Samsung Hub
Singapore 049483

Editor: Becky Taylor
Associate editor: Emma Milman
Production editor: Katie Forsythe
Copyeditor: Sunrise Setting
Proofreader: Philippa Emler
Marketing manager: Camille Richmond
Cover design: Wendy Scott
Typeset by: C&M Digitals (P) Ltd, Chennai, India
Printed and bound by CPI Group (UK) Ltd,
Croydon, CR0 4YY

Library of Congress Control Number: 2014948548

British Library Cataloguing in Publication data

A catalogue record for this book is available from the British Library

ISBN 978-1-4462-5627-5
ISBN 978-1-4462-5628-2 (pbk)

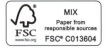

MIX
Paper from
responsible sources
FSC® C013604

At SAGE we take sustainability seriously. Most of our products are printed in the UK using FSC papers and boards. When we print overseas we ensure sustainable papers are used as measured by the Egmont grading system. We undertake an annual audit to monitor our sustainability.

CONTENTS

ABOUT THE EDITORS

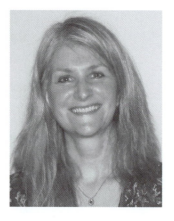

Debbie Wyatt is a Senior Lecturer in the Faculty of Health and Social Care at the University of Chester (UK) and Macmillan Lecturer/Head of Clinical Education at Clatterbridge Cancer Centre NHS Foundation Trust. She qualified as a Registered Nurse at Hammersmith Hospital in 1983 and following a variety of nursing posts moved into nurse education in 1987. She is an NMC registered Lecturer/Practice Educator, and has completed the ENB 237 Oncology Nursing Certificate and Diploma of Professional Studies in Nursing. She holds a BA (Hons) Health from Liverpool John Moores University and an MSc in Nursing from the Royal College of Nursing. Debbie also became an accredited facilitator for the National Cancer Action Team's Connected Advanced Communication Skills Training in 2009 and continues to facilitate communication skills courses for a range of healthcare professionals who work in cancer settings.

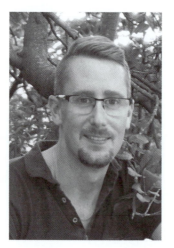

Nicholas Hulbert-Williams is a Coaching Psychologist and Reader in Psychology at the University of Chester (UK) where he is Director of the Chester Research Unit for the Psychology of Health (CRUPH). He holds an undergraduate degree in Psychology from the University of Wales, Bangor, and a PhD from Cardiff University School of Medicine. He is a Fellow of Higher Education Academy and Associate Fellow of the British Psychological Society. He is a member of the NCRI Psychosocial Oncology and Survivorship Clinical Studies Group, IPOS Research Committee and IPOS Early Career Professionals Committees, and was Chair of the British Psychosocial Oncology Society (BPOS) from 2010 to 2014. Nicholas is a member of the Professional Advisory Board (Research Group) for the Maggie Keswick Jencks Cancer Caring Centres Trust, and currently sits on the Editorial Board of the *European Journal of Cancer Care*.

LIST OF CONTRIBUTORS

Victoria Bates, *University of Liverpool, PhD*

Jacqueline Bloomfield, *The University of Sydney, PhD, MN, PGDip (Prof Healthcare Ed), BN*

Mary Boulton, *Oxford Brookes University, BA, PhD*

Hazel Brodie, *Director of Healthcare, 1854 Public Health, BSc, MPH, DFPH*

Leslie Bunt, *University of the West of England, MBE, BA, PGCert, PhD, LGSM (MT), FAMI, FRSA*

Christine Campbell, *University of Edinburgh, BSc (Hons), PhD, MPH*

Mark Cobb, *Sheffield Teaching Hospitals NHS Foundation Trust, BSc, MA, PhD*

Bill Culbard, *Stirling University, MA*

Alison Conner, *Vancouver Coastal Health, Registered Nurse (UK and Canada), MSc Health Sciences, PG Dip in CBT*

Maureen Deacon, *University of Chester, PhD*

Julie Fish, *Director of the Mary Seacole Reearch Centre, De Montfort University Leicester, PhD*

Samantha Flynn, *University of Chester, BSc*

Liz Forbat, *Australian Catholic University, BA (Hons), PG Cert, MSc, PhD*

Claire Foster, *University of Southampton, PhD, MSc, BSc, CPsychol*

George Foster, *Countess of Chester Hospital, MD FRCS*

Margaret Foulkes, *The Clatterbridge Cancer Centre NHS Foundation Trust, BA (Hons), MA, DASS, Home Office Letter of Recognition in Child Care*

Fiona Gibbs

Pat Gillis, *NIHR Clinical Research Network North West Coast, RGN*

Claire Green, *The Christie School of Oncology, PhD, MSc, BSc (Hons) and Adv Dip Counselling*

Anoop Haridass, *The Clatterbridge Cancer Centre NHS Foundation Trust, MSc MBBS MRCP FRCR*

Catherine Heaven, *The Christie School of Oncology*

Gill Hubbard, *University of Stirling, PhD, MSc, BA (Hons), PGCE*

Lee Hulbert-Williams, *University of Chester, BSc, MSc, PhD and AFBPsS*

Nicholas Hulbert-Williams, *University of Chester, BSc (Hons) PhD CPsychol AFBPsS*

Elise Hymanson, *The Christie NHS Foundation Trust, Specialty Doctor Psycho-Oncology, MBChB*

Mark R.D. Johnson, *De Montfort University Leicester, MA, PhD, DipHE*

Daniel Kelly, *Cardiff University, PhD, MSc, BSc, RN, PGCE*

Fiona Kennedy, *University of Leeds, BSc, MSc, PhD*

Alex King, *Imperial College Healthcare NHS Trust, BSc (Hons), MSc, DClinPsy*

Elaine Lennan, *Southampton University Hospitals NHS Trust*

Tina Lightfoot, *Countess of Chester Hospital NHS Foundation Trust, RGN, MS*

Paul Mackenzie, *MSc, BA (Hons), RN*

Paul Mansour, *Southport and Ormskirk Hospital NHS Trust, MBChB, FRCPath*

Ann Maloney, *Western Sussex Hospitals Trust*

Kathryn Mannix, *The Newcastle upon Tyne Hospitals NHS Foundation Trust, MB, BS, FRCP, PGCert, Fellow of BABCP*

Peter McAlear, *Glasgow Area Prostate Cancer Support Group, BEng, CEng, MIMechE*

Alex Mitchell, *Leicestershire Partnership NHS Trust and University of Leicester*

Fay Mitchell, *East Cheshire Hospice*

Helen Neville-Webbe, *The Clatterbridge Cancer Centre NHS Foundation Trust, MBCBH, MRCP, PhD*

Kate Parker, *The Clatterbridge Cancer Centre NHS Foundation Trust*

Ruth Sadik, *University of Chester*

Daniel Seddon, NHS England, *Public Health England, MBChB, MPH, MRCGP, FFPH, PGCert*

Lesley Storey, *Queen's University Belfast, PhD*

Brooke Swash, *University of Chester and University of Cambridge, MEd, BSc (Hons)*

Colin Thain, *University of Central Lancashire, Preston, MA (Hons), MSc, MA, PGDE (Nursing), RN, RNT, FHEA*

Irene Tuffrey-Wijne, *St George's University of London and Kingston University, PhD, RN*

Dale Vimalchandran, *Countess of Chester Hospital, MD, FRCS*

Eila Watson, *Oxford Brookes University, BSc (Hons), PhD*

Jan Woodhouse, *University of Chester, M Ed, PGDE, BN (Hons), DipN, RGN, OND, FETC*

David Wright, *Christie Hospital NHS Foundation Trust, Teenage Cancer Trust and TYAC, BA, BSc*

Debbie Wyatt, *University of Chester and Clatterbridge Cancer Centre NHS Foundation Trust, RGN, DPSN, BA (Hons), Certificate of Education for Nurse Teachers, RNT, MSc*

Emma Whitby, *The Clatterbridge Cancer Centre NHS Foundation Trust, BSc*

FOREWORD

Nearly all health care professionals will come across a person with cancer either in their professional or non-professional lives and by 2030 there will be more than four million people living with a diagnosis of cancer. Nearly half of the population can expect to have cancer during their lifetime; many do not realise how cancer has changed. For some cancers, the majority of patients can expect to live decades after treatment but a significant minority may have unmet needs related to ongoing effects of their treatment; others may live many months or years with incurable but treatable cancer and still others may die within a few months of diagnosis. A holistic approach to treatment and care can make all the difference. We welcome the publication of a book which recognises the importance of understanding cancer in the context of prevailing attitudes as well as how to personalise care for each patient.

Professor Jane Maher, Joint Chief Medical Officer, Macmillan Cancer Support

Cancer is a major cause of mortality and morbidity across the globe. Despite many advances in prevention, screening, detection and treatment, the incidence of cancer is still rising as the population ages, and while some cancers have high cure rates, others are associated with high mortality rates. As treatments improve, the number of people living with cancer, coping with long-term side effects and managing the risk of cancer recurrence is growing. Thus this disease continues to be a major challenge to patients, families, health professionals and healthcare systems.

Cancer is a complex disease that often requires multimodal therapy and the involvement of many different health professionals. Therefore, the multidisciplinary and holistic focus of this book is particularly appropriate and welcome. Decision-making in cancer increasingly involves a multidisciplinary team who meet together and discuss all relevant options, before formulating and presenting a clear recommendation to the patient and family. The optimal combination and timing of treatments often vary from patient to patient. Thus it is critical to have all perspectives, including those of the patient and family, who bring their own values, beliefs, circumstances and goals to the table.

The editors have carefully included chapters on both the physical and psychosocial aspects of the disease, its treatment and care because these aspects are inextricably interleaved in the patient and family experience. For example, patients with worse side effects are known to be at greater risk of anxiety and depression. Conversely high levels of distress can increase the use of pain medication, lengthen hospital stays and increase re-hospitalization rates.

The International Psycho-Oncology Society has set a standard of care that involves monitoring distress as the 6th vital sign, along with temperature, respiration, heart rate, blood pressure and pain. The high rate of distress in cancer patients and family members is well recognized. Patients and their families can be challenged by the stress of diagnosis, the immediate consequences of treatment such as pain, disfigurement and fatigue, existential questions and fear of cancer recurrence, changes to body image, difficulties with sexuality, loss of fertility and interpersonal problems. Thus, psychosocial care is now recognized as an integral part of quality cancer care, and the book includes several chapters discussing different approaches to such care.

Another excellent aspect of this book is its focus on vulnerable and special populations who may need specific care, and can present particular challenges to healthcare staff. These include patients with intellectual disability and mental health issues. Within a busy cancer clinic, these people can cause disruption and confusion if staff do not understand their specific needs and how to ensure they receive appropriate care. The book provides a very helpful perspective on these issues.

In sum, I believe that *Cancer and Cancer Care* will be an invaluable text on cancer for health professionals, researchers and policy makers. The editors have amassed a very expert group of contributors writing on this topic and providing a truly holistic and multidisciplinary view of cancer care.

Phyllis Butow, PhD

Professor and NHMRC Senior Principal Research Fellow, University of Sydney

Centre for Medical Psychology and Evidence-based Decision-making (CeMPED),

Chair, Psycho-Oncology Co-operative Research Group (PoCoG)

PREFACE AND ACKNOWLEDGEMENTS

As a leading cause of morbidity and mortality, cancer continues to be high on the national and global agenda. The impact of the disease and its treatments on individuals cannot be underestimated; cancer has a profound effect on many dimensions of a person's life, including their physical health and their psychological and social wellbeing.

In putting *Cancer and Cancer Care* together we aimed to take an holistic perspective and we purposively emphasize throughout the inter-relationship between biological and psychosocial aspects of the illness experience. Chapters cover fundamental aspects of cancer diagnosis, treatment, survival and aspects of psychosocial support for those affected by cancer. Specialist chapters also focus on the unique challenges of providing cancer care to populations with particular needs, including older adults, children and young people, those with intellectual disabilities and those with mental health problems. The importance of practice is a strong feature of the book, with each chapter illustrating the relevance of the topic to practice. We believe that it is only in taking this holistic, multiprofessional perspective to understanding cancer and its impact that we can provide the best possible cancer care for our patients and those close to them.

Because of the interconnection between the physical and psychosocial, we haven't organized our textbook in formal sections. Rather, we've ordered chapters in a way that (we hope) builds our readers' knowledge from the basics of carcinogenesis and important aspects of diagnosis, risks, screening and detection (Chapters 1–5); through chapters on specific population considerations (Chapter 6–10) and cancer treatments (Chapters 11–16); into a more detailed exploration of psychosocial and survivorship issues for people affected by cancer (Chapters 17–31). We finish with two chapters on research methods in cancer care: one focusing on clinical drug trials, and another on integrating psychosocial perspectives into cancer care research (Chapters 32–33). Readers may engage with the book in its entirety or use it as a reference point or supplementary reading to provide an introduction to any of these specific aspects relating to cancer care.

The book is written from a multidisciplinary perspective and we are delighted to include chapters written by leading experts, practitioners and researchers across the spectrum of subdisciplines within cancer care. We designed the book to be of interest to a wide range of readers, including health and social care practitioners undertaking post-registration oncology education, who may be new to some of the included topics; qualified health and social care practitioners who work with people with cancer (and their families), who may wish to use the book as a resource to refresh their clinical knowledge and skills; managers and commissioners of cancer services, who can consult the book for the latest theoretical and empirical evidence base for cancer care needs and best-practice standards; and researchers who are involved in work with people affected by cancer and their carers, particularly those researching in the field of psychosocial oncology who may lack the biological understanding of a core healthcare practitioner. Whatever reason you've had to pick up this book, we hope that it will provide you with a comprehensive and useful resource to understanding the key factors that influence cancer care, and that you'll be able to use this to positively impact on the experience of those affected by the disease and its treatments.

Undertaking editorship of a textbook of this size and scope was never going to be easy but we are very much in debt to a wonderfully supportive group of people who made the job much easier than it otherwise could have been. We would like to acknowledge the efforts of all of the contributors who have worked with us over the past two years, and who have so eloquently put all of their years of training, experience and expertise into the chapters that follow. We've had some extremely helpful feedback from four anonymous peer reviewers early in the process – thank you for your time, wise words and advice. To the team at Sage – especially Becky Taylor, Emma Milman and Katie Forsythe who have supported this project from its earliest conception – we are grateful for the expertise and encouragement that you've shown to get us to the point of publication. And last, but most certainly not least, we thank our families for the support, patience and forbearance that you've offered whilst we worked on this textbook; we promise not to start another one again *too* soon!

Debbie Wyatt and Nicholas Hulbert-Williams

PUBLISHER'S ACKNOWLEDGEMENTS

The authors and publisher would like to thank the following for their kind permission to republish material:

Figure 3.2 is reprinted from Macmillan Publisher Ltd on behalf of Cancer Research UK: *British Journal of Cancer,* 101(s2): S1-4, copyright (2009).

Table 3.2 is from National Cancer Intelligence Network (2012b) *Routes to Diagnosis.* 2006–2008 NCIN Information Supplement available from: www.ncin.org.uk/publications/routes_to_diagnosis.aspx Republished with permission of National Cancer Intelligence Network (NCIN).

Tables 3.3 and 3.4 are reprinted by permission from Macmillian Publishers Ltd on behalf of Cancer Research UK: *British Journal of Cancer,* 101, S80–S86, copyright (2009).

The example poster: the cough campaign in Chapter 3 is Crown Copyright.

The box in chapter 5 Modified Bloom-Richardson grading of breast carcinoma: Nottingham criteria is reproduced from 'Breast Cancer Grading: Nottingham Criteria' (2005), a publication of the National Office of the NHS Cancer Screening Programmes (operated by Public Health England), with permission.

Table 12.2 Karnofsky scale is republished with permission of John Wiley and Sons. The Zubrod scale is republished with permission of Wolters Kluwer Health.

Figure 13.2 Isodose Distribution is available from: www.jacmp.org/index.php/jacmp/article/view/2060/1216. Republished under a Creative Commons Attribution license.

The patients at East Cheshire Hospice for their permission to republish image in Chapter 26.

1 CANCER IN CONTEXT

DEBBIE WYATT, BROOKE SWASH AND NICHOLAS HULBERT-WILLIAMS

Chapter outline

- Morbidity, mortality and survival
- Lay and professional attitudes to cancer
- Stigma of cancer
- Impact of the media
- Potential impact of lay and professional attitudes to cancer on psychological wellbeing
- Key Government reports
- Relevance of the context of cancer to practice

INTRODUCTION

As a leading cause of morbidity and mortality in the UK (Cancer Research UK, 2014a) and worldwide (Cancer Research UK et al., 2014), cancer continues to have a significant impact on the health of the population and thus remains high on national and global agendas. The effect of cancer and its treatments on those affected by the disease is multidimensional, influencing a person's physical, psychological, social and spiritual wellbeing. Even in the absence of physical symptoms, affected individuals may experience the additional burden of fear, anxiety and depression as a result of negative attitudes towards the disease. Whilst cancer is responsible for significant morbidity and mortality worldwide, myths surrounding cancer and cancer treatments do not reflect improvements in treatment and survival. The high national profile is evident in a range of White Papers, which aim to identify strategies for improvements in prevention, treatment, organization and management of care. It is important for healthcare professionals to be aware of the psychological impact that attitudes to cancer can have on those affected by the disease in order to positively influence the patient and carer experience.

MORBIDITY AND MORTALITY ASSOCIATED WITH CANCER

Although age-standardized **mortality rates** continue to fall, cancers accounted for 29% of all deaths in England and Wales in 2012 (Office for National Statistics, 2013a). In the UK, prostate, lung, breast and bowel cancers account for more than half of all cancers (53%) and almost half of all cancer deaths (46%) (Cancer Research UK, 2014a). This is similar to the global pattern in which the four most common cancers (40% of all cancers) are lung, breast, colorectal and stomach with lung, liver, stomach and bowel cancers accounting for more than half of cancer deaths (Cancer Research UK et al., 2014).

Cancer is a leading cause of death in other economically developed countries where the incidence is also increasing (International Agency for Research on Cancer, 2014). In the UK, 1 in 3 people are expected to develop the disease, and 1 in 4 to die from it (Cancer Research UK, 2014a); these rates are expected to worsen over coming years. In the UK, cancer incidence has increased by more than a third since the mid-1970s (23% males, 43% females) (Cancer Research UK, 2014b). More than two million people in the UK currently have, or have had cancer and this figure is expected to rise to four million by 2030 (Department of Health, 2010b). Current figures estimate that there were approximately 331,000 new cases of cancer (excluding non-melanoma skin cancer) diagnosed in the UK in 2011 (Cancer Research UK, 2014b) and that someone in the UK is diagnosed with cancer every two minutes (Cancer Research UK, 2014c).

THE COMMON CANCERS: BREAST, PROSTATE, LUNG AND BOWEL CANCER

The four **most common cancers** in the UK are breast, bowel, lung and prostate (Cancer Research UK, 2014c). In 2011, breast cancer was the most commonly diagnosed cancer in all persons in the UK, accounting for 15% of the general population incidence (Cancer Research UK, 2014a). Despite it being much more common in women (1 in 8 risk), accounting for 30% of all female cancer incidence, it accounts for only 15% of all female cancer deaths (Cancer Research UK, 2014a).

Lung cancer was the second most common cancer in males and females combined, with 14% incidence in males and 12% in females (Cancer Research UK, 2014a). However, it was the leading cause of mortality, accounting for 22% of all cancer deaths: 23% in men and 21% in women. The rates between the genders are very close, yet Cancer Research UK (2014a) suggests that male mortality rates have fallen to their lowest in forty years, whereas female rates have continued increasing. A large explanatory factor in this is thought to be the increase in female smoking, although the impact of changes in smoking-related UK legislature in recent years are yet to be seen in their full extent.

The third most common cancer in all persons is prostate cancer (13%), although it remains the leading cause of cancer in men (25%) (Cancer Research UK, 2014a). Prostate cancer, being a male-only cancer, is the fourth most common cause of cancer death at 7% when viewed with both sexes combined and is the second most common cause of cancer death in men (13%) (Cancer Research UK, 2014a).

Bowel cancer is the fourth most commonly reported cancer, accounting for 13% of all incidences within the general population, with 14% being diagnosed in men and 11% in women. Incidences are more likely to be in adults over 60 years of age, with cases peaking between 70 and 79 years for men and 85 years onwards for women. By 2011, it had become the second most common cause (10%) of cancer death, accounting for 10% for men and 9% for women cancer deaths in the UK (Cancer Research UK, 2014a).

The 10 most common cancers for males and females in the UK are shown in Table 1.1.

Table 1.1 Ten most common cancers UK 2011

Males		Females	
Prostate	25%	Breast	30%
Lung	14%	Lung	12%
Bowel	14%	Bowel	11%
Bladder	4%	Uterus	5%
Non-Hodgkin lymphoma	4%	Ovary	4%
Malignant melanoma	4%	Malignant melanoma	4%
Kidney	4%	Non-Hodgkin lymphoma	4%
Oesophagus	3%	Brain tumour	3%
Leukaemia	3%	Pancreas	3%
Brain tumour	3%	Kidney	2%
Other sites	23%	Other sites	23%

Source: Cancer Research UK, 2014a.

The **less common cancers** make up approximately 57.5% of all diagnoses (Ferlay et al., 2013) and so are of significant interest. Some of these less common cancers are detailed in the next section.

THE LESS COMMON CANCERS

Head and neck cancers

Head and neck cancers include those arising from the mouth, larynx, pharynx, salivary glands and local structures (International Agency for Research on Cancer, 2014). In total, there are over thirty places for the cancer to be located but around 90% originate in the cells that line the mouth, throat, nose or ear. UK head and neck cancer incidence has not been well profiled (Doobaree et al., 2009); however, The National Head and Neck Cancer audit 2011 (Health and Social Care Information Centre, 2012) reported an incidence of approximately 8100 new cases of head and neck cancers a year (Office for National Statistics, 2011). There is some variation according to anatomical site. Laryngeal cancer, for example, is the fourteenth most common cancer in men with an estimated 157,000 cases worldwide in 2012, but is much less common in women. The incidence of cancers of the lip, oral cavity and pharynx combined, however, are the seventh most common type of cancer with 529,000 new cases in 2012 (International Agency for Research on Cancer, 2014). Smoking tobacco is one of the main causes of head and neck cancers and this, in combination with alcohol consumption, multiplies the risk (International Agency for Research on Cancer, 2014). The symptoms most commonly observed in head and

Brain and central nervous system cancers

This category includes cancers in any part of the brain or the central nervous system (CNS), including the spinal cord. Tumours that originate in the brain are known as primary brain tumours and are more common than cancers of the CNS. Figures from 2011 indicate that CNS and intracranial tumours account for 2.8% of all cancers in the UK, placing it the ninth most common cancer (Cancer Research UK, 2014k). In the UK, around 57% of tumours occur in people aged 65 or less. In 2011, relatively equal numbers of men and women developed a CNS, brain or intracranial tumour (around 4700 men and 4700 women) (Cancer Research UK, 2014l). Symptoms are dependent upon the size and the location of the tumour: those in the frontal lobe of the brain may cause mood disturbances, confusion, disorientation or difficulty concentrating; those in the parietal lobe may cause seizures, numbness, difficulty with handwriting or mathematical calculations and movement difficulties; those in the occipital lobe can affect vision, cause visual hallucinations and seizures; and, finally, those in the temporal lobe cause problems with perception and spatial awareness or difficulty comprehending complex instructions. Frequent headaches may also be present as the growing tumour causes pressure within the skull (Deorah et al., 2006). Survival with these types of cancer is improving, with 4 in 10 surviving one year (compared to 2 in 10 in the 1970s); however, age at diagnosis makes a significant difference to likely outcome. Five-year survival is more than 50% in those aged 15–39 compared to 2% in people diagnosed in their 70s (Cancer Research UK, 2014l). Recurrence is rare outside the CNS and, where it does re-occur, it is generally within this system.

LIFESPAN AND CANCER

There are over 200 different types of cancer but the **incidence** of different tumour types varies across the **lifespan**.

Children and young people

Cancer can occur at any age, but less than 1% of new cancer cases per year occur in children aged 0–14 years (Cancer Research UK, 2014a). Leukaemia is the most common form of childhood cancer and, along with lymphomas, brain and CNS cancers, accounts for more than two-thirds of childhood incidence (Cancer Research UK, 2014m). In the UK, childhood cancer rates have increased over the past forty years, although this is likely to be due to better diagnostic interventions and reporting methods. That said, childhood cancer survival rates have doubled, with three-quarters now being cured when compared to figures from the 1960s. Approximately 1 in 500 children are expected to develop cancer by the time they reach 14 years of age (Cancer Research UK, 2014m). Cancer is also uncommon in young adults, with less than 1% of all cancer diagnoses occurring within the 16–24 year age group (Cancer Research UK, 2014n). The pattern of cancers in this age group changes and more than half comprise lymphomas, carcinomas and germ cell tumours, such as testicular cancer (Cancer Research UK, 2104n). For further details about cancer in children, teenagers and young adults, please refer to Chapter 6.

Adults

The longer a person lives, the higher the risk of them developing cancer. The adult population (25–49 years old) accounted for 10% of cancer incidence, with the most common cancers being breast, malignant melanoma, testes, bowel and cervical cancer (Cancer Research UK, 2014b). There were twice as many cancer diagnoses for females than males between 2009 and 2011 (Cancer Research UK, 2014a). It is likely that this figure is significantly increased in women because of the high incidence rates of breast cancer (Cancer Research UK, 2014a). When sex-specific cancers are controlled for, males were at higher risk of getting cancer than women (White et al., 2009). The highest incidence of cancers occurs in older adulthood (50–74 years old), with 53% of cancers diagnosed in this age group; however, mortality is 44% (Cancer Research UK, 2014a). The most commonly reported diagnoses are breast, lung, bowel and prostate cancer in both the 50–74 age group and elderly aged over 75 years. More than one-third of all cancers are diagnosed in the over 75 age group, with mortality rising to 52% (Cancer Research UK, 2014a). Particular considerations for older adults with cancer are explored in Chapter 7.

The **high national profile** is reflected in a range of White Papers that aim to both identify strategies for prevention and to positively influence the experiences of those affected by cancer through approaches to treatment, organization and management of care. *The Health of the Nation* (DH, 1992), for example, identified cancer as one of five priority areas (coronary heart disease and stroke; cancers; accidents; mental illness; and HIV/AIDs and sexual health) in the first national policy, which aimed to improve the health of the population of England.

Each of the four UK nations have cancer plans (DH, 2011a; Scottish Government, 2008b; Department of Health, Social Services and Public Safety, 2008a; Welsh Government, 2012) that aim to direct improvements in patient outcomes, such as cancer prevention, diagnosis, treatment and support, although each plan is unique and has different timescales (Cancer Research UK, 2014o).

A summary of key reports can be seen in Table 1.2.

Table 1.2 Summary of key cancer reports

Report title	Date	Summary
A Policy Framework for Commissioning Cancer Services	Department of Health, 1995	The expert advisory group on cancer produced a policy framework for commissioning cancer services that aimed to outline the direction of cancer care in **England and Wales** to ensure that all people with cancer had access to a uniformly high standard of care.
		Made recommendation for a new structure for cancer services based on networks of expertise in primary care, cancer units in district hospitals and in specialized cancer centres.

(Continued)

Your list may well have included words such as **death, fear and suffering**, or treatment-related problems such as nausea and hair loss. Cancer continues to be associated with these **negative perceptions** (Kearney et al., 2003; Rowa-Dewar, Kearney, Seaman, 2007; WHO and International Agency for Research on Cancer, 2008; Wyatt and Talbot, 2013) and is considered by the British public to be the number one health priority, over and above any other diseases (Ipsos MORI for Cancerbackup, 2006), and the top priority for the NHS (Featherstone and Whitham, 2010). More than a third of respondents in a survey commissioned by Cancer Research UK (2011) indicated that cancer was the disease they most feared:

> 'cancer is the number one fear for the British public ahead of debt, knife crime, Alzheimers Disease and losing a job' (Cancer Research UK, 2014b: 1)

Individual **attitudes** towards cancer may vary but particular groups such as men and those with lower levels of knowledge and educational attainment are more likely to hold negative attitudes towards cancer and cancer prevention than others (Keeney et al., 2010). Fatalistic attitudes towards cancer are linked to negative attitudes towards early detection and cancer prevention (Schernhammer et al., 2010; Beeken et al., 2011; Befort et al., 2013) and may be more strongly held amongst different cultural groups (Dein, 2005; Saleh et al., 2012; Karbani et al., 2011; Cho et al., 2013).

People with a cancer diagnosis and their carers are confronted with **distressing emotions**, such as fear of death, uncertainty about the future and loss of control over their lives (International Agency for Research on Cancer, 2008; Macmillan Cancer Support, 2011b) but the **stigma** of cancer imposes an additional burden on those affected by the disease (Mosher and Danoff-Burg, 2007; Ferrell and Coyle, 2006). A study by Cataldo et al. (2012), for example, found a positive relationship between lung cancer and depression and an inverse relationship between lung cancer and quality of life. They supported the premise that perceived stigma among people with lung cancer, whether they smoked or not, can lead to negative outcomes such as depression and reduced quality of life.

Fears may relate to **perceptions** around death and dying, perceived limited effectiveness of treatments, disfigurement and symptoms. Furthermore, fear of cancer recurrence is also a commonly reported problem (Befort et al., 2013; Thewes et al., 2011; Taylor S. et al., 2011; Hodges and Humphries, 2009; Skaali et al., 2009). People receiving cancer treatments can, and do, experience side effects, such as nausea, vomiting or hair loss; however, the common misperception that these symptoms are universal can cause additional anguish. Changes in physical appearance, such as weight loss associated with cancer cachexia (Hinsley and Hughes, 2007) and hair loss resulting from chemotherapy treatment (Power and Condon, 2008; Roe, 2011), provide visible cues of a person's cancer or treatment (Harcourt and Frith, 2008) and serve as a reminder of the potential seriousness of the condition.

In addition to fear, diagnosis of a life-threatening illness such as cancer can induce a range of reactions, including anxiety, depression, uncertainty and apprehension (Byrne et al., 2002; Ryan et al., 2005; Saegrov and Halding, 2004; Macmillan Cancer Support, 2011b). **Psychological morbidity** can be particularly prominent at transition points such as diagnosis and commencing or undergoing treatment, although for some, the psychological trauma may even extend into the 'survivorship' phase (International Agency for Research on Cancer, 2008) and lead to post-traumatic stress disorder (Bush, 2009).

The psychosocial impact of cancer and its treatment extends to the **whole family** (Dobbie and Mellor, 2008; International Agency for Research on Cancer, 2008), who not only have their own fears and worries to contend with but who are also expected to support the patient. Caring for a person with cancer can significantly affect the emotional wellbeing and mental health, social lives, relationships and working lives of carers (Cardy, 2006; Macmillan Cancer Support, 2011a). Treatment can also take an emotional and social toll, leading to labile emotions, lack of concentration, altered relationships with family and friends, relationship difficulties, sexual problems, difficulties at work, inability to work and financial hardship (International Agency for Research on Cancer, 2008; Macmillan Cancer Support, 2011b). Patients report difficulties returning to work due to the attitudes of employers and line managers who, although positive about employees returning to work, can hold fearful attitudes towards employees with a cancer diagnosis (Amir et al., 2010).

Psychosocial aspects of cancer will be discussed throughout this textbook; however, an in-depth exploration of some of the primary considerations can be found in Chapters 17 to 31. An awareness that these are not discreet topics and should be considered at all stages of cancer diagnosis and treatment is important, and these impacts should also be considered central to the first few chapters, which focus more predominantly on the medical aspects of cancer care.

Reflective activity

With reference to your own practice, list patients' reactions to

- Their cancer diagnosis
- Their cancer treatment

Describe how this compares to the reactions of their family/friends. Reflect on the implications of these reactions for

- Patients
- Families
- Healthcare professionals

HEALTHCARE PROFESSIONALS' ATTITUDES TO CANCER

The attitudes of healthcare professionals to cancer mirror those of the general public. Nurses working in the community, for example, report cancer as a terrifying disease, dreaded personal diagnosis and perceived limited effectiveness of treatments (Box and Anderson, 1997). In comparison, medical and surgical nurses in a district general hospital in Northern Ireland generally held positive attitudes to cancer, although some, due to deaths of family and friends, were ambivalent about the benefits of treatments (McCaughan and Parahoo, 2000). In contrast, a study of oncology healthcare professionals found that all professional groups revealed persistently negative attitudes towards cancer, regardless of demographics such as gender, profession and clinical experience (Kearney et al., 2003). The beliefs and attitudes of nurses and other healthcare professionals have implications for practice because negative attitudes may be unconsciously conveyed to patients and their families. Healthcare professionals need to understand that people affected by cancer (patients, their families, even other colleagues working in cancer care) may all have different fears, knowledge, perceptions and misperceptions requiring individual assessment and tailored interventions to adequately meet their needs.

WHY MAY CANCER BE ASSOCIATED WITH DEATH AND SUFFERING?

In addition to statistical evidence regarding cancer mortality, there are a number of reasons why cancer, more than other diseases, may be associated with death and suffering:

- Historical context
- Lack of knowledge and understanding
- Media

Cancer through history

Throughout history and up until relatively recently, the outcomes for those with cancer have been poor, with the few treatment options available associated with poor success and major side effects. Surgery, for example, which has been used to treat cancer for centuries, has been associated with high mortality risk and serious complications such as pain, disfigurement and infection (Cancer Research UK, 2014p). It is only in the latter part of the twentieth century that advances in surgical procedures, sometimes in combination with other therapies, have minimized harm and maximized effectiveness of surgical treatments (American Cancer Society, 2014b) (see also Chapter 11). Despite some misperceptions that surgery can hasten the spread of the disease (James et al., 2011; Lord et al., 2012), surgery is now one of the main treatments for cancer (Cancer Research UK, 2014p; WHO and International Agency for Research on Cancer, 2008) and for many, offers the greatest chance of cure (American Cancer Society, 2014a).

Other modalities have been developed more recently. For example, radiotherapy was introduced in the late nineteenth century and chemotherapy in the 1940s, but short- and long-term side effects were severe. Success associated with these modalities has improved over the years, with fewer side effects and improved approaches to managing them, but despite advances made, the experience can be frightening and the side effects remain problematic for some individuals. Developments in cancer treatments and in multimodal approaches have seen significant improvements, particularly with increased knowledge about the molecular biology and the genetic basis of tumours and how this may be used to personalize and target treatments for individuals (International Agency for Research on Cancer, 2014). For some, premature death will be a reality, but others will live many years with the disease or even remain disease free (International Agency for Research on Cancer, 2008).

Lack of knowledge and understanding

Although there have been advances in knowledge and understanding about risk factors for cancer and the development of the disease, there is still much that is unknown. This lack of knowledge may make cancer difficult to conceptualize. It is known, for example, that lifestyle risk factors for cardiovascular disease – a leading cause of morbidity and mortality – are strongly linked to smoking, alcohol, lack of exercise and poor diet (British Heart Foundation, 2012). Reducing these risk factors both before and after cardiac episodes, such as a heart attack, are likely to reduce the chance of such an event occurring again. Cancers are influenced by some of the same lifestyle risk factors (WHO and International Agency for Research on Cancer, 2008), but the evidence to support making lifestyle changes in preventing cancer recurrence is less well established (see Chapter 24).

Media

The media perpetuate the stigma of cancer by associating the disease with death, fear and suffering and by using powerful metaphors that convey frightening messages.

Reflective activity

As you read, watch and listen to media reports about cancer, reflect on the words and metaphors used, and the messages they convey. You may notice the use of such words as 'killer', 'gruelling', 'aggressive' and 'terrifying', for example, that conjure unpleasant images of how cancer affects individuals, or terms related to war, such as 'battle' and 'fight'.

The media could play a vital role in disseminating information about prevention, diagnosis and treatment of cancer, yet coverage tends to focus on personal stories rather than health promotion (Hilton and Hunt, 2010). Partnerships between healthcare professionals and journalists could help to use the media to enhance awareness of cancer and health-seeking behaviours and lessen the stigma of cancer (Williamson, Jones and Hockey, 2011). Instead, such imagery and metaphors perpetuate the myths that death from cancer is inevitable and that treatments are unpleasant. This contrasts to reality that half of the people diagnosed with cancer in England and Wales in 2010–2011 are predicted to be alive ten years after their diagnosis (46% men and 54% women) and either living with their disease or in complete remission (Cancer Research UK, 2014q).

RELEVANCE OF ATTITUDES TO CANCER ON PRACTICE

It is important for healthcare professionals to be mindful of attitudes to cancer because negative perceptions can provoke an array of distressing psychosocial reactions in patients and families. Healthcare professionals can positively influence the patient/carer experience by dispelling any misunderstandings, establishing what impact the cancer diagnosis and treatment will have on each patient and their close family members, and by supporting them with their individual concerns. An awareness of potential psychological distress can prepare healthcare professionals to respond sensitively and effectively to the emotional reactions of those affected by a cancer diagnosis. For example, Stajduhar, Thorne, McGuinness and Kim-Sing (2010) found that acknowledging the fear associated with cancer is helpful to people and highlight that effective communication in facilitating patients' expression of their fears is supportive.

Changing people's behaviour towards cancer requires understanding their beliefs and the factors that influence them (Schernhammer et al., 2010). Negative attitudes of healthcare professionals may create barriers to communication and good quality care (Purandare, 1997), hence the need for cancer care professionals to deal with their own attitudes in case they convey negative non-verbal cues. Good communication is appreciated to be key to delivering high quality cancer care (DH, 2007a; see also Chapter 17).

Key learning points

- Cancer is often associated with death and dying.
- Negative perceptions of cancer can lead to psychological distress such as anxiety and depression.
- Cancer diagnosis and treatment can have a negative psychological and social impact on the lives of patients and families.
- 1 in 3 people in the UK are expected to develop cancer in their lifetime but trends indicate a reduction in mortality and improvements in survival.
- Approaches to prevention, treatment and support are detailed in Government strategies, approaches and targets.
- Healthcare professionals need to establish what impact the cancer diagnosis and treatment have on each patient and their close family members.

Recommended further reading

- International Agency for Research on Cancer. (2014) *World Cancer Report 2014.* Geneva: World Health Organization Press.
- Department of Health, Macmillan Cancer Support and NHS Improvement. (2013) *Living with & Beyond Cancer: Taking Action to Improve Outcomes* (an update to the 2010 The National Cancer Survivorship Initiative Vision). London: NCSI.
- For up-to-date information on cancer incidence, mortality and survival, access the Cancer Research UK website at www.cancerresearchuk.org

2 CANCER RISK AND SCREENING

CHRISTINE CAMPBELL

Chapter outline

- Cancer risk and lifetime risk of most common cancers
- Main risk factors for developing cancer, including genetic risk and lifestyle factors
- Primary and secondary prevention strategies to modify cancer risk
- Effective communication of cancer risk

- Purpose and principles of screening and selected screening terminology
- Current screening programmes in the UK
- Barriers to participation in screening and the importance of informed choice

---

INTRODUCTION

The aim of this chapter is to introduce the reader to concepts relating to the risk of developing cancer and to issues in cancer screening. Cancer screening has an important role in any national strategy to reduce cancer-related mortality. The majority of cancers present symptomatically and, therefore, evidence-based and adequately resourced pathways to diagnosis are essential within the health service. Additionally, effective cancer screening programmes can raise awareness of a particular cancer and associated symptoms, drive improvements in treatment options, and contribute to detection and treatment of early stage disease.

CANCER RISK

What is risk, and how is it quantified?

Within healthcare, risk is the probability of the occurrence of a future adverse event such as death, disease, or a complication of disease. In terms of cancer, the term risk is employed to describe the likelihood of developing or dying from cancer. **Lifetime risk** is a commonly used term, and refers to the likelihood of a person developing cancer in their lifetime (either from birth or during a specified age span): estimates of lifetime risk are usually expressed as the odds of developing cancer ('1 in x') or as a percentage (Cancer Research UK, 2014r; Sasieni et al., 2011).

Risk of developing cancer

The risk of an individual developing cancer is affected by many factors including **genetic** and **lifestyle**, some of which are outlined later. It is estimated that over 1 in 3 people in the UK will be diagnosed with at least one type of cancer during their life. The highest lifetime risks for men are prostate cancer (1 in 8), lung cancer and bowel cancer (both 1 in 14), while for women breast cancer (1 in 8), lung cancer (1 in 18) and bowel cancer (1 in 19) are the most common (Cancer Research UK, 2014r). Fifty-four percent of cancer incidence in the UK is due to cancers at only four sites: breast, lung, bowel and prostate.

CANCER RISK FACTORS

Age

Cancer is largely (though clearly not exclusively) a disease of older age. Although approximately 1 in 3 of the population will develop cancer at some point in their lifetime, over a third are in those aged over 75 years (Cancer Research UK, 2014r). With life expectancy continuing to increase in the UK, cancer in the elderly will become more common. However, cancer is also frequently diagnosed in those aged over 50 years, with 53% of cancers occurring in those aged 50–74 years, and prostate, lung and bowel cancer being most common in men, and breast, lung and bowel cancers being the most frequent in women (Cancer Research UK, 2014s). Screening for breast cancer in women and more recently for bowel cancer in both men and women contributes in part to the high incidence of these cancers in this age group. In adults aged between 25–49 years, breast cancer is by far the most common cancer (Cancer Research UK, 2014s). Cancer is relatively rare in teenagers and young adults (15–24 years), and among children (0–14 years), with less than 1% of total cancers in the UK diagnosed in each of these groups. Leukaemia is the most common childhood cancer (Stiller, 2007; Murphy et al., 2013).

Genetic

Although the majority of cancers are sporadic, a proportion of all common cancers have a familial component, for example between 5–10% of individuals with breast, colorectal or ovarian cancer will have a **family history** of first or second degree relatives with the same cancer, suggestive of an inherited predisposition (American Cancer Society, 2013). Approximately 1% of all cancers are associated with a **high-risk mutation** in one of a number of genes (Garber and Offit, 2005): some of these are associated with very rare familial cancer syndromes, others with common cancers, and many are associated with early onset of the cancer (often below the age of 40). An inherited predisposition to one cancer may also increase the risk of developing other cancers. **Mutations** in BRCA1 (associated with breast ovarian, bowel and prostate cancers) and **BRCA2** (associated with breast, ovarian, prostate and pancreatic cancers) are found in 1 in 850 and 1 in 500 individuals, respectively, although mutations in both are found in 1 in 100 of Ashkenazi Jews, and are also more common in those of African–American and Afro-Caribbean descent (Levy-Lahad and Friedman, 2007; Nelson et al., 2013). **Familial Adenomatis Polyposis** (FAP) accounts for just under 1% of new colorectal cancers, and is caused by mutations in the adenomatosis polyposis coli gene: this mutation has 100% penetrance (Galiatsatos and Foulkes, 2006). **Hereditary non-polyposis colorectal cancer** (HNPCC or Lynch syndrome) is associated with up to 5% of new colorectal cancer cases (Lynch et al., 2009). Specialist cancer genetics clinics provide support to individuals and families: assessing an individual's risk of developing cancer is complex, and has the potential to cause significant distress, including anxiety, depression, and poorer quality of life. Counselling recommendations emphasize the need to carry out a detailed psychosocial assessment, and contextualizing risk communication to the individual's life situation (Trepanier et al., 2004). Key areas relating to psychosocial and behavioural aspects of **genetic counselling** and testing for BRCA1/2 mutations, and for FAP, have been reviewed (Vadaparampil et al., 2006–2007; Douma et al., 2008).

Smoking

Over a quarter (28%) of all cancer deaths in the UK are linked with smoking and, as such, smoking is the single most avoidable risk factor for cancer (Sasco et al., 2004). Smoking is linked with 87% of male lung cancer deaths and 83% of female lung cancer deaths: 10% of these are from exposure to environmental tobacco smoke ('passive smoking') (Parkin et al., 2011; Jamrozik et al., 2005). The link with lung cancer is well established (Doll and Hill, 1950), but epidemiological evidence also demonstrates a link between tobacco consumption and a long list of other cancers, including those of the oral cavity (mouth, tongue and lips), nose and sinuses, the larynx and pharynx, oesophagus, stomach, pancreas, cervix, kidney, bladder and colorectal cancers, as well as some leukaemias (Parkin et al., 2011). Although cigarette smoking rates in the UK have fallen in both men and women in recent decades (Wald and Nicolaides-Bouman, 1991; Office for National Statistics, 2012), smoking prevalence is currently 21% in males and 20% in females, with a strong gradient by socio-demographic group, and by age group (less than 15% of those aged over 60 are current smokers). Globally, cigarette smoking is projected to contribute to cancer in up to 1000 million in the twenty-first century (World Health Organization (WHO), 2011).

Alcohol

Alcohol is one of the most well established causes of cancer, to the extent that it has been rated a 'Class 1' (i.e. the highest category) carcinogen since 1988 (International Agency for Research on Cancer, 1988). Alcohol is associated with 4% overall of cancers in the UK (Parkin et al., 2011). Upper aero-digestive tract cancers (the oral cavity, pharynx, larynx and oesophagus) have the highest alcohol-attributable levels (up to 30%), but even moderate drinking is associated with increased risk of breast and bowel cancer (Corrao et al., 2004; Key et al., 2006; Stickel et al., 2002). Liver cancer is linked to long-term alcohol use (Stickel et al., 2002).

Occupational exposures

It is estimated that over 13,500 cancers are caused in the UK each year due to occupational exposure to **carcinogens** (Parkin, 2011; Baan et al., 2009): this equates to 8% of male cancer deaths and 2% of cancer deaths in women. Occupational exposure to asbestos is attributed to between 80–97% of mesothelioma cases or deaths in men (Rushton et al., 2012) and is particularly common among those who worked in shipbuilding, construction or as carpenters. Lung cancer has also been linked to asbestos exposure, as well as to mineral oils, silica and radon amongst other carcinogens. Other cancers with an occupational link include bladder (e.g. exposure to paint, diesel fumes), larynx (exposure to asbestos), and liver (exposure to vinyl chloride) cancers (Boffetta et al., 2003; Parkin et al., 2011). Shift work has been linked to breast cancer (Megdal et al., 2005).

Infections

Globally, infections by **viruses** are estimated to contribute to 2 million new cancer cases each year (Boyle et al., 2003). The majority of these are in less developed regions of the world (de Martel et al., 2012): in the UK, 3% of new cancer cases per annum are linked to infections (Parkin et al., 2011). Persistent infection with the human papilloma virus (HPV) is a necessary step in the development of cervical cancer (Schiffman et al., 2007). Epstein–Barr virus (EBV) is related to around 45% of Hodgkin lymphomas in the UK; it is estimated that *Helicobactor pylori* infection is linked to just over 30% of stomach cancers in the UK, while approximately 16% of liver cancers were linked to infection with either hepatitis B virus (HBV) or hepatitis C virus (HCV) infection (compared to 85% of all liver cancer cases worldwide) (Parkin et al., 2011; Parkin, 2006). Kaposi's sarcoma is associated with HIV/AIDS (Antman and Chang, 2000).

Diet and body weight

Recent evidence suggests that over 17,000 cancers per year in the UK are linked to being **overweight** (body mass index (BMI) of 25–30) or **obese** (BMI ≥ 30) (Parkin and Boyd, 2011). These include postmenopausal breast cancer (up to 30% increased risk), and colon (particularly in men), endometrial, kidney, oesophagus, gallbladder and pancreas, with weaker evidence for a number of other cancers. Over 65% of men and over 55% of women in the UK are either overweight or obese; however, the links between body weight and cancer are complex and mechanisms of action are not yet fully understood. Body fat becomes an additional source of oestrogen, which increases the risk of selected cancers (Huang et al., 1997). The role of diet and nutrition in cancer causation is similarly complex – although up to 5% of cancers in the UK are estimated to be linked to low intake of fresh fruit and vegetables containing **antioxidants**, their protective effects are likely due to the interactive effect of many different chemicals. The World Cancer Research Fund estimates that about a third (38%) of 12 of the most common cancers in the UK could be prevented through improved diet, physical activity and body weight (World Cancer Research Fund, 2007).

Hormones

Both **endogenous** and **exogenous hormones** have been linked with increased cancer risk. In men, no link has been found between endogenous sex hormones and overall prostate cancer risk, but in women the risk of developing breast, ovarian and endometrial cancers is increased with early menarche and later menopause, and reduced with full-term pregnancy. The risk of breast cancer is reduced with breastfeeding. The risks of endometrial and ovarian cancers appear to be reduced with the use of oral contraceptives containing oestrogen and progesterone, whereas the risks of breast, cervical, and liver cancer appear to be increased (Burkman et al., 2004). Levels of these hormones differ by specific type and formulation of contraceptive, as does the associated risk. Oestrogen-only hormone replacement therapy is associated with a doubling of risk of uterine cancer after five years of use. For ovarian cancer the risk is increased by approximately 25%, which can be associated with use of the combined oestrogen and progesterone HRT (Pike et al., 2004; Lacey et al., 2002; Pearce et al., 2009).

Physical activity

Approximately 1% of cancers in the UK have been linked with physical inactivity, with consistent evidence now emerging that individuals with lower levels of physical activity have an increased risk of cancers independent of body weight. Physical activity seems to have a protective association with colon cancer in both men and women (Wolin et al., 2009), and with both breast and endometrial cancer in women (Moore et al., 2010; Wu et al., 2013).

Sunlight

The incidence rates of **malignant melanoma** have risen dramatically since the early 1970s and this increase is expected to continue for another two decades. Over 85% of new cases are linked to excess exposure to ultraviolet (UV) radiation, either through sunlight or use of sunbeds. Intermittent sun exposure to high-intensity sunlight resulting in sunburn episodes over a lifetime, and use of sunbeds at any age are both linked to increased melanoma risk (Cancer Research UK, 2014t; Cogliano et al., 2011; Parkin, Boyd and Walker, 2010).

MODIFICATION OF CANCER RISK: PRIMARY PREVENTION

Lifestyle measures

Prevention offers the most cost-effective long-term strategy for the control of cancer. **Prevention measures** are required and can be effective at both the individual and the population level (World Cancer Research Fund, 2007). There is good evidence that smoking cessation reduces an individual's risk of lung and other cancers, whilst at a national and global level the tobacco control measures in the World Health Organization Framework Convention on Tobacco Control seek to reduce the prevalence of tobacco use and exposure to tobacco smoke (WHO, 2003). Guidelines have been developed regarding optimal levels of fruits, vegetables and other foods from plant sources, such as whole grains and beans, use of fewer high-fat foods and recommendations on alcohol consumption (World Cancer Research Fund, 2007). Similarly, the UK's Chief Medical Officers provide guidelines regarding physical activity

(DH, DHSSPS, The Scottish Government and Welsh Government (2011)) – although research is ongoing into optimal levels for cancer prevention, at least 30 minutes of physical activity per day is currently recommended. Healthcare professionals are increasingly involved in delivery of these and similar messages, with the aim not just of reducing the risk and rates of cancer but also other non-communicable diseases. *The European Code Against Cancer* (Association of European Cancer Leagues, 2010–2014) promotes the following key **health promotion** messages:

1. Do not smoke. If you smoke, stop doing so. If you fail to stop, do not smoke in the presence of non-smokers.
2. Avoid obesity.
3. Undertake some brisk, physical activity every day.
4. Increase your daily intake and variety of vegetables and fruits: eat at least five servings daily. Limit your intake of foods containing fats from animal sources.
5. If you drink alcohol, whether beer, wine or spirits, moderate your consumption to two drinks per day if you are a man or one drink per day if you are a woman.
6. Care must be taken to avoid excessive sun exposure. It is specifically important to protect children and adolescents. For individuals who have a tendency to burn in the sun, active protective measures must be taken throughout life.
7. Apply strictly regulations aimed at preventing any exposure to known cancer-causing substances. Follow all health and safety instructions on substances that may cause cancer. Follow advice of national radiation protection offices.
8. Women from 25 years of age should participate in cervical screening. This should be within programmes with quality control procedures in compliance with 'European Guidelines for Quality Assurance in Cervical Screening'.
9. Women from 50 years of age should participate in breast screening. This should be within programmes with quality control procedures in compliance with 'European Guidelines for Quality Assurance in Mammography Screening'.
10. Men and women from 50 years of age should participate in colorectal screening. This should be within programmes with built-in quality assurance procedures.
11. Participate in vaccination programmes against hepatitis B virus infection.

Reflective activity

Healthcare professionals are being encouraged to think of all healthcare encounters as potential opportunities to promote healthy lifestyle messages. Reflect on patients you have cared for recently where you recognized that unhealthy lifestyles (e.g. smoking, obesity, etc.) were likely to be contributing to poorer health outcomes. Consider conversational approaches that might have allowed you to sensitively explore patients' own awareness of these risk factors, and their willingness to change.

Consider what might be the sensitivities of these type of conversations and how best to avoid patient distress, embarrassment, or subsequent reluctance to engage with healthcare.

Vaccination

A number of vaccines have been developed or are currently being developed against cancer-causing viruses (Dochez et al., 2014). Prophylactic HPV vaccines have been developed against HPV types 16 and 18 that are based on virus-like particles, induce high titres of neutralizing antibodies and have been shown to be effective in preventing type 16 and 18 cervical intra-neoplasia. The optimal age to vaccinate is pre-adolescence. The UK has a school-based programme of HPV vaccination (Russell et al., 2013).

MODIFICATION OF CANCER RISK: SECONDARY PREVENTION (SCREENING)

The purpose of screening is to identify early disease, or precursors of disease, before it becomes a cancer (i.e. to identify people with an earlier stage of cancer than if they presented with symptoms). The term screening is often used loosely and can refer either to when screening is offered opportunistically to an individual, or in a more systematic approach to a group of people or an individual. Mass screening refers to screening of eligible age groups in the population, and selective screening refers to screening high-risk groups (e.g. those with familial cancer syndromes).

Programmatic **cancer screening programmes** (as carried out in the UK and in many other countries (Benson et al., 2008; Dowling et al., 2010) seek to provide a quality assured and evidence-based service at a population level. The formal definition from the UK National Cancer Screening Committee is given in below.

UK National Cancer Screening Committee

Screening is a process of identifying apparently healthy people who may be at increased risk of a disease or condition. They can then be offered information, further tests and appropriate treatment to reduce their risk and/or any complications arising from the disease or condition (UK National Screening Committee, 2014).

Principles of cancer screening

In the 1960s, WHO commissioned a report on screening that led to the development of screening criteria. These were based, among other factors, on the capacity to detect the condition at an early stage and the availability of an acceptable treatment, and have become the standard screening criteria to guide decision-making in establishing cancer screening programmes (Wilson and Jungner, 1968).

More recently, these criteria have been updated to reflect the now widespread screening for genetic conditions, as well as newer issues that have emerged over the last four decades that have shaped both Western medicine and society more generally, including trends such as increased consumerism, the emphasis on informed choice and on evidence-based healthcare, and the rise of healthcare systems where cost-effectiveness, quality assurance, and accountability of decision makers are recognized (Andermann et al., 2008). The use of potential biomarkers for cancer screening will also become more commonplace in the next decade. The new criteria are:

- The screening programme should respond to a recognized need.
- The objectives of screening should be defined at the outset.
- There should be a defined target population.
- There should be scientific evidence of screening programme effectiveness.
- The programme should integrate education, testing, clinical services and programme management.
- There should be quality assurance, with mechanisms to minimize potential risks of screening.
- The programme should ensure informed choice, confidentiality and respect for autonomy.
- The programme should promote equity and access to screening for the entire target population.
- Programme evaluation should be planned from the outset.
- The overall benefits of screening should outweigh the harm.

Screening should never be considered as merely the provision of a test, rather as a system where improved cancer outcomes are achieved through earlier detection by means of the test, coupled with the provision of effective and available treatment options ('sieving and sorting').

Terms used in cancer screening

A number of terms are commonly used when describing the evaluation of screening services and the effectiveness of specific screening modalities (see Raffle and Gray, 2007: 86–96 and Bhopal, 2008: 178–90 for detailed descriptions).

Selection bias – people that choose to take part in screening differ from those that don't. Individuals who participate in screening – the 'healthy screenee' tend to be healthier than those who do not, for many reasons (see 'Barriers to screening participation' below).

Lead time bias – apparent improvement in survival due to earlier date of diagnosis by screening compared with the usual time of diagnosis by symptomatic presentation.

Length time bias – screening more likely to pick up slower growing tumours with better prognosis (screen-detected cancer cannot be assumed to be directly comparable to those that present symptomatically).

Overdiagnosis bias – detection of pre-invasive disease that would not have progressed to invasive disease (e.g. *ductal carcinoma in situ*), although in reality it is not possible to distinguish for any one individual whether this applies.

Sensitivity – the ability of a test to detect the condition that the test is measuring for when the condition is actually present (i.e. the proportion of people who have the disease that have a positive test).

Specificity – the ability of the test to detect that the condition being measured for by the test is not present when it is, in fact, not present (i.e. the proportion of people who do not have the disease that have a negative test).

True positive – the individual has the condition, and the test result is positive.

True negative – the individual does not have the condition, and the test result is negative.

False positive – the individual does *not* have the condition, and the test result is positive.

False negative – the individual *has* the condition, and the test result is negative.

Positive predictive value – the proportion of people with a positive test that have the disease.

Negative predictive value – the proportion of people with a negative test that don't have the disease.

A variety of study designs are used to evaluate screening (see Raffle and Gray, 2007 and Bhopal, 2008). Cohort studies can compare survival in screen-detected and non-screen-detected (i.e. symptomatic) cases. Time-trend studies compare trends in incidence and death before and after the introduction of screening, but this method is prone to bias from changes in diagnosis or treatment. Case-control studies to compare screening history are useful particularly to examine the impact of different policies and protocols, but they cannot reliably measure the differences between screened and not-screened population. Well-conducted and adequately powered randomized control trials (RCTs) are the only rigorous way of evaluating the effectiveness (and if designed well, the cost-effectiveness) of a new screening modality.

Current screening modalities within the UK

Cervical screening

The UK had a longstanding cervical cytology programme, which underwent a major upgrade around twenty years ago. The programme is estimated to save around 4500 lives per year, and the number of cervical cancer cases has decreased by about 7% each year since the 1980s (Sasieni et al., 2003). In England, all women aged between 25 and 64 are invited for cervical screening. Women aged between 25 and 49 are invited for testing every three years, and women aged between 50 and 64 are invited every five years. Currently, cervical screening is based on **liquid-based cytology** (National Office of the NHS Screening Programme, 2014a). More recently, in England, HPV triage has been introduced into the cervical screening programme based on evidence of effectiveness in sentinel sites (Kelly et al., 2011). If a conventional smear is found to have borderline changes or low-grade dyskaryosis, the sample is tested for human papilloma virus (HPV). If this is HPV positive, the woman is invited to attend a colposcopy; if negative she returns to a regular screening invitation every 3–5 years (dependent on age). There are some differences across the UK: in Scotland and Wales, cervical screening is offered to eligible women aged 20–60 every three years, but this will change to 25–64 years from 2015 (Cancer Research UK, 2014u). In England, cervical screening coverage (the proportion of women who have been screened within the past five years) is approximately 80%, with variation by socio-economic status and ethnicity, and markedly lower coverage in younger women from more deprived areas (National Office of the NHS Screening Programme, 2014b). Trials are ongoing to examine whether self-sampling will be effective in increasing coverage (Szarewski et al., 2011).

Breast screening

Two-view mammography is used in all national breast-screening programmes across the UK. **Digital mammography** is currently being introduced nationally (National Office of the NHS Screening Programme, 2014c). Across the UK, women aged 50–70 are invited for breast screening with mammography every three years. Women over 70 are eligible for breast screening but are not automatically invited, although a trial is underway examining the potential benefits of extending breast-screening age to women aged 47–49 and 71–73 (Moser et al., 2011). Of the 2.3 million women aged 50–70 years invited for a mammogram in 2010–2011, the average attendance was 73.4%, with variation by geographical region, ethnicity and by socio-economic status (National Office of the NHS Screening Programme, 2014d).

Bowel screening

Following large-scale pilots of the feasibility and acceptability of screening with the guaiac-based **faecal occult blood test** (FOBT) (Moss et al., 2011), roll-out of routine FOBT for men and women aged 60–69 years began in England from 2006 (Cancer Research UK, 2014v). Screening is administered through five screening 'hubs' with around 100 centres where colonoscopy and any required treatment takes place. Participation in bowel screening is lower than for either breast or cervical screening at approximately 55%. In Scotland and England, 50–74-year-olds are invited; in Northern Ireland the age range is between 60 and 71 with extension up to 74 from mid-2014, while in Wales the age range is 60–74 years, with plans to reduce the age to those aged 50 over the next few years (Cancer Research UK, 2014v). There is good research evidence that the use of immunochemical FOBT kits, which have more acceptable modes of stool sampling, has the potential to increase uptake and may be introduced into the programme. Results of the major RCT of **flexible sigmoidoscopy** (FS) together with clinical and cost-effectiveness modelling suggests that a one-off FS could reduce incidence of colorectal cancer by 33% and mortality by 43% in the screened population (Atkin et al., 2010), and the UK National Screening Committee has recommended that FS be introduced. Pilots are underway of a one-off FS at 55 years, followed by a FOBT from 60–69 years (National Office of the NHS Screening Programme, 2014e).

PSA testing

There is currently no screening programme in the UK for prostate cancer. Although one European study has shown deaths from prostate cancer could be reduced by 20% if there was a screening programme using the **prostate specific antigen** (PSA) test, only one additional life would be saved for every 48 men treated, and a North American study demonstrated no reductions in prostate-specific mortality (Andriole et al., 2009; Schröder et al., 2009). However, rather than a national screening programme, there is an informed choice approach called 'prostate cancer risk management' where the benefits and harms of PSA testing are presented (National Office of the NHS Screening Programme, 2014f).

Barriers to screening participation

Uptake is the most important factor in determining the success of any screening programme. As described earlier, uptake in the three screening programmes in the UK varies considerably. This is particularly true for bowel screening. The reasons are complex, and are often underpinned by a range of health beliefs and cultural attitudes. Generic factors across all cancer sites include a perceived lack of clinical support (for some, this is especially so if no primary care provider is involved in the screening process), fear of a cancer diagnosis or of treatment and side effects, a lack of understanding of the nature of screening (e.g. in the absence of symptoms), or embarrassment at the procedure. For many, conflicting priorities, including lack of time to attend a screening appointment, caring responsibilities, and existing poor physical or mental health, are important deterrents to screening participation. For some, cultural concerns, such as taboos around handling and storing faecal matter, fatalistic beliefs, poor understanding of the health system, and concerns around cost and access, may play a role. The importance of poor health literacy is increasingly being acknowledged as a barrier (Weller and Campbell, 2009; Power et al., 2009; Weller et al., 2009).

Considerable research efforts seek to address these barriers to participation, even whilst acknowledging the need to respect the principle of informed choice. Examples include the introduction of more acceptable screening modalities, such as a one-sample immunochemical FOBT and HPV self-sampling tests. Another strategy involves improving access through extended screening facility hours, more convenient locations and reducing or eliminating direct costs. Adapting recruitment materials by development of targeted and tailored materials to meet the information needs of specific communities has been adopted. There is good evidence that use of pre-notification letters and reminders can improve uptake. Primary care can play a role through endorsement of invitations, contacting non-responders and general practice-based promotion of screening (Weller and Campbell, 2009).

Benefits and harms of screening

No screening test or procedure is perfect, and screening therefore has the potential to benefit an individual, but also to harm him/her (Raffle and Gray, 2007). Benefits may include improved prognosis for some cases, less radical treatment, resource savings and the reassurance for negative test results. Disadvantages may include longer morbidity where the prognosis is unaltered, over-treatment of abnormalities that would not have progressed to become malignant, resource costs, false reassurance for false negatives, adverse effects of false positives including psychological distress and unnecessary testing, and exposure to hazards of a test (such as colon perforation with colonoscopy). A review of the psychological sequelae following a false positive mammogram found that studies using disease-specific measures (such as the Psychological Consequences Questionnaire, PCQ) suggested that negative psychological impact can last up to three years, with the degree of distress related to the extent of invasiveness of the investigation (Bond et al., 2013). High distress levels have also been associated with false positive bowel screening results (Denters et al., 2013).

Mr Murray, a 62-year-old man, is visiting his general practice nurse for routine diabetes checks. The general practice takes a proactive approach to encouraging patients to consider all relevant screening invitations, and the practice nurse sees in Mr Murray's notes that he has not taken part in bowel cancer screening despite repeat invitations. The practice nurse decides to explore this decision, and it quickly becomes clear that Mr Murray has received and read the invitations but is very concerned that treatment for any cancer detected might be ineffective – he lost a friend to advanced bowel cancer despite chemotherapy. The nurse and Mr Murray then spend some time discussing the purpose of screening to detect early bowel cancer, where survival outcomes are higher. They also discuss the pros and cons of screening, including the potential for distress caused by an abnormal test result, as well as the need to be vigilant for symptoms.

Informed choice in cancer screening

There has been controversy about the balance of harms and benefits for breast screening over recent years, leading to an expert panel Breast Screening Review in the UK in 2011/2012 (Independent UK Panel on Breast Cancer Screening, 2012). The Report estimated that although screening prevents about 1300 breast cancer deaths per year, it can also result in about 4000 women aged 50–70 in the UK having treatment for a problem that would not have troubled them (i.e. overdiagnosis). This has led to a renewed emphasis on informed choice and provision of clear and adequate information to women (National Office of the NHS Screening Programme, 2014g; Forbes and Ramirez, 2014). Informed choice principles involve recognition of the ethical underpinnings to any screening provision (autonomy, non-maleficence, beneficence, justice). It is clear, however, that although most people value information on the limits of screening, provision of information and education alone are not sufficient to facilitate an informed choice, and rather an individual's personal experience, values, and health and social contexts are equally or more important. The potential tension between personal autonomy and public health benefit is also recognized because facilitating informed choice does not necessarily increase uptake. However, autonomous decision-making does not preclude provider input: there is evidence that the UK public would welcome a recommendation from the NHS – not as an alternative to information, but as an *adjunct* to it, consistent with a 'consider an offer' approach (Waller et al., 2012; Entwistle et al., 2008).

Screening for other cancers

Policy documents emphasize strong commitments to cancer screening and prevention. The *Cancer Reform Strategy* (DH, 2007a: 47) stated 'We will extend and widen our existing screening programmes and continue to investigate opportunities for new screening programmes for other cancers', while the 2011 *Improving Outcomes: A Strategy for Cancer* had a strong public health focus particularly in areas such as diet, obesity, smoking and on screening participation across all communities (DH, 2011a).

There is currently no national screening programme for lung cancer in the UK; however, a recent trial in the USA has shown that screening individuals aged 55–74 who have cigarette smoking histories of 30 or more pack years with low-dose helical computed tomography (spiral CT) reduces lung cancer mortality by 20% and all-cause mortality by 6.7%. Screening would lead to false-positive test results in approximately 25% of those screened (Oken et al., 2011). Research is underway in the UK to examine how lung cancer screening may be introduced in the future for selected populations.

Randomized controlled trials are currently underway in the UK to assess the effectiveness of screening in high-risk women and in the general population for ovarian cancer with the tumour marker CA125 and transvaginal ultrasound (Institute for Women's Health, 2014). Results from the UK Collaborative Trial of Ovarian Cancer Screening (UKCTOCS) will be available after 2015.

COMMUNICATING RISK TO PUBLIC AND PATIENTS

Communicating risk, whether to an individual and/or their family and carers, to other health professionals, or to a wider lay or professional audience, is an important skill. Effective risk communication needs to be transparent, understandable and meaningful to those receiving it and clear enough to allow others to make appropriate decisions based on the information received if necessary.

Cancer risk communication requires a balanced summary of available evidence of the potential benefits, and the potential harms, associated with participating in an activity (e.g. smoking cessation, participating in screening) or undertaking a course of treatment (e.g. chemotherapy). Provision of information should improve the recipient's perception and understanding of their own risk, enable a discussion and, where appropriate, ensure shared decision-making consistent with the patient's values (Ahmed et al., 2012).

There are a number of reasons why effective risk communication can be difficult, not least because many health professionals, as well as patients, have trouble interpreting health statistics (Gigerenzer et al., 2007). Low health literacy is also recognized as a contributing factor to cancer health inequalities because patients with low health literacy are less likely to participate in cancer screening, have less understanding of cancer susceptibility and the importance of early detection of a cancer, and may also lack numeracy skills to inform and guide their decisions (Dewalt et al., 2004; Davis et al., 2002).

A number of strategies have been developed to help address these and similar challenges. These include the use of **Framing manipulation**, where logically equivalent information can be provided in different ways, positively or negatively (e.g. 'screening will improve your chance of survival from cancer' versus 'not participating in cancer screening will reduce your chance of survival from cancer'). Presenting risk reduction (i.e. relative risk reduction, absolute risk reduction or number needed to treat), personalizing risk information (based on the individual's own risk factors), the use of natural frequencies (rather than percentages) and the use of decision aids (interventions designed to aid shared decision-making) have also been advocated (Ahmed et al., 2012). Recommendations have been developed to guide risk communication to patients: some of the most salient for cancer are provided below.

Recommendations to guide risk communication

- Use plain language to make verbal and written materials more understandable
- Present data using absolute risks
- Present information in pictographs if using graphs
- Present data using frequencies
- Use incremental risk to highlight how treatment can change risk from the pre-existing baseline level
- Recognize that the order in which potential benefits and harms are presented can affect risk perception
- Consider providing only the information that is most critical to the patient's decision-making, even at the expense of completeness

Source: Fagerlin et al. (2011).

Although challenging, early studies that explicitly apply these principles in cancer treatment contexts have encouraging initial results (Korfage et al., 2013).

Communicating uncertainty

There are times when the evidence base regarding risk information or treatment options is limited and/or ambiguous, presenting considerable challenges in how to communicate risk or the balance of potential benefits and harms in a meaningful way. Responding to uncertainty is influenced by both the clinician's and the patient's personal characteristics and values (Politi et al., 2007) – clinicians modify their risk communication strategies depending on their own perception of the patient's ambiguity aversion (Portnoy et al., 2013), while communicating uncertainty in shared decision-making can lead to less patient decision satisfaction (Politi et al., 2011).

Other sources of cancer risk information

Increasingly, the general public and patients and their families will make use of the vast array of health websites on the Internet to learn more about cancer risk and to inform their healthcare decisions. Clearly, there are many excellent health websites providing accurate and evidence-based information, but equally there are many that do not and not only provide inaccurate or out-of-date information but also cause unnecessary anxiety and fear. There is a need for health professionals to signpost patients and their families to reliable, high-quality online sites.

Key learning points

- Although there are no proven ways to prevent cancer, individuals can reduce their risk of developing this disease through healthy lifestyle choices.
- Cancer screening has the potential to reduce an individual's risk of developing cancer through detection of pre-neoplastic or early disease.

- Cancer screening is a process and, to be effective and efficient, each step should be underpinned by evidence.
- In the UK, screening programmes have been established for cervical, breast and bowel cancer. Reducing inequalities in participation across socio-economic and minority ethnic groups remains a challenge.
- Effective communication with patients and with the public about cancer risk, and about the potential benefits and harms of cancer screening, is an essential skill for healthcare providers to cultivate.

Recommended further reading

- World Cancer Research Fund/American Institute for Cancer Research. (2007) *Food, Nutrition, Physical Activity, and the Prevention of Cancer: a Global Perspective* (www.dietandcancereport.org/er)
- Raffle, A. and Gray, M. (2007) *Screening: Evidence and Practice*. Oxford: Oxford University Press.
- Bhopal, R. (2008) *Concepts of Epidemiology: Integrating the Ideas, Theories, Principles and Methods of Epidemiology*. 2nd edn. Oxford: Oxford University Press.
- Chamberlain, J. and Moss, S. (eds) (1996) *Evaluation of Cancer Screening*. London: Springer.
- NHS Cancer Screening Programmes (www.cancerscreening.nhs.uk/)

Examples of online resources

- Cancer Research UK (www.cancerresearchuk.org)
- Macmillan Cancer Support (www.macmillan.org.uk/Home.aspx)
- National Cancer Institute (www.cancer.gov) Although not a UK site and therefore some terminology and healthcare options are US-specific, this is a very helpful and comprehensive resource for both professionals and patients.
- American Cancer Society (www.cancer.org) Again, not a UK site, but a well-designed and informative resource for patients.

3 CANCER DETECTION AND DIAGNOSIS

DANIEL SEDDON AND PAUL MACKENZIE

Chapter outline

- Detecting and diagnosing cancer
- Approaches and challenges to early detection
- Routes to diagnosis
- The role of the Primary Care team in the UK:
  - Risk Assessment Tools
  - The National Primary Care Audit
  - NICE referral guidelines
- Raising public awareness of potential signs of cancer and when to seek help
- Barriers to earlier detection of cancers
- English Awareness and Early Detection Initiative

INTRODUCTION

Cancer must be diagnosed before any effective advice, treatment or support can be given to an affected individual; however, the diagnostic process itself is not straightforward. Diagnosis of cancer occurs in many different ways following, for example:

- An investigation for a **'red flag' symptom**, such as a persistent cough in a smoker. ('Red flag' symptoms are symptoms and signs that should lead to urgent investigation/referral to exclude or confirm a cancer diagnosis) (National Institute for Health and Clinical Excellence (NICE), 2005b).
- **Screening** such as at a colonoscopy after a positive screening test for blood in faeces.
- Emergency admission to hospital with a complication of an unrecognized cancer such as lung, bowel or blood cancer (leukaemia).

Diagnosis is generally assumed to be a good thing; however, it may not always be in an individual's best interests if the underlying natural history of that condition is not understood.

Neuroblastoma screening programmes introduced in Japan, for example, increased the number of positive diagnoses, but did not change population outcomes, such as mortality. This means that cancer was diagnosed when it would otherwise have caused no harm (Raffle and Gray, 2007). A similar paradox exists for prostate cancer in the UK: the number of diagnoses of prostate cancer is rising dramatically year on year, but mortality is static or falling. Advances in treatment do not explain the apparent improvement in survival. What is actually happening is that more men have prostate cancer detected who would never have been harmed by the cancer had it not been found.

Diagnosis describes the process of understanding and correctly defining the cause and nature of an illness, i.e. the correct identification of the **occurrence** of cancer. There is no rigorous definition of *cancer detection,* although 'detection' and 'diagnosis' are often used interchangeably, as in 'early detection' and 'early diagnosis'. It is sometimes helpful to use the two words differently because detection has more of a sense of a first recognition that something is wrong compared to diagnosis, which has a sense of understanding and labelling.

DIAGNOSING CANCER IS NOT ALWAYS EASY

Cancer incorporates a large number of diseases that can affect any body system. Whilst some presentations, especially of advanced cancer, may be more obvious, many early symptoms and signs are non-specific, subtle or vague. There are several tools and advisory guidelines available to aid the decision to investigate for cancer and these are appropriate for the majority of cancer most of the time. However, cancer is often detected in people without the classic 'red flag' symptoms and only a small minority of those with classic symptoms actually have a cancer. For example, a middle-aged woman presenting to her doctor with new symptoms of abdominal distension and pain (these are 'red flag' symptoms) has a 2.5% chance of being diagnosed with ovarian cancer (Hamilton, 2009). Figure 3.1 illustrates the paradox.

There are three main challenges to diagnosing cancer:

1. How to order tests or refer to specialists speedily, whilst avoiding the harm of 'over-investigating' or wasting resources.
2. How to get individuals with symptoms to consult their GP or other health advisor in the first place. Some people do not recognize serious symptoms, some people do recognize them and are afraid to act, and some people experience organizational barriers to consulting their GP (Robb et al., 2009). Robb found that awareness of 'cancer warning signs' was lower in those from lower socio-economic groups and in males. Awareness was also lower in younger and older people versus a middle-age range.
3. Understanding and overcoming delays in the journey to a diagnosis. The National Awareness and Early Detection Initiative (NAEDI) pathway for England provides an excellent map of this journey (Richards, 2009; Figure 3.2). NAEDI is a partnership of Government, charities and academic bodies in England, set up to understand and to remedy England's high cancer mortality and relatively poor survival (DH, 2007a). Similar initiatives exist in other UK countries.

A simplistic interpretation of cancer detection would place diagnosis as the first stage in any individual's cancer pathway; however, careful consideration of health-related behaviours,

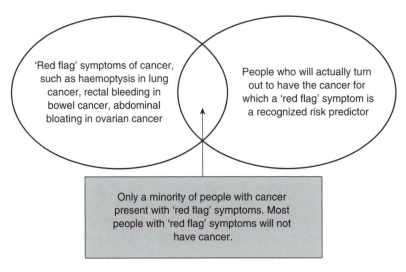

Figure 3.1　How helpful are early symptoms and signs of cancer?

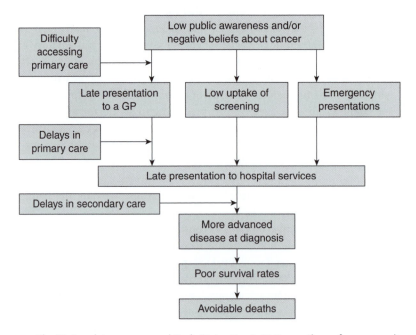

Figure 3.2　The National Awareness and Early Detection Initiative pathway for cancer diagnosis
Source: Richards (2009).

patterns of consultation and the role of lay health experts supports a more sophisticated model of cancer detection. The NAEDI pathway presents such a model.

The pathway acknowledges the key role of the general practitioner (GP) in the UK health system, but highlights that delays can occur both before and after GP consultation. It also illustrates the alternative routes to a diagnosis of cancer through screening and emergency admissions.

The pathway demonstrates the individual's process from recognition that something might be wrong, through consideration of whether to act, investigation of sources of advice, and then consultation with a health expert. This first stage of the process, from recognition to a decision to consult, may be completely outside any healthcare system. Only after this stage will a GP or alternative be encountered. The National Primary Care Cancer Audit (Rubin et al., 2011) has shown that most cancers are referred on speedily by GPs.

WHERE IS CANCER DETECTED?

It is tempting to assume that cancer is always recognized in a clinical or professional setting; however, cancer may be recognized initially by a wide range of people, in a variety of settings. Cancer awareness and early detection campaigns promote the recognition of warning signs by families or individuals. Table 3.1 shows some of the settings where cancer can be detected.

Table 3.1   Where is cancer detected? Not just the doctor's surgery ...

Cancer type	Where might it be first detected?	Notes
Skin cancer: melanoma, basal or squamous cell cancer. These cancers begin with small changes to appearance or feel	In the supermarket queue, at the swimming pool or on the beach	Guides to recognizing suspicious skin lesions are widely available.[a]
Breast cancer: may present as a lump, hardening or irregularity in one breast or a discharge from the nipple	Most breast cancers present symptomatically: breast lumps are likely to be found at home by a woman or her partner	There are about 48,000 new cases of breast cancer each year in the UK; 16,500 are diagnosed through screening.[b]
Bolorectal cancer: sometimes the first warning is blood passed in or with faeces	Someone notices blood in the toilet or on toilet paper after they have passed faeces	The most common cancer in the UK, after breast and lung. In people over 50 years, rectal bleeding has a predictive value of nearly 7% for bowel cancer (Hamilton, 2009).
Lung and bowel cancers	Accident and Emergency department: a quarter of all colorectal cancer is diagnosed via an emergency route	Both bowel and lung cancers are commonly detected when an individual goes to the hospital acutely ill, not suspecting that they may have cancer
Cervical cancer	A colposcopy clinic: colposcopy will be used to investigate an abnormal cervical smear test	About half of all invasive cervical cancer occurs in women who have not attended their smear test (Sasieni and Castanon, 2012)

Notes:
[a]There are a number of guidelines for the public and for professionals. For example, NHS Choices at www. nhs.uk/Conditions/Malignant-melanoma/Pages/Symptoms.aspx
[b]Cancer Research UK. Figures are for 2009 for new cases; 2007/8 for screen detected. Web resource accessed July 2012 at http://info.cancerresearchuk.org/cancerstats/types/breast

THE ROUTES TO DIAGNOSIS

Just as the NAEDI pathway helps to measure timelines and consider where delays to diagnosis and detection of cancer occur, study of the various routes that people take to diagnosis helps to illustrate where change is needed.

The **Routes to Diagnosis** project, led by the National Cancer Intelligence Network (NCIN) in England, is a NAEDI work stream (National Cancer Intelligence Network, 2010a). The project analyzes six possible routes to a cancer diagnosis in the English health system, plus two categories where information is lacking. The six routes are:

- *Screen detected*: at the time of the analysis, two cancer screening programmes were in place across England, for cervical cancer between ages 25 and 64 and for breast cancer between ages 50 and 69. Colorectal cancer screening was introduced in England between 2006 and 2009.
- *Two-week wait*: the English NHS provides a facility for GPs to urgently refer those with 'red flag' symptoms to a specialist to be seen within two weeks.
- *GP/outpatient referral*: referrals to a specialist labelled routine or urgent, but not under the two-week rule.
- *Other outpatient*: where an outpatient referral to a specialist doesn't fit the previous categories.
- *Inpatient elective*: where a cancer diagnosis is made at a pre-booked, planned hospital admission.
- *Emergency presentation*: this includes a first presentation to Accident and Emergency (casualty/emergency room), emergency GP referral to a specialist, or other emergency route.

Two further categories reflect the realities of routine data collection and analysis:

- *Death certificate only*: some cancer diagnoses are made after death, or the cancer registry is unable to find any more information than on a death certificate.
- *Unknown*: in these circumstances, healthcare data describe a cancer diagnosis but no other information can be obtained.

The first *Routes to Diagnosis* briefing published for cancers diagnosed in 2007 revealed that:

- Less than 1 in 20 (5%) of all cancers were diagnosed through *screening programmes* in 2007 in England.
- More than 1 in 4 (25%) were diagnosed via an urgent referral, for suspected cancer, to a specialist.
- Just less than 1 in 4 (24%) were diagnosed through a specialist referral that did not use the two-week cancer rule.
- Just less than 1 in 4 (23%) were diagnosed following an emergency presentation to hospital (GP referred or not).
- Most cancers were not diagnosed via the urgent route designated for suspected cancer.

Table 3.2 shows the routes to diagnosis for selected cancers.

Table 3.2   How cancer is diagnosed in the English health system: the *Routes to Diagnosis* findings for selected cancers

	Screen detected	Two-week wait	GP referral	Other outpatient	Planned inpatient	Emergency presentation	Death certificate	Unknown	Number of new cases
Bladder	–	32%	28%	15%	2%	18%	O	4%	2551
Breast	21%	42%	12%	9%	O	4%	O	12%	34,232
Cervix	14%	16%	25%	16%	2%	12%	O	13%	2085
Colorectal	–	26%	24%	15%	4%	25%	1%	6%	27,903
Kidney	–	20%	29%	1%	18%	24%	1%	6%	5172
Lung	–	22%	10%	13%	1%	38%	1%	5%	29,420
Melanoma	–	41%	29%	11%	1%	3%	O%	16%	8117
Oesophagus	–	25%	21%	17%	10%	21%	1%	4%	6001
Prostate	–	20%	38%	16%	3%	9%	O%	14%	28,362
Stomach	–	17%	21%	16%	7%	32%	1%	5%	5841
Testis	–	48%	14%	16%	2%	10%	O%	10%	1569
All cancers	3%	25%	24%	14%	2%	23%	1%	8%	225,965

Notes

Excludes non-melanoma skin cancers.

Colorectal cancer screening was introduced in England from 2007/8.

Source: National Cancer Intelligence Network, 2012b.

THE ROLE OF THE PRIMARY CARE TEAM

Summerton (1999) described the 'tight rope' that the primary care doctor walks between harmful and expensive over-investigation, and a failure to act on warning symptoms. However, in 2012, because of the policy emphasis on early diagnosis, the UK GP is more of a gateway to diagnosis and treatment than a gatekeeper of scarce resources.

Three particularly useful resources that support GPs in their role in diagnosing cancer include the Risk Assessment Tool, the National Primary Care Cancer Audit and referral guidelines from NICE.

The Risk Assessment Tool

The **Risk Assessment Tool** (RAT) is a decision aid for cancer diagnosis (Hamilton et al., 2009). It uses evidence collected from primary care settings to estimate the chance of a cancer diagnosis, given one or more **'red flag' symptoms**. This approach quantifies estimates of risk, is tailored to particular cancers and can consider individual risk factors such as age, sex and smoking status.

The 'score' that the tool gives is a positive predictive value (PPV)[1] (as a percentage) for a cancer diagnosis within a defined time period. Confidence intervals can be calculated for the estimates of risk. For example, if a woman over the age of 50 presents in middle age with new symptoms of abdominal distension alone, there is about a 2.5% (confidence intervals 1.2%, 5.9%) risk of ovarian cancer being found on investigation.

Evidence for the risk scores was gathered by analyzing symptoms reported to GPs before cancer was diagnosed, including matched controls that did not develop cancer. The original work was part of the CAPER (Cancer Prediction in Exeter) study of colorectal, lung, prostate and brain cancer symptoms (Hamilton, 2009). A predictive tool for ovarian cancer was also published in 2009 as a separate study. In the CAPER study, rectal bleeding and haemoptysis both had positive predictive values of 2.4% for colorectal and lung cancer, respectively. In contrast, the predictive value of headache for brain cancer was 0.01% (1 in 1000).

Reflective activity

In order to illustrate the tool, refer to the lung cancer assessment tool for non-smokers (Table 3.3) and for colorectal cancer (Table 3.4). Here's how to look up a risk:

1. Choose the symptom 'haemoptysis' along the top line of Table 3.3.
2. Look down the final column for 'risk as a single symptom'.
3. Read off the risk 'positive predictive value' as a percentage from the box.
4. You will see that 2.4% of non-smokers over 40 in England, presenting to a doctor with haemoptysis, will turn out to have a lung cancer. (For smokers, a separate tool shows the risk as 4.5%.)
5. Now look up the risk for rectal bleeding in Table 3.4.

Note that it is possible to look up the same symptom on both row and column headings. This allows a risk calculation of the same symptom occurring twice over a period of time.

The Risk Assessment Tool supports risk-based referral decisions based on presenting symptoms. It allows a doctor to discuss the actual likelihood of a cancer diagnosis with the patient, and provides information to the patient so that they are informed about why they are being referred and what the possible outcomes of that referral are. The list of symptoms and signs may act as a prompt to the diagnostician.

The National Primary Care Cancer Audit

Scotland was ahead of England in auditing the diagnosis of cancer in primary care. Baughan et al. (2009) published the results of an audit of 16,475 cancer diagnoses made in Scotland during two years from 2006 to 2008 and reported variability between tumour groups in the time between symptoms and first consultation with a GP, and in time from presentation to referral.

---

[1]Positive predictive value (PPV) is a measure of risk (the likelihood of a particular disease, given a test result or other set of circumstances). It is commonly used to describe screening and diagnostic tests. The PPV value is highly dependent on the background incidence of a disease.

Table 3.3 Lung cancer assessment tool for non-smokers[a]

	Cough	Fatigue	Dyspnoea	Chest pain	Loss of weight	Loss of appetite	Thrombocytosis	Abnormal spirometry	Haemotpysis
Risk as a single symptom	0.4	0.4	0.7	0.8	1.1	0.9	1.6	1.6	2.4
Cough	0.6	0.6	0.8	0.8	1.8	1.6	2.0	1.2	2.0
Fatigue		0.6	0.9	0.8	1.0	1.2	1.8	4.0	3.3
Dyspnoea			0.9	1.2	2.0	2.0	2.0	2.3	4.9
Chest pain				0.9	1.8	1.8	2.0	1.4	5.0
Loss of weight					1.2	2.3	6.1	1.5	9.2
Loss of appetite						1.7	0.9	2.7	>10
Thrombocytosis								3.6	>10
Abnormal spirometry									>10
Haemoptysis									17

Notes: [a]Dark grey and black suggest two-week wait referral; white does not, but use your clinical judgement. Use to supplement NICE guidance. For patients aged 40 and over. For multiple symptoms, read cell with worst symptoms.
Source: Hamilton, 2009 (simplified).

Table 3.4 Colorectal cancer assessment tool[a]

	Constipation	Diarrhoea	Rectal bleeding	Loss of weight	Abdominal pain	Abdominal tenderness	Abnormal rectal examination	Haemoglobin 10–13 g/dl	Haemoglobin <10 g/dl
Risk as a single symptom	0.4	0.9	2.4	1.2	1.1	1.1	1.5	0.97	2.3
Constipation	0.8	1.1	2.4	3.0	1.5	1.7	2.6	1.2	2.6
Diarrhoea		1.5	3.4	3.1	1.9	2.4	11	2.2	2.9
Rectal bleeding			6.8	4.7	3.1	4.5	8.5	3.6	3.2
Loss of weight				1.4	3.4	6.4	7.4	1.3	4.7
Abdominal pain					3.0	1.4	3.3	2.2	6.9
Abdominal tenderness						1.7	5.8	2.7	>10

Notes: [a]Dark grey and black suggest two-week wait referral; white does not, but use your clinical judgement. Use to supplement NICE guidance. For patients aged 40 and over. For multiple symptoms, read cell with worst symptoms.
Source: Hamilton, 2009 (simplified).

A similar audit tool was undertaken across England (see box). The audit tool is still available and is now actively promoted by the Royal College of General Practitioners and cancer networks as a tool for all GPs (Rubin et al., 2011). There are two aspects: a retrospective timeline of the pathway to diagnosis for recently diagnosed cancers (excluding those identified though screening programmes), plus a practice team discussion akin to significant event analysis.[2]

The National Primary Care Cancer Audit in England in 2010

This was conducted during 2009 and 2010 and sponsored by the English Department of Health, National Cancer Intelligence Network and the Royal College of General Practitioners.

A total of 1170 general practices participated in the audit (14% of all general practices in England), from 20 out of 28 local cancer networks. 18,879 patient journeys were recorded.

GPs looked back at their records of the most recent 15 people diagnosed with cancer (excluding those diagnosed through screening; non-melanoma skin cancer and carcinoma in situ). They recorded when the first symptom was recognized by the patient, when first reported to the doctor, and key milestones thereafter. This created a timeline of the pathway to diagnosis for each patient.

The profile of patient characteristics in the audit closely matched that of routine reports to cancer registries, which support the generalizability of the findings.

Two out of three (66%) patients consulted their GP once or twice before being referred on. One in 20 (4%) consulted more than four times. One in 10 (9.5%) did not see their GP before cancer had been diagnosed. Younger males were more likely to have multiple consultations prior to referral, as were patients who developed cancer of the lung, ovary, pancreas, stomach and lymphoma.

The two-week urgent pathway for cancer referral was used in more than half of patients, and about 1 in 8 (12.9%) patients were referred as emergencies. Emergency presentation was more likely in those under 25 years old, and for cancers of the brain, blood, liver and pancreas.

In 6% of cases, the GP believed that better access to investigations would have reduced delay in diagnosis.

The National Primary Care Cancer Audit (NPCCA) has made two particularly important contributions to understanding how cancer is diagnosed in England.

First, individual practices undertaking the audit identified specific measures that could improve their timely recognition of cancer. GPs, for example, found that they referred most people with significant symptoms speedily; however, where the appropriate advice was to return if symptoms did not improve, GPs learned that this could be interpreted too often as reassurance. A better way would be to suggest that the patient made a follow-up appointment, and only cancelled it if their problem had resolved. This approach to 'failsafe' was a key learning point for audit participants. Second, the NPCCA showed prompt onward referral to be a hallmark of GP practice.

---

[2]Significant Event Analysis (SEA) is a recognized technique of enquiry and discussion of events of interest (for example, a missed diagnosis or other adverse event). In SEA, practice staff gather the key facts and their reflections. In England, SEA is part of the Quality Outcomes Framework that rewards general practitioners for meeting quality standards.

The NPCCA is now a recognized quality improvement tool for primary care teams and is endorsed by the Royal College of General Practitioners in the UK.

Using the NPCCA in a local cancer network

During 2009/10, a tenth of practices (N=33) in seven Primary Care Trusts in Merseyside and Cheshire (North West England) volunteered to conduct the Cancer Audit and report results for local and national analysis. Each nominated a lead person (doctor, nurse or manager) for the audit.

Practices were reimbursed in line with nationally agreed rates, dependent on their active participation, reporting data and confirmation of a practice significant event discussion having taken place.

A series of meetings were held with the practice leads where experience could be pooled.

A local report based on the findings in Merseyside and Cheshire was produced by the Cancer Network and shared widely across all local practices (Seddon et al., 2010). Merseyside and Cheshire data was shared with the national team and formed part of the final report (Rubin et al., 2011).

Reflections:

- Congruence between local findings and national work was strong.
- Local practices reported high satisfaction with their involvement, and most practices committed to action within their teams to improve failsafe mechanisms, actively manage referrals and explicitly trust their own clinical judgement when faced with negative results or specialist assessments.
- The cohort of practices who were involved have become key partners in establishing a network of primary care teams interested in improving cancer outcomes.

Referral guidelines from NICE

In 2005, NICE published their *Clinical Guideline 27*, directed towards NHS primary care, about GP referrals to specialists for suspected cancer (NICE, 2005b). In 2011, they updated the ovarian cancer elements, as *Guideline 122* (NICE, 2011). The guidance covers adult cancers in eleven groups, and cancers in children and young people as a separate topic.

Like all NICE guidance, the level of evidence behind recommendations is made explicit, with almost all specific recommendations having an evidence base of strength C, D or less ('expert committee reports, opinions and/or clinical experience of respected authorities').

The guideline provides an accepted and explicit manual to inform cancer diagnosis in primary care. It describes standards for speed of referral and information to patients and relatives, and acknowledges that cancer diagnosis can be difficult. Algorithms for each tumour group summarize the guidance, as shown in Figure 3.3. In contrast with Hamilton's Risk Assessment Tool (RAT), there is no quantification of risk; however, it is a simple format, and easy to follow.

Both the RAT and the NICE guidelines are specific for particular cancer types; however, patients present with symptoms rather than a diagnosis, and so the diagnostician needs skill, knowledge and experience to match symptoms with suspected cancer.

NICE guidelines in England and Wales give clear instructions about acceptable practice, which health service clinicians are consistently expected to follow.

Guidance from other organizations such as Macmillan Cancer Support is also relevant for frontline NHS staff. Macmillan Cancer Support have extended their support to local GPs over recent years by, for example, funding part-time lead cancer GPs in many local areas. This new generation of 'Macmillan GPs' are working to improve early detection of cancer in primary care.

Macmillan Cancer Support also produces written guidance for practices on cancer topics, such as haematuria and ovarian cancer, using the strapline '10 top tips' (Macmillan Cancer Support, n.d.). The top tips are written by Macmillan GPs for GPs. In addition, *Improving the Quality of Cancer Care in Primary Care'* (Macmillan Cancer Support, 2012c) is a toolkit arranged into five work modules, three of which are relevant to detection and diagnosis. Although addressed principally to GPs, any primary care health worker could use the toolkit to improve their awareness, confidence and skills in detecting cancer earlier.

DEVELOPING PUBLIC AWARENESS: HELP FOR LAY PEOPLE

A number of cancer charities also produce quality information about the detection and diagnosis of cancer that is suitable for a lay audience, for example the NHS Choices and Cancer Research UK websites, and NAEDI-sponsored cancer awareness campaigns in England, which use the strapline 'catching cancer quicker'.

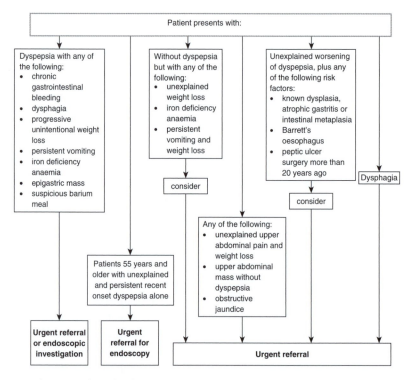

Figure 3.3   The NICE algorithm for upper gastrointestinal cancer diagnosis

Source: National Institute for Health and Clinical Excellence (2005b). Reissued 2011.

NHS Choices

NHS Choices is an information centre about NHS treatments and how to use the NHS for any illness, including cancers. It also provides information to help people recognize symptoms such as skin cancer.

Cancer Research UK

Cancer Research UK resources are comprehensive, balanced and accessible to the reader. Their website has separate tailored sections for professionals and patients, including information on cancer detection and diagnosis in the 'spot cancer early' pages.

Cancer awareness campaigns

Cancer awareness campaigns geared to earlier recognition of symptoms or to reducing risk factors for cancer also help to raise the profile. The theme '**Be clear on cancer**' runs through all the current national campaigns. Campaigns on lung cancer during 2012 and 2014, for example, make use of doctors as informants by suggesting that if someone has had a cough for three weeks, their doctor wants to see them.

Example poster: the cough campaign

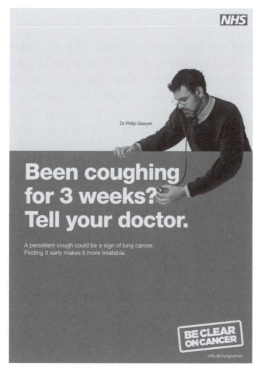

Source: www.nhs.uk/be-clear-on-cancer/lung-cancer/home

The first campaign to be tested regionally and rolled out nationally was for bowel cancer awareness. Messages focused on persistent loose poo and blood in the poo as reasons for a visit to the doctor.

The four findings of the evaluation in pilot areas were:

- People's behaviour changed – 50% more people over 50 with the publicized symptoms went to their doctor.
- More bowel cancer screening kits were returned for testing in the areas where the campaign was run.
- On average there was one additional consultation per GP per week during the pilot.
- Urgent referrals (known as 'two-week wait referrals') went up, with the biggest increase in the areas with the most intensive campaigning.

BARRIERS TO EARLIER DETECTION

Detection and diagnosis of cancer is delayed if individuals do not go for advice promptly when symptoms occur. This is the first part of the 'NAEDI pathway' referred to earlier. Individuals may delay because of

- Attitudinal barriers
- Service barriers
- Cultural barriers
- Emotional barriers

It is important to understand these barriers in order to target interventions that improve earlier presentation and also encourage the public to access services as early as possible. The NAEDI and the associated **National Cancer Equality Initiative** (NCEI) were developed to begin to address some of the issues around late presentation and to reduce cancer inequalities (DH, 2007a). NCEI is a partnership of the voluntary sector, academics and advocates for equality that was set up under the English Cancer Reform Strategy. It drives an action plan to reduce inequalities in cancer care in deprived groups and across the six equality strands of race, gender, disability, religion or belief, sexual orientation and age. Similar initiatives exist in other UK countries (for further detail on inequalities in cancer, please refer to Chapter 8).

Barriers that stop people going for help arise from a lack of knowledge, an attitude of hopelessness, a practical difficulty in access to a service or cultural and emotional factors.

A lack of knowledge about signs and symptoms

People with low literacy, sensory impairment, learning disabilities and severe mental health problems, as well as the travelling communities, may not hear, see or understand traditional advertising and cancer awareness messages. Some awareness campaigns may systematically exclude people. For example, the 2011 and 2012 bowel cancer awareness campaigns emphasized the importance of blood in poo as a significant symptom. This was irrelevant for people with severe vision impairment.

Another barrier in the past has been inconsistent health messages. For example, a change in bowel habit has been identified as a potential key symptom of bowel cancer; however, conflicting and contradictory messages have been given to the public about how long they should delay seeing the doctor, whether that is six weeks, four weeks or three weeks. The English 'Be clear on cancer' initiative aims to reduce these disparities by agreeing consistent messages at a national level (currently three weeks).

Three reports by the same group of researchers describe public understanding of cancer symptoms and help-seeking behaviours. Report one describes the development of the first validated **Cancer Awareness Measure** (CAM) as an interview tool for describing awareness of cancer risks and symptoms (Stubbings et al., 2009).

Report two describes how the tool was applied using traditional survey methods, and studied awareness of cancer warning signs, perceived barriers to seeking medical advice and anticipated delay (Robb et al., 2009). The findings indicated that awareness of cancer signs was lower amongst those who were male, younger and those from lower socio-economic groups or ethnic minorities. Reported barriers to seeking help included:

- Not wanting to 'waste the doctor's time'
- Worry about what would be found
- Difficulty making an appointment

These concerns were more reported by men than by women. The researchers also elicited emotional barriers such as fear, fatalism and worry about what would be discovered. Some practical barriers reported were difficulty obtaining an appointment and being too busy.

Report three describes the CAM used for 1500 members of ethnic minority communities using quota sampling (Waller et al., 2009). They concluded that awareness of the warning signs of cancer was low amongst all the ethnic groups, with lowest awareness amongst the African group. Men were less likely to seek help and women identified emotional barriers. The study concluded that culturally sensitive and community-based interventions should support awareness of cancer warnings and promote earlier presentation by patients. The important message is that healthcare professionals should not assume that 'one size fits all' and need to engage with communities in order to best facilitate and enhance understanding of the awareness of warning signs of cancer and to ensure that barriers to access to services are removed.

This raises a question about whether knowledge translates into behaviour. An example can be illustrated in respect of the CAM in Merseyside and Cheshire Cancer Network in 2010 (Flynn and Quinn, 2010). In Merseyside and Cheshire Cancer Network, awareness of the national bowel cancer screening programme amongst participants was nearly double that of the national omnibus CAM survey, yet uptake rates in Merseyside and Cheshire Cancer Network differed very little from anywhere else in the country. This could highlight a disparity between intention to act and actually 'doing'.

Table 3.5 Relevance to practice: who, what and why?

Who	What	Why
A primary care centre receptionist	Their role is a facilitator of access to the expert resources and advice of the doctor, practice nurse or other health professions.	Awareness and confidence about some of the common cancers and how they present will enable this health worker to encourage a reluctant patient to consult or advise a family friend to get a suspicious mole checked out.
	They may well act as a lay health expert to family and friends.	Familiarity with cancer screening programmes will enable the receptionist to explain to a woman what will happen at a breast screening appointment.
A dentist or dental hygienist	These professionals see healthy people regularly over long periods of time. They have a unique opportunity to discuss other health issues such as cancer (including oral cancer), cancer screening and cancer prevention.	The dentist or hygienist screens for oral cancer as part of the regular check-ups that they offer.
A GP	Sees people with an illness who are worried about that illness, and sees their family members.	The GP has a big challenge to recognize cancer early.
	The GP may audit their own practice and the processes in their team.	By reviewing practice and being aware of current guidelines, they can be confident that they are making a difference.
A practice nurse	The practice nurse sees patients for routine treatments and may also see patients with new problems in some practice teams.	The nurse may be seen as more approachable than the doctor. They may be able to spend time with someone frightened of a smear test or who has been referred for an urgent specialist appointment.
A pharmacist or pharmacy technician	The pharmacist dispenses prescribed medicine but also gives advice and sells 'over the counter' products	When a middle-aged man consults a pharmacist with a persistent cough, the pharmacist may be seen as a legitimate advisor about the need to seek help.
Another healthcare professional	*Think of other ideas*	*... and here.*

Coleman et al., 2011). The result is that individuals with cancer in the UK are less likely to be alive one or five years after diagnosis, than individuals in comparable other countries, such as Scandinavian countries, Australia or New Zealand (see box).

The EUROCARE studies and the International Benchmarking of Cancer Survival Programme

The EUROCARE studies are a collaboration between European cancer registries to provide comparative cancer survival reports. EUROCARE 4 included more than 13 million cancer diagnoses from 93 population-based cancer registries in 23 countries in Europe. The study centre is in Italy at the Cancer Epidemiology Unit and Data Analysis Centre, Istituto Superiore di Sanità, Rome. EUROCARE publishes sequential analyses of one and five-year survival estimates for 42 types of cancer in 23 countries in Europe. Countries are compared and ranked to show those with survival in the top quartile (coloured green) and lowest quartile (red). The biggest differences between countries are for one-year survival. Differences in survival between one and five years are much less. In the latest (EUROCARE 4) study, all four UK countries have lower survival than Norway, Finland and Sweden.

The International Benchmarking of Cancer Partnership unites academics, clinicians and policymakers from six nations with comparable health systems (Australia, Canada, Denmark, Norway, Sweden and the UK). The Partnership aims to provide up-to-date and accurate cancer survival statistics so that differences can be agreed and explored. In January 2011, they published findings showing survival from four common cancers: colorectal, lung, breast and ovarian. Survival had increased in all countries since 1995 and, for breast cancer, there was a closing of the gap between best and worst. The six countries were ranked into high survival (Australia, Canada, Sweden), intermediate (Norway) and lower survival (Denmark, England, Northern Ireland, Wales). Technical discrepancies in cancer registration did not account for the survival differences. There is a stronger case for real differences in timeliness of diagnosis or in treatment effectiveness to be the cause.

Two contrasting explanations for the findings have been postulated:

1. The UK picture is no worse than other comparable health systems – it is the statistics that are spurious and it has been suggested that the UK approach to population cancer registration captures information unavailable in other healthcare systems.
2. The statistics are valid, and an explanation of the difference in survival is due to:

    - Fewer available tests or lower technology tests available
    - Less effective treatments for cancer: related to quality of care, use of cancer drugs, high-tech treatment options, etc.
    - More aggressive cancers
    - Less healthy individuals with more co-morbidities
    - Delays in recognition of serious symptoms or signs and late diagnosis of cancer

The spurious statistics argument is generally refuted, but real delays in presentation of symptoms, or in the process of primary or secondary care, lead to more advanced disease at diagnosis and subsequent reduced survival (Richards and Hiom, 2009).

Compared with the best countries in Europe for cancer survival, England has 10,000 excess cancer deaths each year (Abdel-Rahman et al., 2009). This is solely related to the excess deaths attributable to later diagnosis.

Three examples of practical ways that seek to reduce cancer deaths due to late diagnosis

Example one: the 424 lives primary care project

Merseyside and Cheshire Cancer Network serves a population of little over two million people. In the network, there are at least 424 avoidable deaths from cancer. These deaths could be avoided if the best survival rates in European countries applied in Merseyside and Cheshire. This is the same as one or two people for each general practice. A small team of project managers work with GPs, pharmacists, primary care staff and the new Clinical Commissioning Groups (CCGs) to ask every practice to develop an action plan for detecting cancers earlier in their own patients. Two senior clinicians are available to help with training events and to work with the Boards of the CCGs.

Individual practices have appointed cancer champions, run cancer awareness events, trained receptionists, followed-up cancer screening non-attenders, used RATs and undertaken cancer event audits.

Example two: the iVan cancer awareness vehicle

This 27-foot long, bright yellow van is accompanied by a small team of trained cancer health workers. The van is kitted out as an information point and can provide a small confidential discussion area. The team visits events, workplaces, shopping centres and other gatherings across Merseyside and Cheshire. The team, though not the van, has also visited secure settings such as prisons. Four levels of contact with people are recorded, from a simple visit to a one-to-one discussion about concerns. Two things stand out from the evaluation. First, many people don't visit their GP despite their specific concerns about cancer symptoms. Second, there are now dozens of case studies where an individual has gone on to get a cancer diagnosis, after approaching the iVan team for advice. IVan has become an important brand for raising cancer awareness in Merseyside and Cheshire. Find out more at www.mccn.nhs.uk/index.php/about_us_ivan

Example three: the Lancashire and Cumbria staff awareness training online

Lancashire and South Cumbria Cancer Network developed a cancer awareness training package. It has been used by frontline staff in councils and in the health service to improve knowledge about cancer symptoms and signs. Find out more at www.cancerresearchuk.org/cancer-info/spotcancerearly/naedi/local-activity/getting-results/interventions-services-and-service-change-public/staff-awareness/

CHAPTER SUMMARY

Although early detection and diagnosis of cancer are not desirable in every situation, evidence suggests that early diagnosis improves survival. This is not always easy to achieve due to symptomatic patients presenting late to health professionals and also to delays during pathways to diagnosis. The general aim should be to diagnose cancer earlier, when it is easier to treat and there are better outcomes.

The UK lags behind the best in terms of timely diagnosis and cancer survival but everyone can make a difference by promoting people's awareness of cancer and by addressing the barriers that prevent people bringing their symptoms for diagnosis.

Key learning points

- Early diagnosis and detection is important in reducing the number of deaths from cancer.
- We should be careful to do more good than harm in our efforts to catch cancer earlier.
- Cancer may be diagnosed via a range of routes, for example following investigations, screening or emergency admission to hospital.
- Understanding delays in diagnosis and detection involves examining individual cancer journeys, from initial recognition that something is wrong through to consultation with a healthcare professional and referral for investigations.
- Individuals might not come forward with symptoms out of fear rather than ignorance.
- The Primary Care Team plays a key role in detection and diagnosis.
- Risk assessment tools and referral guidelines facilitate speedy referral of symptomatic patients for investigations and specialist support.
- Attitudinal, service, emotional and cultural barriers may obstruct early detection.
- Raising awareness of potential signs and symptoms of cancer is likely to encourage people to access Primary Healthcare providers for advice.
- The UK lags behind the best in terms of timely diagnosis and cancer survival.
- The general aim should be to diagnose cancer earlier when it is easier to treat and has better outcomes.

Recommended further reading

- Richards, M.A. and Hiom, S. (eds) (2009) 'Diagnosing cancer earlier: evidence for a National Awareness and Early Detection Initiative', *British Journal of Cancer*, 101(Suppl. 2): S1–S129. This is a comprehensive and detailed evidence review, which underpins the English National Awareness and Early Detection Initiative.
- Willie Hamilton's slim and readable book *Cancer Diagnosis in Primary Care* (2007) and the 'CAPER' studies by the same author (2009) are also excellent resources.

(Continued)

(Continued)

- Cancer Research UK (www.cancerresearchuk.org). This site has a wealth of data, information and advice. In particular, their 'catching cancer earlier' pages are very helpful and interesting.
- We also recommend the *Routes to Diagnosis* website (www.ncin.org.uk/publications/routes_to_diagnosis), which makes fascinating reading, as well as Macmillan Cancer Support (www.macmillan.org.uk).

4 THE BIOLOGY OF CANCER

DEBBIE WYATT AND VICTORIA BATES

Chapter outline

- Normal cell division
- DNA replication
- Cell cycle
- Carcinogenesis
- Genetic basis of cancer

- Cell mutation and role of carcinogens
- Oncogenes and proto-oncogenes
- Cancer genes
- Properties of cancer cells
- Relevance to practice

INTRODUCTION

Cancer is not, as commonly believed, one single disease, but a term used to describe more than 100 different diseases that share common features (Almeida and Barry, 2010). **Carcinogenesis** is the process by which cancer develops (Yarbro et al., 2011). In order to understand carcinogenesis, it is necessary to understand how normal cells behave and how this changes in cancer. This chapter describes the crucial role of DNA (**deoxyribonucleic acid**) in maintaining cell function and cell reproduction, and explains how changes to the DNA in cancer lead to the uncontrolled growth of abnormal cells, which have the potential to spread to distant parts of the body.

DNA forms the basis of genes and as genes direct cell function, faulty DNA causes cells to behave in abnormal ways. This chapter focuses on how the genetic basis of cancer explains the differences between normal cells and cancer cells. It also describes the properties of cancer cells and how these properties result in the uncontrolled growth of malignant tumours.

It is important for healthcare professionals to understand the biological basis of cancer in order to inform their practice.

NORMAL CELL DIVISION

In order to understand cancer, it is useful to comprehend the difference between normal and cancer cells. The human body is composed of many millions of cells, each of which has a specific function (Van Putte et al., 2014). From birth to adulthood, the number of cells is constantly increasing, but from maturity to death, there is a balance between cells dying and those being produced. Some cells divide frequently, such as the epithelial cells of the skin and blood cells formed in the bone marrow; others, such as bone cells, reproduce much more slowly (Gould and Dyer, 2011). DNA is found in the nucleus of cells and is responsible for both initiating and maintaining cell reproduction and cell function (McConnell and Hull, 2011). Cells are only stimulated to reproduce when another cell dies, following trauma or when growth factors are produced (Porth, 2011). **Growth factors**, chemicals produced by a variety of cells in the body, are capable of stimulating the proliferation of cells that they target. Cells only reproduce, therefore, when new ones are needed. Two other processes – contact inhibition and cellular senescence – also contribute to these safe guards. **Contact inhibition** is a process that stops cells dividing when they come into contact with each other. **Cellular senescence** is a process whereby cells that are old and worn out lose their ability to reproduce (Porth, 2011).

DNA REPLICATION

DNA forms **chromosomes**, which are thread like structures located in the nuclei of cells. Cells in humans have 46 chromosomes (23 pairs), except for ova and sperm, which have only 23 and red blood cells, which have none. The structure of DNA can be described as two long strands lying side by side and coiled as a pair into a spiral or double helix (see Figure 4.1). The two strands are held together by weak hydrogen bonds, which means that the two strands can separate when needed during the process of cell reproduction. The strands of DNA consist of four nitrogenous **bases** called adenine, thymine, guanine and cytosine, lined up in different combinations like coloured beads along a thread. Now imagine the two parallel strands of DNA lying side by side. The pattern of bases (or beads) along each strand is specific in that adenine is only ever paired with thymine (AT or TA) and guanine with cytosine (GC or CG). In other words, if thymine is found on one strand of DNA, adenine will be found at the same point on the opposite strand. Similarly, if guanine is found on one strand, cytosine will be found at the same point on the other.

Genes are made up of DNA and act as an instruction manual to make up different molecules of a cell. In other words, genes are sections or stretches of the chromosomal DNA and can be compared to a book of rules that each cell must follow to ensure they behave in an orderly and controlled way. The exact number of genes is not known, but it is estimated that it may be between 20,000 and 25,000 (Almeida and Barry, 2010).

In normal cells, the products of genes (**proteins**) are very tightly regulated and these products must be made in the correct amount. Genes must be 'switched on' and 'switched off' at the correct time because genes have specific roles at specific times. The set of genes that are 'on' at any given time is critical. Different genes need to be 'on' at different times depending on the needs and functions of any particular cell.

DNA has three main roles: to sustain the life of the cell, initiate and maintain cell function, and initiate and maintain cell reproduction. In simple terms, DNA is the life force of cells, controlling what they do, when they do it and when and how they reproduce. When a cell divides

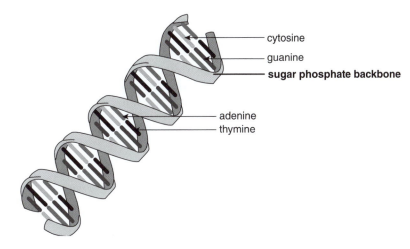

Figure 4.1 Structure of DNA

during the process of mitosis, a new cell is produced to form an exact copy of the original. This includes the creation of new DNA, which is formed when the paired strands of DNA separate and free floating bases found in the nucleus of the cell pair up with their matching base along each separated strand. This forms two sets of new DNA, which are an exact copy of each other (Figure 4.2).

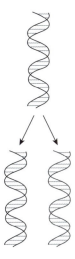

Figure 4.2 DNA replication

THE CELL CYCLE AND GROWTH

The right number of cells is required for organs and systems to function correctly. To do this, cells undergo a cycle of events known as the **cell cycle**, i.e. the different stages of development a cell goes through during its life (International Agency for Research on Cancer, 2008). Cancer cells go through the same phases of the cell cycle. This involves both cell division (called mitosis) and the period between two successive divisions (a period called interphase), which is the period that most people associate with being 'the cell cycle'. Mitosis, the end result of the cell cycle, is when the cell divides. Some cells, such as the gametes (the female ova and the male sperm), do not divide by mitosis but divide by a different process called meiosis (Marieb and Hoehn, 2013).

The phases of cell growth and proliferation in the cell cycle of reproduction are described next.

Interphase – the 'cell cycle'

This is a very active phase of cell growth and proliferation made up of Gap phase 0 (G_0), Gap phase 1 (G_1), Synthesis (S), Gap phase 2 (G_2) and Mitosis (M). Gap phase can also be known as growth phase. A cell that is in the process of preparing for cell division or is dividing is said to be in the cell cycle of reproduction and consists of the G_1, S, G_2 and M phases.

G_0 is described as the resting phase and has no time limit. People often refer to this stage as being inactive, which isn't entirely true. The cell is not preparing to divide, but it continues to perform normal metabolic functions in order to survive. Cells in G_0 require growth factors (naturally occurring substances that are able to fuel cellular growth) to instruct the cell to enter the next stage of the cell cycle, G_1. Some cells, such as epithelial cells, are in the resting phase for relatively short periods of time because they continually need to be replaced, whereas nerve cells, for example, do not need to be replaced as regularly so remain in G_0 for long periods of time.

G_1 is the first step a cell makes to undergo cell division. At the end of the cell cycle, there will be two identical cells instead of one, and therefore it is important that there are sufficient numbers of organelles (a cellular 'organ' or subunit that has a specific function within a cell) to meet the demands of the two cells. To accommodate the extra organelles, the cell increases in size. To make these duplicate organelles, proteins and lipids are transported across the cell membrane into the cell and RNA (**ribonucleic acid**) is synthesized. DNA contains genes that are transcribed into RNA and then RNA can be translated into a protein. The standard information flow is:

DNA → RNA → Protein

RNA is important in the generation of proteins and is made up of one single strand of nucleic acids (unlike DNA which is double-stranded). The generation of new proteins demands a lot of energy, which requires the use of glucose as fuel for these processes. This stage must be complete before the next stage commences and usually takes around 8 to 12 hours (Martini et al., 2012), although in cells that divide slowly, this phase may last from days to years (Marieb and Hoehn, 2013).

During S phase, a completely new and identical set of DNA is produced and all of the chromosomes have been replicated. During this process, DNA is particularly vulnerable to damage from external carcinogens. A slightly shorter phase than G_1, S lasts around 6 to 8 hours (Martini et al., 2012).

During G_2, the cell continues to grow and synthesize much-needed proteins, such as microtubules (tube-like filaments), which help to support and maintain the structure of the cell. These are required for cells to undergo mitosis. This phase is shorter again, lasting around 2 to 5 hours (Martini et al., 2012).

Mitosis, where one cell becomes two, involves a process called nuclear division (karyokinesis). It consists of four distinct phases: prophase, metaphase, anaphase and telophase. The whole process of mitosis lasts around 1 hour in a typical human cell (Marieb and Hoehn, 2013).

1. *Prophase:* This is the longest phase of mitosis. **Chromatin** (replicated DNA and protein) threads condense into chromosomes. The nucleoli (found within the cell's nucleus and made up of proteins and nucleic acids), becomes invisible and the nuclear membrane disappears. Just like the organelles, centrioles (small organelles found in the cytoplasm that aid division) are replicated, begin to migrate to opposing sides of the cell and project radiating fibres. Mitotic spindles (protein framework) then develop on both sides (Van Putte et al., 2014). The chromosomes come between the spindles in the centre of the cell and attach to both halves of the spindle via the chromosomal centromeres – the area where chromatid pairs (chromosomes) are linked.
2. *Metaphase:* This is the lining-up phase, which is a shorter phase than prophase. Chromatid pairs line up along the centre of the cell. Each chromosome attaches to its own spindle fibre.
3. *Anaphase:* Chromatid pairs separate and are drawn to opposite sides of the cell by shortened mitotic spindles. This is another short phase.
4. *Telophase:* The chromatid strands become invisible as they uncoil. Spindle fibres detach from the chromatids. The nuclear membrane is formed around each complete set of chromosomes, creating two nuclei, ready for the cell to divide.

Finally, in a process called cytokinesis, spindle fibres are degraded and the cytoplasm and organelles divide so that each new cell contains equal and sufficient numbers of each (International Agency for Research on Cancer, 2008). Figure 4.3 represents the stages of the cell cycle.

WHAT IS CANCER?

Cancer is a disease in which DNA changes. Normal cells function and reproduce in a very controlled manner and work on a 'supply and demand' basis (Porth, 2011). Cells will only

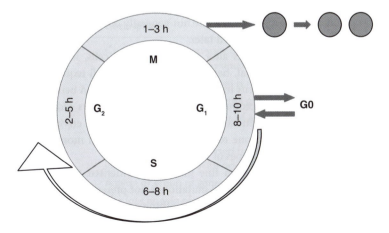

Figure 4.3 A diagram representing the stages of the cell cycle of a normally functioning cell

Table 4.2   Types of cancer genes

Type of gene	Normal function	Mutated function	Types of proteins
Tumour supressor gene	Suppresses cell division	Fails to suppress cell division	Cell cycle checkpoint molecules
Oncogene	As proto-oncogene, promotes cell division	Promotes cell division – abnormal time or cell type	Growth factors
DNA repair gene	Repairs DNA mutations	Fails to repair DNA mutations	Enzymes for DNA repair

Tumour suppressor genes

When functioning normally, tumour suppressor genes will act to prevent cells with mutated DNA from completing the cell cycle, therefore preventing them from passing their errors onto other cells. When a tumour suppressor gene acquires a mutation, it can no longer perform this function, and cells with DNA mutations are able to pass through the cell cycle undetected (Hesketh, 2013). The most common tumour suppressor genes to be mutated are cell cycle checkpoint genes, such as p53 mentioned earlier. Other common tumour suppressor genes that are mutated in cancer include RB and VHL (see Table 4.3).

Table 4.3   Examples of tumour suppressor genes, oncogenes and DNA repair genes

Example	Normal function	Cancer
Tumour suppressor genes		
APC	Scaffold protein[a]	Colorectal
CDKN2A	Regulates cell division	Melanoma
RB	Regulates cell division	Retinoblastoma
TP53	Regulates cell division and apoptosis	Lung
VHL	Regulates cell division and angiogenesis	Kidney
Oncogenes		
B-RAF	Intracellular signalling	Melanoma
HER2	Growth factor receptor	Breast
MYC	Transcription factor	Neuroblastoma
RAS	Intracellular signalling	Colorectal
VEGF	Angiogenesis promoter	Metastatic colorectal
DNA repair genes		
ATM	DNA repair	Leukaemia
BRCA1/2	DNA repair	Breast
MLH1	DNA repair	Colorectal
MSH2	DNA repair	Colorectal
XPA	DNA repair	Lung

Notes:
[a]Important in the regulation of signalling pathways.

Proto-oncogenes and oncogenes

Proto-oncogenes are genes that promote cell growth. Proto-oncogenes have one of four main functions:

1. Growth factor: a protein or hormone that can stimulate cell growth and proliferation.
2. Growth factor receptor: binds to the growth factor.
3. Signal transduction: once the growth factor binds to the receptor, the receptor is activated, allowing the signal to grow or proliferate to be passed to the cell.
4. Transcription factor: binds to DNA and 'reads' the genetic information from DNA to RNA, which is vital for the production of proteins required for normal cellular behaviour.

When a proto-oncogene becomes mutated, it becomes an **oncogene** (see Table 4.2) (Marieb and Hoehn, 2013). An oncogene also promotes cell growth, but this time in an unchecked, uncontrolled manner. It can cause cells to send and receive signals to divide even if it is not required. As these mutated cells continue to grow, they can acquire more mutations, causing them to behave even more abnormally. Examples of oncogenes include human epidermal growth factor 2 (HER2), rat sarcoma (Ras) and vascular endothelial growth factor (VEGF).

DNA repair genes

These are genes that ensure each strand of genetic information is accurately copied during cell division of the cell cycle. Mutations in DNA repair genes lead to an increase in the frequency of mutations in other genes, such as oncogenes and tumour suppressor genes (International Agency for Research on Cancer, 2008). Breast cancer susceptibility genes (BRCA1 and BRCA2) and hereditary non-polyposis colon cancer susceptibility genes (MSH2, MLH1, PMS1, PMS2), for example, have DNA repair functions. Their mutation will lead to a significantly increased chance of carcinogenesis.

PROPERTIES OF CANCER CELLS

The most significant change in cancer is to the DNA, and therefore to the genes. If the DNA changes, so does the set of rules by which the cell is programmed to behave. These changes to the DNA are called mutations and several mutations are needed in order for cancer to develop.

Cancer cells have different properties to normal cells and they behave in different ways, but it is important to remember that cancers do not necessarily grow any faster than normal cells. Just as in a normal healthy body when some cells divide frequently and others less often, some cancers grow quickly and others slowly.

The original six **hallmarks of cancer** (Hanahan and Weinberg, 2000) and the recent addition of two further hallmarks described by Hanahan and Weinberg (2011) help to provide a framework for understanding neoplastic disease.

Mutations in **growth factors** such as VEGF signal angiogenesis and blood vessels grow towards the site of the tumour. Some cancer cells may then break through the basement membrane and enter the blood or lymphatic vessels. From here, they have the potential to travel anywhere around the body. Not all cancer cells that enter blood vessels will survive – in fact only 2% of circulating cancer cells escape to form micrometastases and only 1% of these develop into tumours (Hesketh, 2013). They are either damaged when entering through the blood vessels, the immune system may detect and destroy them, or they may become damaged whilst travelling along the blood or lymphatic vessels. For cancer cells that do survive, they can attach to the blood vessel wall in a new location and squeeze through the vessel walls into the surrounding tissue where they can begin to proliferate and create a new generation of cancer cells (secondary tumour). This process is called the **metastatic cascade** (Figure 4.5).

7. Reprogramming of cellular energy metabolism
    Altered energy metabolism in cancer cells leads to continuous cell growth and proliferation. Normal cells need oxygen (aerobic respiration) to survive and proliferate. Cancer cells can switch to anaerobic respiration, which means they no longer need a regular supply of oxygen. Instead, they increase uptake of glucose, which provides enough energy to survive.

8. Evading immune destruction
    The immune system recognizes and eliminates many cancer cells. Some cancer cells, however, can evade attack by the immune system by disguising themselves as normal cells and becoming invisible to the immune system.

A summary of the hallmarks of cancer can be seen in Table 4.4.

Table 4.4   Summary of hallmarks of cancer

Hallmark	Mechanism
1. Sustaining proliferative signalling	Cancer cells do not need to receive growth signals to grow and proliferate. Some cancer cells actually generate their own growth signals. Some cells have too many growth factor receptors (over-expression) and are able to grow and proliferate more often than they should.
2. Evading growth suppressors	Cancer cells are able to ignore these signals and carry on dividing despite them. This commonly occurs due to mutation in the retinoblastoma (RB) gene.
3. Resisting cell death	Cancer cells can evade cell death, allowing cells to carry on dividing, passing on mutations to other cells.
4. Enabling replicative immortality	Cancer cells evade 'old age' and can live for greater periods of time. This is usually caused by mutations of the RB or p53 genes or the production of telomerase, which enable cells to survive for longer.
5. Inducing angiogenesis	Cancer cells can send signals to allow new blood vessels to grow towards the tumour, providing the tumour with more oxygen and nutrients to survive. This is usually caused by a mutation or over-expression of VEGF.

Hallmark	Mechanism
6. Tissue invasion and metastasis	Invasion of cancer cells into blood vessels and surrounding tissues is essential for a tumour to grow and metastasize. They are able to do this by mimicking and altering proteins that normally prevent metastases.
7. Reprogramming of cellular energy metabolism	Cancer cells have a greater uptake of glucose due to adjustments in their metabolism of energy. This provides cancer cells with enough energy to survive and reproduce.
8. Evading immune destruction	The immune system is very good at detecting and destroying many cancer cells. Some cancer cells can evade the immune system by disguising themselves as normal cells and becoming invisible to the immune system.

Source: Hanahan and Weinberg, 2000; Hanahan and Weinberg, 2011.

RELEVANCE TO PRACTICE

It is important for healthcare practitioners from a variety of professional backgrounds, including nursing, allied health professionals and psychosocial care, to understand the effects of carcinogenesis for a number of reasons. These range from recognizing physical symptoms to facilitate early detection and prompt treatment, through to providing psychosocial support around the physical and psychological impact of cancer on the individual (see Table 4.5).

Table 4.5 Importance of knowledge of carcinogenesis on practice

Benefit	Rationale	Example
	Knowledge and understanding of the biology of cancer:	
Early detection of cancer	Raises awareness of potential physical symptoms associated with cancer, such as lumps, bleeding, fatigue	A practice nurse reviewing a patient's blood pressure notices that the patient's skin is covered in small bruises. She is aware that bruising can be a symptom of haematological cancers and organizes a full blood count and appointment for the patient to see his GP.
	Enhances opportunities for healthcare professionals to recommend that patients seek advice for such symptoms Facilitates early referral of patients to relevant healthcare professional e.g. GP	

(Continued)

Table 4.5 (Continued)

Benefit	Rationale	Example
	Knowledge and understanding of the biology of cancer:	
Prompt treatment of physical symptoms experienced by people with a diagnosis of cancer	Promotes effective assessment through anticipation of potential symptoms	During a physiotherapy-led breathlessness management clinic for people with lung cancer, the patient divulges that he has also developed severe back pain. The physiotherapist is aware of the potential for spinal cord compression as a result of metastases and refers the patient to his oncologist.
	Leads to early referral for appropriate interventions, such as treatments and/or symptom management	
Meets patients' information needs about their cancer and symptoms	Facilitates effective explanations and responses to questions that are tailored to the level of patient need	A patient who has just received a diagnosis of ovarian cancer asks the nurse to explain what cancer is and how it leads to symptoms. The nurse explains the biology of cancer at a pace and depth guided by the patient.
Effective monitoring of progression or remission of disease	Raises awareness of potential physical changes (and their implications), which can be promptly communicated to patients/relevant healthcare professionals	A patient diagnosed with prostate cancer 18 months ago informs the urology nurse specialist at clinic that frequency of urination has increased over the last few weeks. The clinical nurse specialist is aware that this may be due to growth of the prostate cancer and orders further investigations.
	Promotes effective treatment and support	
Promotes patient safety	Enables healthcare professionals to understand the action of treatments on cancer and anticipate potential side effects	A community occupational therapist undertaking a home visit discovers that severe fatigue is negatively impacting on the patient's ability to cope with everyday life. The occupational therapist is aware that this may be a result of the cancer or cancer treatments and refers the patient to her oncologist, physiotherapist and social worker.
	Promotes effective assessment and management of potential side effects	
	Informs decisions that underpin practice	

Benefit	Rationale	Example
	Knowledge and understanding of the biology of cancer:	
Meets patients' and carers' information needs about the effect of treatments on cancers	Facilitates effective explanations and responses to questions that are tailored to the level of patient need	A patient admitted to a chemotherapy unit for adjuvant chemotherapy treatment for breast cancer, asks the nurse what effect the chemotherapy will have on her cancer. The nurse, guided by the level of the patient's information needs, explains the effect of chemotherapy on normal cells and cancer cells.
Promotes effective multiprofessional team working	Promotes effective communication of clinical information between members of the multiprofessional team	A dietician giving dietary advice to a patient with tonsillar cancer discovers that the patient is very low in mood because he is unable to swallow. The dietician is aware that this may be a symptom of the cancer or treatment but is a serious consequence of either. She informs the multiprofessional team for review and referral to the clinical psychologist.
	Informs discussions around clinical decisions and patient care	

Reflective activity

- Reflect on your practice and identify situations where knowledge of the biology of cancer has been important.
- Consider why and how your understanding impacted positively on patient care.
- Compare your experiences to those suggested in Table 4.5.

CHAPTER SUMMARY

This chapter emphasizes the crucial role that DNA plays in cell life, function and reproduction. Inherited or acquired mutations in DNA can lead to the formation of cancer cells characterized by different properties that cause them to behave in abnormal ways. The mechanisms by which this occurs are complex but the eight hallmarks of cancer identified by Hanahan and Weinberg (2011) help to explain how cancers grow and have the potential to spread to other parts of the body. Insight into these mechanisms helps to inform practice on a number of levels and is therefore an important requirement for those working in cancer care.

Key learning points

- DNA sustains the life of a cell, initiates and maintains cell function, and maintains cell reproduction.
- In normal tissues, new cells are only produced when they are needed (e.g. following trauma, cell death or in response to stimulation by a growth factor).
- Cancer is a disease in which DNA changes.
- Genetic mutations can be inherited or acquired after birth.
- Cancer cells continue to proliferate regardless of whether new cells are needed.
- Cancer cells behave differently to normal cells and

  o Have a reduced need for growth factors to stimulate cell reproduction,
  o Produce their own growth factors that stimulate the division of cells,
  o Lose the restriction point in their cell cycle, which contributes to excess proliferation of cells,
  o Resist cell death by avoiding apoptosis,
  o Produce significant amounts of the enzyme telomerase, which prevents shortening of telomeres and leads to cancer cell immortality,
  o Switch on angiogenesis in order to grow their own blood supply when a collection of cancer cells grows to about 1-2 mm in size,
  o Can invade local tissues and metastasize to distant parts of the body,
  o Can increase their uptake of glucose, which provides them with enough energy to survive,
  o Can evade cells of the immune system that would normally destroy them.

- Knowledge and understanding of carcinogenesis enhances cancer care.

Recommended further reading

- Almeida, C.A. and Barry, S.A. (2010) *Cancer: Basic Science and Clinical Aspects*. Oxford: Wiley-Blackwell.
- Hanahan, D. and Weinberg, R.A. (2011) 'Hallmarks of cancer: the next generation', *Cell*, 144: 646–74.
- Hesketh, R. (2013) *Introduction to Cancer Biology*. Cambridge: Cambridge University Press.

5 TUMOUR PATHOLOGY: CLASSIFICATION, GRADING AND STAGING

PAUL MANSOUR

Chapter outline

- Tumour classification
- Tumour grading
- Tumour staging
- Tumour markers
- What happens in a cellular pathology laboratory?

- The nature of histopathological diagnosis
- The role of the pathologist
- The role of the autopsy

INTRODUCTION

The role of the **pathologist** is to give the rest of the clinical team the information they need to decide how best to manage the patient. Everything that goes on in the laboratory, from receipt of the specimen to signing the final report, happens (or should happen) with that aim in mind. An important part of that role is to explain the content and significance of their reports to their clinical colleagues, but it is easy for pathologists to assume that the rest of the team is as familiar with the technical terms used as they are. It is, therefore, important that clinicians have some idea of what is meant by such concepts as grade, stage, differentiation, **immunohistochemistry** and so on. Furthermore, patients are increasingly likely to see their pathology reports, and frontline clinicians must be prepared to explain at least the more common terms to them.

It is tempting to view the pathology laboratory as a 'black box' into which specimens are fed and out of which reports are issued. However, although a detailed knowledge of how a laboratory works is not necessary, it is vital that clinicians have a general idea of how specimens move through the laboratory, the timescales involved and what tests are likely to be done on them. They can then use the laboratory in an efficient way that maximizes the amount of information extracted from each specimen.

different characteristics, and it is important to recognize and diagnose these variants because they behave differently and may respond differently to treatment.

Furthermore, besides its own characteristic epithelium, the breast is made up of many different types of mesenchymal tissue including fibroblasts, blood vessels, smooth muscle, fat, nerves and lymphocytes, none of which is specific to the breast. Both benign and malignant tumours can arise from each of these different tissues, although much more rarely than does carcinoma.

Therefore, although the term 'breast cancer' without further qualification is taken to mean adenocarcinoma of the breast, strictly speaking it could also equally mean an **angiosarcoma** or **lymphoma** of the breast. Of course, this situation is not unique to the breast – although every organ has one or two common primary malignancies, all have the potential to give rise to a wide range of tumour types.

TUMOUR GRADING

The **grade** of a tumour is a measure of its degree of **differentiation**, which reflects how closely it resembles the normal tissue from which it arose. Higher grade (poorly differentiated) tumours will tend to behave more **aggressively** (grow faster and metastasize earlier) than lower grade tumours. Well-differentiated cancers can resemble benign tissue so closely that it can be difficult (and sometimes extremely difficult) to tell whether it is actually a cancer at all, or just a reaction to inflammation or injury. This problem is even more difficult in small biopsies. At the other end of the spectrum, a poorly differentiated cancer can show so few identifying features that it can be difficult to tell what tissue type it arose from. Deciding the grade of a tumour usually involves assessing a combination of its architecture, its functional activity (in terms of what substances it produces), the size and shape of its nuclei and how frequently its cells divide.

Tumour architecture

Cancers generally try to form the same structures as the benign cells from which they arise. For example, adenocarcinomas arise from glandular epithelium and therefore tend to form glands or tubules, made up of cells arranged around a central space or lumen. Well-differentiated adenocarcinomas form more tubules than less well differentiated tumours; some poorly differentiated adenocarcinomas form solid cords or sheets of cells without any gland formation, and their nature may only be evident from other glandular features such as secretion of mucus (see later), or by identifying specific proteins within the tumour cells.

Cell secretions

Just as normal cells produce substances characteristic of each different cell type, so too do cancer cells, depending on their degree of differentiation. Benign glandular cells often produce mucus, and carcinomas arising from glandular cells (adenocarcinomas) will also tend to do so. This can be demonstrated by staining the cells with chemicals that react with specific types of mucin. Normal squamous cells (such as on the surface of the skin) produce a protein called **keratin**, which forms a protective outer layer; squamous carcinoma cells also produce keratin, which can be seen microscopically as pink, slightly shiny material within the cancer cells.

Nuclear features

Cancer is the end result of a series of mutations in the DNA within genes (Hanahan and Weinberg, 2000), and it is therefore not surprising that visible changes indicating cancer are most obvious within cell nuclei. Cancer cells tend to have larger, darker and more irregular nuclei than benign cells, with poorly differentiated tumours showing more nuclear abnormality than well-differentiated ones.

Frequency of cell division

Mitosis is the process by which cells divide and can be recognized microscopically, with individual chromosomes visibly separating into two new clusters as the cell splits apart. A histological section of a tumour is, in effect, a snapshot taken at the moment of fixation, at which time its cellular processes are 'frozen'. The rate of cell division (which usually reflects how fast the tumour is growing) therefore cannot be measured directly, but counting the number of mitoses in a given area of the tumour is an indirect way of doing so. Poorly differentiated cancers therefore typically have more numerous mitoses per square millimetre than well-differentiated tumours.

These different features do tend to vary in step with each other: a well-differentiated adenocarcinoma, for example, will tend to show well-formed glands, fairly regular nuclei and few mitoses, and produce mucin. This is not always the case, however, and more sophisticated grading systems (such as that used for grading breast cancers) assess each of these factors separately (see box below).

There comes a point in the most aggressive tumours where the type of cell from which they arise can no longer be identified by routine microscopy, and such very poorly differentiated tumours are sometimes described as 'undifferentiated' or **'anaplastic'**. It is in this group that **immunohistochemistry** (see later) is of most use in identifying the type of cancer.

Modified Bloom-Richardson grading of breast carcinoma: Nottingham criteria

Gland formation (proportion of tumour made up of well-formed glands)

> **75%** of the tumour:	Score	1
10-75% of the tumour:		2
< **10%** of the tumour:		3

Nuclear atypia/pleomorphism (compared with adjacent benign nuclei)

Slightly enlarged; minor variation in size, shape and chromatin pattern:	Score	1
Enlarged; nucleoli visible; distinct variation in size, shape and chromatin pattern:		2
Markedly enlarged and vesicular; marked variation in size, shape and chromatin pattern:		3

(Continued)

(Continued)

Mitotic count per 10 high-power fields (adjusted for each individual microscope)

< 10:	Score	1
10-20:		2
> 20:		3

FINAL GRADING: add all three scores together:

Total score:	
3-5 = **grade 1**
6-7 = **grade 2**
8-9 = **grade 3**

Reproduced from *Breast Cancer Grading: Nottingham Criteria* (2005), a publication of the national office of the NHS Cancer Screening Programmes (operated by Public Health England), with permission.

TUMOUR STAGING

The **stage** of a tumour is a measure of how large it has grown and how far it has spread. It is important not to confuse the stage of a tumour with its grade, although they are associated to some extent: a poorly differentiated tumour will generally grow faster and metastasize earlier than a well-differentiated tumour.

TNM staging system

The commonest international staging system is the TNM system, in which the primary **T**umour, lymph **N**ode involvement and the presence (or absence) of **M**etastases are assessed separately (Sobin et al., 2010). This general approach to staging is applicable to all tumours, although the details differ for each. As an example, the TNM system for carcinoma of the bladder is given in the following box.

TNM staging for carcinoma of the urinary bladder

T: PRIMARY TUMOUR

TX	Primary tumour cannot be assessed
T0	No evidence of primary tumour
Ta	Non-invasive papillary carcinoma
Tis	'Flat' carcinoma in situ
T1	Tumour invades subepithelial connective tissue
T2	Tumour invades muscle:
T2a	– inner half of muscle of bladder wall
T2b	– outer half of muscle of bladder wall

T3	Tumour invades perivesical tissue:	
T3a	- microscopically	
T3b	- macroscopically (with extravesical mass)	
T4	Tumour invades any of the following:	
T4a	- prostate stroma, seminal vesicles, uterus or vagina	
T4b	- pelvic wall or abdominal wall	

N: REGIONAL LYMPH NODES

NX	Regional lymph nodes cannot be assessed
N0	No regional lymph node metastasis
N1	Metastasis in a single lymph node in the true pelvis (hypogastric, obturator, external iliac or presacral)
N2	Metastasis in multiple lymph nodes in the true pelvis (hypogastric, obturator, external iliac or presacral)
N3	Metastasis in one or more common iliac lymph node

M: DISTANT METASTASES

M0	No distant metastases
M1	Distant metastases present (including distant lymph node metastases)

The pre-treatment or clinical classification, based on clinical examination and/or imaging, is designated TNM (or cTNM). The post-treatment classification, based on pathological examination of resected tissue, is designated pTNM.

Reproduced from Sobin et al. (2010) under STM copyright permission guidelines.

Dysplasia

An epithelium is described as **dysplastic** when it has undergone some, but not all, of the genetic changes needed to become fully malignant. In some organs, the term 'dysplasia' has been replaced by '**intra-epithelial neoplasia**'. In the uterine cervix, for example, mild, moderate and severe dysplasia have been replaced respectively by Cervical Intra-epithelial Neoplasia grades 1, 2 and 3 (CIN 1, CIN 2 and CIN 3). High-grade dysplasia is more likely to progress to invasive carcinoma than low-grade dysplasia.

Inherent in the concept of epithelial dysplasia is the fact that, although neoplastic (because the cells have escaped the normal control mechanisms that usually govern their proliferation), the proliferating cells are still confined within the basement membrane that separates the epithelium from the underlying connective tissue stroma and are therefore still 'non-invasive'; therefore, because there are no blood or lymphatic vessels within the epithelium, neoplastic cells limited to the epithelium cannot metastasize. Complete excision of the dysplastic area will therefore ensure complete 'cure', at least of that particular dysplastic area.

Micro-invasive carcinoma

Recognizing the role of the basement membrane in defining the presence of invasion also intro-duces the idea of 'micro-invasive carcinoma', that is, a carcinoma that has invaded through the basement membrane to such a limited extent that the risk of metastasis is virtually non-existent, so that (in at least some organs) it can be treated in the same way as a non-invasive tumour (Bianchi and Vezzosi, 2008; Mota, 2003).

Sentinel node staging

It is important to know if a cancer has spread to the local **lymph nodes** or not because, depending on the organ involved, this may indicate whether or not the cancer is still cur-able by surgery or whether radiotherapy or chemotherapy are needed as well. **Sentinel node biopsy** is a technique used to identify and remove the first node that the cancer would spread to (instead of randomly sampling several nodes). If this first, or 'sentinel', node is negative, it is highly likely that all the other nodes will also be negative. If positive, then all the local lymph nodes can be removed. The sentinel node is identified by injecting both a coloured dye and a radioactive liquid into the tumour some hours before surgery and removing the first node encountered that is either coloured, radioactive or both. Sentinel node biopsy is currently used in staging breast cancer (Kumar et al., 2012) and skin melanoma (Stebbins et al., 2010), and its use is being investigated in cancers of other organs.

TUMOUR MARKERS

Tumour markers are substances, often proteins, secreted by tumours and detectable in the blood that can be used to diagnose tumours or to monitor their response to treatment, or both (Table 5.2). They can be raised in a number of cancers, as well as in many benign conditions, and are most useful in monitoring previously diagnosed tumours by serial measurement rather than in primary diagnosis.

The need for informed consent should be considered before requesting tumour markers to diagnose cancer, especially in a screening context. For example, screening men for prostate cancer by measuring blood levels of **prostate specific antigen** (PSA) is not currently recom-mended in the UK (UK National Screening Committee, 2010; Hummel and Chilcott, 2013), partly because a raised level does not necessarily indicate the presence of cancer, but also because even if cancer is diagnosed by prostate biopsy following a raised PSA result, it is not currently possible to tell whether that cancer would ever require treatment or not. Indeed, some authorities question whether small, low-grade prostate tumours currently regarded as cancers are, either biologically or clinically, actually malignant at all (Ahmed et al., 2012). Furthermore, both diagnosis and treatment carry significant complications: trans-rectal pros-tate biopsy is unpleasant and carries a risk of infection of about 4%, serious enough to need admission in 0.8% (Loeb et al., 2012), and radical surgery for prostate cancer causes erectile dysfunction in one-third of men and incontinence in one-fifth, with a risk of post-operative death of 0.5% (Chou et al., 2011). These complications may well be considered acceptable if the patient is cured of a potentially lethal cancer, but not if the cancer was known in advance to be unlikely to shorten the patient's life. These issues should be fully discussed with men who ask for a PSA test so that they are fully aware of the possible consequences of a 'positive' result.

Table 5.2 Tumour markers

Marker	Raised in cancers of:	Also raised in:	
		Benign	Cancers of
PSA	Prostate	Benign prostatic hyperplasia; urinary tract infection; catheterization	None known
CA125	Ovary	Pregnancy; menstruation; endometriosis; hepatitis; kidney and heart failure	Breast; uterus; liver; lung; pancreas
CA19–9	Pancreas	Pancreatitis; inflammatory bowel disease	Bowel; bile ducts
CEA	Large bowel	Irritable bowel syndrome; jaundice; hepatitis; kidney failure	Breast; stomach; lung; thyroid; oesophagus; pancreas
AFP and ß-HCG	Testis	Hepatitis; benign liver disease; pregnancy	Liver; bowel; lung; stomach
Paraproteins	Myeloma; lymphoma	Autoimmune and infective conditions, especially in old age	None known
Hormones	Endocrine organs	Benign endocrine conditions	Lung

Source: Information derived from Pathology Harmony (2012); Lab Tests Online UK (2014).

WHAT HAPPENS IN A CELLULAR PATHOLOGY LABORATORY?

The range of specimens received by a diagnostic histopathology laboratory will naturally depend on the type of hospital it serves, but samples typically vary in size from endoscopic biopsies only 2–3 mm in diameter to mastectomy and total colectomy specimens. Most laboratories deal with general gastrointestinal, breast, lung, skin, urological and gynaecological specimens, while more specialized laboratories may also receive paediatric, bone and eye cancer, and neuropathological specimens. The ultimate purpose of each laboratory, however, is the same: to produce one or more **glass slides** from each specimen that the pathologist can examine microscopically to make a diagnosis.

It is recommended that slides be kept for at least 10 years, and blocks for at least thirty years (Royal College of Pathologists, 2009). This allows slides to be reviewed for comparison with subsequent specimens or for quality purposes and audit. It also allows further sections to be cut and stained if necessary.

Fixation

The first step in this process is **fixation,** that is, the use of chemicals to preserve (or 'fix') the tissue in a condition as close as possible to how it was when it was removed from the patient. The most common fixative in routine use is formalin, an aqueous solution of formaldehyde gas. Formalin is toxic and carcinogenic, and both skin contact and inhalation should be avoided.

a tumour's behaviour and response to treatment. For example, a common test is the use of fluorescent *in situ* hybridization (FISH) to identify whether breast cancer cells contain multiple copies of the gene that codes for the HER-2 protein. Those cancers in which this gene is amplified in this way behave more aggressively, but are also sensitive to drug treatment with the monoclonal antibody trastuzumab (Herceptin) (Higgins and Baselga, 2011). Similarly, drugs are now available that are effective only if specific genetic mutations are either present, as in the EGFR gene in lung cancer (Lyseng-Williamson, 2013), or absent, as in the KRAS gene in colorectal cancer (Malapelle et al., 2014), and these cancers are now routinely tested for these mutations. The use of molecular genetics is now in the process of transforming the practice of diagnostic histopathology as radically as immunohistochemistry did thirty years ago.

Cytopathology

In contrast to histology, **cytological** diagnosis usually involves assessing the characteristics of individual cells or groups of cells and does not allow assessment of tissue architecture. This is compensated for by the greater detail in which the cells can be examined, and in particular the clarity of the chromatin pattern of the cell nuclei. This reflects the amount and distribution of chromosomal DNA within the nucleus and is often deranged in malignancy. Furthermore, it is often less invasive (and less painful) to obtain cytological specimens and, with almost instant fixation and without the need for tissue processing, results can be available within a few minutes of the sample being taken. Nevertheless, particularly in doubtful cases, a histological diagnosis is generally taken as definitive.

The three common types of cytology samples received are **exfoliative** specimens (where cells are either shed spontaneously from the surface of an organ, as in urine cytology, or scraped from it, as in smears from the uterine cervix); **aspiration** specimens of serous cavity effusions (such as pleural or ascitic fluid); and **fine needle aspiration** samples of solid organs or tumours. Samples can be spread directly onto glass slides, or collected into a variety of fluid fixatives and then centrifuged onto slides. Special stains (including IHC) can also often be performed on cytology specimens.

THE NATURE OF HISTOPATHOLOGICAL DIAGNOSIS

In some pathology disciplines, such as clinical chemistry, the pathologist's role is to interpret the numerical values produced by blood analyzers in the context of the patient's clinical condition. Histopathological diagnosis, on the other hand, is much more subjective and mainly involves recognizing patterns revealed by staining tissue with a variety of dyes.

A useful analogy is that of an art expert asked to decide whether a particular painting is a true masterpiece, the work of a pupil working under the Master, or a modern forgery. The expert will form their opinion largely by assessing quite subjective characteristics of the painting. What is the picture of? Is the general style appropriate for the period? Are the pattern and thickness of brush strokes similar to those in known genuine works? The expert may assess each characteristic individually and systematically, especially if they are not as familiar with that particular painter as with others, but in more straightforward cases they will come to a conclusion almost subconsciously, without even necessarily being aware of the steps they have taken to reach that conclusion. One or more technical investigations may be of help: chemical analysis of the paint, for example, may reveal modern pigments not in use in the sixteenth century, or X-rays might show a modern painting beneath the forged 'masterpiece'. But if the results are not clear cut, then these technologies will merely help to guide the expert, rather than provide an unequivocal answer.

In pathological terms, the question being posed is usually, 'Is this cancer or some benign mimic?' Most cases are relatively straightforward, and the standard H&E stain will be sufficient to reach a confident diagnosis based on pattern recognition. In more difficult cases, technology may be called upon, in the form of special stains such as immunohistochemistry, but this often merely helps guide the pathologist rather than giving a definitive answer.

It is important to be aware of the subjective nature of a histopathology diagnosis, and to recognize that what is offered is no more than an opinion, albeit one based on many years of experience. Indeed, even experienced breast pathologists examining the same slides can disagree over whether a sample is benign or malignant in a number of cases (Stang et al., 2011). It is therefore common for pathologists to seek opinions from colleagues, either within the same department or in other hospitals, and in some laboratories a second pathologist must formally confirm all new diagnoses of cancer.

THE ROLE OF THE PATHOLOGIST

Pathologists are usually medically qualified doctors, whose medical training allows them to interpret a patient's pathological diagnosis in the context of the clinical situation as a whole. In some pathology disciplines, especially biochemistry and genetics, consultant clinical scientists are trained to a high degree (at least to doctorate level) and fulfil the same role as their medical colleagues. Their training gives them a similar degree of clinical insight within their specialty, but perhaps without the broad overview that medical training provides. In cellular pathology, almost all consultants are still medical doctors, but this is likely to change in the future as more scientists take on extended roles.

Pathology reports are necessarily of a technical nature: they are written with the clinical team in mind to guide treatment and predict prognosis; however, patients are increasingly likely to ask for a copy of their reports, and will need guidance from their cancer team in understanding them. Most cancer organizations have produced leaflets to help patients make sense of their pathology reports (Breast Cancer Care, 2013; Prostate Cancer UK, 2012).

Multidisciplinary cancer teams

One of the most important recent changes in the way that UK pathologists work has been in the establishment of multidisciplinary cancer teams (MDT), which arose out of concern in the 1990s that the outcomes of patients with cancer in the UK did not match those elsewhere in Europe or in the USA. Largely as a result of this initiative, pathologists today are core members of the clinical team, participating fully in weekly MDT meetings along with the surgeons, oncologists, radiologists, specialist nurses and the palliative care team, and are able to explain the pathology report, including importantly, any areas of pathological uncertainty. When the pathology report is inconclusive, additional clinical information may become available at the MDT meeting and allow a definite diagnosis to be made. The pathologist is also able to advise on any further investigations that may be needed. Alternatively, if it is clear at the meeting that

(Continued)

- Read a pathology report of a cancer specimen. Reflect on how well you understood it and how you would explain it to a patient in your care.
- Attend a multidisciplinary cancer team meeting at which a patient of yours is discussed. Reflect on the roles of the different participants and how the discussion might have improved your patient's clinical care.
- Read the case study about a malignancy of unknown origin. Reflect on the importance of a multidisciplinary approach to cancer diagnosis and the value of seeking second opinions.
- A patient in your care has died and their relatives ask you if they should agree to a hospital autopsy. Consider what issues you might discuss with them.

Key learning points

- Tumours can be classified in several ways, each of which gives useful information about a tumour's likely behaviour and response to treatment.
- The grade (or differentiation) of a tumour is a measure of how closely it resembles the normal tissue from which it arose.
- The stage of a tumour is a measure of how big it is and how far it has spread.
- Tumour markers are generally more useful in monitoring the progression of known tumours than in their diagnosis.
- A pathological diagnosis depends primarily on a subjective assessment of various tumour characteristics, and should be regarded more as an opinion than as necessarily a statement of fact.
- A pathology report should always be interpreted in the light of all available clinical information. If the report does not fit with the clinical picture, then discuss the case with the pathologist.
- Accurate pathological assessment of a specimen is impossible without full clinical information: always provide this on the request form. This information will govern how a sample is dealt with in the laboratory.
- Rapid fixation is essential: specimens must be sent in a large volume of fixative, and large specimens must reach the laboratory as soon as possible.
- The interpretation of special stains, especially immunohistochemical stains, is not necessarily straightforward.
- Histology and cytology each have their own advantages and disadvantages, and in general are complementary.
- Molecular genetic techniques are revolutionizing the practice of pathology, and are paving the way to an era of 'personalized medicine' where treatment is individualized to each patient's specific tumour.
- The autopsy is an invaluable tool for audit, teaching and research. Relatives are likely to agree to an autopsy if asked in the right way.

Further reading

- For a general introduction to cellular pathology, *Muir's Textbook of Pathology* can be recommended as a standard textbook aimed at undergraduate medical students: Herrington, C.S. (ed) (2014) *Muir's Textbook of Pathology*. 15th edn. Boca Raton, FL: CRC Press.
- For a more detailed but still general textbook: Kumar, V., Abbas, A., Fausto, N. and Aster, J.C. (eds) (2010) *Robbins & Cotran Pathologic Basis of Disease*. 8th edn. Philadelphia, PA: Saunders Elsevier.
- For a detailed but concise description of specific diseases, and a fairly accessible, standard reference work used by practising histopathologists: Rosai, J. (ed) (2012) *Rosai and Ackerman's Surgical Pathology*. 10th edn. St Louis, MO: Elsevier.

6 LIFESPAN PERSPECTIVES: CHILDREN, TEENAGERS AND YOUNG ADULTS

RUTH SADIK AND DAVID WRIGHT

Chapter outline

- Why cancers may occur in infants, children, teenagers and young adults
- Incidence, aetiology and survival related to the most common cancers among infants, children, teenagers and young adults (ICTYA)
- Cancer prevention initiatives

- Psychosocial impact of cancer on ICTYA and their family members
- Role of the multiprofessional team in supporting children, teenagers and young adults through their cancer and treatments

---

INTRODUCTION

This chapter will explore issues surrounding malignancies in infancy, childhood, teenage and young adulthood and the impact this can have on the family. It will do this by examining the following concepts:

- Incidence
- Aetiology
- Survival
- The physical, psychological and social impacts of a cancer diagnosis
- Challenges to promoting quality cancer care
- Support for families

In order to add further clarification to the remit of this chapter, the terms infancy (under 1 year old), children (under 13 years of age), and teenagers and young adults (TYA) (15–24) will be adopted to describe the transition from birth to 24 years of age and are in keeping with the 2005 guidelines from NICE.

For brevity, the abbreviation ICTYA (infants, children, teenagers and young adults) will be used throughout this chapter where the concept under discussion applies to all.

In order to fully comprehend the needs of ICTYA, the professional needs a full understanding of the underpinning issues that lead to malignancy in this age group and the ways in which they manifest.

Reflective activity

- How confident are you in caring for ICTYA with cancer?
- Who could you ask for help if you came across a caring issue you were unsure of?

BIOLOGICAL BASIS OF CANCERS IN INFANTS, CHILDREN, TEENAGERS AND YOUNG ADULTS

Unlike adult malignancies, which histologically resemble the mature tissue or organs from which they arise, ICTYA cancers frequently come from **embryonal tissue** normally seen in the foetus (Dixon-Woods et al., 2005). The failure of genetic safeguards against unregulated cell growth and proliferation means that malignancies of infancy and young childhood are fast growing and most resistant to treatment (Stiller and Shah, 2012).

Biologically, cancer can be built into cells via various mechanisms that occur from conception onward. The billions of cells that undergo **mitotic** change mean that there is a high probability of error happening, either through increased replication or decreased cell death. According to Federico et al. (2011), this can result in either failure to turn off the division trigger, or lack of ability to repair or replace DNA in the correct sequence, leading to an increase in cell mass and tumour formation. This mutation occurs on a grand scale and has been estimated to affect 2.4×10^{10} cells every day (Kovar and Izraeli, 2012). To counteract this, there are in-built safeguards through a complex system of intracellular and immune surveillance mechanisms. As the 'safeguards' themselves are encoded with the same genome, under certain circumstances they also may fail at any stage of cellular growth and regeneration, increasing the likelihood of tumour formation (Kovar and Izraeli, 2012; Lanzkowsky, 2011; Virshup and McCance, 2010).

In contrast with those found in infants and young children, molecular, epidemiological and therapeutic outcome comparisons offer clues to the distinctiveness in most of the common cancers of TYA. The rationale for this, according to Bleyer et al. (2008), is attributable to surges in the reproductive hormones during puberty in both males and females. This hypothesis is partially based on work carried out by Weir et al. (1998) and Coupland et al. (1999) that suggested that late puberty had been found to have a protective effect.

INCIDENCE AND CAUSES OF CANCERS IN ICTYA

Childhood cancer in all its forms is extremely rare, with Stiller and Shah (2012) indicating that in the UK, one child in every 484 will develop some form of malignancy prior to their fifteenth birthday, leading to approximately 1550 new diagnoses per year, or 0.5% of all cancers diagnosed (Cancer Research UK, 2013a). This figure is significantly lower in developing countries.

According to an American study by Yang et al. (2006), malignancies occurring in the first year of life are the most prevalent, representing 10% of all malignancies diagnosed in the 0–14 year age group and the only time in life when the incidence is equal between girls and boys, after which incidences in childhood in females is lower (Barr et al., 2007). This decreases markedly in 15–24-year-olds when, in the UK, just 961 females and 1061 males per year were diagnosed in the period 2007–2009 (Cancer Research UK, 2012a). This illustrates just how rare cancer is in ICTYA.

Despite its overall rarity, incidences in the white ICTYA population across the UK and Europe are increasing annually by 1–2% (Hemminki and Mutanen, 2001), a finding endorsed by data recently released by the Childhood Cancer Research Group (Stiller et al., 2012). Causes for such an increase are tentatively attributed to changes in lifestyle and diet (Steliarova-Foucher et al., 2005) and the impact of these on the individual's genetic pre-disposition (Stiller, 2009). Whilst any definitive cause remains elusive, factors that are thought to potentially have an adverse impact on cellular abnormality and malignancy formation appear to be rooted in these postulations. According to various authors (Stiller, 2009; Terracini, 2009; Lanzkowsky, 2011; Stiller and Shah, 2012) obesity, infections, trauma, ionizing radiation, infectious organisms, toxic substances, other genetic abnormalities and a positive family history have all been identified. Additionally, Gilham et al. (2005) postulate that excessive hygiene and domestic cleaning can denude the environment of the microorganisms that challenge the immune system of very young infants and children and may have an impact on cancer development in later life.

Although approximately thirty ICTYA per week are diagnosed with some form of malignancy, the number presenting with any one specific type is very small. This can lead to challenges for **epidemiologists** in gaining cohorts to study that are sufficiently large enough to yield valid and reliable results on which to base present and future treatments (Stiller, 2009; Terracini, 2009). As a result of these difficulties, countries have collaborated in research leading to the formation of National, European and worldwide cancer research – The Childhood Cancer Research Group, Children's Cancer and Leukaemia Group, UK Children's Cancer Study Group, Childhood Cancer Nurse's Research Group, International Childhood Cancer Cohort Consortia, Teenage Cancer Trust and so forth – which all orchestrate treatment trials for different variants of cancer. According to Cancer Research UK, using the ICC-D classification (Cancer Research UK, 2012a), the three most common cancers of childhood are leukaemias, brain and central nervous system (CNS) tumours and lymphomas, accounting for almost three-quarters of all cases (see Figure 6.1).

Typically, teenagers and young adults sit at the interface between child and adulthood cancers and as such present with tumours that would be seen in both specialities. The three most common cancers seen in this age group are also lymphomas with the addition of carcinomas and germ cell tumours, which account for over 50% of all cases (see Figure 6.2; Cancer Research UK, 2014s). As such, these are the malignancies that will be addressed in some detail.

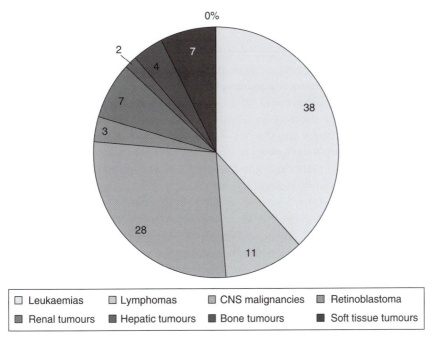

Figure 6.1   Incidence summary children aged 0-14 in Great Britain 1996-2005

Source: Cancer Research UK, 2012a

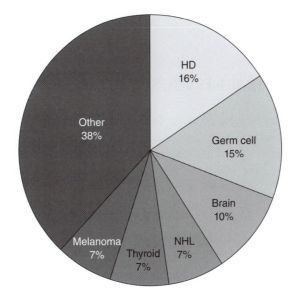

Figure 6.2   Incidence summary of TYA aged 15-24 in Great Britain 2014

Source: Adapted from Cancer Research UK, 2012a

LEUKAEMIAS

In the UK, in 2009, 460 children under the age of 15 years were diagnosed with some form of leukaemia, the most common type of childhood cancer. **Acute lymphoblastic leukaemia** (ALL) is the most common form and accounts for almost three-quarters of all cases, with **acute myeloid** (AML) and **chronic myeloid** (CML) accounting for the remainder.

As the leukaemias are the most prevalent, they are the easiest to study and consequently have a better-informed causal base than any of the others.

The incidence of childhood leukaemia, in keeping with cancers in general, has been rising steadily over the last 30 years (Shah and Coleman, 2007; Stiller, 2007; Kaatsch et al., 2008; Hagopian, 2010), with slightly different rates according to ethnicity, age and gender (Forsythe, 2010). Like most malignancies, boys considerably outnumber girls.

Leukaemias diagnosed in the first 12 months of life are the most virulent and account for approximately 5% of ALL and up to 14% of AML (Chung-Hon and Evans, 2006). There are slightly more girls than boys with infant leukaemia, and the majority of cases (20%) appear to be genetic and linked with the TEL-AML1 gene (Greaves and Wiemels, 2003). For cases diagnosed in the first year of life, the chances of a twin developing the disease is particularly high because precursor leukaemia cells can transfer from one twin to the other during pregnancy (Greaves et al., 2003). Children with chromosomal abnormalities such as **Down's syndrome**, **ataxia telangiectasia** and **Noonan syndrome** are also at greater risk of developing leukaemia, with most studies reporting an increased risk of between 10- and 20-fold (McCance and Huether, 2010; Lanzkowsky, 2011). According to the Childhood Cancer Research Group (2012) there are typical surges in ALL at 2–3 years of age and again in teenage years, whilst AML has almost certainly presented by the age of 2 and can present at any age up to teenage.

BRAIN AND CENTRAL NERVOUS SYSTEM TUMOURS

In the UK, primary brain tumours affect approximately 350 children and their families each year (Cancer Research UK, 2012a), and around one-third of all cancer deaths in children are from a brain tumour. The incidence of childhood brain tumours in the UK has risen by almost 3% a year, mainly in those under 2 years of age (Cancer Research UK, 2012a; Stiller and Shah, 2012). CNS malignancies represent approximately 15% of all childhood malignancies: 40% of which are astrocytomas, 15% gliomas and 9% ependymomas (Arora et al., 2009). The incidence of CNS tumours tends to be higher in boys than girls and higher among white children than black, although brain tumours in African children are now becoming more common (Idowu and Idowu, 2008). According to Gurney et al. (2012), young children have a relatively high occurrence of malignancies in the cerebellum and the brain stem, and older children have higher rates in the cerebrum. In children between the ages of 5 and 9, brain stem malignancies are nearly as common as cerebral malignancies. The pattern shifts among young people between the ages of 10–19, when brain stem and cerebellar cancer incidence decrease and cerebral malignancies increase slightly (Fleming and Chi, 2012).

LYMPHOMA

This refers to a group of malignancies characterized by a proliferation of abnormal lymphocytes (Heath and Ross, 2010) and affects the bone marrow, thymus, spleen and lymph nodes (Marieb and Hoehn, 2013). Although thought to be mainly genetic in origin, the alterations underlying **Hodgkin lymphoma** and **non-Hodgkin lymphoma** are not well understood. Incidence rates of Hodgkin lymphoma in identical twins are around 99 times higher than in the general population, whereas non-identical twins have no increase in risk (Mack et al., 1995). The incidence rates increase with age, and although boys outnumber girls in the 10–14-year-olds, this disappears in the 15–19-year-old groups where affected males and females are equal (Clavel et al., 2004). The main classifications of non-Hodgkin lymphoma in ICTYA are, according to Cancer Research UK (2014x): **Burkitt** and **atypical Burkitt**; **lymphoblastic**; **diffuse large B-cell** and **anaplastic large cell**, together accounting for 10% of all cancers in this group.

One difference in these four groups tend to exist in their anatomical involvement, with Burkitt's lymphoma being diffuse and involving extranodal sites such as the gastrointestinal tract, kidneys and ovaries, whilst large B-cell lymphoma usually occurs in a single site, with mediastinal and abdominal primary sites being most common (Martelli et al., 2013). Anaplastic lymphoma affects the T-cell line, is seen predominantly in males over 10 years of age and is associated with both extranodal involvement and lymphadenopathy (Hochberg et al., 2009).

GERM CELL TUMOURS

As **germ cells** are the basis of ovum and sperm production, tumours in this category tend to develop in the ovaries or testes (Bleyer et al., 2008; Stiller, 2009). However this is by no means exclusive because during embryological development, **primordial** germ cells (precursors to sperm and ova) have to migrate across the embryo to reach somatic gonadal precursors, where they carry out their function (Marieb and Hoehn, 2013). Richardson and Lehmann (2010) found that residual germ cells could be misplaced during this process, resulting in benign or malignant growths occurring in diverse anatomical locations later in life. According to Cancer Research UK (2014s), the most predominant extragonadal tumours tend to appear in the brain, abdomen or thorax but remain extremely rare, accounting for approximately 3% in under 10 years and 14% of all cancers in 14–19-year-olds (Cancer Research UK, 2014s).

OSTEOSARCOMA

Osteosarcoma is a **mesenchymal** malignancy in which the neoplastic cells synthesize and secrete the organic components of bone matrix (Ritter and Bielack, 2010). It accounts for almost 50% of the malignant tumours in bones and joints, followed in order of frequency by **Ewing sarcoma** and **chondrosarcoma** (Bleyer et al., 2008; Stiller, 2009).

Males are 1.5 times more likely to develop this malignancy compared to their female counterparts and incidence peaks during the 15–19 year age group (Ritter and Bielack, 2010). Although the aetiology of osteosarcoma is obscure, osteosarcoma arises most often in long bones, especially the distal femur, proximal tibia and proximal humerus during the height of the body's growth spurt. It is for this reason that authors (Bleyer et al., 2008; Beckingsale and Gerrand, 2010; Ritter and Bielack, 2010) have speculated that the hormonal chaos of this transitional period may be a major causative factor. Conversely, the Ewing sarcoma family of tumours preferentially affects the axial skeleton, as does chondrosarcoma, and are characterized by the reciprocal translocation $t(11;22)$ (q24; q12) in the great majority (Bleyer et al., 2008; Stiller, 2009).

INCIDENCE OF OTHER CANCERS

In addition to these more specialized malignancies, professionals working with TYA may also come across tumours that are more readily associated with older adults. Whilst a single cause for ICTYA cancer is both unlikely and elusive, the plethora of research implicating environmental triggers continues to grow, leading the UK Government to take rigorous cross-party steps in producing environmental health guidance (DH, 2004b, 2007a, 2009c; NICE, 2005a) in an effort to decrease the incidence.

PREVENTATIVE INTERVENTIONS

Tobacco consumption in adults who are either trying to or who have conceived is recognized as the most important human **carcinogen**, causing between 30 and 35% of all cancers in developed countries (Peto, 2011). The regulation and control of places that cigarette smoking and advertising can take place is thought to have a greater impact on reducing cancer incidence and mortality than any other known strategy in children, young people and adults (Public Health England, 2010). Benefits to ceasing the inhalation of cigarette smoke begins as soon as an individual stops smoking. The UK's ban on tobacco advertising resulted in an estimated 3% reduction in smoking (Crosier, 2005), and it is hoped that the ban on smoking in public places should further reduce the prevalence of smoking by an estimated 4% (Dalgleish et al., 2004); however, this is yet to be measured. In recent attempts to identify the impact of smoking bans, Roberts (2012) and Roxby (2012) both identify that although smoking by adults has marginally decreased overall, there is still no legislation to decrease pregnant women smoking at all, nor adults smoking within the house where children are present.

Increasing fruit and vegetable consumption is seen by the Government as the second most effective strategy for reducing the risk of cancer (Committee on Medical Aspects of Radiation on the Environment (COMARE), 2005), and the Government's 'five-a-day' policy directly addresses this. An estimated two million children had benefited from its school fruit and vegetable schemes up to 2004 (DH, 2004b); however, with the change of Government, these schemes have now ceased in many cities (Her Majesty's Government, 2011).

The public policy debate around food labelling is also pertinent and it is thought that there is some potential to reduce obesity by raising awareness of food components, although the relative impact of this on ICTYA cancer incidence is as yet unknown (Cancer Research UK, 2012a; Eastwood, 2011).

With regard to cancers in TYA specifically, the Department of Health (Department of Health, 2007a) made the decision to offer all 12–13-year-old females the opportunity to receive the human papilloma virus (HPV) vaccination in an attempt to reduce the incidence of cervical cancer. Early results of an evaluation of the programme carried out by Schiffman and Wacholder in 2012, indicate that the vaccine is having a positive impact on the development of cervical cancers in later life.

Other public health initiatives aimed at reducing cancer have included campaigns about the risks of prolonged sun exposure or, more worryingly, sunbed use, and national screening programmes through local healthcare initiatives; yet despite these efforts the increasing incidence continues. Chapter 24 of this book discusses lifestyle in cancer survivorship, although many of the themes and frameworks discussed are also relevant to changing behaviour to reduce onset of cancer.

DIAGNOSIS

The diagnosis of cancer in ICTYA is subject to the same procedures and processes as in adults and much of the radiological imaging techniques used to confirm and identify the degree of spread has now been manufactured to cater specifically for even the smallest of infants (Rajaraman et al., 2011). In TYA, however, Fern et al. (2013) identify myriad factors that can adversely impact the early diagnosis of cancer that would benefit from more detailed study and could lead to stronger links between delayed diagnosis and subsequent outcome. In a meta-analysis of barriers to trial recruitment Mills et al., (2006) identified three main factors: patient related, physician related, or protocol related. These findings were endorsed by a recent trial when it was found that concerns also related to a distrust of medical research, which is described in a disparaging way, as being when 'doctors prescribe medication as a way of experimenting on unknown patients' (Shewale and Parekh, 2013: 173). Whilst this is fundamentally true, in this study participants and their families appear unwilling to countenance the benefits of research into cancer treatments with their specific relatives. Both papers identified that a more successful trial recruitment strategy would include having a dedicated trial manager, being a cancer or drug trial, and having interventions only available inside the trial, which may alleviate the belief that doctors were immune to the impact of blind control trials. The most commonly reported strategies to improve recruitment were newsletters and mailshots, but it was not possible to assess whether they were causally linked to changes in recruitment. The analyses suggested that successful trials were those addressing clinically important questions at a timely point. The investigators were held in high esteem by the interviewees, and the trials were firmly grounded in existing clinical practices. The implications of this for practitioners is to ensure that all clients and their families are not only provided with information, but also that their perceptions are questioned repeatedly during the lead up to trial recruitment.

Once diagnosed, treatment can be determined and recruitment to trial if appropriate. This is important because cancers in children have been found to be more sensitive than adults to cytotoxic chemotherapy, which in multimodal medication is the mainstay of treatment, alongside radiotherapy and surgery. However, in keeping with the crossover from childhood to adulthood, TYA malignancies are more variable in their responses.

TREATMENTS AND OUTCOMES

According to Verschuur et al. (2012), cells, both normal and abnormal, proliferate and fall victim to the effects of the various drugs. Pharmacological developments in use for all age groups have increased the survival rate to the point that by 2050, 1 in 1000 people in the UK will have survived childhood cancer (Stiller et al., 2012).

Although the pharmaceutical companies have made considerable efforts to reduce the toxicity of drugs without compromising the impact of cure, given current data according to the Childhood Cancer Research Group (Stiller et al., 2012) 50% of long-term survivors of childhood cancers will have or will develop disabilities that impact their quality of life.

Late effects depend on the initial treatment protocol but include secondary malignancies, **endocrinopathies**, growth failure and skeletal anomalies, learning difficulties, **cardiopulmonary disease** and **neurocognitive impairment** (Butler and Haser, 2006; Temming and Jenney, 2011). This is especially so following treatment for brain tumours or cancer regimens requiring high-dose chemotherapy. Replacement of **prednisolone** with **dexamethasone** has, according to Temming and Jenney (2011), been showing some positive comparisons in guarding against neurocognitive development, height and length disparities and skeletal anomalies, whilst systematic surveillance and management of these late effects has become the focus of many specialist children's cancer services.

Whilst survival has unarguably improved in recent years due to better treatment, it does have a tendency to depend on the type of cancer (Johnston et al., 2010), the stage it has reached prior to diagnosis and the country that the child lives in (Trigg et al., 2008; Linabery and Ross, 2008; Baade et al., 2010; Couto et al., 2010; Kulkarni and Marwaha, 2011). From the UK Childhood Cancer Study (UKCCS) (Johnston et al., 2010), the current five-year survival rate is 72.7% for all childhood cancers, dropping to 67.9% at fifteen years from diagnosis. Hidden within these statistics, however, are dramatic inequalities, for example 96% of children with **retinoblastoma** will survive compared to only 53% with **neuroblastoma**.

The overall survival rates across all TYA is about 80% at five years; however, some disease groups have found survival rates to be static over the last few years, whilst others have almost a 100% survival rate (Cancer Research UK, 2014s). To highlight this, germ cell tumour survival at five years is approximately 96%, according to 2005 figures published in 2013 by Cancer Research UK (2014s) whilst bone cancer survival remains static at 56%.

The lack of progress with regards to survival for the TYA age group has primarily been put down to a lack of clinical trials and recruitment into the trials that exist (Fern and Whelan, 2010). The benefit of trials and trial entry has been seen in childhood cancer survival rates, which have continued to grow up to the present day. It was alluded to earlier that all children with cancer are treated by principal treatment centres and this makes the running of trials easier and ensures that all children receive access to trials. Unfortunately this is not the case for TYA and forms a large part of the ongoing work to improve TYA cancer care.

In order to improve access to healthcare and decrease inequalities in outcomes, *The Cancer Reform Strategy* (DH, 2007a) was created as a progression to the *NHS Cancer Plan* (DH, 2000). It sought to increase and improve services over the next five years by offering guidance to the changing commissioning bodies about high quality prevention, detection, treatment and care of all client groups with cancer (DH, 2007a). In reviews carried out in 2010 (National Audit Office) and 2011 (Her Majesty's Government) findings identified that although healthcare for ICTYA with cancer has become more localized, there remained significant gaps in information about important aspects of cancer services, such as information on chemotherapy, follow-up treatment and on the stage that a patient's cancer has reached at the time of diagnosis. The House of Commons report (Her Majesty's Government, 2011) went on to identify that although great strides have been made, the impact of the Cancer Reform Strategy could not be measured against key outcomes such as survival rates and 'does not know if it is commissioning cancer services cost-effectively, due to poor data on costs and because outcomes data are not sufficiently timely' (2011: 2). The implication of this for stakeholders, is to ensure that robust mechanisms are in place to collect high quality, comprehensive and timely data; raise awareness of cancer; provide transparency in the performance of commissioning consortia; and ultimately drive improved outcomes for cancer patients (Her Majesty's Government, 2011).

Reflective activity

- How may a cancer diagnosis impact on the lives of ICTYA and their families?
- What may be the different needs of this age group compared to those of the adult population?

THE PSYCHOSOCIAL IMPACT OF ILLNESS AND TREATMENTS

In recent years there has been an increasing recognition of the significance of understanding the psychosocial issues associated with ICTYA cancer. Research on the psychosocial aspects of the ICTYA cancer experience provides important insights to inform the development of supportive care services that help families cope with the considerable impact of diagnosis and treatment.

Social isolation has the potential to have the greatest impact on a young person because treatment can be profoundly isolating. Physical side effects, such as fatigue, nausea and vomiting and diarrhoea, may prevent a young person from being able to meet up with others, and psychological distress may leave the young person unable to face mixing with friends and relatives. This isolation can result in a fear of rejection from peers and difficulties with returning to school or work, which can increase psychological distress and further disrupt peer relationships and normal socialization (Elwell et al., 2011; Rowland, 1989).

According to Decker (2006b) and Li-Min et al. (2009), adolescence is a crucial time of identity formation and emerging independence, two developmental processes that can be disrupted significantly by cancer treatment lasting from months to several years. Potentially including repeated rounds of medical and or surgical procedures and treatments forces teenagers to depend more on parents or other caretakers than is developmentally normative (Decker, 2006b). Jones et al. (2013) go on to identify that loss of independence, isolation from peers, changes in family and peer interactions, and the stark unpredictability of the illness can all have lasting emotional effects on the patient and other family members.

The impact of having a dependant with cancer is far reaching and takes an enormous toll on the family. Eiser and Upton (2007) identified that additional financial expenditure could be as great as £100 per week and, despite assistance from charities, almost 70% of families worried about money. ICTYA cancer has an impact on all family members as individuals, as well as on the family as a unit (Clarke-Steffen, 1997; Scott-Findlay and Chalmers, 2001). The diagnosis of a serious illness represents a crisis for the family (McCubbin et al., 1998) because parents often have to cope with reactions from the rest of the family, which can be an additional burden and occurs when parents are most vulnerable in terms of lacking control and in emotional turmoil (McGrath and Phillips, 2008). Another crisis occurs when the individual's treatment is complete (Labay and Walco, 2004), and Haase and Rostad's study in 1994 identified that parents whose children were completing cancer treatment experienced two sets of emotions: one of celebration and hope, and one of uncertainty and fear. Hope that the pain and drudgery of treatment regimens is over and fear of relapse or disability. McGrath and Phillips' study (2008) identified that mothers and fathers experience stress reactions, including anxiety and depression, for up to two years after diagnosis and found it extremely stressful to establish limits on both the child they are with and the one(s) left at home. Once initial treatment had been completed, parents found that they felt pressurized to return to work, which also increased stress and anxiety.

Research into the impact on siblings of having a brother or sister with cancer has increased greatly over the years and is now very well documented (Dixon-Woods et al., 2005). They note that siblings suffer loss and separation for both their sibling and main carer, and roles and relationships frequently change as the older sibling takes on additional domestic responsibilities, which causes social relationships to suffer. Malone and Price (2012) identify that siblings require mechanisms to develop coping strategies to help them to deal with their brother or sister having cancer, assistance with carrying out their everyday lives, such as school attendance, whilst the main carer may be absent, and someone to help regain a sense of normality in their lives. For more about the impact of cancer on families, see Chapter 20.

In the current healthcare environment, support services come in a variety of guises and represent voluntary, independent, governmental and quasi-governmental agencies (see Table 6.1).

Table 6.1   Providers of support services for parents and siblings

Environment	Resource
Primary healthcare team	General practitioner, community children's nurse, health visitor, social worker, voluntary/charity organization staff, spiritual support, pharmacist, dietician, physiotherapy, speech and language
Local hospital team	Children's nurses, paediatrician, play leader, dietician, outpatients service, pharmacist, activity and social spaces, spiritual support, physiotherapy, speech and language
Specialist regional hospital	Children's nurses, paediatrician, play specialist, clinical psychologist, child psychiatrist, dietician, outpatients service, pharmacist, complementary therapists, counselling services, school and educational provision, activity and social spaces, radiotherapy and diagnostic imaging, occupational therapists, spiritual support, parental support services, sibling support services, speech and language, physiotherapy
Hospice care	Children's nurses, paediatrician, play specialist, clinical psychologist, child psychiatrist, dietician, pharmacist, complementary therapists, counselling services, school and educational provision, activity and social spaces, occupational therapists, spiritual support, parental support services, sibling support services, speech and language, physiotherapy, music therapy, hydrotherapy

Reflective activity

How can infants, children, teenagers and young adults with cancer, and their families, be supported through their cancer diagnosis and treatments?

APPROACHES TO SUPPORTING ICTYA AND THEIR FAMILIES

The report, *Improving Outcomes in Children and Young People with Cancer* (NICE, 2005a) provides guidance on how healthcare provision should be tailored to meet the needs of children and young people and recognizes that needs are different to those of adults with cancer. It highlights the need for specialist multiprofessional teams made up of a collection of professionals, including specialist medical staff, nurses, youth workers, social workers, psychologists and wider allied health professionals. The aim is to help and support a young person to overcome a cancer diagnosis and to enable them to live the life they desire during treatment, after treatment and at the end of life. This team is there to ensure that young people:

- Have opportunity for social interaction with other young people
- Are treated in age-appropriate environments, whether that be in TYA units or in general oncology wards that have facilities for young people (such as Internet access so that they can keep in touch with friends whilst in hospital)
- Have access to trials
- Have the most appropriate treatment
- Receive age-appropriate psychological support to help them adjust to and cope with their diagnosis
- Are supported in a smooth transition to end-of-life care (where relevant), with the young person retaining as much control as possible.

In addition, those that surround a young person, whether that be family, friends or partners, should also be supported.

Specialist TYA services are neither mandatory nor widespread and a large-scale evaluation study (The Brightlight Project) is currently underway, financed by the Government and carried out independently. Brightlight aims to explore the experiences of young people with cancer over a three-year period to establish if their quality of life is affected by the specialist care they receive. The findings (due for publication circa 2017) will be used to help shape the future of cancer services for young people.

CHAPTER SUMMARY

There are clearly challenges to treating and supporting ICTYA with cancer that range from correct treatments to the issue of small patient numbers, from the impact of diagnosis to the issue of survival. It would be too easy to suggest that having all children, teenagers and young adults referred to an appropriately qualified team would solve these issues, but it would be a good start. Young children are frequently disenfranchised and left to be cared for by professionals that are not optimally informed about their biological, psychological or social needs (NICE, 2005a; Her Majesty's Government, 2011), whilst the TYA team is charged with easing the transition from paediatric and adult services in order to ensure that young people are receiving the correct treatments. Addressing these challenges can ensure that trial entry is as high as it can be, and it can lead to the development of best practice with separate services learning from each other. Although there is scope for improving support for this population, services for all children, teenagers and young adults, whilst relatively new, continue to improve with direction from NICE guidelines and peer reviews. The benefits of specialist services in achieving quality care cannot be underestimated, but further research into *how* they work to improve the lives of all children and young people with cancer is needed to inform further development and delivery of services to this vulnerable group.

Key learning points

- As cells proliferate rapidly to enable growth of an individual from conception to adulthood, the chances of faulty DNA production is high. Faults in genes that normally programme the destruction or repair of faulty DNA increase the likelihood of tumour formation.
- Cancers in ICTYA are rare and survival in these groups is increasing.
- The three most common cancers found in infants and children are leukaemias, brain and central nervous system tumours, and lymphomas. In teenagers and young adults, they are lymphomas, germ cell tumours and carcinomas.
- Cancer prevention strategies focus on health behaviour change and HPV vaccination may be beneficial.
- Cancer diagnosis and treatments can have profound psychosocial effects on the individual and their family.
- Healthcare provision should be tailored to meet the specific needs of children and young people through specialist multiprofessional teams.

Recommended further reading

- Carroll, W.L. and Finlay, J.L. (2010) *Cancer in Children and Adolescents*. London: Jones and Bartlett Publishing.
- Smith S., Case L. and Waterhouse K. (2012) *A Blueprint of Care for Teenagers and Young Adults with Cancer*. London: Teenage Cancer Trust and TYAC.
- Stevens, M.C.G., Hubert, C.N. and Biondi, A. (eds) (2012) *Cancer in Children: Clinical Management*. 6th edn. Oxford: Oxford University Press. pp. 1-13.

7 LIFESPAN PERSPECTIVES: OLDER ADULTS

HAZEL BRODIE

Chapter outline

- Life expectancy and lifespan
- The physiology of ageing
- Epidemiology and aetiology of cancer in older age
- Treatment considerations in the context of ageing
- Ageism, age discrimination and age equality legislation
- Stereotypes and attitudes to ageing
- Delivering age-friendly services
- Common medical, functional and social support needs of older adults

---

INTRODUCTION

The UK population is ageing, and cancer is predominantly a disease of older age. Consequently, the number of people in the UK aged 65 and over living with a cancer diagnosis is set to treble by 2030 (Maddams et al., 2012). Concerns regarding the ability of cancer services to cater for the needs of an ageing population have prompted a rise in interest in the topic of cancer and ageing over recent decades. Challenges faced by current day services must be addressed in the context of increasing numbers of older patients, with many older people being diagnosed late, under-diagnosed, and undertreated, thus leading them to experience poorer cancer outcomes than their younger counterparts. Cancer survival rates tend to decrease with increasing age, and mortality rates for older people in the UK are improving at a much slower rate than in the younger population (National Cancer Intelligence Network, 2010b). Older people also face cancer **inequalities** in terms of their experience of care (Quality Health, 2013a).

The extent to which age discriminatory practice contributes to the observed inequalities experienced by older people is a source of much debate. Nonetheless, recent years have seen the introduction of legislation and policy that have addressed the issue of age discrimination, not only in cancer care, but also in health and social care in general. In October 2012, the provisions within the Equality Act (2010), which prohibit age discrimination, were extended to the field of goods and services (Home Office, 2010). This means that health and social care services, including cancer services, are now required to eliminate unequal treatment on the grounds of age. Prior to this change in the law, the Department of Health published key policy documents that promoted age equality. The *National Service Framework for Older People* (DH, 2001b) focused on rooting out age discrimination, providing person-centred care, promoting older people's health and independence, and fitting services around people's needs. The *Cancer Reform Strategy* (DH, 2007a) clearly stated that age should not be a barrier to treatment and this was echoed by the 2011 *Improving Outcomes: A Strategy for Cancer* (DH, 2011a).

This chapter will discuss some of the complex challenges that face cancer care providers when striving to provide high quality care to an ageing population. The scope of this topic is broad, so this chapter will focus mainly on access to cancer treatment because many would argue this is where the most complex challenges lie. The term 'older people' is a subjective one. Older age is categorized using a number of cut off points, depending on the context. It is often defined as age 65 and over, 70 and over, or 75 and over. Age 85 and over is commonly used to describe the 'older old'. For the purpose of this chapter, we will cite the most readily available evidence.

Key concepts

- **Ageism:** an unjustifiable prejudicial attitude of mind towards older people.
- **Age discrimination:** discriminatory actions, made purely on the basis of age that can be observed and sometimes even measured.
- **Direct age discrimination:** *Direct* age discrimination treats two individuals with similar needs differently purely on the basis of their age.
- **Indirect age discrimination:** *Indirect* age discrimination treats people of all ages the same, not recognizing the greater needs of particular age groups so those age groups are disadvantaged.
- **Equality:** *Equality* is the state of being equal, especially in terms of health outcomes, status, rights or opportunities.
- **Equity:** *Equity* is the fair distribution of benefits across the population.

Reflective activity

- Read the Centre for Policy on Ageing (2010) briefing on discrimination in health and social care in the UK.
- Think of an example, relevant to your practice, for each of the key concepts.

LIFE EXPECTANCY AND LIFESPAN

Western society is ageing, and it is estimated that 1 in 4 children born in the UK today will become centenarians (Department of Work and Pensions, 2010). Life expectancy at birth in England and Wales in 2009–2011 was 78.7 years for males and 82.6 years for females (Office for National Statistics, 2011); however, this does not mean that when a female born today reaches 70, she can only expect to live another 12.6 years. There is an important distinction that should be made between **life expectancy** and **lifespan**. Life expectancy is the approximate amount of time an individual ought to live, based on the average life expectancy of the population. Lifespan is how long an individual actually lives. Another consideration that should not be ignored is how many of those years the individual will spend in good health. According to the World Health Organization (WHO), **healthy life expectancy** is the 'average number of years that a person can expect to live in "full health" by taking into account years lived in less than full health due to disease and/or injury' (WHO, 2013b). In 2005, 65-year-old males in the UK had an *average* life expectancy of 17 years, with an expected 13 of those years spent in good health (Office for National Statistics, 2013b). Females of this age could expect to live an *average* of 20 more years, with 14.5 of these years spent in good health.

PHYSIOLOGY OF AGEING

As the physiological ageing process occurs, there are a number of characteristics that are experienced by each of the body's systems. As the body ages, it has diminished capacity to regenerate cells and lost tissues, which leads to systems becoming less effective. Older people are more likely to have co-morbidities and geriatric syndromes such as incontinence, falls, functional decline, poly-pharmacy and delirium. These age-related factors may affect treatment tolerance and hence which cancer treatments and supportive therapies are most appropriate to give (Repetto, 2003).

- Decline in renal and hepatic function can increase risk of chemotherapy toxicity.
- Decreased haemopoietic bone marrow reserve increases the risk of myelosuppression.
- Body composition changes, such as an increase in percentage body fat, can affect the distribution of lipid-soluble and water-soluble drugs.
- A reduction in gastrointestinal absorption may reduce the bioavailability of oral cancer drugs and supportive therapies.

Clinical guidelines, which take into account biological ageing processes, are being developed by organizations such as the International Society of Geriatric Oncology (SIOG) and the EORTC Cancer in the Elderly Task Force. A number of studies are being undertaken (post-licensing) to observe the effects of treatments in older people. In 2012, there were eight UK cancer trials specifically recruiting older people (National Institute for Health Research, 2013).

When taking these physiological factors into consideration, it is important to remember the **heterogeneity** of the older population – as a *population,* older people are more likely to experience these issues, but that does not mean that every *individual* within that population will. Age alone is a poor predictor of treatment tolerance. Due to a unique profile of genetic and environmental factors, every individual experiences ageing differently: striking differences can be observed between older individuals in terms of lifespan and experience of health and well-being. Some older patients tolerate chemotherapy, radiotherapy or surgery well, whilst others experience severe toxicity, post-operative complications and functional loss. In the context of cancer care, it is important that people are viewed in terms of their biological age, as opposed to their chronological age.

EPIDEMIOLOGY, AETIOLOGY AND TREATMENT OF CANCER IN OLDER AGE

Cancer is a disease of older age (see Figures 7.1 and 7.2). Between 2008 and 2010 approximately 160,000 new cancers were diagnosed in people aged over 70 in the UK (Cancer Research UK, 2013a), approximately half of all newly diagnosed cancers (see Figure 7.2). There are a number of factors that increase our risk of cancer in later life. Older tissues have been exposed to carcinogens for a longer period of time, and there is evidence to suggest that older tissues are more susceptible to environmental carcinogens (Balducci and Ershler, 2005). The increased risk of developing cancer with increasing age is particularly marked for certain cancer types. The most commonly diagnosed cancers amongst the UK 70+ population are prostate, lung, bowel, bladder and stomach cancers (in males), and breast, bowel, lung, pancreas and non-Hodgkin lymphoma (in females) (Cancer Research UK, 2013a).

Survival rates for many types of cancer decrease with older age (see Figures 7.3 and 7.4) and cancer mortality rates for older people in the UK are improving at a much slower rate than in the younger population. From 1995–97 to 2003–05, cancer mortality rates fell by 16–17% for those under 75, but increased by 2% in those aged over 85 (National Cancer Intelligence Network, 2010b). Three-quarters of all cancer deaths occur in the 65+ age group (Cancer Research UK, 2013b).

A number of factors contribute to the poorer cancer outcomes observed in the older population: the clinical characteristics of cancers experienced by older people are often different from that of younger people; the physiology of the aging process alters the environment in which that cancer is present; and older people often receive different therapies to younger people (Hurria and Balducci, 2009). Late diagnosis is thought to play a significant role for some tumour types. Breast cancer in older people tends to be diagnosed later; however, this is not the case for lung cancer (Lyratzopoulos et al., 2012). Despite this, lung cancer outcomes are still poorer for older people than their younger counterparts.

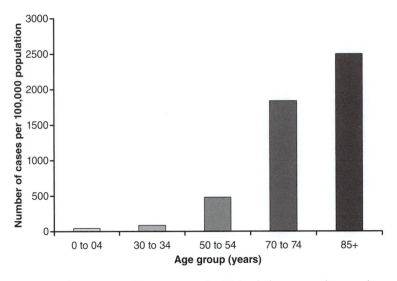

Figure 7.1 Age specific cancer incidence rates in the UK (excluding non-melanoma skin cancer) 2008–2010

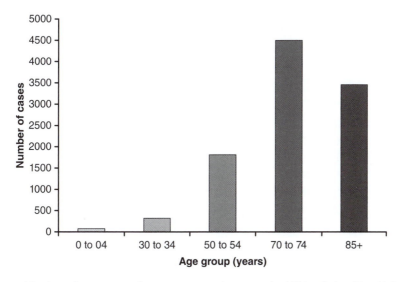

Figure 7.2 Number of new cases of cancer per year by age in the UK (excluding Non-Melanoma Skin Cancer) 2008–2010

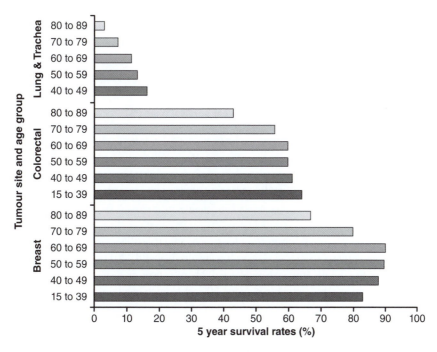

Figure 7.3 Five-year survival rates by age in England (females) 2004–2008

For some cancer types, the prognosis is actually better in older people than younger people; for other cancer types the contrary is true. Some tumour types, such as ovarian cancers and malignant brain tumours, become more aggressive and lethal with ageing. For example, acute myeloid leukaemia is usually more aggressive in older people due to changes in the biology of the disease, which include a higher prevalence of multi-drug resistant, non-Hodgkin lymphoma (Roellig et al., 2010). On the other hand, breast cancers often become less aggressive, and this is thought to be due to the increased prevalence of hormone receptor-rich tumours (Carlson et al., 2008). It is important to note that these generalizations may be applied to the population, but are not always observed on an individual case-by-case basis.

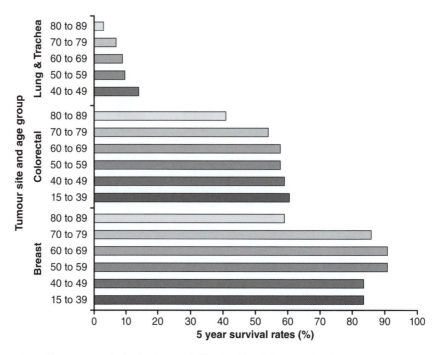

Figure 7.4   Five-year survival rates by age in England (males) 2004–2008

Access to cancer treatment

The most compelling example of age-related inequality in access to cancer treatment is variation in access to surgery. Surgery is widely accepted to be the most clinically effective treatment for most solid cancer tumours; however, older people are far less likely to receive surgery than their younger counterparts (National Cancer Intelligence Network, 2011a). In women in the UK diagnosed with symptomatic (not screen detected) breast cancer in 2007, there was a significant relationship between age and access to surgery: 90% of women aged under 50 received surgery, compared to only 39% of patients aged 80 and above (National Cancer Intelligence Network, 2011b). There is long-established evidence to show that older people are less likely to access chemotherapy and radiotherapies (National Cancer Intelligence Network, 2010b; Turner et al., 1999).

Reflective activity

Do you think that the observed variation in access to cancer treatment by different age groups is due to age discrimination?

The challenges cancer clinicians face when advising the best course of treatment for many older patients are complex, and the extent to which lower clinical intervention rates in the older population are appropriate is a source of much debate. In 2012, a report by the Royal College of Surgeons (Royal College of Surgeons, 2012), categorized the reasons for lower surgical intervention rates in older adults into:

- Clinical reasons;
- Clinical approaches; and
- Patient awareness and preference.

Reflective activity: chemotherapy equity audit

Your department has just undertaken an audit of adjuvant chemotherapy in women aged over 70 who had early stage breast cancer (EBC). It appears there is a significant variation practice between the four oncologists who work in your department.

	Total cases EBC (females aged 70+)	% given adjuvant chemotherapy
Oncologist 1	10	50.0%
Oncologist 2	45	15.6%
Oncologist 3	32	31.3%
Oncologist 4	35	8.6%

- What additional information would you require to explore this variation further?
- What factors could explain the observed variation in chemotherapy usage?
- Read the *Adjuvant Chemotherapy in Elderly Women with breast cancer (AChEW)* study (Ring et al., 2013).

Clinical factors and treatment

Physiological consequences of ageing have implications when prescribing cancer therapies, as does the biology of cancer in older people, which is often different to that of younger people. Furthermore, older patients may present with more advanced disease where radical therapies are deemed ineffective. For example, women aged 75–79 are 46% more likely to be diagnosed with stage III or IV breast cancer than those aged 65–69 (Lyratzopoulos et al., 2012).

In many cases it is medically justifiable to not offer aggressive treatments due to patients not being able to tolerate the treatment, or the treatment being of limited benefit to the patient. When doctors take the Hippocratic Oath they vow to 'keep them [their patients] from harm' and as such, are duty bound to avoid interventions where the harms significantly outweigh the benefits. There are significant risks associated with certain treatments in frail older patients, or those with complex co-morbidities. Surgical complications and inherently toxic anticancer drugs can lead to life-threatening clinical events in patients of all ages.

Clinical factors and patient choice do not fully account for the variation in access to cancer treatment experienced by older patients in the UK. Detailed studies relating to breast cancer treatment have shown chronological age as a major factor in determining treatment, even when tumour characteristics and co-morbidities are accounted for (Lavelle et al., 2007).

Patient choice and treatment

Patient experience, knowledge, beliefs and communication with clinicians are all factors that influence treatment decisions. Complex factors, in particular the impact on quality of life versus survival advantage, must all be taken into account. It is important that all patients are supported to make informed decisions about their cancer treatment; however, this is not always the case:

● Physicians spend shorter time with individual older patients and provide less encouragement to take an active role in decision-making (Radecki et al., 1988).
● Many older people perceive themselves as less capable of communicating their preferences to physicians, and take a more passive role in treatment decision-making (Singh et al., 2010).
● Older people are more likely to follow their doctor's recommendation, yet are less likely to receive appropriate information (Cox et al., 2006).
● *The National Cancer Patient Experience survey* found that older patients were less likely to be given the name of a clinical nurse specialist and were also less likely to be provided with understandable and written information about possible side effects of treatment (Quality Health, 2013a).

Reflective activity

If older people are supported to make informed decisions about cancer treatment, do you think more, or less, older people will access treatment?

Poor communication is recognized as a significant barrier to treatment (Thorne et al., 2005). Mandelblatt et al. (2010) found that the higher the older breast cancer patients rated the quality of communication with their oncologist, the more likely they were to consent to chemotherapy. Chouliara et al. (2004) criticized that the research into the experiences of older people with cancer is inadequate, particularly relating to their experience of the way treatment decisions were made. Between 2005 and 2013, less than ten studies specifically examining cancer treatment decision-making in the older age group are recorded in the National Center for Biotechnology Information (NCBI) PubMed database (2013). Further research is urgently required to look at the treatment decision-making process for older people with cancer.

Clinical attitudes and approaches

A number of studies have examined the impact of age in oncology decision-making. In 2012, the Department of Health commissioned an international study, which used patient scenarios across a number of cancer types, to examine the way in which clinical attitudes inform oncology clinical decision-making (DH, 2012e). The results showed that chronological age played a significant role in oncology decision-making, even though many of the participating clinicians stated that chronological age was not a factor in their decision-making. This suggests that much age discriminatory practice is covert, and that clinicians may be using chronological age as a proxy for factors such as co-morbidity and life expectancy. A similar study investigating the treatment of HER-2 positive breast cancer patients, presented oncologists with various scenarios and found that of 101 oncologists, 81% would prescribe chemotherapy for a high-risk patient aged 68; however, only 47% would recommend chemotherapy for an otherwise identical patient aged 73 years old (Ring, 2010).

The lack of clinical guidelines and trial evidence to support clinicians to manage older cancer patients with complex health needs leaves a wide margin for clinical judgement. It is reasonable to suggest that some clinicians adopt a more risk adverse approach than others, in fear of causing harm to their patients with aggressive therapies. Furthermore, many oncologists in the UK receive little training on the specific needs of older people with cancer and this may affect their confidence in prescribing therapies to frailer older adults and those with complex needs.

Clinicians at the Massachusetts General Hospital published a paper in *The Oncologist* that summarized the discussion of a Schwartz Center Round, which specifically focused on age bias (Penson et al., 2004). Staff who participated in the 'Round' spoke candidly about their own attitudes and assumptions about older patients. One discussion point focused on a case study of an elderly lady who wished to start chemotherapy. Clinicians perceived her to be too frail and unsuitable for this type of treatment, but were pleasantly surprised when she tolerated the treatment well.

STEREOTYPES AND ATTITUDES TO AGEING

Ageism presents itself in many ways, not just in cancer care, but also in society at large. Health and social care services exist within this very same society and it stands to reason that the same negative beliefs about older people are held by some health and social care staff. In giving evidence to the Joint Committee on Human Rights in 2007, the National Director for Older People's Services is quoted as saying 'although overt age discrimination is now uncommon in our care system, there are still deep-rooted negative attitudes and behaviours towards older people' (Joint Committee on Human Rights, 2007: 21). Some would argue that most age discriminatory behaviours amongst health and social care staff are covert, arising from subconscious attitudes, well-meant paternalism and feelings of protectiveness to frailer older people. Common misconceptions about older people that may lead to substandard cancer care include: people aged over 70 have a short life expectancy; older people can't tolerate aggressive cancer treatments; older people are not interested in sexuality or body image; and people regress to a child-like state in old age.

Sexuality in older age

A review by Taylor and Gosney (2011) explores health professionals' beliefs, attitudes and behaviour regarding sex and the older person and makes recommendations for improving practice. If healthcare professionals do not accept that older people enjoy sex and sexual

(Continued)

(Continued)

intimacy, then it is unlikely that sexual problems will be effectively explored, diagnosed and treated.

Many cancer treatments have both temporary and long-term consequences that can make it physically difficult to have sexual intercourse and engage in sexual intimacy. Furthermore, some treatments can damage confidence and lower body image. Misconceptions about the body image needs and preferences of older women may lead to health professionals not even raising the topic of breast reconstruction. In 2007 only 1% of women in their 70s had immediate breast reconstruction following their mastectomy, compared to 20% of women in their 40s (National Cancer Intelligence Network, 2011b). Research supports this hypothesis with many older women expressing that they would like the option of reconstructive surgery, and many reporting that this option was rarely discussed (Fenlon et al., 2012).

Reflective activity

- Read the review by Taylor and Gosney (2011).
- What other aspects of cancer care could be affected by misconceptions about sexuality in older age?

It is difficult for anyone to fully appreciate the realities of older age until they have experienced it themselves. As such, it is only natural that many younger people have misconceptions about the ageing process. People often get defensive when this topic is raised; however, it is important that everyone undertakes reflective practice to become aware of their own attitudes to older people, so that these attitudes do not translate into age discriminatory practice. Undertaking an objective assessment of an older person's needs and preferences, as opposed to making assumptions, may minimize the impact of ageist assumptions on the care of older people.

DELIVERING AGE-FRIENDLY SERVICES

The NHS spends 80% of its resources and 80% of its time on people aged 65 and over (NHS Southwest, 2010), yet services are not designed with older people in mind. Addressing these challenges may seem like an insurmountable task; however, there are practical, cost-effective steps that can be taken to equip services to meet the individual needs of older patients:

- Assessment plays a vital role in identifying individual needs and preferences, and facilitating personalized care.
- It is important to ensure the cancer workforce is equipped with the right skills.
- Commissioners must ensure services are available in a timely manner to address identified need.
- Older people should be engaged in the design and delivery of services.

Experienced-based co-design, Kings Fund

Experience-based co-design (EBCD) is an approach that enables staff and patients to work in partnership to co-design services and care pathways. It uses qualitative methods, such as in-depth interviews and focus groups to gather experiences from patients and staff. Emotionally significant points (referred to as 'touch points') in the patient pathway, which provoke either negative or positive feelings, are identified. A short impactful film is then created to convey to staff how patients experience their service. Staff and patients will then work together to agree areas of the service to redesign. They then come up with design solutions to make improvements to those areas of the service. One patient involved in EBCD said, 'I often feel that my experience isn't reflected on [surveys] … I want to tick a box that's not there and this gave [me] a chance to say what's actually happening.'

When talking about 'experts in older people's care', it's important not to forget about older people themselves.

Reflective activity

- Think of your work over the past year. List any potential opportunities to engage older people in either the design or delivery of services (e.g. staff training, clinic refurbishment).
- What are the barriers to engaging older people, and how would you overcome these?
- Draw out an example of a patient cancer pathway. What points in the pathway do you think are associated with particularly good or poor experience for older patients?
- Access the experienced-based co-design toolkit (Kings Fund, 2013).

Assessment and care planning

The International Society of Geriatric Oncology (SIOG) recommends the use of comprehensive geriatric assessment (CGA) prior to medical or surgical intervention for older people with cancer (Extermann et al., 2005). SIOG argues that this evidence-based assessment, which looks at domains of health and wellbeing (including medical assessment, psychological assessment, assessment of functioning, social assessment and environmental assessment), should lead to:

- Better, more informed treatment decisions;
- The early identification and treatment of problems such as malnutrition;
- Better tolerance of treatment; and
- Improved outcomes.

Gosney (2005) discusses in detail some of the screening tools utilized to assess the aforementioned domains of health. In 2012, the Department of Health (2012d) published the findings of a project that tested the use of CGA in 14 cancer centres across England. Key recommendations focus on the importance of ensuring assessment findings are acted upon, providing practical support and routinely engaging geriatricians in the care of older cancer patients.

Workforce considerations

Assessment of any patient can often identify complex needs. Simply putting an assessment process in place alone is not enough – the wider system must be able to meet the needs identified by the assessment. Services should maximize opportunities for multidisciplinary and multi-agency working in order to address these needs. Working in partnership with elderly care teams, therapists, community and primary care, voluntary sector organizations, care homes and social services to name a few, can all support the delivery of improved cancer care to older people. This relationship should be reciprocal, with cancer services staff enhancing their skills relating to care for older people, and the generalist workforce increasing their knowledge and skills in relation to cancer care.

Geriatricians in particular can provide invaluable input as part of the cancer multidisciplinary team. Many older people have additional needs, which must be co-managed with their cancer, and geriatricians have the expertise to manage these multiple health issues. In a 2011 study, Cesari et al. concluded,

> The combination of expertise from oncologists and geriatricians is likely to result in (1) an improved selection of candidates for interventions aimed at increasing disability-free life expectancy and/or overall survival, and (2) a more rational exclusion of patients at higher risk of toxicity or with poor prognosis (Cesari et al., 2011: 153).

Other services, such as orthopaedics, recognize the benefits of engaging geriatricians as part of the multidisciplinary team. Ortho-geriatrics is now a growing speciality in the UK.

Developing an evidence base

Clinicians have a limited evidence base to draw upon when treating older patients. There is a paucity of trial data and clinical guidelines to inform evidence-based cancer treatment in this age group. Prescribers must decide whether to prescribe a drug, even though they may only have limited knowledge of its effects and side effects in older people. One systematic review of colorectal cancer treatment trials showed the average age of the participants was 62, despite the fact that the median age of people diagnosed with this type of cancer is 72 (PREDICT, 2008). Researchers face a challenge to address this gap in evidence because many frail older patients are often excluded from clinical trials on health grounds. PREDICT (**PaR**ticipation of the **El**Derly **I**n Clinical Trials) claims that older people are systematically excluded from research, and purports that this lack of trial data is a clear example of age discrimination (PREDICT, 2013). Practical advice to help increase participation of older people in clinical trials can be found on the PREDICT website.

COMMON NEEDS OF OLDER CANCER PATIENTS

In the context of cancer care, age equality isn't about treating everyone the same; it is about providing equal care for equal need. Many older people have complex needs, which, if not met, may present a barrier to accessing cancer treatment. Failure of services to put measures in place to meet these needs could be construed as an act of indirect age discrimination (see the earlier Reflective Activity). These needs are not just medical – social, environmental, psychological and functional issues can also present difficulties when undergoing cancer treatment.

Medical and psychological needs

Many older patients have other medical and psychological needs in addition to their cancer. Geriatric syndromes, such as falls, incontinence, sleep disorders, confusion, skin breakdown and problems with eating, are common in the older population (Sleeper, 2009). Extermann et al. (1998) estimates that people aged over 70 are likely to suffer from an average of three co-morbid conditions in addition to their cancer. It is important that these issues are managed effectively to maximize a patient's capacity to tolerate treatment and their ability to benefit from that treatment.

Poor nutritional status increases the risk of postsurgical complications and can also affect the way drugs are processed by the body. For example, **hypoalbuminaemia** affects distribution of drugs that bind to albumin (Medscape, 2013). In 2011, 38% of people aged 65 and over who were admitted to hospital in the UK were found to be malnourished at the time of admission (BAPEN, 2011).

With the prevalence of **dementia** increasing (Dementia UK, 2013), it is important that cognitive function is appropriately assessed and mental capacity is taken into account when making treatment decisions. The British Medical Association has produced a Mental Capacity Toolkit, which clinicians may find useful (British Medical Association, 2013).

Poly-pharmacy often results from having many health problems. A 2011 systematic review by Lees and Chan discussed in detail the impact of poly-pharmacy in cancer, and highlights that one-third of patients aged over 70 have problems with their existing medication regimens upon cancer diagnosis (Lees and Chan, 2011). They recommend that a review of patients' medications before cancer treatment is an integral part of the assessment, and that such reviews should identify potential pre-existing drug-related issues.

Psychological issues, such as depression and anxiety, affect older cancer patients; however, there is conflicting research as to whether the psychological impact of a cancer diagnosis is greater or less in the individuals (Roth and Modi, 2003; Kua, 2005). Nonetheless, the prevalence of depression and anxiety in the older population in general is significant (Royal College of General Practitioners, 2011). Older people are more likely to receive medication for psychological issues and are less likely to access talking therapies (Mind, 2013). It is important that older people are given the same access to psychological support services as younger people.

Hearing loss

Mr Adams is 82 years old and has been diagnosed with colorectal cancer. He has come into the clinic to discuss options for surgery with his consultant. His daughter, who is accompanying him, says 'Dad can't hear very well, so you can talk to me and I'll explain everything to him later'. The healthcare assistant, who has escorted Mr Adams and his daughter into the

(Continued)

CASE STUDY

(Continued)

consulting room, notices that Mr Adams is wearing hearing aids in both ears. The health-care assistant asks, 'Can't he hear at all? He's wearing two hearing aids'. The daughter replies, 'They haven't been working for a while now'.

The healthcare assistant replaces the batteries in both hearing aids to see if this makes any difference. It does – both hearing aids now work. He also sets up an induction loop system in the consulting room. At the start of the consultation, the surgeon asks Mr Adams if he is happy for his daughter to stay in the consultation. Mr Adams replies 'no', and later explains that he is worried his daughter will pressurize him to have an operation and that he doesn't want to have surgery. When asked why, he says he is worried it will result in having a colostomy bag. The surgeon reassures him that his cancer is treatable, and it is highly unlikely he will need a colostomy bag. Mr Adams is reassured at the end of the consultation and decides to have the recommended surgery.

Reflective activity

- Does your clinic have access to hearing aid batteries and loops systems?
- Do your staff know how to work hearing aids?
- What could have been the consequences if the healthcare assistant hadn't changed the batteries in the hearing aid?

Functional, social and environmental needs

There is a wide range of functional, social and environmental issues that can present a barrier to older people receiving appropriate cancer treatment. Effective assessment and care planning can minimize the impact that these issues have. It is essential that cancer services providers are aware of the most common needs, and have access to services that can provide appropriate support.

Due to the ageing process, many older people already experience functional limitations in personal tasks, such as bathing and dressing, and in instrumental tasks, such as housework and shopping. General mobility is also an issue, with 1 in 5 older people reporting they have difficulty getting to and from their hospital appointments (Department For Transport, 2011). These limitations may be exacerbated by cancer and cancer treatment. For example, fatigue is the most common side effect of chemotherapy, and is known to interfere with patients' activities of daily living. Simple assessment tools, such as the Barthel Index (Royal College of General Practitioners, 1993) can identify functional limitations quickly and effectively. Establishing functional status is essential in order to determine if an individual can seek medical attention if they develop cancer symptoms or adverse treatment side effects. Once an assessment is undertaken, a care plan can be developed and delivered with support of stakeholders such as Occupational Therapy and local voluntary sector organizations. Formal social care packages may be required. Referral into fatigue services, or physical activity programmes may also be of particular benefit.

Social isolation is commonplace in the UK older population. Half of all people aged 75 and over in the UK live alone, and 1 in 10 people have less than monthly contact with friends, family and neighbours (Office for National Statistics, 2012). Individuals experiencing isolation are less likely to access cancer treatment (Cavalli-Bjorkman et al., 2012). Many voluntary sector agencies provide 'befriending services', which aim to reduce social isolation. Encouraging participation in groups, such as exercise classes, can also reduce feelings of isolation and loneliness (Social Care Institute for Excellence, 2011).

Caring responsibilities can limit access to healthcare, with one-third of older carers in the UK reporting they have delayed or cancelled treatment for a health condition due to the demands of their caring responsibilities (The Princess Royal Trust for Carers, 2011). Over half a million people aged 65 and over have caring responsibilities that take up at least 20 hours per week (Carers UK, 2013a), and increasing numbers of families now rely on grandparents for informal childcare. Social services and the voluntary sector may be able to provide support to carers and carers support groups have good nationwide coverage. A directory of carers support groups is provided online by Carers UK (2013b).

Despite the fact that 1 in 6 pensioners in the UK live below the poverty line (Joseph Rowntree Foundation, 2012), the National Cancer Patient Experience Surveys report older people are less likely to be signposted to financial advice following their cancer diagnosis (Quality Health, 2013a). Poverty may lead to a number of issues such as poor heating, poor diet, lack of access to transport services, lack of telephone access and home disrepair (which can increase the risk of falls). These issues can all raise concerns about the safety and practicality of commencing cancer treatment. As such, it is important that people of all ages are given access to financial advice and support. Organizations such as the Citizens Advice Bureaux and Age UK are often able to provide these services.

Care planning

Mrs McDonald has been diagnosed with breast cancer and has been referred for surgery. Her assessment identifies the following issues:

- Mrs McDonald is widowed and lives on her own in a high-rise block of flats, which has lift access. She owns a small terrier dog. She gets the bus to and from the hospital independently. She does not have a telephone. Her home electricity is powered by a key card, which she tops up every week. She complains that her weekly pension is only £70 per week, which 'doesn't leave much after rent and bills'. Mrs McDonald's only son visits twice a week and takes care of the grocery shopping and all finances. You suspect that she may have been struggling financially because her clothes are threadbare and she appears unkempt.
- Mrs McDonald is on medication for hypertension, which is well controlled. She reports no other significant health problems. She is slightly underweight, and reports that her weight hasn't changed over recent months. Mrs McDonald's assessment of cognition raises concerns. Possible causes such as infection or medication side effects are ruled out. You are concerned she may have early stage dementia. Mrs McDonald was admitted to hospital last year with a broken wrist, which she sustained as a result of a fall in the home.

CASE STUDY

Reflective activity

- Which of these issues could impact on Mrs McDonald's successful recovery from surgery?
- What services could you refer Mrs McDonald to? What might her care plan look like?
- Does your service have links with the relevant agencies and services to deliver an appropriate care package for a patient with needs similar to Mrs McDonald?
- Would you consider referring Mrs McDonald to the local Safeguarding Adults team?

Key learning points

- Cancer is predominantly a disease of older age. The population is ageing and the number of older people with a diagnosis of cancer is set to rise dramatically over the coming decades.
- Older people typically experience poorer cancer outcomes than younger people in terms of survival and experience.
- Age equality legislation in the UK prohibits age discriminatory practice in the delivery of cancer care.
- The older population is a heterogeneous population and chronological age is a poor predictor of treatment tolerance and ability to benefit from treatment.
- Effective assessment and care planning is essential to ensure all patients are offered appropriate treatment options and their support needs are met during and after treatment. This is particularly important in the older population, due to its heterogeneity and the increased likelihood of individuals in this age group to have complex support needs.
- Elderly care specialists can play an important part of the cancer care team to support the delivery of care to an older population.

Recommended further reading

- Bellizzi, K.M. and Gosney, M.A. (2012) *Cancer and Ageing Handbook: Research and Practice.* 1st edn. Hoboken, NJ: Wiley-Blackwell.
- Nolan, M., Davies, N. and Grant, G. (2001) *Working With Older People And Their Families: Key Issues in Policy and Practice.* 1st edn. Buckingham, UK: Open University Press.
- Department of Health (2012) *Cancer Services Coming of Age* [Online] Available from: www.gov.uk/government/publications/improving-older-peoples-access-to-cancer-treatment-services [accessed 9 December 2013].

8 DIVERSITY AND EQUALITY IN CANCER CARE

MARK R.D. JOHNSON AND JULIE FISH

Chapter outline

- The context of health inequalities, with specific examples from relevant population groups.
- Exploration of epidemiological, knowledge, care and treatment differences among minority groups or other strands of legally recognized diversity.

- Differing understandings of causes/effects, values and terms such as 'family' or partner, among people from diverse culturally defined groups.
- Improving the knowledge, attitudes, behaviour and clinical practice of health professionals dealing with cancer in diverse groups.

INTRODUCTION

Tackling health inequalities is crucial to improving outcomes and achieving cancer survival rates which 'equal the best performing countries in the world' (DH, 2011a). Cancer inequalities, including differences in cancer outcomes (e.g. mortality) and in user or carer satisfaction of cancer care, affect a range of groups including socio-economically disadvantaged groups, black and minority ethnic groups (BME), older or younger people, men or women, people with disabilities, people from particular religions, and the lesbian, gay, bisexual and transgender (LGBT) community.

Inequalities can occur at any stage of the patient pathway, including awareness of the signs and symptoms of cancer, beliefs about susceptibility to cancer, or post-diagnosis outcomes and experiences. The NHS Constitution clearly outlines that there is a core duty to 'promote equality' (of access and outcome in health). The *Cancer Reform Strategy* (DH, 2007a) highlighted the significance of cancer inequalities in both morbidity and mortality, including survivorship, and in the experience of health services for cancer, noting that a major challenge to addressing this concern was the lack of evidence. Subsequently, the National Cancer Action Team published its National Cancer Equality Initiative (NCEI) (2010), which summarized the available evidence. They suggested a series of initiatives to reduce cancer inequality, whilst noting that there was still little reliable evidence on the causes of inequality (in any of the equality strands examined), or on effective interventions to reduce inequality.

Inequalities in health are an acknowledged fact, highlighted by reports such as the *Marmot Commission* (Marmot, 2010), which focused primarily on socio-economic aspects. The policy context also includes the growing political and strategic importance of the UK Equality Act (2010), which came into full effect in 2012. Policy concerns being articulated at a European level must also be acknowledged, as must the effects of the possibility of multiple discrimination or impact of membership of more than one disadvantaged category (for example, migrant women, older people with a disability, or LGBT minority ethnic people), known as **intersectionality** (Fundamental Rights Agency, 2013).

This chapter summarizes the key dimensions of cancer inequality, extrapolates from other sources some of the reasons for these inequalities and suggests ways in which these might be addressed. It also illustrates examples of good practice and interventions or projects that appear to have promise. The chapter aims to provoke reflection on the issues and to stimulate professionals to take action and report their findings, to reduce cancer inequality in future.

A POLICY CONTEXT

The existence of inequality in health status and in the experience of receiving healthcare has become, despite the intentions of the founders of the NHS, both an established fact and a matter for policy concern. New dimensions of inequality, going beyond the poverty that informed Beveridge's reforms, have become increasingly recognized.

The first major inquiry into **health equity**, commissioned by the Labour Government of 1974–79, (Black, 1980) demonstrated that while the introduction of the NHS had improved the overall health of the nation, there remained widespread inequalities. It concluded that the main cause was economic inequality. Some startling gradients were noted, for example the overall death rate for men in social class V (unskilled manual workers) was twice that for men in social class I (professional and managerial) and the gap between the two was increasing, not reducing as was expected. This was controversial because the founding principle of the NHS was that cost and income should not be a barrier to healthcare, which was to be 'free at the point of need'.

These findings were reinforced and reiterated in subsequent Government commissioned reports, particularly the *Whitehead Report* (1987), the *Acheson Report* (1998), and the *Marmot Review* (2010), and in each of these, key mechanisms or dimensions of inequality were found to be socio-economic gradients (i.e. being poor was bad for health) and ethnicity. BME groups consistently showed worse outcomes than white people, even when socio-economic status was taken into account, recognizing that their income was likely to be lower and their residential concentration was highest in areas of deprivation. It does not, however, appear that ethnicity can be simply reduced to a marker of socio-economic deprivation: both issues are important because 'being Black' has effects on poverty as well as beyond (Williams and Johnson, 2010).

Cancer inequalities are differences between people's cancer experience and/or outcome that result from their demographic or social characteristics (All Party Parliamentary Group on

Cancer, 2009). These social inequalities are collectively known as the **social determinants** of health (Navarro, 2009; Wilkinson and Pickett, 2010; Marmot, 2010) and include:

- Age
- Class
- Disability
- Gender
- 'Race' and ethnic origin
- Religion
- Sexual orientation
- Gender identity

The NHS of the twenty-first century, under the terms of the guiding NHS Constitution, has a responsibility to ensure that such inequalities are addressed and, insofar as possible, removed. The Care Quality Commission, which is responsible for enforcement of quality standards, explicitly places 'equity' under the headings of quality and safety in its guidance, and states,

> Equality, diversity and human rights ... Providers must consider equality, diversity and human rights in every aspect of their work. You should consider the needs of each person using a service against six key strands of diversity: Race, Age, Gender, Disability, Sexual orientation, Religion or belief. We sometimes refer to this as identifying a person's 'diversity' or 'diverse needs'. (Care Quality Commission, 2011: 38).

EPIDEMIOLOGICAL INEQUALITIES

These national studies referred to earlier were unable to focus on other 'protected characteristics' (Equality Act, 2010) recognized as affecting inequality, beyond noting the well-established fact that men and women tend to have different life expectancies. However, a more detailed analysis of cancer statistics, undertaken for the National Cancer Action Team (National Cancer Equality Initiative, 2010), reported that both cancer incidence and mortality were generally higher:

- In deprived groups compared with affluent groups;
- In older compared with younger people; and
- In men compared with women.

These pictures were more complicated when considering specific cancers: breast cancer is known to have higher incidence in more affluent groups, but mortality is actually higher in less affluent women, including BME women.

It is also apparently well established among health professionals, on the basis of nationally available epidemiological data (Gill et al., 2004), that cancer is less of a threat to people of a minority ethnic background than to the majority ('white') population. Why, therefore, is it considered important to examine issues of biopsychosocial welfare in relation to cancer and ethnicity?

Reflective activity

Consider your initial training and understanding of the biology of cancer: how far were issues of genetically defined 'race' and socio-cultural aspects of 'ethnicity' highlighted in the course texts and lectures?

It appears from closer scrutiny of the data that the prognosis for people from BME groups varies according to both the site of cancer and between ethnic groups. In general, incidence of cancer as a total cause of ill health and death is lower amongst ethnic minority groups (possibly because of their lower average age), although there are some important exceptions. These are reviewed next, using data from the National Cancer Intelligence Network (NCIN) review (2009).

Ethnicity

Incidence of prostate cancer is greater amongst Black African and Black African–Caribbean men and appears to progress faster, starting at a younger age. There is more liver cancer in South Asian groups as a whole, whilst mouth cancer is more common specifically in Bangladeshi men and women, both of whom have higher rates of tobacco use than average. Chinese groups have a higher overall expectation of cancer, but there are few robust data on specific cancers.

The reason behind this lack of specificity is that the quality of data recording in relation to ethnic groups is poor and this affects the ability of service providers to plan and deliver suitable services (Iqbal et al., 2008, 2009). The situation is even worse in terms of describing the specific needs and experiences of people in terms of their religious beliefs, sexual orientation or any disabilities, largely because such data are not routinely recorded in NHS data in a format that permits analysis (Johnson, 2008, 2012); however, data on age, sex and place of residence are routinely collected and can be used to look at variations in terms of gender, age group and poverty (indirectly) by association with area-base deprivation index scores.

More specifically, the following key facts or 'headline risks' can be deduced from the latest data (National Cancer Intelligence Network, 2009), in relation to minority ethnic groups:

- Black males of all ages were more likely to have a diagnosis of prostate cancer than white males (age-standardized Relative Risk (RR) between 1.26 and 2.48, based on different assumptions regarding 25% of patients with unknown ethnicity).
- Black and South Asian males and females had a higher rate of liver cancer than white males and females. (Black ethnic groups: RR 1.47–2.67, South Asian ethnic groups RR 1.47–2.43.)
- Black males and black females had a higher rate of myeloma than white males and females (RR 1.79–2.80).
- South Asian females 65 and over had an increased risk of cancer (compared to white females) of the mouth (RR 1.18–1.97), whereas South Asian men may have a lower risk of cancer of the mouth than white men.
- South Asian females aged 65 and over had a higher risk of cervical cancer than white females (RR 1.15–2.29).

It is not always possible to link rates and established patterns of cancer risk to lifestyle and behavioural patterns associated with ethnicity or specific ethnic groups, beyond the data on smoking and use of oral tobacco. There are few reliable data on lifestyle and diet that can be linked to clinical outcome data; however, early detection has been identified as a national priority, and although levels of public awareness of cancer signs and symptoms are generally low, they are known to be even lower in groups such as deprived communities, some BME groups and men. This may contribute to lower uptake of screening and later presentation when symptoms arise, and hence to poorer outcomes.

Sexual orientation

Differences between the health and other behaviours of LGBT people and the general population may also lead to differences in cancer incidence associated with sexual minority status. There are some forms of cancer that have much higher incidence in LGBT groups, such as anal cancer, which is 31 times more common in gay men who may practice penetrative sex (Frisch et al., 2003). Conditions related to HIV–AIDS, such as **Kaposi's syndrome** (Frisch et al., 2003), are significantly more common among gay men, while some lesbians may have made life choices (including reduced likelihood of giving birth and breastfeeding), which raise the risk of breast cancer (Zaritsky and Dibble, 2010). It is believed that lesbian, gay and bisexual people are more likely to smoke (Tang et al., 2004), increasing their risk of lung cancer. A recent UK study found a two-fold increased likelihood of a smoking history among 18–19-year-old LGB young people (Hagger-Johnson et al., 2013).

Some health professionals and lesbians themselves believe that lesbians are at a lower risk of cervical cancer due to a lower perceived risk of **human papilloma virus** (HPV) infection because they do not have sex with men (Fish, 2009); however, reported rates of HPV infection among lesbians range from 3.3–30%, with a prevalence of 19% for lesbians with no reported history of heterosexual sex (see Fish, 2009). Campaigners at one time objected to the fact that although vaccination for HPV was being actively promoted for young women to prevent cervical cancer, it was not being made available to sexually active gay men, where they argued that it might help prevent anal cancer (*The Guardian*, 13 June 2012, Society Supplement: 34). The National Cervical Screening Guidelines now recommend that lesbian and bisexual women should be offered routine screening tests on the same basis as other women.

INEQUALITIES IN ACCESS TO CARE AND TREATMENT

There are geographical variations in the accessibility and availability of certain services, as is widely debated in terms of media coverage. This includes the willingness of local healthcare bodies (led by the local Clinical Commissioning Groups that replaced the former Primary Care Trusts) to set local priorities and limits on the funding of treatment within the general parameters set by NICE. There are few sources of data, however, that can be relied on to debate this issue, apart from difficulties caused by income, education and language ability (which specifically may affect access to information, depending on the availability of interpreter support: see Kai et al., 2011). It behoves all practitioners and policymakers to reflect on their responsibilities in this respect, and to create and examine local data to ensure they are not discriminating against any of the 'protected characteristics' and that their locality represents 'good practice'.

In general, a poorer experience of care is reported by members of black and minority ethnic groups, men with prostate cancer, and people living in London. This has important consequences, since some analysts suggest that part of the striking variations in mortality can be attributed to later presentation for care, arising from delayed diagnosis amongst deprived groups, older people (at least for breast cancer) and certain BME groups. However, the contribution of any delay in diagnosis to poorer outcomes such as survival rates, and the observed higher mortality amongst men than women, is still uncertain (NCEI, 2010).

While there is little published evidence of discrimination in terms of clinical care, access to drugs and surgical interventions, or other aspects of medical care delivery, it seems that people living with cancer do feel that their identity in terms of ethnicity, gender and sexual orientation – and membership of other 'protected characteristics' – might affect the way they are treated or viewed by professionals. This comes out very clearly in terms of the way they feel they have been communicated with. A UK National Cancer Patient Experience Survey (NCPES, 2013) reports that there are consistent patterns of inequality across the data collected. White people, especially those living in less-deprived areas and reporting heterosexual orientation, (sometimes described as the 'generic majority' population), consistently felt happier about their treatment than members of the 'at risk' groups designated by membership of one or other of the 'protected characteristics'. In particular, they highlight the following differences.

Differences between ethnic groups

Communication: Cancer patients from all minority ethnic groups were consistently significantly less likely to be positive about some aspects of communication and how they were treated as patients by NHS staff compared to white patients. This key finding replicates the findings of surveys of NHS patients in other patient pathways, as reported in the annual GP Patient Surveys and other official NHS national surveys of mental health service users and hospital inpatients (see https://gp-patient.co.uk/about). This suggests that rather than something specific in the delivery of cancer services, there may be aspects of healthcare in general, less well-experienced or more heavily criticized by some ethnic minority patients. Throughout the NCPES, where there are statistically significant differences between white patients and patients from ethnic minority groups, white patients are almost always the most positive, with black patients being the least positive on six items; Asian patients least positive on six items; and Chinese/other ethnic group patients being the least positive on nine items (NCPES, 2010). Those questions covered a wide range of issues, from information giving (such as whether they received 'understandable answers' to their questions), to confidence and trust in nurses, the control of pain and assessment of primary care support. Communication is clearly a crucial part of the process and key to many inequalities (Johnson, 2012a). It is worth noting that subsequent rounds of the NCPES have found very similar differences: in the 2011/12 round, 25 statistically significant differences were found between 'majority' and minority ethnic groups, all in the same direction and pattern as in 2010 (Macmillan Cancer Support, 2013a; National Cancer Intelligence Network, 2012a).

Patient information: Access to culturally relevant information about cancer and its signs and symptoms has also been recognized as an issue. There may be an unmet need from BME communities for cancer awareness outreach that is not at present being met through initiatives such as the Ethnic Minority Cancer Awareness Month (EMCAM) or the work of minority-led initiatives such as Cancer Black Care, Cancer Equality and BME Cancer Communities (www.bmecancer.com). Existing cancer information may not always reflect multi-ethnicity in terms of images and language (e.g. patient information stating that skin might appear red after radiotherapy) (Hill, 2003). Very few 'generic' mainstream information resources include details of foods that appear more frequently in minority ethnic diets (such as *saag*, *naan*, or *ackees*).

Religion and spirituality: There is very little information on differences in cancer incidence, treatment or outcomes by religion, and none at a national level other than what can be inferred from the 2009 National Cancer Intelligence Network report (2009) about incidence and survival by ethnic group. Some equality issues that are explicitly related to religion may be identified. Patients may find it difficult to access health services during religious festivals, for example the Muslim holy month of fasting (Ramadan) can have substantial impact on attendances at cancer clinics. It is important that NHS services work with local communities to address these issues. Similarly, practices such as fasting (which is not confined to Muslim groups) may impact upon cancer treatment and interfere with medication regimes. Many of the issues faced by different religious groups are closely related to ethnicity and culture, and therefore action on many of the issues identified in this section on ethnicity will also have a positive impact on tackling inequalities according to religion.

There is also evidence that religion and spirituality affect psychosocial adjustment to cancer. Research conducted with Black Caribbean and White British patients living in South London boroughs with advanced cancer explored how religion and spirituality influenced their self-reported cancer experience (Koffman et al., 2008). In this group, Christianity was the only religion referred to. Strength of religious belief appeared to be more pronounced among Black Caribbean patients. Three main themes emerged from patients' accounts: the ways in which patients believed religion and belief in God helped them comprehend cancer; how they felt their faith and the emotional and practical support provided by church communities assisted them to live with the physical and psychological effects of their illness and its progression; and Black Caribbean patients identified the ways in which the experience of cancer promoted religious identity. Patients from both ethnic groups appeared to derive benefit from their religious faith and belief in God, but the manner in which these were understood and expressed in relation to their cancer was culturally shaped (Koffman et al., 2008).

Culture and lifestyle: A study of breast awareness among women from different BME groups living in London and Sheffield suggests that Asian and Arab women share much in common with the White British socially disadvantaged women, in terms of general poor level of knowledge about breast cancer, notions of breast cancer, personal susceptibility and pessimism about prevention; however, distinct cultural differences were observed between these groups. For the Asian and Arab women, their frame of reference was firmly embedded in a specific socio-cultural–economic context, including cancer beliefs held in their ancestral country and the experience of being a migrant being of particular relevance. These contributed to the development of cultural constraints over the discussion of cancers, engagement with preventative behaviours and with healthcare services (Scanlon, 2004).

Reflective activity

Consider your own lifestyle and 'frames of reference' and discuss with a friend from a different background (ethnic, social class, religious, language or other) what their 'points of reference' might be. How might this lead to a professional needing to give you different advice?

Differences in relation to sexual orientation

In the 2010 NCPES, respondents were asked to indicate their sexual orientation (as hetero-sexual, bisexual, gay or lesbian, or other sexual orientation) for the first time. Significant numbers of respondents (5%) said they preferred not to answer (a specific answer option) and a more substantial number than usual did not answer the question at all (8%) – this compares to only 3.7% who failed to answer the question on gender. It is possible that sig-nificant numbers of people who were not heterosexual reacted in this way to the question, and that cancer patients who were not heterosexual are undercounted in the data. Only 800 patients (1.1%) overall chose one of the response options other than heterosexual. Analysis showed significant differences in the experiences of cancer services between LGB and het-erosexual patients, and again the minority – LGB – patients reported less positive views in relation to 15 questions, specifically those which asked about communication and the way they were treated by staff, such as 'Did you get understandable answers from the Clinical Nurse Specialist all/most of the time' and 'Did you feel Hospital staff always did everything they could to control (your) pain' (Quality Health 2013a: 116–117). Worryingly, many LGBT patients felt depersonalized and were significantly more likely to reply negatively to statements such as:

- Patient was told sensitively that they had cancer.
- Doctors/nurses did not fail to tell patient things they wanted to know.
- Patient never felt treated as a set of cancer symptoms rather than as a whole person.

It is possible that there is a strong association between those respondents who defined themselves as non-heterosexuals and other variables known to influence patient opinion. For example, non-heterosexuals are significantly younger than the heterosexual respond-ent group. It is also possible that in 2010, which was the first time on any NHS survey that this question has been asked, people may have been reluctant to answer (as was the case when the census first asked about 'race'). It takes time for survey participants to feel assured that their confidentiality cannot be compromised. An alternative explanation is that they were uncertain how to answer the question: it appears that the London Metropolitan police attempted to monitor sexual orientation among staff, and significant numbers of respondents did not understand the term 'heterosexual' (personal communication, 2006). Nevertheless, it is important to recognize the differences of view between heterosexuals and non-heterosexuals and to note that 11 of the 15 questions on which non-heterosexuals have less positive views on cancer treatment relate to communication and (broadly) the respect and dignity with which the patient was treated.

The subsequent rounds of the NCPES, as with the analysis by ethnicity, found a continued pattern of relative disadvantage affecting those classified as 'non-hetero-sexual'. Although in 2011/12, response rates had improved slightly for questions on sexual orientation, the propor-tion belonging to non-heterosexual categories was the same, and the reported analysis shows only a collapsed 'non-heterosexual' category without differentiating between groups (National Cancer Intelligence Network, 2012a). One factor of relevance that does emerge from the new questions asked in 2011 was that lesbian/gay and other sexual minority groups were signifi-cantly more likely to express a willingness and enthusiasm for participation in cancer research studies, suggesting at least that they appreciated the opportunity to express their views, and perhaps reflecting an awareness that research can lead to improved treatment.

Differences between age groups

People with cancer in both the youngest and oldest age groups (16–25 and 76+, respectively) often have less positive views about their treatment than those in the middle-age groups. There are 42 separate issues on which there are significant differences between age groups as a whole in the NCPES survey and there are clear themes in relation to young patients, related specifically to ensuring that explanations of treatment, condition, tests and so forth are given in a fashion that recognizes the lack of hospital experience which many of this age group will have at the time they start treatment. As far as older people are concerned, there is strong evidence that fewer of them have easy access to clinical nurse specialists and fewer of them receive information about financial help and benefits than is the case for other age groups. In other respects, there are few definite areas of inequality in cancer attributable to age differences that could be addressed by health practitioners or policymakers, except to ensure that any assumptions about the natural history or likelihood of disease, or worth in terms of need for treatment are not based on preconceptions relating to the age of people at risk.

Patients with long-term conditions or disabilities

Disability encompasses a wide range of issues from mental health to learning disability and sensory impairment, as well as physical disability. There is no national information on variations in cancer incidence, treatment and outcomes for people with a disability, although there is some evidence for increased incidence of cancer associated with some mental illnesses (although people living with schizophrenia may have a lower incidence of respiratory cancers). This is associated with increased cancer mortality. People with intellectual disabilities appear to have a similar age-standardized incidence to the general population, although patterns of incidence may be different and screening uptake for those with learning disabilities and mental health needs seems to be lower than the general population. People with physical disabilities may also experience barriers to screening and those with learning difficulties or other communication impairments may struggle to express changes to their health, potentially complicating and delaying diagnosis. (Issues relating to intellectual disabilities and mental illness are more fully discussed in Chapters 9 and 10.)

Cancer patients taking part in the NCPES survey were asked if they had other long-term health conditions (LTC). On 48 questions there were statistically significant differences of opinion between those patients with a long-term condition or conditions and those without one. In almost all cases the patients with long-term conditions were less positive. Insofar as is possible to look at individual long-term conditions, it is clear that patients with mental health conditions and those with intellectual disabilities were very much less positive than cancer patients without long-term conditions of any kind, and less positive than patients with other kinds of long-term conditions. Again, there were complaints about depersonalization: people felt that they were being treated as a set of cancer symptoms rather than as a whole person, and that communication and respect were lacking in their treatment. People with disabilities, especially those characterized as having intellectual disabilities, are at particularly high risk.

Reflective activity

Look for examples of 'Easy Read' documentation designed for people with an intellectual disability and consider whether this style of approach would help with your practice, or in informing other so-called 'hard-to-reach' groups, especially across language barriers. Good practice examples can be found on the website of the charity Action for Real Change (www.arcuk.org.uk).

DIFFERENCES IN ATTITUDES OR BEHAVIOURS AMONG PATIENTS

A key element in understanding inequalities and variations in uptake or response to treatment and prevention programmes is that people do not all have the same values or understandings. Ethnicity is a complex concept, which includes elements of a number of ways in which people think of themselves and live. These include language, religion and culture – and that last concept might include different understandings of what is meant by 'family' and the responsibilities or roles of family members, as well as drawing on different musical or artistic traditions and having access to different pools of knowledge. For minority groups defined by a history of migration (e.g. 'South Asian' peoples), this will include awareness of patterns of diseases and treatments or outcomes drawn from other countries. This is also true for people whose migration (or parents) came from other European countries, as well as the more usually described 'BME' groups.

Similarly, people defined by their sexual orientation or age will have different understandings of family relationships and different experiences that will affect the way they think and behave, or indeed, the ways in which professionals may respond to and treat them. For example, for LGBT people, some research has suggested that their partner or carer was not seen as a legitimate person to be involved in decision-making about treatment and care, and were often overlooked by clinicians and other health professionals (Fish, 2010; BRAP, 2010).

An under-reported issue in relation to cancer treatment is the potential threat to **fertility**, which has very specific implications for younger women, but has also been raised in controversies relating to men's ability to store gametes (semen) for future use. Treatment, especially with toxic drugs or radiation therapies, can lead to infertility, and beliefs (or values), stereotypes and knowledge all affect the way this may be discussed and resolved. A study specifically looking into this issue (Chattoo et al., 2010) found that gender was seen as an important consideration, as was life stage, in discussing treatment options. When ethnicity was discussed, it was often in terms of generalized assumptions, assuming homogenous communities, in addition to a strong sense of minorities being the 'other'. Professionals could interpret similar responses very differently according to the cultural and ethnic background of the patient and often felt ill-equipped to respond to the needs of a multicultural society.

This issue can become even more salient within the context of families of South Asian origin due to the assumptions professionals have about their family culture being patriarchal, oppressive and intrusive. In fact, people from minority cultures exhibit considerable flexibility and sophistication in approaching such concerns. For example, Islam does not in fact prevent men from using sperm-freezing, although South Asian families may have different understandings of kinship roles and expectations, and sometimes feel exposed to greater peer pressure (see Culley et al., 2009). For women, **gamete storage** is a more complex and time-consuming procedure that could significantly affect onset of treatment and it is important that these matters are raised early and discussed sensitively. It is also important to note that similar issues (and problems of professionals' feelings of comfort in discussing them) arise in relation to people in LGBT relationships (Hinchliff et al., 2005). Although that paper relates primarily to sexual health, it may be that cancer professionals need to discuss with LGBT patients how their cancer might impact on their sexual health (e.g. lesbian sex following cervical cancer, or sex between men following anal or prostate cancer).

As people face cancer and the end of life, the social, cultural and therapeutic role of food takes on an increasing significance. This has not been widely researched, or reported, but one small study by Payne et al. (2008) involving older Chinese people resident in the UK investigated their beliefs about the influence of food on cancer and its role in supportive cancer care. The analyses revealed four main themes: (1) food as 'therapeutic'; (2) food as 'risky'; (3) food as supportive and comforting; and (4) beliefs about the lack of culturally appropriate and acceptable food in hospitals. Expectations about the lack of Chinese food and the poor quality and perceived unsuitability of 'Western' food were regarded as major concerns in relation to hospital admission (Payne et al., 2008). It can be assumed that similar beliefs and feelings may also be expressed by members of other groups used to a distinctive 'traditional' diet.

RELEVANCE TO PRACTICE

It is important to recognize that although much of the earlier text reports concerns, inequalities and feelings of exclusion associated with belonging to BME and LGBT (and other 'at risk' minority) groups, there have also been a number of examples of 'good practice' and interventions designed to address these and provide an improved experience and outcome for members of these groups. At present, most of these are still only at the stage of being researched or evaluated in pilot sites, but as they are increasingly reported in appropriate formats, providers and commissioners of services will find pressure to adopt them into regular provision (e.g. Nottingham City and County PCT, 2011; Fish, 2012). Readers, therefore, should seek out newly reported research and evaluation studies, and ensure that their practice is able to reflect the lessons learned. Specialist journals, such as *Diversity & Equality in Health and Care*, or relevant charities like Stonewall will probably be the first place to report these, and may also note new studies as they start. Key to this will be ensuring collection of appropriate data relating to ethnicity, sexual orientation, disability and other 'risk factors' for inequality, and performing audits to ensure that differences are *not* invariably associated with inequalities.

Reflective activity

Consider any research activity or audit that you are involved in or have the opportunity to conduct. Would it be possible to include ethnicity or sexual orientation in this? What would you expect to find?

A number of Government initiatives have been introduced following the *Cancer Reform Strategy* (DH, 2007a) that aim to reduce cancer inequalities and improve the survivorship of patients with the poorest outcomes. In 2010, the NCEI produced a principles and practice guidance document for good equality working, which outlined ten good practice principles:

Principles for good equality working (NCAT/NCEI 2011)

1. There is an evidence base
2. Work is targeted and specific
3. There is community engagement
4. There is service improvement and innovation
5. Interventions are tested and refined
6. There is a process to measure effectiveness
7. The work is led by champions working in partnership with others
8. The work is evaluated
9. Sustainability is built-in
10. Learning is shared

Since the NCEI was established in 2008, a number of good practice examples can be found:

- NCAT Cancer Awareness newspapers targeted at African and African–Caribbean, South Asian and Irish communities, along with guidelines for Wellbeing Boards and GP Commissioners have been uploaded and published through their website (www.ncat.nhs.uk/our- work/improvement/equality)
- Other NCAT campaign materials developed as part of the 'Cancer Does Not Discriminate' programme can be found on the websites of partner agencies (see Principles for good equality working 7) such as:

  - the RAFFA site working with faith communities (www.raffa.org.uk/health-and-wellbeing)
  - Stonewall (www.stonewall.org.uk for LGBT groups)
  - Breast Cancer Care (www.breastcancercare.org.uk) and Cancer Research UK (www.cancerresearchuk.org)

CHAPTER SUMMARY

Equality issues should be embedded throughout cancer services rather than being a token gesture. Taking three of the principles as exemplars, we highlight the developments made in efforts to reduce cancer inequalities. These identify the need for robust research evidence and, to this end, the NCEI has been instrumental in developing the evidence base for cancer among groups who experience inequalities.

1. The National Cancer Intelligence Network (NCIN), for example, has recently produced a report about ethnicity and lung cancer, which shows that Bangladeshi and white men have higher rates of lung cancer than Indian and Pakistani men (Jack et al., 2011). The data will enable targeting campaigns within these communities to raise awareness of risk factors and reduce smoking.

2. Engaging with communities and diverse groups to understand the reasons underlying poorer experiences of care is essential. NCAT has established the national *BME Cancer Voice*, which incorporates both Asian and black groups to support improvements in the experience of those affected by cancer in BME communities and develop more personalized interventions. It aims to raise awareness of cancer and its signs and symptoms, and access to screening programmes by people from all BME communities through carefully targeted campaigns, including the NCAT Cancer Does Not Discriminate campaign, aimed at raising awareness of cancer in BME communities.

3. With regards to service improvement and innovation, there is a project funded by the Economic and Social Research Council (ESRC), which aims to develop knowledge among cancer and social care professionals about breast cancer in lesbian and bisexual women. Working alongside the charities Breast Cancer Care and Macmillan Cancer Support, the project aims to develop organizational cultures and practices in cancer and social care services. Breast Cancer Care produced a policy briefing document, which raises awareness about risks, diagnosis and time of presentation, access to information and treatment and access to emotional support (Dhami, 2011). It makes recommendations for Cancer Charities, professionals and commissioners of cancer care and policymakers. As a result, Breast Cancer Care now collects sexual orientation data for their volunteers and plans to do so for everyone that uses their services. They will use these data to see patterns of service usage and if there are any differences that can be attributed to equality issues, and implement the recommendations in their policy work. In the work with Macmillan Cancer Support, cancer and social care professionals attended a seminar that examined differences in the research evidence about any form of cancer in LGBT people, and included a Macmillan GP-led discussion about differences in cancer experiences. A service user and carer also spoke about their cancer journey. In workshop sessions, a number of case studies were discussed and these were developed to form a new resource for professionals working in cancer (Fish, 2012). Most cancer professionals are committed to promoting equality, but in order to do so they need resources to support them in delivering good practice and an evidence base on which to underpin their interventions.

Reflective activity

Consider the relationship between cancer care and the social inequalities:

- Age
- Class
- Disability

(Continued)

(Continued)

- Gender
- 'Race' and ethnic origin
- Religion
- Sexual orientation
- Gender identity

What can be done about health service providers' lack of knowledge about LGBT and BME issues?

What might LGBT people or those from religious and cultural minority backgrounds fear about health professionals?

What concerns do professionals have about LGBT or religious-distinctive patients?

Are differences between 'diverse' groups (whether defined by sexual orientation/sexuality, gender, age, disability, ethnicity or faith) the result of accident, an artefact of the data or due to discrimination?

What is the responsibility of the individual practitioner to understand the needs of members of groups, as defined by these dimensions of inequality?

Key learning points

- The incidence of some forms of cancer is lower among BME groups; however, the prognosis may be worse than for other groups – some cancers are much more common in certain groups of LGBT people.
- BME patients report less positive care in relation to information giving, confidence and trust in nurses, control of pain and assessment of primary care support.
- LGBT patients are more likely to report that they are not treated with dignity and respect and that they felt depersonalized in healthcare interactions.
- Older patients are less likely to say that they had received information about financial help and benefits than their younger counterparts.
- Patients with mental health conditions and those with learning disabilities were less positive about their care and reported feeling depersonalized.
- The cancer care community needs to create a healthcare environment that is welcoming of diversity and includes training in effective communication with inequality. As such, diversity should be integral to Continuous Professional Development.
- It is important to develop a knowledge base of local and national resources for inequality groups in order to signpost people with cancer, their families and carers to longer-term support through treatment and follow-up.

Recommended further reading

- Lethborg, C. and Posenelli, S. (2010) 'Improving psychosocial care for cancer patients', in P. Bywaters, E. Mcleod and L. Napier (eds.), *Social Work and Global Health Inequalities*. Bristol: The Policy Press. pp. 198–208.

Navarro, V. (2009) 'What we mean by social determinants of health?', *International Journal of Health Services*, 39 (3): 429–441.

Wilkinson, R. and Pickett, K. (2010) *The Spirit Level: Why Equality is Better for Everyone*. Harmondsworth, UK: Penguin.

Williams C, and Johnson M.R.D. (2010) *Race and Ethnicity in a Welfare Society*. Maidenhead, UK: Open University Press/McGraw Hill.

Note: selected 'grey literature' reports about cancer inequalities on open access can be found at the CERP Portal (www.cancerinfo.nhs.uk/healthcare-professional/cerp).

Selected websites exhibiting Good Practice/ Further online resources

- www.cancerblackcare.org.uk/
- www.bmecancervoice.co.uk/
- www.ncin.org.uk/about_ncin/default.aspx
- www.bmecancervoice.co.uk/images/ncat%20health%20supplement%20issue%201. pdf
- www.cancerinfo.nhs.uk/

9 CANCER AND MENTAL ILLNESS

MAUREEN DEACON AND ELISE HYMANSON

Chapter outline

- Relationship between cancer and mental illness
- Barriers to cancer screening and diagnosis experienced by people with a mental illness
- Challenges associated with cancer treatments among people with mental illness
- The implications of caring for a person with cancer who also has a mental illness
- Best care practice in situations that can be complex and challenging

---

INTRODUCTION

The initial challenge is to define the population described as the 'mentally ill'. This requires clarity both in relation to the evidence base and when considering how different forms of mental illness may inter-relate with the experience of cancer. Conventionally, this population tends to be simplistically divided into those with **serious mental illness** (SMI), those with **common mental health problems** and those who have **problematic substance misuse**. The former is generally taken to refer to people with a diagnosis of **psychosis, schizophrenia, schizoaffective disorder** or **bipolar disorder** (DH, 2011b) but can also include people with **personality disorder** who are disabled to the extent that they frequently use mental health services (DH, 2003). Those with common mental health problems include people with anxiety disorder and mild-to-moderate depression (DH, 2011b) who are generally treated – if treated at all – within primary care. Like SMI, these mental health problems also tend to recur. In this chapter, the population who have mental illness prior to developing cancer will be considered.

The evidence base from research concerning the complex relationships between different forms of mental illness and different forms of cancer is conflicting, but this field of research is developing. More broadly, there is growing concern about the physical ill health and early death of people with SMI, and Thornicroft (2011) calls this, 'the scandal of premature mortality' (p. 441). Mentally ill men are likely to die about 20 years earlier than their counterparts; mentally ill women die about 15 years earlier than their peers (Thornicroft, 2011). It has been suggested that the stigma attached to SMI has meant that this situation has gone largely unnoticed and that a similar mortality difference in any other population would have been met with horror (Gray, 2012).

Unravelling the relationships between SMI and physical ill health is a work in progress and we remain largely ignorant of the micro processes involved in more carefully defined cases. Clearly there are decades of research still ahead; however, the probable underlying causes of reduced life expectancy in people with SMI are largely agreed upon internationally (Chadwick et al., 2012). These are summarized by Thornicroft (2011) as an increased risk of death by suicide and accidents; high risk factors for long-term conditions such as a lack of exercise and smoking; social disadvantage generally and specifically in accessing and receiving physical healthcare; and side effects of some psychiatric drugs.

Depression and **anxiety** have been related to cancer and an increased risk of premature death, although these are not consistent findings across different studies (Russ et al., 2012). Having established that both SMI and common mental health problems are associated with higher morbidity and mortality when compared to the general population, the reasons for this will now be explored.

FACTORS THAT MAY INFLUENCE THE PHYSICAL HEALTH AND MORTALITY OF PEOPLE WITH MENTAL ILLNESS

Taken as a whole, people who are mentally ill are at higher risk of dying from unnatural causes, that is, from suicide, violence and accidents. Thornicroft (2011) observes that 20% of people with schizophrenia die from such causes compared to 3% of the general population; however, Bradshaw and Pedley (2012) note that death by natural causes is a bigger factor overall. These causes include cardiovascular disease, metabolic syndrome, cancer and respiratory disease (Drake, 2013). Unhealthy lifestyles are understood to play a significant part in these excess deaths, including a lack of exercise, smoking, high levels of obesity and a poor diet.

Mental illness can go hand-in-hand with **social disadvantage**. People may be poor, isolated and badly housed and such social factors are unequivocally implicated in health inequalities and health behaviour (Street, 2013). The latter is often associated with the notion of lifestyle *choices*, but choice may not be relevant to some people with mental illness. For example, Cormac et al. (2005) found that people with schizophrenia who were hospitalized gained weight. Similarly, morbid weight gain is caused in some people by anti-psychotic drugs (Vandyk and Baker, 2012).

Social disadvantage is evident in relation to accessing physical healthcare and there are four elements to this. First, people with mental illness may not seek out physical healthcare because of their mental illness (Robson and Gray, 2007). For instance, a person with highly unstable bipolar disorder may be too fatigued when depressed to make the effort or too chaotic when **hypomanic** to be organized enough. Second, the mentally ill may experience **diagnostic overshadowing**, whereby any health complaints they have are seen through an unhelpful and biased lens by healthcare professionals (Jones et al., 2008). For example, a person with schizophrenia who is obese and on anti-psychotic medication is advised to lose weight when they complain of a change in bowel habit, rather than being properly investigated. Third, people with mental illness suffer from **social stigma**, which may result in their concerns just not being taken seriously (Deacon, 2013b). Finally, the organization of healthcare may act as a barrier to people accessing effective care. For instance, some insurance-based systems are not well set up for people with co-morbidity, and just making an appointment to see a GP requires social resources. Chadwick et al. (2012) reviewed studies that explored service users' experiences of attempting to access physical healthcare. Service users cited practical and interpersonal problems, including long waiting times and feeling disrespected during consultations. A growing awareness and a developing evidence base of all these factors have led policymakers to attempt to positively influence physical healthcare for the mentally ill.

HEALTH POLICY AND THE PROMOTION OF THE PHYSICAL HEALTH OF THE MENTALLY ILL

In the UK, policymakers have been acting on these matters for some time. From 2004, GPs have been encouraged to develop case registers of their patients with SMI and to offer them annual check-ups (Bradshaw and Pedley, 2012). The Chief Nursing Officer's strategic review of mental health nursing (DH, 2006) recommended that mental health nurses fully engage in promoting the physical health of service users and that their competence to do this should be developed. Evaluation of the impact of implementing this review found that NHS Trusts were giving greater priority to this aspect of healthcare (Hardy and Thomas, 2012).

No Health without Mental Health was published by the UK Department of Health in 2011. It sets out several objectives, including that people with mental illness should have good physical health. This was followed by an implementation plan (DH, 2012a), the success of which is to be reviewed via a national mental health dashboard.

In relation to cancer, the Department of Health has published *Improving Outcomes: A Strategy for Cancer* (2011a). Aiming to improve outcomes across the cancer trajectory, it emphasizes the need to reduce all inequalities. Furthermore, the provision of psychological care for all cancer patients is receiving growing attention in the UK; *Psychological Support Measures* (National Cancer Peer Review–National Cancer Action Team, 2010) describes a workforce strategy and implementation plan for its provision. Having knowledge and understanding of relevant health policy can enable healthcare practitioners to advocate on behalf of the people they care for.

THE INCIDENCE AND MORTALITY OF PEOPLE WITH SMI AND CANCER

The relationship between SMI and the incidence and mortality rates of cancer is a difficult one to ascertain and this has long been the case. For example, there has been research carried out on schizophrenia and bipolar disorder and their association with cancer, and the results of this research are conflicting (De Hert et al., 2011; Hodgson et al., 2010). For a century at least there was the idea that people with schizophrenia have a lower incidence of cancer than the general population (Hippisley-Cox et al., 2007) and these matters remain opaque. It has been speculated that those with schizophrenia may have genetic protection (Howard et al., 2010) or that anti-psychotic medication may inhibit cell mutation (Hippisley-Cox et al., 2007). On the other hand, Howard et al. (2010) and Kisely et al. (2008) have found higher levels of death from cancer in patients who are mentally ill. As indicated earlier, the whole basis of such research evidence is problematic because it has been carried out using assorted populations and methods. Given that these mental illness diagnoses are themselves subject to debate (Barker and Buchanan-Barker, 2012), this is not that surprising. Adding to this fundamental uncertainty and research limitations, such as underpowered studies and the use of biased populations, it is possible to understand why this is such contested territory. In an effort to avoid such limitations, Hippisley-Cox et al. (2007) analyzed data about six common cancers: breast, colon, rectal, gastro-oesophageal, prostate and respiratory malignancies. By using the QRESEARCH general practice database from 454 sites, they were able to examine 40,441 cases of these cancers and compare them with matched controls, that is, they compared people with and without schizophrenia and with and without bipolar disorder. The study demonstrated that those with schizophrenia had a significantly higher risk of colon cancer and a lower risk of respiratory cancer. The risk of colon cancer was particularly high in people prescribed anti-psychotic drugs. This study found no such differences identified for patients with bipolar disorder – a population less likely to be prescribed long-term anti-psychotic drugs. Conversely, a study in Israel by BarChana et al. (2008) found an enhanced risk for cancer among both male and female Jewish–Israeli patients with bipolar disorder. Overall, it has been noted that older studies have been more likely to show a reduced incidence of cancer in patients with schizophrenia, whereas contemporary studies demonstrate a higher than expected incidence of mortality in these patients (Hodgson et al., 2010).

With regards to mortality rates, Harris and Barraclough (1998) conducted a Medline search over the period 1995–8. They established no significant differences in cancer mortality between the general population and patients with bipolar disorder. The same search demonstrated significant differences for people with the diagnosis of schizophrenia, namely evidence for increased risk of death due to breast cancer in women with schizophrenia. One proposed theory is that this increased risk is related to lower fertility rates in this cohort of women or the use of anti-psychotic drugs (Howard et al., 2010). There was also shown to be a decrease in lung cancers in men. This was believed to be related to the limit on cigarettes for inpatients during the 1950s (Harris and Barraclough, 1998).

Using the UK GP database, Osborn et al. (2007) examined seven of the most frequently acquired cancers: respiratory, colorectal, breast, prostate, stomach, oesophagus and pancreas. They compared people with serious mental illness with the general population. There was no difference found in mortality rates for non-respiratory cancers. There was a statistically significant increase in mortality from respiratory tumours for those aged 50–75. This disappeared when adjustments for smoking and social deprivation were made. Kisely et al. (2008) studied cancer incidence and mortality in psychiatric patients in an area of Canada and found a higher mortality rate from cancer (29%), which could not be explained by a higher incidence of cancer in their study population. Work by Kisely et al. (2008) and Howard et al. (2010) led them

than recognizing it as part of their underlying psychiatric illness. This could act as a barrier to their care (Lawrence and Kisely, 2010). Furthermore, once a diagnosis has been established, there is some evidence that psychiatric service users do not always receive the same level of care as the rest of the population (Jones et al., 2008). According to Jones et al., (2008), there are two studies that have demonstrated that patients with mental illness and cardiovascular disease are less likely to receive revascularization treatment and diabetic patients are less likely to be admitted to hospital if they have a mental illness. This may also be true of cancer patients and can be understood to be a consequence of diagnostic overshadowing. This negative social process may also impact on the promptness of diagnosis, potentially affecting treatment options and prognosis.

Organizational issues

Organizational models for mental health and medical services may be contributing to the lack of integrated care for people with mental illness and cancer. Traditionally psychiatric services have been run separately from other healthcare providers, both geographically and financially (Druss, 2007). This can result in poor sharing of information and ineffective collaboration overall. Service users may be called to numerous appointments at different sites and this may affect their level of concordance. Clearly, rapid and accurate diagnosis of cancer is of the same critical importance to people with mental illness as it is to anybody else, yet the matters discussed earlier may have negative ramifications for achieving this.

TREATMENT CHALLENGES

Cancer patients with SMI may experience many difficulties surrounding their treatment. The first hurdle that they have to navigate is consenting to treatment, and this relies on both good dyadic communication and **shared decision-making** (Charles et al., 1997; see also Chapter 17). In order to make an informed decision, patients require **mental capacity** and must be able to:

- Understand the information pertaining to this specific decision;
- Retain that information and use it as part of their decision-making process; and
- Communicate their decision (whether by talking, using sign language or any other means) to the relevant caregivers.

It is the responsibility of the medical team caring for the patient to determine whether or not they have the capacity to make decisions about their cancer treatment. If it is deemed that they do not, a decision needs to be made in the patient's best interest and this process should include all those involved in the patient's care. Healthcare professionals need to be knowledgeable and up-to-date concerning the Mental Capacity Act 2005 (DH, 2005a) including their local organizational procedures. Mental capacity can be compromised by many aspects of mental illness, but a lack of capacity should not be assumed. For example, consider Joan, a 52-year-old woman who is severely depressed and refuses treatment for breast cancer on the basis that she is suicidal and hopes that it will kill her. This raises **ethical**, **legal** and **medical dilemmas**.

She may be well able to articulately demonstrate her understanding of her diagnosis and the treatment proposed, but is her capacity to make a decision compromised by her mental illness? We will return to this question later.

Cancer treatments can involve many hospital appointments and unpleasant routines that have to be followed if the treatment is to be potentially successful. This can require a certain degree of organizational ability, practical resources, stamina and resilience. In some cases, patients with SMI do not possess the necessary skills and resources and will require intensive support during this time. These resources should not be assumed and a raised awareness of the individual needs should be sought.

Many cancer treatments are extremely arduous and this is the case for all who experience them. Some cancer patients are exposed to treatments that can induce feelings of anxiety, low mood and helplessness. For example, some radiotherapy treatments require patients to be in isolation, unable to leave a room or have people entering for over 24 hours; other radiotherapy treatments may require patients to wear a tight-fitting mask whilst receiving their treatment; chemotherapy treatments on haematology wards can involve long stays in one room, with limited visits to reduce infection risk. For patients with SMI, who already may experience disturbing thoughts or hallucinations, this may be too much for them to bear without carefully managed and creatively delivered care.

Drug treatment also requires consideration. It is important that people with SMI continue to take their prescribed psychiatric medication because any decline in their mental health may affect their ability to comply with their cancer treatment. Some **psychotropic drugs** can interact with chemotherapy regimes. They may enhance or oppose each other or affect their **metabolism** and **excretion** (Howard et al., 2010). Another concern is the effect that chemotherapy and some psychotropic medication can have on the blood cells in the body. These effects can lead to overwhelming infections or clotting disorders, which can prove fatal. A **collaborative approach** between oncologists and mental health teams would be advisable, with close monitoring of patients' blood results and mental health.

Other medications that are prescribed alongside the chemotherapy can have a detrimental effect on patients with SMI. **Steroids** may be prescribed, sometimes in very high doses to reduce side effects from the chemotherapy. Steroids may exacerbate some psychiatric symptoms such as anxiety, agitation and mania. Anti-sickness medications, such as **metoclopramide** and **haloperidol**, when dispensed alongside anti-psychotic drugs can lead to disabling movement disorders. Again, a joint approach for these patients would be advisable to try to minimize these issues.

As discussed, there is some evidence to suggest that patients with SMI have a worse outcome than the general population following cancer treatment (Howard et al., 2010). They are more likely to have concomitant medical problems, such as cardiovascular and respiratory disease, and have poor lifestyle factors (see earlier). This puts them at risk of a poorer outcome post-treatment (Howard et al., 2010). These factors illustrate that patients with SMI have specific increased risks and treatment requirements when compared to the general population. In addition, they may have multiple health and social care professionals involved in their care, dispersing overall responsibility for who takes the lead in regards to their physical health and potentially leading to missed opportunities and poor communication.

CASE STUDY EXAMPLES OF CASE MANAGEMENT

Essentially, reaching the best standard of care requires the healthcare team to factor in the mental health needs of the person requiring high quality cancer care. The following two case studies exemplify best care considerations and processes.

CASE STUDY

Joan

Joan discovered a painless lump in her right breast whilst in the shower. Coincidentally her mental health was deteriorating. She felt worthless and had suicidal thoughts, having made suicide attempts in the past. The breast lump offered her some relief; perhaps she would die of cancer. She kept the lump secret and Joan became increasingly depressed. She was highly anxious and was physically agitated. Her very concerned and loving husband, Dennis, observed that she unusually kept feeling her right breast. When he commented on this she denied that there was a problem and became angry with him. Eventually, he took Joan to visit her GP to discuss her depression. Dennis mentioned this new 'breast checking' behaviour, thinking that it might be another sign of her terrible agitation. However, the GP observed that this would be very unusual and asked Joan if she could examine her breast. Tearfully, Joan capitulated to the persuasion of both Dennis and her GP. Having felt the lump, the GP referred her to the local breast clinic, increased the dose of her anti-depressant medication and referred her back urgently to the local community mental health team (CMHT). Joan fully cooperated with the investigations at the breast clinic but appeared distant, distracted and preoccupied with her own thoughts. Following the investigations, she was sensitively given, in Dennis's presence, a diagnosis of breast cancer by a breast surgeon and breast care nurse. She was advised that in the first instance she would need to have the lump surgically removed and that what followed from this would depend on tests carried out on the removed tumour. During this consultation, Joan sat wringing her hands. When asked if she understood what she was being told and given the opportunity to ask questions, she stood up, said 'don't worry, I'm just getting what I deserve' and left the room. Dennis, who was very shocked and frightened by the cancer diagnosis, apologized and ran after her.

Case considerations and questions:

- Joan is severely depressed and has been treated by the CMHT in the past. Joan may be a high suicide risk and she may have depressive delusions. Has the GP explained this to the breast care team in the referral?
- Joan has been referred back to the CMHT. Does the breast care team know this? Do the CMHT know about the referral to the breast clinic?
- Have the breast care team realized that Joan is mentally unwell? The staff carrying out the investigations may have thought that she was just a bit 'odd' and not communicated any concerns to the surgeon and nurse.
- Joan has breast cancer and needs to commence potentially life saving investigations and treatment. Early indications are that she is refusing treatment. Does Joan have the mental capacity to either refuse or consent to cancer treatment? How urgently does Joan require cancer treatment? Can Joan be treated for cancer whilst her mental state is so acutely disabled?

- Joan has a devoted and caring husband, but Dennis is now very distressed and worried about Joan's condition. There is evidence that Dennis can persuade Joan to 'comply' with healthcare. Should the breast care team take advantage of this relationship for the sake of Joan's health?
- Does the oncology service have access to a psycho-oncology team?

Reflective activity

Consider this scenario from the perspectives of the different people involved: what are they likely to be thinking and feeling? What will each of them believe that they are responsible for and what might the implications of this be?

What should happen next? What are the priorities and who should take responsibility for organizing Joan's care?

The current key issues around decision-making

Joan requires treatment for breast cancer *and* for depression – the simultaneous presence of both leads to 'more than the sum of their parts'. That is, Joan's depression complicates any cancer treatment in terms of her capacity to consent and cooperate, and her breast cancer may become enmeshed in her depressive state. Furthermore, the 'cancer diagnosis shock' that Dennis has experienced, in addition to his own distress and concern, leads to his greater vulnerability and threatens his health and capacity to be Joan's carer.

There are four initial priorities:

- To urgently assess and treat Joan's mental illness. This can either be done by the CMHT or, if available, the psych-oncology team (although such teams are rare) in collaboration with the CMHT.
- To decide how urgent her breast treatment is and to consider if this can wait until her mental state has improved. The breast care team will need to seek advice from their oncology colleagues.
- For all staff to support, inform and collaborate with Joan *and* Dennis.
- For the whole of this particular care system to effectively communicate and collaborate.

Mental health services in England and Wales operate the Care Programme Approach (DH, 2008b). This means that Joan would be allocated a care coordinator within the CMHT. Their role is to ensure that potentially fragmented services work together with the service user to provide them with the best possible care. Staff working within cancer services can find out who Joan's care coordinator is by contacting the relevant CMHT.

Joan's treatment

The joint care team (including Dennis) decide that the treatment priority is Joan's mental health. Whilst treating her cancer is important, their reasoning is that currently Joan does not have the capacity to consent to cancer treatment; that the tumour appears small and there is no indication of lymph node involvement; and that Joan's distress and ill health is caused first and foremost by her depressive disorder. They agree that as soon as Joan has recovered sufficiently to have the mental capacity to consent to cancer treatment, they will progress that as quickly as possible. During this decision-making phase, Joan's mental health has deteriorated further and the consultant psychiatrist successfully recommends that Joan be legally detained in a psychiatric ward for assessment and treatment under the Mental Health Act, 2007 (DH, 2007b). Her care coordinator contacts the breast care nurse to enquire if the mental health team need to do anything in particular with regard to her breast cancer. They are advised to promote her physical health as much as possible, in preparation for cancer treatment. The care coordinator agrees to communicate with the breast care nurse regarding Joan's progress. The care coordinator does some background reading about breast cancer and advises and informs the mental health team what is likely to happen to Joan. The mental health team decide on a drug treatment regime based on Joan's past history and discuss how to respond to Joan's depressive thinking about her cancer: to respect her views but to offer optimism and accurate information about the treatment she will have and its likely positive outcome. Given that Joan's appetite is poor (a common feature of depression), the ward nurses take care to ensure that Joan is regularly encouraged to eat and drink. They engage Dennis in these efforts and monitor her weight. The ward nurses are less concerned about physical exercise because, ironically, Joan's level of agitation is such that she frequently paces the ward.

After five weeks, Joan is considered well enough to be discharged from the ward, with regular follow-ups from her care coordinator. Joan makes the case that she would like a week at home before having surgery. This will help her prepare and catch up with important matters in her life. A date for admission to the surgical ward is agreed. The breast care nurse seeks advice from the care coordinator regarding the care of Joan's mental health. The care coordinator stresses the importance of ensuring that Joan continues to receive her anti-depressant medication correctly and informs the breast care nurse about Joan's **relapse signature**. This describes a set of signs that may indicate relapse that are both general to depressive disorder and specific to Joan (Birchwood et al., 2000). The breast care nurse is advised that the cancer care team should proactively and privately ask Joan and Dennis about how Joan's mental health is, rather than ignoring it. The care coordinator agrees to visit Joan post-surgery and to keep in touch.

Joan, who is now in a position to give informed consent, commences her cancer treatment. Dennis and the care coordinator are concerned that fear of cancer and post-surgical debilitation might impact negatively on Joan's mental health. Together, they vigilantly monitor her mental health.

Case considerations

- Severe depression requires a sustained recovery period. How can the risks between relapse and the need for cancer treatment be balanced?
- Should the whole system care team have considered applying to use the Deprivation of Liberty Safeguards (DH, 2007b) whereby Joan could have been treated simultaneously for breast cancer and depression within the surgical setting? Would the surgical setting have had the resources to contain and care well for a person who was acutely mentally ill?

- Organizational practices may make the whole care team approach described impractical. The staff involved will work in different settings with an expectation that their work is bounded within certain types of activities. Will they be willing and able to work differently for Joan's benefit?
- Is it realistic to expect practitioners to 'research' other unfamiliar aspects of healthcare? Is this what should be expected from an accountable professional?

Reflective activity

- Think about what you consider to be the hallmarks of good practice from the description of Joan's care.
- Discuss your views with a colleague on whether the team made the right decisions.

CASE STUDY

George

What follows is a shorter case study, based loosely on a real case involving the work of a psycho-oncology team. George was a 60-year-old man with a recent diagnosis of pancreatic cancer. In the previous few months, he was noted to have started to exhibit bizarre beliefs and behaviours. He had been referred to the local mental health crisis intervention team and had been prescribed anti-psychotic medication. Not long after this, he was admitted to a cancer hospital for a paracentesis (a procedure to drain fluid that has accumulated within the abdomen) and chemotherapy treatment. During his admission, his psychotic symptoms worsened. He was agitated and upset, believing that he was receiving commands from the television and the radio advising him not to trust hospital staff. He refused to have any clinical observations done and he refused any tests related to his treatment. He was having difficulty sleeping.

The hospital psycho-oncology team were asked to review George. It became apparent that he had been developing these symptoms gradually over the last six months. Since his admission, they had become worse. On assessment, George was defensive and did not initially wish to see the psychiatrist/nurse. When asked why he was refusing his treatment, he stated that he did not need any because he did not have pancreatic cancer and he wanted to know when he could be discharged home. He did not feel at ease on the ward and believed that his food was being tampered with. He disclosed that he was being spoken to by the television but that these voices were not disturbing to him.

It was judged that George probably had an underlying psychotic illness with a possible acute confusion, which had culminated in further deterioration of his mental state. His anti-psychotic medication was increased. The nursing staff were advised by the psychiatric team how best to manage his behaviour. For example, it was discussed whether placing him in a single side room might help to keep him calmer and protect other patients from his disturbance. They were helped to find a consistent way of responding to his paranoid ideas and enlisting his family in supporting him. An organic cause

(Continued)

(Continued)

needed to be excluded for George's behaviour and he consented to bloods being taken and a brain scan. No organic cause was found and his behaviour continued to worsen. It was becoming increasingly difficult to manage his behaviour on a general ward and he had begun to wander off the ward at times. He was still not consenting to any cancer treatment.

The psychiatric team discussed the situation with George's family and the medical team caring for him. It was judged that it was not possible to treat his cancer until the mental health problems had been treated. He was, therefore, detained under Section 2 of the Mental Health Act and transferred to his local psychiatric hospital. Regular review of his physical health was arranged.

After a few weeks, George's psychotic symptoms were successfully treated. He was discharged home with psychiatric follow-up care in the community. He was now able to consent to his cancer treatment and plans were made for his readmission back to the cancer hospital with supportive psychiatric care.

Reflective activity

During the initial phase of his care within the cancer setting, George gave intermittent consent to undergo investigative cancer-related procedures. Do you think that the team should have considered the use of the Mental Capacity Act?

Consider the challenges involved in caring for a person who is acutely mentally ill on a medical ward. Reflect on your experience of this.

Why do you think that George's mental health deteriorated further on the medical ward?

CHAPTER SUMMARY

It has been argued that **best care principles** for a person with cancer and mental illness need to take into account all the individual factors involved, with a particular focus on the ramifications of a 'mix' of symptoms. We have shown how the consequences of co-morbidity can increase both physical and mental risks and distress. The two case studies presented are acute cases. Many people with a history of mental illness may cope sufficiently well with their cancer but will benefit, like all patients, from sensitive, person-centred care. All people with cancer should be asked routinely about their mental health at initial assessment because understanding their history of mental illness is key to putting an effective care plan in place. People do not appear to take offence at this in the slightest, particularly if approached by the healthcare professional as a normal and natural part of the conversation. The patient's family can be involved in this conversation as appropriate.

Example questions to ascertain prior mental health history

- Have you ever had any problems with your mental health?
- How is your mental health now?
- How do you think that might affect your treatment? What can we do to help you with that?
- Are you under the care of a mental health service?
- Would it be okay if I contacted them to discuss how best to care for you? I'll let you know what we talked about and check that you are okay with what we decided.

What becomes clear is that the first three principles of best care are (1) sensitive and dexterous information gathering; (2) taking responsibility for effective communication; and (3) contributing proactively to effective teamwork. It is critically important for all members of the care team to take responsibility for these matters.

Principle 4 is taking responsibility for in-context learning. For example, learning about the Mental Capacity Act and its implications for care provision is imperative for all health and social care professionals because it provides a legal context for their work (Deacon, 2013b). Finding out a little more about different types of mental illness will enhance confidence in collaborative care. Moreover, work-based learning such as this will help the practitioner to meet their professional Continuing Professional Development (CPD) requirements.

The overarching fifth principle is person-centred care. Delivering this can be challenging within, but will prove to be the most efficient and effective type of care in the longer term. This, of course, is the same for all patients within the cancer care setting.

In this chapter, we have examined the evidence concerning the relationships between cancer and mental illness. From this, we have drawn out the implications of providing the best standard of care for such patients and have used practice-focused case studies to demonstrate these ideas in action. It is clear that the research evidence base in this field is quite limited and we have discussed why this might be the case. We like to envision a time when every person with SMI and cancer has as good a prognosis as anybody else, and when their experience of care leads the way in showing how caring for people with co-morbidity can and should be done.

Key learning points

- People who are severely mentally ill die earlier than the general population: cancer is implicated in this excess mortality.
- The severely mentally ill are socially disadvantaged, vulnerable and stigmatized. This contributes to them being at high risk of diagnosis and treatment overshadowing.

(Continued)

(Continued)

- Healthcare services tend to be fragmented. This has implications for the care of people with co-morbid health problems. Healthcare professionals are personally accountable for effective cross-boundary communication and teamwork.
- There are particular diagnostic and treatment challenges involved in the care of this group. Practitioners need to think beyond matters that they may normally take for granted, such as patients having particular social resources and accessing physical health services.
- Giving the best standard of care requires the healthcare team to factor in the mental health needs of the person requiring high quality cancer care: in short this means the provision of person-centred care.

Recommended further reading

- Collins, E., Drake, M. and Deacon, M. (eds) (2013) *The Physical Care of People with Mental Health Problems. A Guide for Best Practice.* London: Sage Publications.
- Department of Health (2005) *Mental Capacity Act 2005 Code of Practice.* (www.dh.gov.uk) Note: there are many supplementary guides about implementing this policy.
- Department of Health (2009) *Reference Guide to Consent for Examination or Treatment.* 2nd edn. (www.dh.gov.uk)
- Charities such as The Mental Health Foundation (www.mentalhealth.org.uk) and Mind (www.mind.org.uk) have also produced useful resources on this topic.

10 CANCER AND INTELLECTUAL DISABILITY

IRENE TUFFREY-WIJNE

Chapter outline

- What is intellectual disability?
- Cancer incidence and profile in this group
- Health inequalities
- Cancer prevention, screening and issues of late diagnosis
- Communication: understanding cancer and treatment decisions
- Coping with cancer for the patient and their family

INTRODUCTION

This chapter explores the issues for people with intellectual disabilities who have cancer, and people with intellectual disabilities who are affected by the cancer diagnosis of a relative. This was a previously hidden population, but with the closure of many long-stay hospitals, people with intellectual disabilities are now reliant on mainstream services to meet their health needs. This is an ageing population with a rising incidence of cancer.

People with intellectual disabilities form a significant minority group, but many general healthcare professionals are unfamiliar with this group of patients. They may be apprehensive about their ability to provide adequate treatment and care to a patient who may not be able to communicate in conventional ways.

This chapter is based on research evidence and the wider literature, and contextualizes key issues, including the current state of knowledge about health, cancer and intellectual disability. It addresses issues that are of relevance to the care of people with cancers who have intellectual disabilities, including communication, understanding and treatment decisions. When properly supported, many people with intellectual disabilities cope remarkably well with cancer and this chapter will provide strategies to harness their resilience. Many people with intellectual disabilities are affected by cancer because of the diagnosis of a relative or friend – their needs are also given attention.

WHAT IS INTELLECTUAL DISABILITY?

The definition of **intellectual disability** (also sometimes referred to as **learning disability** in the UK) includes three aspects, all of which must be present (Schalock et al., 2010):

1. Impaired intelligence
2. A reduced ability to cope independently, with significant limitation in their conceptual, social and practical skills
3. Starting in childhood, with a lasting effect on development.

An intellectual disability occurs when brain development is affected either before birth (e.g. maternal illness or genetic disorders, such as **Down syndrome** or **Fragile X syndrome**), during birth (e.g. oxygen deprivation) or in early childhood (e.g. childhood illness). Many people with intellectual disabilities also have other physical and emotional conditions, and some have complex multiple medical conditions. Examples of common associated medical conditions include **autism**, **epilepsy**, **cerebral palsy** and mental health conditions. It must be noted, however, that not all people with intellectual disabilities have these other conditions, and not all people with other conditions (such as cerebral palsy or autism) also have intellectual disabilities.

The following groups of people are among those *not* necessarily classified as having intellectual disabilities:

- People with dementia or people who sustained brain injuries in adulthood (their cognitive limitations did not start in childhood)
- People with **dyslexia**, or **Asperger's syndrome** (they may have average or above-average intelligence)

The term 'intellectual disabilities' covers a very wide range of people with a wide range of different needs. A distinction is often made between mild, moderate, severe and profound intellectual disabilities.

Mild and **moderate intellectual disabilities** are likely to result in learning difficulties in school and possible developmental delays in childhood. Most people can learn to develop some degree of independence, and will be able to live and work in the community with varying levels of support, and many will be able to maintain good social relationships. Most will acquire adequate communication skills. Not all people with mild or moderate intellectual disabilities will have a carer with them when they access cancer services; some may never have been diagnosed as having intellectual disabilities. People with mild intellectual disabilities present a particular challenge to cancer services because they may be difficult to identify within the population. Most are not known to any service providers.

Severe and **profound intellectual disabilities** are likely to result in continuous need for support, and possible severe limitations in self-care, continence and mobility. Communication skills will be severely limited. This group of people will depend on carers to access cancer services and communicate their needs.

Prevalence figures for intellectual disability vary markedly, depending on the different methodologies and population parameters used. The World Health Organization (WHO) estimates a prevalence between 1% and 3% of the population (WHO, 2001). Most of these have mild intellectual disabilities. The prevalence rate for moderate, severe and profound intellectual disabilities is 0.3%.

People with intellectual disabilities find it much more difficult to understand new or complex information, or to learn new skills. It is not difficult to see how this makes coping with cancer much harder because so much of the life changes implicit in a cancer diagnosis are complex and involve new, unfamiliar territory.

> ## Reflective activity
>
> - Have you ever encountered a patient or relative with intellectual disabilities?
> - How easy or difficult is it for you to know whether or not someone has intellectual disabilities?
> - Who could you ask for help if you are not sure about someone's intellectual disabilities?
> - Do you know how to find the intellectual disability professionals in your area?

CANCER INCIDENCE AND PROFILE

The population of people with intellectual disabilities is ageing. Better healthcare has led to reduced childhood mortality, and mortality patterns of those living into adulthood are now approaching those of the general population (Haveman et al., 2009).

A review of the state of knowledge around cancer and intellectual disabilities found a lack of firm evidence or figures around incidence and prevalence (Hogg and Tuffrey-Wijne, 2008). Methodological problems make comparisons with the general population difficult. Many studies have used institutional populations, whereas nowadays many people with intellectual disabilities live in the community and are exposed to a different range of cancer risk factors, such as smoking, poor nutrition and low levels of exercise.

Cancer incidence

Despite this lack of reliable data, some research evidence has been fairly consistent. Cancer is a major cause of death among people with intellectual disabilities, although the reported incidence of cancer deaths among this population is lower than that of the general population. In England and Wales, cancer is the most common cause of death (29% in 2012) (Office for National Statistics, 2013a). An in-depth investigation of the deaths of 247 people with intellectual disabilities found that heart and circulatory problems were the most common cause of death (22%), followed by cancer (20%). Cancer occurred at a much younger age than in the general population (median age of death: 55–59 years) (Heslop et al., 2013). Rates of cancer-related deaths among people with intellectual disabilities in previous studies include 16% in a population-based study in Finland (Patja et al., 2001), and 16% in a study of death certificates in London (Hollins et al., 1998).

Cancer profile

Some types of intellectual disability have a **chromosomal** or **genetic** cause, and it may be that this cause leads not only to intellectual disability but also to a predisposition to certain types of cancer. Patja et al. (2006) found that people with Down syndrome have a ten-fold increased risk of leukaemias, most clearly in childhood. Men with Down syndrome have a five-fold increase in risk of testicular cancer. There is a lower risk of solid tumours (Satgé and Vekemans, 2011). Breast cancer is rare among women with Down syndrome. It is worth noting that the incidence of breast cancer in all women with intellectual disabilities (not just those with Down syndrome) is less than half of that of the general population (Sullivan et al., 2003).

Lymphomas are more common among people with intellectual disabilities. Gastro-intestinal cancers account for over half of all cancer deaths in people with intellectual disabilities, as opposed to 25% in the general population (Cooke, 1997; Jancar 1990; Patja, Eero, and Iivanainen 2001). Possible reasons for this include high levels of **Helicobacter pylori** infection in institutionalized populations (Duff et al., 2001); chronic constipation among people with intellectual disabilities, as well as the ever-present possibility that symptoms may be over-looked until treatment is impossible (Hogg and Tuffrey-Wijne, 2008).

HEALTH INEQUALITIES

People with intellectual disabilities are at much higher risk than the general population of undiagnosed health problems, and are therefore at higher risk of dying from preventable causes. One study, which screened the health of 190 people with intellectual disabilities, found that over half had undiagnosed health problems and 9% of the study group had previously undiscovered serious morbidities (Baxter et al., 2006).

Since the 1990s, there have been reports in the literature that people with intellectual disabilities are more likely to die young than the general population. The UK Department of Health (2009b) quotes figures drawn from Hollins et al. (1998), estimating that people with intellectual disabilities are 58 times more likely to die prematurely than the population as a whole. The Health Service Ombudsman for England (Parliamentary and Health Service Ombudsman, 2009) highlighted distressing failures in the quality of health and social care, and found patients with intellectual disabilities were treated less favourably than others, resulting in prolonged suffering and inappropriate care. When relatives complained, they were left drained and demoralized and with a feeling of hopelessness. An Independent Inquiry into healthcare for people with intellectual disabilities (Michael, 2008) found that they 'appear to receive less effective care than they are enti-tled to receive. There is evidence of a significant level of avoidable suffering and a high likelihood that there are deaths occurring which could be avoided' (p. 53). An inquiry into premature deaths of people with intellectual disabilities in England found that 42% of deaths were premature, and that this was mostly due to failings of the healthcare system; conversely, premature deaths in comparator cases without intellectual disabilities were mostly due to lifestyle factors (Heslop et al., 2013).

Reasons for such avoidable deaths include:

- Failure to recognize pain
- Poor communication
- Diagnostic overshadowing (where the symptom or behaviour is attributed to the intellec-tual disability itself, rather than to the underlying health problem)
- Delays in treatment
- Lack of basic care
- Lack of 'reasonable adjustments' to help people with intellectual disabilities access healthcare services
- Poor staff understanding of the laws on mental capacity (Mencap, 2012; Heslop et al., 2013)

Some of these issues are explained further later.

One case example highlighted in Mencap's report is that of Emma, who died of cancer in 2004. She had a severe intellectual disability, which meant that she sometimes exhibited challenging behaviour and had difficulty in communicating how she felt. The hospital delayed treating her because they said she would not cooperate with treatment and therefore could not consent to treatment.

Emma

Emma's mother first took her to her GP because Emma had not eaten for eight days. While she was in hospital for investigations, Emma was distressed and in pain. She was not eating and couldn't take a painkiller orally. The hospital found Emma's behaviour very difficult to manage. Emma was discharged from the hospital on the grounds that there was nothing more they could do for her. She was sent home without any help to control her pain.

When Emma was eventually diagnosed with Lymphoma B1 type cancer, the family was told that, with treatment, she had a 50:50 chance of survival. But the doctors decided not to treat her, saying that she would not cooperate with the treatment. This included a lack of treatment for pain relief. Emma and her mother were sent home with no advice about Emma's care needs and still no way of dealing with her pain. Pain relief was only started following an action in the High Court.

A second medical opinion was sought and this doctor said that as the cancer had advanced, she now had only a 10% chance of survival with treatment. It was decided that palliative care was now the only course of action to take.

A few days later Emma was moved to a hospice where she received excellent care. She started drinking again and her pain was well controlled until she died. Emma was just 26 years old.

Source: Mencap (2007: 7).

It is unlikely that a 26-year-old woman without intellectual disabilities would have been sent home without treatment if she had presented with the same problems as Emma. In Emma's case, there was a lack of staff understanding and compliance with the laws on mental capacity. In England and Wales, the Mental Capacity Act (Department for Constitutional Affairs, 2005) states that if the patient is unable to consent to treatment, decisions need to be made in his or her best interest (see Mental capacity box). For Emma, there should have been a clear weighing up of the pros and cons of treatment – it seems that healthcare staff made assumptions about her ability to comply with treatment, rather than listening carefully to those who knew Emma well. In particular, it is hard to see how a lack of pain relief could be in Emma's best interest. It may be that staff unfamiliarity and lack of understanding of people with intellectual disabilities leads to fear and even avoidance of this group of patients (Tuffrey-Wijne et al., 2013).

Mental capacity

The Mental Capacity Act in England and Wales (Department for Constitutional Affairs, 2005) stipulates that neither professionals nor family or carers have the right to make healthcare decisions on behalf of an adult, if that person has the capacity to make the

(Continued)

treated. One study, which used focus groups of people with intellectual disabilities who had a relative or friend with cancer (most of whom had died of the disease), found that many had a rather black-and-white view of cancer. They thought that cancer inevitably leads to death. They wanted to know how people get cancer and were unsure whether or not you can catch it. They thought that doctors and nurses had the answer to everything, and found it hard to believe that outcomes could be uncertain (Tuffrey-Wijne et al., 2012).

In helping people cope with cancer, it is often best to stick to explanations of those things that will have an immediate effect on the person's life. Someone who needs to undergo a colectomy does not necessarily need to understand exactly what part of their intestines are being removed and why, but he does need to understand that he will wake up from the operation with a colostomy. Preparations, therefore, may involve looking at colostomy bags and a visit to the recovery room where he will wake up from the operation. How much of this you explain in one session, and when you explain it, will depend on the person's ability to understand complex information. Some people want to know well in advance what is going to happen, whereas others cope best if they are helped to understand changes as they occur.

TREATMENT DECISIONS

Far too often, decisions are made for people with intellectual disabilities without involving them or listening to their wishes. This includes treatment and non-treatment decisions. A study of 13 people with intellectual disabilities who had cancer found that healthcare professionals often rely on (family) carers to guide them in their decision-making (Tuffrey-Wijne, 2010). Whilst it is crucially important to listen to families and consider their views, it is also important to make sure that the family's preferences are based on what is best for the person, not on what is best for them, and also that assumptions about what the person can and cannot cope with are substantiated. It is easy to make assumptions about someone's ability to understand or cope.

Dimas

Dimas Ferreira was 47 and had profound learning disabilities. His understanding of abstract concepts was severely limited. He communicated with sounds rather than words. He lived in a residential care home. When Dimas was diagnosed with cancer of unknown origin that had spread to his lymph nodes, it was incurable, but the doctors proposed a course of radiotherapy treatment in order to prolong his life. His next of kin was his elderly aunt, Mrs Lopez, who had been visiting him for the past 14 years - before that, his grandmother used to visit. Mrs Lopez did not think Dimas should be put through the pain and distress of treatment. He greatly disliked hospitals and she didn't feel he would be able to understand. What was the point of prolonging his life and making him suffer? The doctors went along with her decision and sent Dimas back to his residential home. He died nine months later.

Source: Tuffrey-Wijne (2010: 70).

Reflective activity

- Dimas clearly lacked the capacity to make his own treatment decisions. Do you think it was right that his aunt took this decision for him? If yes, why? If no, why not?
- What information do you think you need to have in order to make the right treatment decision for Dimas?

Reflection: mental capacity

Dimas' case happened before the Mental Capacity Act became law in England (see earlier). Nowadays, his doctors should not simply follow Dimas's aunt's view. As in Emma's case, there should be a 'best interest' meeting involving those who cared for him on a daily basis, possibly an intellectual disability expert, as well as his family. They should consider carefully what the benefits and drawbacks of palliative radiotherapy might be for Dimas. How has he coped with hospitals and treatment in the past? What is important to him in his daily life? Would the advantages of the treatment (extended life and possible control of his symptoms) outweigh the disadvantages? Or would he simply be too distressed by the radiotherapy treatment? How could the radiotherapy be explained to him? Might there be a way in which he could cope with it, and lie still for long enough?

Sometimes tests or treatments that are in someone's best interest can only be endured with sedation. This is perfectly acceptable as long as there is a clear and documented rationale for it. In fact, it may be negligent to withhold treatment that is in someone's best interest simply because the patient has not consented to it or because there have been no 'reasonable adjustments' (which can include sedation) to help the patient cope.

It is possible that the decision not to give Dimas radiotherapy was the right decision; however, it was not made in the right way because the decision had not been carefully considered with the involvement of everyone involved in Dimas's life and care.

COPING WITH CANCER

Given the right levels of support, people with intellectual disabilities are no worse at coping with cancer than the general population (Tuffrey-Wijne, 2010). Such support may have to be extensive, particularly for people who find change difficult. Mostly, support will come from families, carers or the person's usual paid care staff. It is important to remember that these people are not skilled or experienced in coping with cancer. Most paid care staff, although professionals, are not used to giving physical care and don't know what to look out for. They should be given support and encouragement by general healthcare professionals, including GPs, district nurses, hospital nurses and specialist cancer professionals.

Dimas spent the final days of his life in hospital. His care home staff made a rota so that someone could be with him at all times; however, they felt very unsure and were upset about the fact that the hospital nurses often passed by Dimas's room. Similar problems of hospital staff expecting too much of carers were reported by carers in a study of the safety of patients with intellectual disabilities in acute hospitals (Tuffrey-Wijne et al., 2013).

It can be hard because we are not nurses, we are carers, but we are left to do the nursing with him. They don't always come into the room. I think they expect that they don't need to see to him, because we are here. But we are not nurses. (Tuffrey-Wijne, 2010: 145–146).

Resilience

A study of 13 people with intellectual disabilities who had cancer found that given the right levels of support, they could be remarkably resilient in the face of illness and declining health. The following aspects were identified that helped them to cope with their illness (Tuffrey-Wijne, 2010: 203):

- They were 'experienced sufferers' with a lifelong training in coping with adversity. Cancer seemed just one more misfortune in a long life of hardship.
- They were skilled at 'taking each day as it comes'. Those with more severe intellectual disabilities were particularly good at living in the present moment.
- People with intellectual disabilities were realistic about their immediate future. For example, they understood the need to go into a nursing home when they were unable to look after themselves. Most people coped best with realistic short-term goals.
- Terminal illness often means a loss of independence. All the people with intellectual disabilities, including those who had gained a degree of independence, already had extensive experience of being helped and cared for.
- Being a person with cancer meant that people were identified as part of a group of 'people with cancer' (which consisted of people in the general population) rather than just as 'people with intellectual disabilities'. This could be empowering for some.
- The presence of one or two trusted, loving carers or relatives was important in harnessing people's resilience.
- People with intellectual disabilities wanted to 'keep going' with routines and familiar activities, right up to their final days. They coped best if they were enabled to hold on to their routines and activities.

Family members with intellectual disabilities

Even cancer professionals who have never had a patient with intellectual disabilities will usually have had patients who have had a son, daughter, sibling, partner or other relative or friend with intellectual disabilities. A study of the needs of these relatives or friends had a number of striking findings (Tuffrey-Wijne et al., 2012).

- Those who had not been told about the patient's illness felt excluded. Being told that someone had cancer did not necessarily mean that the person with intellectual disabilities understood the implications.
- People with intellectual disabilities had vivid memories of events and feelings, even many years later. They worried about their families and felt protective towards them. Several had become carers themselves, but their caring role had not been recognized or supported.
- People with intellectual disabilities lacked knowledge about cancer and wanted to know more. Many worried that they themselves would get cancer.
- The people in the study would have liked to share their feelings and questions with family, friends or professionals, but most had not done so. Many felt unable to ask their family

for support because they were acutely aware of their relatives' distress. They did not know what support could be offered by cancer professionals (including nurses) and would not ask them any questions.

The people with intellectual disabilities who took part in the study suggested the following helpful support strategies, and ranked them in order of importance as follows:

1. Someone to talk to about my feelings and worries
2. Someone to support the rest of the family
3. My family, carers and doctor should tell me everything
4. Someone I can ask questions about cancer
5. A support worker to be with me
6. Other people with intellectual disabilities to talk together about our experiences
7. Easy words and pictures to explain cancer
8. Photos of the ill person to help me think and talk about them
9. Someone to help look after the ill person.

Breaking bad news and communicating with people with intellectual disabilities about illness and death can be extremely challenging. The publication of a new model and guidelines for breaking bad news to people with intellectual disabilities may help in supporting this (Tuffrey-Wijne, 2013).

CONCLUSION

Cancer professionals are usually highly trained, and this includes training in communication skills. Caring for a very wide and diverse range of patients and relatives will have given them the skills to provide truly patient-centred care. Supporting patients and relatives who have intellectual disabilities should therefore not be outside their capabilities. Some additional knowledge and skill may be needed, particularly around issues of capacity and communication. Most important, however, is a willingness to engage with the patient, whatever his or her level of understanding, way of communicating or coping strategies. This involves engagement with the family and other carers, who will know a lot about the person and about intellectual disabilities, but probably not very much about cancer. Together with the cancer expertise from all relevant professionals, it is possible to provide excellent, sensitive and patient-centred care. Like all other patients, people with intellectual disabilities deserve nothing less.

CHAPTER SUMMARY

- Avoidable deaths are more common in people with an intellectual disability as a result of failings in the healthcare system, such as poor communication, diagnostic overshadowing and lack of basic care.
- Although the reported incidence of cancer deaths among people with an intellectual disability is lower than that of the general population, cancer is a major cause of death.
- People with an intellectual disability may have a late diagnosis of cancer for a variety of reasons including lack of adequate cancer screening, inaction in addressing complaints of symptoms and misinterpretation of behavioural changes resulting from pain or discomfort.

- People with intellectual disabilities are often reliant on others to help them access cancer screening, recognize symptoms and receive prompt medical attention.
- Carers do not always know enough about cancer and cancer risk to support their relatives/clients.
- Reasonable adjustments may be required within healthcare services to improve the patient experience. Tools are available to help carers and professionals pick up early signs of illness and ensure that people with intellectual disabilities receive adequate and timely interventions.
- Communication should be tailored for each individual, including the use of simple language and checking understanding. The person with an intellectual disability should be involved in decision-making whenever possible.
- Given the right levels of support, people with intellectual disabilities are no worse at coping with cancer than the general population

Recommended further reading

- Tuffrey-Wijne, I. (2010) *Living with Learning Disabilities, Dying with Cancer: Thirteen Personal Stories*. London: Jessica Kingsley Publishers.
- Tuffrey-Wijne, I. (2012) *How to Break Bad News to People with Intellectual Disabilities: A Guide for Carers and Professionals*. London: Jessica Kingsley Publishers.
- Satgé, D. and Merrick, J. (eds) (2011) *Cancer in Children and Adults with Intellectual Disabilities: Current Research Aspects*. New York, NY: Nova Science Publishers.

Useful websites

- The *Books Beyond Words* series tells stories in pictures rather than words (www.booksbeyondwords.co.uk).
- The Disability Distress Assessment Tool (DisDAT) (www.disdat.co.uk).
- The Anticipatory Care Calendar is a simple tool for social care staff to improve the daily surveillance of health for adults with intellectual disabilities and dementia (www.anticipatorycarecalendar.org).
- This website (www.intellectualdisability.info/) is about intellectual disability and health. It is an ideal learning resource for medical, nursing and other healthcare students, and contains valuable information for anyone working in healthcare services.
- This website (www.easyhealth.org.uk/) brings together a wide range of accessible health resources for people with intellectual disabilities, including a wealth of cancer related leaflets. Many are downloadable.
- The Palliative Care for People with Intellectual Disabilities Network website (www.pcpld.org) contains a useful resources page.
- This website (www.breakingbadnews.org) has guidelines and practical tips for breaking bad news to people with intellectual disabilities.

11 SURGERY

GEORGE FOSTER, TINA LIGHTFOOT AND DALE VIMALACHANDRAN

Chapter outline

- Introduction
- The role of surgery in the treatment of cancer
- Factors influencing the decision to operate
- The principles of oncological surgery
- Risks of surgery
- Decision-making in cancer surgery
- Support for people undergoing surgery for cancer
- Beyond surgery

INTRODUCTION

Over the last thirty years, there have been significant improvements in the surgical treatment of cancer, ranging from detection, staging and surgical technique through to **adjuvant treatment** and follow-up. Surgery is **evidence-based** with underpinning principles advocated by national bodies such as NICE and speciality associations. Surgical **resection** for cancer is generally (but not exclusively) employed for **solid organ cancers** (i.e. skin, breast, lung, gastrointestinal, gynaecological, prostate, pancreas, renal, thyroid and selected bony and neurological tumours). There is also an increasingly transparent approach to data management and accessibility within the NHS, and this recent change brings about further, previously unseen issues for patients and clinicians alike, for example patients can now access information about their surgeon's mortality rate before they perform major surgery (Yi et al., 2013). Clearly, the data available are only as good as the data that have been inputted, but in the modern era of cancer surgery this may add to the psychological burden of a patient who is already swamped with information and decisions (Ganai, 2014).

This chapter will outline the principles of surgical resection for these tumours because other cancers, such as those of the haematopoietic system, are usually treated medically. Important issues in **decision-making** and consequences of surgical resection will also be covered. Given the variety of organs involved and the increasing complexity of treatment algorithms, underlying principles will be illustrated using specific examples.

THE ROLE OF SURGERY IN THE TREATMENT OF CANCER

Surgery for cancer has been in existence for many centuries, but the first cancer operation using anaesthesia was thought to have been undertaken in the nineteenth century (Cancer Research UK, 2014v). Pioneer surgeons realized that resection offered the only hope of cure, although in this era the intent was often palliation from symptoms of the primary tumour. Modern cancer surgery has a number of intentions: (1) removal of primary tumour and its draining lymphatic basin; (2) accurate pathological assessment and hence staging of the disease; and ultimately (3) prevention of disease recurrence (may be local or systemic).

Different solid organs present different challenges to clinical teams with respect to the diagnosis, surgical treatment options and psychological consequences of such resections. For example, diagnosis of pancreatic cancer can be extremely difficult due to symptoms appearing at a late stage and in a variable manner. In addition, the **retroperitoneal** location of the pancreas renders it easily visualized only with cross-sectional imaging such as **computerized tomography** (CT) (Soriano et al., 2004). Consequently, the disease very often presents at a late stage, making any possible surgical resection extremely complex with poor long-term patient outcomes (Koh et al., 2014). Conversely, other tumours, for example those of the thyroid gland and testes, present at an early stage due to their **subcutaneous** situation, making surgical resection generally more straightforward. This often leads to better long-term patient outcomes (Lang et al., 2007; Yoshida et al., 2009). Breast cancer and pelvic cancers, such as those of the rectum and anus, offer a variety of complex surgical approaches, but, importantly, are most often associated with significant patient **morbidity** due to body image consequences and resultant functional deficits following surgical procedures (Mols et al., 2014; Montazeri, 2008).

Surgical resection is underpinned by increasingly accurate preoperative staging techniques. This has led to (1) a decrease in the resection of some cancers (e.g. oesophageal) as a result of the improved ability to detect advanced disease (Torrance et al., 2013); and (2) expansion in the number of surgical techniques employed, often with the intent of organ preservation to reduce the psychological and/or functional sequelae of such major surgery. For example, breast cancer was historically treated with major resection of the breast, chest wall and **axillary lymphatics** but can now be treated with a combination of **breast conservation** and **reconstruction**, with selective sampling of involved (**sentinel**) **lymph nodes** determining the need for further **axillary surgery** (Galimberti et al., 2013). More recently, there is growing interest in organ preservation of early rectal cancers and the avoidance of a **permanent stoma** with advances in **minimally invasive** rectal cancer surgery and **endoluminal radiotherapy** (Neary et al., 2003; Myint, 2013).

Laparoscopic minimally invasive surgery (otherwise known as minimal access surgery or keyhole surgery) has been in regular use by gynaecologists since the 1980s for the removal of ovarian and some endometrial cancers. Keyhole surgery first came into use in general surgery in 1990 for the removal of the gall bladder. Laparoscopic techniques have significant advantages due to the reduction in the size of the surgical access wound and subsequent reduction in post-operative pain. This results in quicker ambulation and a lower complication rate. These techniques are now routinely employed in colorectal cancer surgery, after a number of trials demonstrated equivalence to open surgery (Colon Cancer Laparoscopic or Open Resection Study Group et al., 2009; Green et al., 2013). Currently, minimally invasive surgery is employed in approximately 40% of all colorectal cancer resections. In addition to the short-term benefits,

there is also the important potential that with an accelerated recovery compared to open surgery, patients are, where necessary, fitter for earlier adjuvant therapy (Poylin et al., 2014), which has recently been shown to be associated with improved survival (Des Guetz et al., 2010).

Minimally invasive techniques are also used in liver, renal, prostate and pulmonary surgery with similar benefits. Keyhole techniques have also been described in superficial surgery such as breast and thyroid, although the benefits in these patients are less clear. This type of surgery can be technically demanding for the surgeon, particularly in the narrow confines of areas such as the pelvis, where the limitations of rigid hinged instruments cannot match those of fingers. However, **robotic surgery** can match and supersede this, and in some centres, **radical prostatectomy** (Health Quality Ontario, 2010) is regularly performed by robotic techniques. The current costs of robotic surgery are, however, so high as to limit their use to only the wealthiest healthcare systems.

Surgery may be used alone or in combination with other modalities, such as cytotoxic chemotherapy and/or radiotherapy to treat cancers (see Chapters 12 and 13 for discussions of these treatments). For many cancers, such as breast, colon and pancreas, surgery is only the first stage of cancer treatment. Following accurate pathological staging, for example, many patients will receive adjuvant chemotherapy (chemotherapy *following* surgery) to reduce the levels of circulating **micrometastatic tumour cells** (Eguchi et al., 2008). Micrometastases are cancer cells that have spread to other parts of the body but which cannot be detected by usual screening or diagnostic tests.

Other treatments can also be given prior to surgery (**neoadjuvant therapy**). Neoadjuvant treatment, for example, is given for many gastric and oesophageal cancers (Moorcraft et al., 2014) and is the focus of new clinical trials in colon and rectal cancers (FOxTROT Collaborative Group, 2012; Glynne-Jones et al., 2014). Neoadjuvant radiotherapy may be used for cancers of the rectum, which on initial presentation are not resectable with a clear **margin** (Glynne-Jones et al., 2014). Radiotherapy is, however, not without its risks, with short-term **toxicities** that may affect the surgical procedure and long-term risks to cardiovascular systems.

Surgery also plays an increasing role in the management of advanced and/or metastatic disease where it may be **palliative** (for example, in the case of advanced obstructing colon cancer or fungating breast tumours) or **potentially curative** when liver or lung metastases are resected.

FACTORS INFLUENCING THE DECISION TO OPERATE

An operation, in its purest sense, is a legal form of assault (battery) on an individual: the decision taken to operate is, therefore, not to be taken lightly and must demonstrate positive benefit to the patient. Any health professional who deals with a patient with cancer must constantly bear in mind the principles of **beneficence** (an action that is done for the benefit of others) and **non-maleficence** (to do no harm). In the past, this decision was often taken by a single person (the surgeon); however, this meant that crucial decisions were often made on the basis of personal experience rather than evidence base or consensus.

Today, most decisions on operative strategy involve a **multidisciplinary team** (MDT) including the surgeon, oncologist, radiologist, specialist nurse, the patient and their family. NICE, for example has published quality standards related to the diagnosis and management

Early disease

Whilst surgery for early disease has long been established for some cancers (e.g. certain skin cancers), it is relatively new to others (e.g. rectal cancer). For early disease, the patient may simply require a **limited resection** with a margin of healthy tissue, which results in fewer functional or cosmetic defects if performed expertly.

The real development has come in those tumours where minimally invasive and/or radio-therapy approaches offer the chance to preserve the entire cancer-bearing area and avoid consequences of major resection, such as a stoma. It must be stressed, however, that in the case of rectal cancer, many of these treatments can only be offered within the context of a clinical trial before becoming adopted into mainstream practice. For other cancers, such early disease has the opportunity to allow the surgeon to tailor the surgery to the least invasive options, such as laparoscopic surgery for early colon cancer, or to offer immediate reconstruction in early breast cancers.

Incurable disease

For some cancers, such as those of the pancreas and oesophagus, patients more frequently present with incurable disease. Whilst surgery cannot cure the disease, it is often employed to palliate the symptoms. Formal surgical procedures to bypass an obstructed duodenum, bile duct or colon, for example, are still used, but such surgery is still a major undertaking in patients who have other complex co-morbidities, such as **cachexia** and malnourishment. Developments in the field of **endoluminal stenting** have enabled an obstructed lumen to be dilated and kept open by the passage of a self-expanding metallic stent, thereby avoiding a formal open surgical procedure. Formal palliative surgery may still be required in the event that luminal stenting is not possible or for debulking of tumours such as those of ovarian origin (Greimel et al., 2013).

PRINCIPLES OF ONCOLOGICAL SURGERY

The surgical approach for each solid cancer is unique by virtue of its organ of origin, anatomical location, physiological function and the behaviour of the cancer; however, the principles underlying surgical resection of solid cancers are similar. All cancer surgery requires the following:

1. Accurate diagnosis, assessment and staging of the disease
2. Careful preoperative assessment of fitness for surgery
3. Fully informed and valid consent in a timely fashion
4. Meticulous surgical resection respecting anatomical tissue planes, lymphatic drainage, blood supply and surrounding tissues, and incorporating where necessary reconstruction
5. Careful perioperative management
6. Accurate pathological assessment examining not only stage of tumour to prognosticate but also assessing quality of surgery
7. Reliable follow-up.

Although these key components underlie all oncology surgery, some will have a greater relevance for certain cancers. Broadly speaking, surgery for cancer can be divided into procedures entering a body cavity (abdomen, pelvis, thorax, cranium); operations on superficial structures (skin, testicular); and intermediate operations (thyroid, breast). Surgery that enters a body cavity is inevitably more complex, with a higher risk of complications from the stress of the surgical access and the problems that may result from the loss of the organs removed. In these cases, it is imperative that the patient is fully assessed to determine whether they can undergo rigorous and often lengthy surgery. This may include more formal physiological assessment such as **cardiopulmonary exercise testing** (CPET) in the preoperative assessment of many patients with gastrointestinal cancer who are often elderly (Moyes et al., 2013; Junejo et al., 2014; West et al., 2014), or nutritional assessment to identify which patients require preoperative nutritional support.

Having established that a patient is fit enough to undergo surgery, the patient must be consented for the procedure. Obtaining fully informed consent is a process rather than a single event (Anderson and Wearne, 2007). Information regarding consent is often given at multiple intervals and in different formats, for example information sheets, CDs and web-based advice, which ensures that the patient and their family have plenty of opportunity to ask questions and obtain clarification. Risks and complications are discussed, but many units now provide prewritten consent forms with all the common complications and their incidence rates included.

Whilst the clinical and MDT decision may be to operate, the final decision will always lie with the patient. The **clinical nurse specialist** plays a pivotal role in helping the patient and their family assimilate the information given and come to a decision regarding surgery. Many cancer operations are complex procedures and it is important that patients fully understand the short-term immediate risks and the longer term, often more functional risks or side effects. Importantly, for some cancers, these long-term side effects may have a greater role in affecting the quality of life of the patient than the initial cancer diagnosis itself.

Whichever surgical approach is employed, structures should be mobilized and removed by dissecting in the appropriate **embryological** and **anatomical plane**. This ensures that the operative field is as bloodless as possible, and that anatomical tissue planes are not breached, compromising oncological quality. There is increasing recognition that, for many cancers, adherence to this **oncological plane** is critical and is strongly associated with long-term outcomes (Søndenaa et al., 2014). For some cancers, however, such as breast, liver, and cranium, such embryological planes do not exist and surgery is performed within anatomical planes with the intention of preserving function in the residual organ that remains. In order to achieve this, careful and meticulous pre- and perioperative imaging is used to either determine functional capacity of the residual liver in the case of liver surgery, or to ensure that critical nearby structures remain unharmed in the case of stereotactic neurosurgery. For some organs, such as the thyroid, ovary or testicle, limited resections for cancer are not possible and the whole organ(s) needs to be removed. In the case of a total thyroidectomy, great care is needed to preserve nerves to the laryngeal muscles and the important parathyroid glands. For some cancers (colon and breast) surgical resection of the involved organ together with its lymphatic drainage is mandatory.

For other cancers, reconstruction is also required to restore continuity of a **luminal organ** (e.g. gastrointestinal tract) or to correct the **deformity** caused by surgery (breast, limb, head and neck). A variety of techniques may be employed to restore gastrointestinal continuity (**anastomosis**); however, the principles underlying the techniques are similar: tension-free anastomosis, good blood supply and absence of adjacent inflammation. For gastrointestinal surgeons, one of the most dreaded complications of cancer surgery is failure of this anastomosis. Reconstruction to restore deformity can be broadly divided into tissue implants, such as those used in breast surgery, and **native tissue flaps** used in breast and head and neck cancers. Such tissue flaps are moved from one part of the body to restore the defect left by surgical resection or, in the case of breast surgery, to cosmetically simulate breast tissue. Such flaps may be moved to a nearby area whilst leaving the tissue attached to its native blood supply (**pedicled flap**) or may be fully removed to a distant site (**free flap**). These flaps require delicate microsurgical anastomoses of tiny blood vessels, failure of which leads to the devastating complication of flap failure.

For many patients, the greatest risk of their cancer surgery lies not on the operating table but in the immediate post-operative period – this is the critical time when serious physical complications are most likely. Whilst those complications related directly to the surgical procedure cannot be altered, close observation and early detection of an impending complication can prevent a rapid irreversible deterioration following surgery for cancer.

Surgical nurses should be aware of potential complications and times that they are likely to occur in order to identify those patients whose clinical state moves outside the expected recovery envelope. Complications, particularly in the context of body cavity surgery, may relate to both the stress of the surgical insult and the resulting associated impairment (e.g. gastrointestinal and respiratory function).

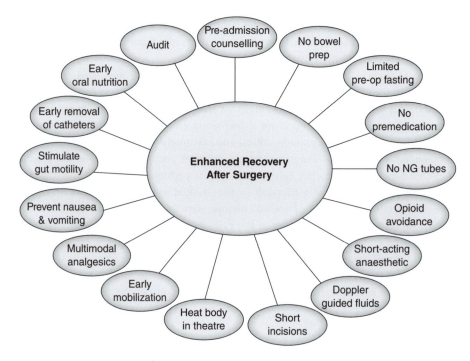

Figure 11.1   Key components of an enhanced recovery programme in colorectal surgery

Source: Adapted from Fearon et al. (2005).

Henrik Kehlet from Denmark has for many years worked in the area of **pre-emptive analgesia** (pain relief before a painful stimulus) and **enhanced recovery** (Kehlet and Wilmore, 2008), such that today these programmes are now part of standard care in many cancer units throughout the UK (Hjort Jakobsen et al., 2014; Lee et al., 2014). Enhanced recovery incorporates a number of elements from the point of diagnosis through to the immediate post-operative period (Ljungqvist, 2014). These elements prepare the patient psychologically for surgery, as well as to physiologically attenuate the stress response to surgery via specific mechanisms. The diagram below illustrates the key components of an enhanced recovery programme in colorectal surgery.

Following surgical resection, the resected specimen is immediately placed in fixative and transferred to the pathology laboratory for assessment (see Chapter 5). In some cancers, such as breast and small rectal cancers, the specimen is marked and orientated to ensure that if a resection margin is involved microscopically with cancer it is easy to identify. Pathological assessment examines both the quality of the surgery and provides very important prognostic information, such as TNM staging (refer to Chapter 5). In the context of surgical resection, it is critical that the pathologist determines whether or not cancer has been left behind at either a macroscopic or microscopic level. If this is the case, for many tumours the likelihood of recurrent disease is extremely high and there is rarely a second chance to go back and remove more tissue. In these cases, reliance will be placed on adjuvant therapies such as radiotherapy.

THE RISKS OF SURGERY

The potential risks of surgery can be classified in a number of ways. Complications are most often classified into either general complications or those specific to a particular procedure. They may also be classified on a temporal basis as immediate (within 24 hours), early (first week) or late (weeks to months). Late complications generally relate to specific procedures, but in the long term, may cause the biggest detriment to quality of life once the initial risks have passed. This classification helps clinicians to discuss issues of consent with patients and their families, and for patients and families to understand what can often be very significant, even life-threatening complications.

Immediate complications

Immediate complications generally relate to major bleeding or problems with the cardiorespiratory systems. The risk of bleeding may be greater for a number of reasons, including:

- Location of tumour in an anatomically inaccessible location (e.g. thorax or pelvis)
- Effects of previous surgery or neoadjuvant therapies (e.g. adhesions or radiotherapy)
- Bleeding diathesis (e.g. warfarin or antiplatelet therapy)
- A greater inherent risk of bleeding with certain procedures such as liver resection; however, modern anaesthetic and surgical techniques have now ensured that major liver resection is associated with very low mortality rates (Simillis et al., 2014; Dunne et al., 2014).

Cardiorespiratory complications most often occur in patients with pre-existing disease, although some types of procedure or surgery (e.g. thoracic) may be associated with higher rates.

debilitating and disfiguring surgery with the patient and their family (as applicable to each patients' own situation). It cannot be assumed that an individual wishes to be cured of cancer at any price. Neither can the healthcare professionals categorize such patients according to age, gender or social circumstance. This is a purely individual experience and time must be given for the patient to consider what lies ahead in order for them to make an informed decision.

Preoperative assessment is important in order to explore what the patient understands and how they feel about their diagnosis, proposed treatment and its implications. The period from diagnosis to surgery is very short, during which time the patient has not only to contend with the psychological impact of their cancer diagnosis, but also with a plethora of information about their treatment and potential side effects. The cancer specialist nurse should, where possible, be involved from diagnosis through to the pre- and post-operative phases in order to provide a consistent support for the patient (and their family) with their different needs at different points in time. Assessment should identify patients' specific needs, problems and potential problems so that a post-operative care plan can be developed jointly with the patient, which also includes discharge planning and referral to other members of the multiprofessional team where appropriate.

HOLISTIC NEEDS ASSESSMENT

There are specific challenges when considering the needs of patients undergoing surgery with either curative or palliative intent. Adopting an **Holistic Needs Assessment** (HNA), the first guidance for which was published in 2007 by the National Cancer Action Team (2007) and complemented by National Cancer Action Team in 2013, ensures a consistent approach to assessing patients' physical, psychological, social and spiritual issues, which then informs a care plan in partnership with the patient. Patient's needs cannot be compartmentalized, however, because there is so much overlap with one issue or concern influencing another. For this reason, it is better to describe a patient as having holistic needs. A fundamental role of the cancer specialist nurse is to be aware of all the patient's concerns whether they are:

1. Physical, such as problems with pain control or difficulty with natural functions (e.g. bowel or bladder control);
2. Psychological, such as difficulty adjusting to the diagnosis (see also Chapter 18);
3. Social, such as financial concerns if employment is threatened; and
4. Spiritual, such as fear of dying, no chance to make amends (see also Chapter 27).

It is also important to understand how one concern may influence or impact on another, and that assessment should be an ongoing and dynamic process.

Reflective activity

- What concerns may a patient admitted to a ward for surgical treatment of their cancer have about their operation, post-operative recovery and long-term future?
- Why is it important for the surgical nurse to be aware of these concerns?

A patient admitted for surgery will not only have concerns about their imminent surgery, but also fears regarding its outcome. For them, this might be a matter of life or death, and for this reason, the nurse may find some patients more anxious than others or possibly more withdrawn. It takes time to adjust to a life crisis and, therefore, a patient arriving on the ward will not only have received a cancer diagnosis in the preceding weeks, but will also have undergone staging investigations with all the fear and hope that those involve. The surgery will have been explained to them along with the risks, the implications and the possibility of success. By this point, few have had a chance to fully psychologically adjust to all that has happened and the nurse receiving the patient on the ward must be prepared to meet someone whose life is in turmoil.

The time a patient spends in hospital undergoing and recovering from surgery is extremely short when compared to the time they will spend visiting the hospital for appointments, investigations and ongoing treatments. Although short, for most patients this is an important part of their treatment pathway because the surgery may represent the only hope of a cure for their cancer. A surgical ward nurse must be able to demonstrate empathetic understanding for the patient's situation and must be knowledgeable with regard to the patient's diagnosis and their treatment plan. Similarly, there must be engagement with the patient's carers or family who will also be individually affected (see Chapter 20) because they also play an important role in the adjustment of the patient (see Chapter 18). Sensitive communication skills will help to elicit a patient's concerns and enable information to be tailored to individual need regardless of age, gender, ethnicity, sexuality or disability (see also Chapter 17).

BEYOND SURGERY: LIVING WITH THE CONSEQUENCES OF SURGERY FOR ANY CANCER

Surgery is physically traumatic and there are often long-term consequences for the patient. Long after the cancer has been removed and the patient has been cured, the consequences of their diagnosis and treatment, such as a change in appearance or loss of function (see also Chapter 21), remain with them as a daily reminder that they once had cancer.

Examples of change to appearance (body image) may include:

- Amputation of limb
- Facial disfiguration
- Wide excision of skin lesion with grafting
- Faecal/urinary stoma

Examples of loss of function may include:

- Loss of speech
- Sexual dysfunction
- Urinary dysfunction
- Bowel dysfunction
- Mobility

HOW DOES CHEMOTHERAPY WORK?

The aim of chemotherapy is to kill cells by interfering with cell replication through a variety of mechanisms (Gabriel, 2007). One of the limitations of cytotoxic chemotherapy, however, is that it cannot distinguish between normal and malignant cells. Normal cells are inevitably destroyed during treatment and it is for this reason that some patients experience side effects such as **neutropenia**, nausea and vomiting, **stomatitis** and **alopecia**.

Normal cell division

Understanding normal cell division and the cell cycle is key to understanding the approach to treating cancer with chemotherapy.

Figure 12.1 shows how one cell divides to become two, a process which is replicated throughout the billions of cells in the body. The time it takes each cell to divide varies depending on the cell function, for example cells in the gastrointestinal tract (GIT) replicate much more frequently than bone cells. Rapidly dividing cells are most sensitive to chemotherapy and are, therefore, also the site of many side effects. The normal process of cell division is often referred to as the cell cycle and can be seen in Figure 4.3, earlier on in this book.

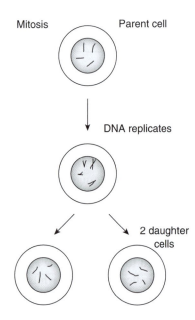

Figure 12.1   Cell division

Source: US National Library of Medicine

The cell cycle

Cells that are not dividing are said to be in G0 phase and will be resistant to chemotherapy. The first stage of cell reproduction is G1 when the cell enters a growth phase, which lasts for a varying length of time in different tissues. After G1, the cells move into the phase of DNA synthesis, the S phase, in which the amount of chromosomal material is doubled. The cell then passes through a pre-mitotic or pre-division phase, G2, and then into mitosis, M, in which the pairs of chromosomes separate and the cell divides (Lennan, 2011).

The rate of cell division both in normal cells and in human tumours varies considerably from one anatomical site or cancer type to another. The speed at which tumour cells grow also varies depending on the original cell type, and although proliferation in a normal cell remains controlled and regulated, tumour cell proliferation becomes uncontrollable and deregulated (for further detail on the cell cycle and the properties of cancer, see Chapter 4).

Reflective activity

- List parts of the body where normal cells divide rapidly.
- Now make a list of side effects that patients may experience as a result of cytotoxic chemotherapy.
- How would you explain the relationship between the two lists?

CLASSIFICATION OF CYTOTOXIC DRUGS

Knowledge of cell division and the cell cycle promotes understanding of how each cytotoxic drug works to kill cells and treat tumours. There are several ways to classify cytotoxic drugs, but the one most frequently used is the biochemical classification, which also outlines the major modes of action (see Table 12.1).

Table 12.1 Classification of anticancer drugs

Drug name	Mechanism of action	Cell phase specific	Uses in practice
Alkalating agents			
Cyclophophamide	Breaks the DNA strands		Breast, gynae, lymphoma
Carmustine	Cross-links DNA, preventing replication		Brain, lymphoma
Temozolomide			Brain
Treosulfan	Cross-links DNA, preventing replication		Ovary
Ifosphamide	Damages DNA, thus interfering with cell replication		Sarcoma, testes, lymphoma
Vinca alkaloids			
Vincristine	Inhibits assembly of equipment for replication	M phase	Lymphoma, leukaemia, lung, sarcoma
Vindesine	Inhibits assembly of equipment for replication	M phase	Breast, melanoma

(Continued)

Table 12.1 (Continued)

Drug name	Mechanism of action	Cell phase specific	Uses in practice
Vinerelbine	Inhibits assembly of equipment for replication	M phase	Breast, lung
Platinum			
Carboplatin	Cross-links DNA, preventing replication		Ovary, lung
Cisplatin	Cross-links DNA, preventing replication		Bladder, testes, ovarian, lung, cervix
Oxaliplatin	Cross-links DNA, preventing replication		Colorectal, pancreas
Taxanes			
Paclitaxel	Promotes equipment assembly, and then prevents de-assembly		Ovary, breast
Docetaxel	Promotes equipment assembly, and then prevents de-assembly specifically G2 phase	G2 phase, M phase	Breast, lung, prostate
Antibiotics			
Epirubicin	Intercalates DNA/RNA, causing free radicals – cell bursts		
Mitomycin C	Binds to DNA, inhibits DNA synthesis and function		Breast, bladder, colorectal, ovarian, sarcoma
Mitoxatrone	Causes DNA cross-linking, resulting in strand breaks		Breast, leukaemia
Doxorubicin	Intercalates DNA/RNA, causing free radicals – cell bursts		Leukaemia, breast, lymphoma, sarcoma
Antimetabolites			
Methotrexate	Inhibits synthesis of ribonucleosides	S phase	Breast, lymphoma
5Fluorouracil	Prevents DNA synthesis	S phase	GI tract, breast, head and neck
Gemcitabine	Prevents DNA synthesis by replacing one of the building blocks of nucleic acids	S phase, G1 phase	Pancreas, lung, breast, bilary tract
Cytarabine	Acts by interfering with pyrimidine synthesis	S phase	Leukaemias
Topoisomerase inhibitors			
Irinotecan	Inhibits topisonomerase1	S phase	Colorectal
Topetecan	Inhibits topisonomerase1	S phase	Colorectal, ovary

Drug name	Mechanism of action	Cell phase specific	Uses in practice
	Miscellaneous		
Etoposide	Inhibits topisonomerasell	S phase, G2 phase	Lymphoma, lung
Erubilin	Inhibits growth of microtubles	G2 phase, M phase	Breast

Source: British National Formulary, 2012.

Combination chemotherapy

Combination chemotherapy refers to treatment that involves a combination of two or more different cytotoxic drugs. Chemotherapy may be cell-specific (toxic to the cell as a whole) or phase-specific (damaging cells whenever they are in a particular phase of the cell cycle) (see Table 12.1). Prescribing a combination of drugs promotes greater cell kill than using one alone. This happens for two reasons. First, because different drugs act on cells that are in different phases of the cell cycle: each time a cell passes through a particular phase of the cell cycle, it will be damaged by the drug acting on that phase of the cycle. A combination of drugs, therefore, may be prescribed to damage cells in G1, S and M to achieve greater cell death and also to reduce the risk of drug resistance. Drugs may also be synergistic, interacting with each other to produce increased activity, which is greater than the effect achieved by giving the same drugs separately. Second, a combination of drugs with different cell toxicity can be given to a maximum tolerated dose without causing unacceptable or irreversible toxicity.

SCHEDULING OF CHEMOTHERAPY TREATMENTS

Chemotherapy is not a one-off event and usually involves a course of treatment. The length of the course and schedule is determined though clinical trials. Different drugs have different schedules and durations of treatment. Irrespective of the specifics of treatment, each treatment is known as a cycle and several cycles make up a regimen or course. Prescribing cycles of chemotherapy in pulses over a period of time maximizes cancer cell death whilst allowing normal cells to recover between cycles (see Figure 12.3). The interval between treatments is very important: too short an interval and normal cells do not have sufficient time to recover and repair; too long an interval and cancer cells have more time to replicate and the tumour may grow. The exact interval between treatments or cycles varies depending on the drug combination, as does the duration of treatment or course.

A **maximum tolerated dose** is given at each cycle, which results in the death of a proportion of cancer cells. An interval, such as three or four weeks, is required to allow normal cells that have been inadvertently killed, time to recover between cycles: tumour cells are unable to recover at the same rate. Figure 12.2 illustrates how at Treatment 1, the number of both normal and cancer cells decreases, but that by Treatment 2, the normal cells have recovered, and the cancer cells have recovered at a reduced rate. If this process is repeated with further cycles, normal cells continue to recover, but the pattern of tumour cell death continues until the course of chemotherapy has been completed.

When therapy is successful, cancer cell killing is greater than cell regrowth. Drugs should, therefore, be scheduled in such a way as to produce maximum killing. This will depend on the rate of recovery of the normal tissues that have been most damaged by the drug. These sensitive tissues are usually the gut and bone marrow, which regenerate quickly in comparison to most cancer tissue.

Although reduced doses and delays in treatment can occur due to the toxicity of treatment or health of the patient, it has become more important in recent years to understand the significance of administering planned doses on time because there is evidence to suggest that optimal timing and dose results in improved outcomes for patients. As early as 1995, Bonadonna et al. (1995) noticed improved outcomes in patients who received a full dose of chemotherapy on schedule, that is, the maximum dose of drugs at the planned points in time. Fifty-two percent of those receiving 85% or more of the planned dose were alive at 20 years, compared to 35% of those that received less than 85% (Young et al., 2009). It was also noted that patients who continued with treatment but received less than 65% of that which had been planned did not derive any benefit from the chemotherapy. It remains important, therefore, to aim to give the planned dose on time in order to maintain dose intensity and prevent suboptimal outcomes.

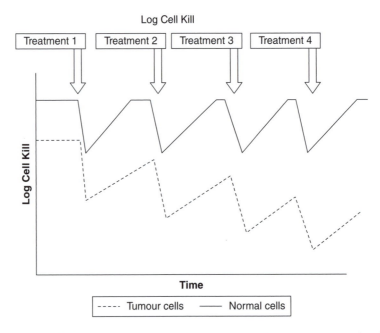

Figure 12.2   Log cell kill graph – cancer cell death and normal cell recovery over cycles of chemotherapy

TREATMENT INTENTIONS

Whilst each individual patient needs to be carefully assessed regarding their suitability and desire to receive treatment, it is also important to think about the potential outcome of that treatment. As chemotherapy is toxic, careful consideration should be given to the purpose of treatment. For some, the treatment aims to cure, but for others prolonged symptom control might be all that can be achieved. The success or impact of any course of treatment is classified as either complete response (CR), stable disease (SR) or partial response (PR). Both SR and PR in metastatic disease would be considered a good outcome. Aggressive management of metastatic disease must be carefully considered against the predicted side effects of chemotherapy that would have a significant effect on quality of life.

Choice of chemotherapy should always be determined by the aim of the treatment, but a patient's age, performance status and stage of disease are also important factors to consider (National Institute for Health and Clinical Excellence, 2009a). Chronological age should not be used as a parameter for withholding chemotherapy, although ageism in chemotherapy does exist (Dockter and Keene, 2009; see also Chapter 6).

The *National Confidential Inquiry into Patient Outcome and Death* (2008) undertook a review of the care of patients who died within 30 days of receiving chemotherapy. The findings revealed that many patients were in poor health just prior to their last cycle of chemotherapy, which highlights the need for an increased focus on an individual's performance status before and during treatment. Assessment of performance status using standardized scales helps to quantify a person's overall health, which can then guide health professionals to make an informed decision regarding fitness for treatment. Commonly used scales are the Karnofsky Scale and the Zubrod Scale (see Table 12.2), although psychosocial issues should also always form part of the overall assessment. Living alone is a clear risk factor in terms of toxicity management and psychological wellbeing, for example, and partners or significant others will also have psychosocial needs whilst they support their loved one undergoing chemotherapy treatment (Ream et al., 2013; see also Chapter 20).

Table 12.2 Karnofsky and Zubrod Scales of performance status

Karnofsky Scale		Zubrod Scale	
Normal activity, no evidence of disease	100	Normal activity	0
Able to perform normal activity with only minor symptoms	90		
Normal activity with effort, some symptoms	80	Symptomatic and ambulatory	1
Able to care for self but unable to do normal activities	70	Care for self	
Requires occasional assistance, cares for most needs	60	Ambulatory for >50% of time	2
Requires considerable assistance	50	Occasional assistance	
Disabled requires special assistance	40	Ambulatory for <50% of time	3
Severely disabled	30	Nursing care needed	
Very sick, requires supportive treatment	20	Bedridden	4
Moribund	10		

Source: Svirbeley, 2009.

Reflective activity

- Consider patients in your care and assess their current status using both the Karnofsky and Zubrod Scales.
- Which tool did you find most useful and why?
- What implications does assessment of performance status have on treatment intent and patient support?

CURRENT CHEMOTHERAPY APPROACHES

Neoadjuvant chemotherapy

The usual aim of neoadjuvant chemotherapy is to shrink, prior to surgery, very large tumours or those wrapped around complicated structures such as the aorta, renal arteries or neck. Neoadjuvant treatment can change an inoperable tumour into one that is operable (Mansi et al., 1989) or can reduce the extent of surgery required (see also Chapter 11). The intention would be curative if the cancer is confined to the primary site.

Primary chemotherapy

Primary chemotherapy is when chemotherapy is the only treatment required to treat the cancer (i.e. no surgery is necessary). This term only really relates to lymphomas and leukaemias – cancers that are present throughout the body. In these cases, surgery would be unlikely to remove all the tumour burden. The intention may be curative or palliative.

Adjuvant chemotherapy

This approach involves the administration of chemotherapy following an alternative primary cancer treatment, such as surgery. The aim of adjuvant chemotherapy is to reduce the risk of recurrence by killing any undetectable or subclinical disease. The intention of adjuvant chemo-therapy is usually to cure the patient.

Palliative chemotherapy

Metastatic cancer is *generally* incurable but chemotherapy has a role in controlling the disease and or associated symptoms. Several lines of treatment are now common and many patients are in and out of treatment for several years. The intention of palliative chemotherapy is to improve quality of life and the benefits must always outweigh potential side effects.

DRUG ADMINISTRATION

Dose calculation

There is no standard dose of chemotherapy: each prescription is individualized for each patient based on body surface area. A particular drug will be calculated, for instance, at 60 mg per metre squared. This will be, for example, 108 mg for a person with a body surface area of 1.8 metres squared. The patient's body surface area is determined by a height and weight nomogram (chart) (DuBois and DuBois, 1916). These are readily available in electronic prescribing systems and drug texts. There remains a debate around whether to treat obese patients with a dosage calculated on an actual weight or on an ideal weight and often the decision is instead based on other factors such as renal function, general fitness of the patient (i.e. performance status) and any co-morbid conditions. The American Society of Clinical Oncologists guidelines indicate that in most cases the actual body weight should be used (American Society of Clinical Oncologists, 2012).

Routes of administration

The Department of Health (2011c) states that the administration of chemotherapy should only be undertaken by nurses with the skills and qualifications to do so (competency frameworks are available from the Skills for Health website at http://skillsforhealth.org.uk). Chemotherapy is commonly administered via the intravenous route. This is the most reliable method of drug delivery because absorption rates are predictable and administration is the responsibility of the nurse. Oral chemotherapy has also been developed over recent years, but the administration responsibility shifts from the healthcare professional to the individual. The responsibility of the nurse here is to ensure that patients understand the safety aspects, for them and their family (Oakley et al., 2010). The various routes of administration are outlined in Table 12.3.

Table 12.3 Various routes of chemotherapy administration

Route	Advantages	Disadvantages
Intravenous	Rapid and reliable delivery of a cytotoxic drug to the tumour site	Lengthy treatment
	Rapid dilution of a drug, which reduces local irritation and the risk of tissue damage	Potential for **extravasation**
	Accurate titration of drug to achieve desired effect	More time spent in hospital
		Intravenous access needed
		Labour intensive
Oral	Ease of administration	Potential **poly-pharmacy**
	Avoids cannulation	Reliance on patient for concordance and compliance
	Less time spent in hospital	A misbelief that tablets are less toxic
	Patient preference	
Subcutaneous	Administering therapy in the community	The irritant nature of the drugs and/ or tissue damage
	For patient convenience	Incomplete absorption may occur
	Quick	Bleeding as a result of **thrombocytopenia**
		Discomfort of regular injections
Topical	Ease of administration	Leakage on clothing
Intrathecal	Gives direct access to the central nervous system and some drugs, given via other routes, are unable to cross the blood–brain barrier	Requires lumbar puncture
		Strictly controlled procedures

(Continued)

Table 12.3 (Continued)

Route	Advantages	Disadvantages
Intravesical (into the bladder)	Direct contact with tumour	Requires **cystoscopy**
	Very little systemic absorption, therefore less side effects	Labour intensive
	Reduces cytotoxic exposure to patients and their carers because excretion of the drug is quicker than when administered systemically	
Intraperitoneal	Direct access to tumour	Requires abdominal **paracentesis**
	Very little systemic absorption, therefore less side effects	Occasionally needs radiology placement of catheter
		Labour intensive
Intrapleural	Direct access to the pleural space	Requires pleural tap
	Very little systemic absorption therefore less side effects	Labour intensive
	Can often be used as a way to sclerose pleural space, therefore preventing further accumulation of malignant fluid	May require radiological placement
Intra-arterial	Facilitates the delivery of high concentrations of drug to the primary or secondary tumour mass	Very high levels of drug in a perfused organ may result in excessive tissue damage
	A reduction in systemic circulating levels of drugs has been shown to occur in many circumstances, resulting in a corresponding reduction in side effects to the patient	Requires access device

Source: Doherty and Lister (2012)

Venous access

As the majority of chemotherapy is given intravenously, it is important for the nurse to undertake a venous assessment based on the individual drugs planned, the condition of the veins, patient preference and the longevity of treatment. Most treatment is given via **peripheral cannula** but also via tunnelled **central lines, implanted ports** and **peripherally inserted central catheters** (PICC). The advantages and disadvantages of each are outlined in Table 12.4.

Some drugs must be given centrally due to their toxic effects on peripheral veins and, there-fore, a central access device is required. The choice of device will depend on patient choice and lifestyle, the availability of equipment and expertise. Some patients experience needle phobia and others can develop significant fear and anxiety in relation to repeated cannulation, which must be acknowledged in the assessment process (Anxiety UK, 2010; Dorrell, 2005).

Table 12.4   Common access devices

Device	Advantages	Disadvantages
Peripheral cannula	Convienient	Pain on insertion
	Cheap	Scarring
	Several sizes available	Short term
		Easy dislodgement
Tunnelled central line	Single or double lumen	Radiology placement
	Self-care possible	Requires maintenance if not in use
	Indefinite use	Thrombus/infection risk
		Possibility of inadvertent damage / dislodgement
		Surgical procedure to remove
PICC	Can be placed at bedside though often in radiology	Self-care difficult
	Single or double lumen	Requires maintenance if not in use
	Quick central access	Thrombus/infection risk
	Can be used for several months	Possibility of inadvertent damage / dislodgement
	Easily removed	
Implanted port	Hidden under skin	Self-care difficult
	Quick central access	Requires maintenance if not in use
	No dressing required	Thrombus/infection risk
	Indefinite use	Surgical procedure to place and remove
	Single of double lumen	

Reflective activity

- Reflect on patients currently under your care who have venous access devices.
- Is the choice of device appropriate for the patient's individual need or the convenience of the organization? Discuss with your colleagues.

Extravasation

It is the responsibility of the nurse administering each drug to ensure that the access device is **patent** and that the entire drug enters directly into the vein (European Oncology Nursing Society, 2010). Extravasation literally means 'leaking into the tissues'; however, in cytotoxic therapy it is the term used to describe the inadvertent leakage of vesicant drugs into the tissue surrounding the vein.

Cancer drugs can be grouped into three broad categories, based on their potential to cause tissue damage upon extravasation:

- Non-vesicants
- Irritants
- Vesicants.

Non-vesicant drugs generally cause little injury, although irritants can cause pain and inflammation that can lead to ulceration. **Vesicant** drugs, however, can lead to **necrosis** and serious tissue injury that requires plastic surgery. All chemotherapy units are required to have extravasation guidelines and all staff administering chemotherapy should have received training in prevention and management of extravasation. Guidelines should include a step-by-step guide of what to do for each group of drugs, including the administration of any antidotes to prevent further tissue damage. In the context of the tens of thousands of chemotherapy doses given each day, the incidence of extravasation remains low; however, it can have devastating consequences when it does happen. Management of any extravasation event depends on the drug and the volume in the tissue, but might include administration of antidotes, flushing the area through with saline, or plastic surgery and skin grafts. The National Extravasation Information Service provides accessible and useful information on the prevention and detection of extravasation (see end of chapter).

PATIENT INFORMATION AND INFORMED CONSENT

All patients undergoing a course of chemotherapy should consent to treatment. The consent procedure should include information about the likely benefits, as well as the common side effects or toxicities of treatment. The *Manual of National Cancer Standards* (DH, 2011c) specifies that all patients must be given written regimen-based information and that they should be offered an opportunity to discuss this in a pre-treatment consultation. This consultation, often with the chemotherapy nurse, should ideally be on a different day to that of the first treatment because patients and families need time to reflect on the verbal and written information provided. This can be a very stressful time for patients, who may need to assimilate the potential implications of both their cancer and treatment. The consultation should also include an holistic assessment of needs, venous access assessment (when appropriate) and advice regarding benefits and wigs where needed.

One useful resource is *Macmillan Cancer Care*, which hosts a comprehensive list of such information sources that has been validated by patients through a peer-review process (see www.macmillan.org.uk/Cancerinformation/Cancertreatment/Treatmenttypes/Chemotherapy/Chemotherapy.aspx). In addition, all patients should be given access to a 24-hour helpline and should rehearse with the nurse what actions should be taken in the event of problems, based on what is available in the locality. In response to the National Confidential Inquiry into Patient Outcome and Death (2008) audit, which highlighted that many patients are confused about the severity of side effects and often contacted the cancer centre for help only when the symptoms were severe or even life threatening, the National Chemotherapy Advisory Group (NCAG) (2009) recommends a proactive monitoring of patients on chemotherapy.

COMMON TOXICITIES OF CANCER CHEMOTHERAPY

The tolerability of chemotherapy is largely dependent on managing unwanted side effects. Patients are reviewed prior to each cycle in order to determine both response to treatment and fitness to receive the next cycle. Physical response to treatment is frequently confirmed by intermittent scans. It is often not possible to determine response to treatment at every cycle, but indications of effectiveness include reduction in:

- Size of cancer *in situ* (i.e. inflammatory breast lump, reducing lymph nodes);
- Symptoms associated with presenting cancer (i.e. pain, less reliance on analgesia, improved swallowing, etc.); and
- Tumour marker levels (for example for ovary, colorectal, testicular, prostate and pancreatic cancers).

From a psychological perspective, establishing how patients are coping with treatment and adopting approaches to boost their ability to cope is equally as important as physical considerations (see also Chapters 18, 19 and 22).

In relation to determining fitness to receive the next cycle of treatment, the nurse needs to assess any signs and symptoms associated with the cancer and any side effects of the drugs.

The common side effects or toxicities of anticancer cytotoxic agents used to treat cancer are classified using common toxicity criteria and are generally graded on a scale of 1 to 5, with 5 always referring to death (National Cancer Institute, 2010). A snapshot of common toxicity criteria are included in Table 12.5, although the full guidance covers every system (National Cancer Institute, 2010).

Bone marrow depression (myelosuppression)

Myelosuppression is is the most common dose-limiting side effect of chemotherapy, but also potentially the most life threatening (Zitella, 2013). All blood cells (**leucocytes, erythrocytes and platelets**) derive from a **single stem cell**. This is a regulated process and is determined by need (i.e. the haemopoietic process aims to keep the mature blood cells within normal levels); however, the process adapts to need and so more white cells are produced in response to infection, for example, or more platelets are formed as a result of bleeding. Immature red cells, white cells and platelets are formed in the bone marrow and then enter the blood stream as mature cells. Chemotherapy damages these rapidly dividing cells in the bone marrow, which results in a fall in circulating mature cells in the blood known as myelosuppression.

Neutropenia

Neutropenia, an abnormally low level of **neutrophils** in the blood, is a serious consequence of chemotherapy and may be mild, moderate, severe or life threatening (see Table 12.5). Neutrophils constitute around 70% of all the white blood cells and form a main defence against infection. As it takes approximately 10 days for a neutrophil to develop in the bone marrow before entering the blood stream, the lowest number of neutrophils (known as the

Table 12.5 A sample of common toxicity criteria

	1 Mild	2 Moderate	3 Severe	4 Life threatening
Neutrophils	$<1.5 \times 10^9$/L	<1.5-1.0×10^9/L	<1.0-0.5×10^9/L	$<0.5 \times 10^9$/L
Platelets	$<75 \times 10^9$/L	<75-50×10^9/L	<50-25×10^9/L	$<25 \times 10^9$/L
Hair loss	Thinning or patchy	Complete	–	–
Nausea	Loss of appetite without alteration in eating habits	Oral intake decreased without significant wt loss, dehydration or malnutrition	Inadequate oral calorific or fluid intake, IV fluids, tube feedings or TPN indicated	Life-threatening consequences
Vomiting	1 episode in 24 hours	2-5 episodes in 24 hours – IV fluids indicated	>6 episodes in 24 hours – IV fluids indicated or TPN	Life-threatening consequences
Hyperpigmentation	Slight or localized	Marked or generalized	–	–
Palmar-plantar erythrodysaesthesia (PPE)	Numbness, dysaesthesia/ paraesthesia, tingling, painless swelling or erythema of the hands and/or feet and/or discomfort which does not disrupt the patient's normal activities	Painful erythema and swelling of the hands and/or feet and/ or discomfort affecting the patient's activities of daily living	Moist desquamation, ulceration, blistering and severe pain of the hands and/or feet and/or severe discomfort that causes the patient to be unable to work or perform activities of daily living	–
Nail changes	Discolouration, ridging, pitting	Partial or complete loss of nail(s), pain in nail bed	Interfering with activities of daily living (ADL)	–
Peripheral neuropathy	Asymptomatic; loss of tendon reflexes or paraesthesia (including tingling) but not interfering with function	Sensory alteration or paraesthesia (including tingling) interfering with function but not interfering with ADL	Sensory alteration or paraesthesia interfering with ADL	Disabling
Stomatitis	Erythema of the mucosa	Patchy ulcerations or pseudomembranes	Confluent ulcerations or pseudomembranes bleeding with minor trauma	Tissue necrosis, significant spontaneous bleeding, life-threatening consequences
Diarrhoea	Increase of <4 stools per day over baseline, mild increase in ostomy output compared to baseline	Increase of 4-6 stools per day over baseline, IV fluids indicated; moderate increase in ostomy output compared to baseline not interfering with ADL	Increase of >7 stools per day over baseline; incontinence; IV fluids, hospitalization severe increase in ostomy output compared to baseline. Interfering with ADL	Life-threatening consequences i.e. haemodynamic collapse
Constipation	Occasional or intermittent symptoms; occasional use of stool softeners, laxatives, dietary modification or enema	Persistent symptoms with regular use of laxatives or enemas indicated	Symptoms interfering with ADL, manual evacuation required	Life-threatening consequences i.e. obstruction, toxic megacolon

nadir) typically develops 7–14 days post-chemotherapy, with recovery generally less than 7 days post-treatment (Zitella, 2013). Neutropenia renders a person susceptible to infection and the presence of an oral temperature of greater than 38°C makes this situation an oncological emergency (Zitella, 2013).

Patients with fever and presumed neutropenia must attend the hospital immediately for assessment. They will require broad-spectrum intravenous antibiotics within 1 hour from 'door-to-needle' and urgent assessment of vital signs (DH, 2009a). Left untreated, a fever in neutropenia leads to **septic shock**, which will most likely be fatal. Mortality rates ranging between 2% and 21% have been reported in adults with neutropenia and a fever. Aggressive use of inpatient intravenous antibiotic therapy has helped reduce mortality, and intensive management for sepsis is now needed in fewer than 5% of cases in England (NICE, 2012c). Sometimes it may be necessary for the patient to be prescribed a **granulocyte colony stimulating factor** (GCSF) to promote the production of neutrophils by the bone marrow. This is used to prevent or recover low neutrophil counts and may contribute to the reduction of febrile episodes during neutropenia (Aapro et al., 2006).

Whilst neutropenia is predictable, neutropenic sepsis needs effective management strategies that begin with good patient education and vigilance. Patients at home should be advised to monitor themselves for signs of infection, such as fever, sore throat, dysuria or productive cough. If a patient has any sign of infection, they should be advised to contact the hospital chemotherapy unit immediately. Rehearsals with patients about what to do should this situation arise is a clear recommendation of national policy (DH, 2009a).

Anaemia

Anaemia is a deficiency of red blood cells or **haemoglobin** in the blood. It is common and generally worsens as more treatment is given (i.e. towards the end of a course of treatment). As circulating red cells have a lifespan of around 120 days, a reduction in the number of these cells produced by the bone marrow is less noticeable until numbers decrease sufficiently to cause anaemia. Most patients can function and manage with low haemoglobin levels and generally transfusions are only given if patients are symptomatic.

Thrombocytopenia

Thrombocytopenia is a reduction in **platelet** count in the blood. Although common, a considerable drop in platelet levels (i.e. less than 20×10^9/L) requiring intervention is uncommon. Lower than normal platelets (i.e. grade 2–4; see Table 12.5) may cause a delay in treatment until levels return to normal

Alopecia

Alopecia is where hair loss has been caused by chemotherapy – it is temporary and reversible. Hair is constantly growing and because chemotherapy affects dividing cells, hair is a target for cell death and therefore hair loss. It is a distressing side effect of treatment, but does not affect all patients. Some drugs will always cause hair loss, some may cause hair to thin and others have no effect on hair at all. Although not a life-threatening event, loss of hair has a profound social and psychological impact on individuals and their acceptance of treatment (Callaghan and Cooper, 2013). Efforts to prevent hair loss have been made using a technique known as scalp cooling, although results have been variable. The theory suggests that freezing the scalp protects the hair from being killed by reducing blood supply to that area, and temporarily inhibiting cell division whilst chemotherapy is administered (Callaghan and Cooper, 2013).

Hair contributes greatly to body image and, consequently, the loss of hair can have a devastating emotional impact on a patient (see also Chapter 21). In the absence or failure of hair-preserving techniques, more emphasis needs to be placed on the psychological support of the patient and on creative measures to preserve self-image. This may take many forms including advice on wigs. Wigs, whilst available through cancer centres, are not free of charge unless the individual is on low income; however, many centres have organized charitable funds to help with costs. Other approaches to enhance self-image may include referral to organizations such as Headstrong, which offers hair loss support for men and women.

Nausea and vomiting

Chemotherapy-induced nausea and vomiting (CINV) is a recognized adverse effect of cytotoxic cancer treatment, and one that is consistently cited by patients as one of their greatest fears (Tipton, 2013; Hesketh, 2008; Miller and Kearney 2004; Grunberg et al., 2004; Hickok et al., 2003; Roscoe et al., 2002; Eckert, 2001; King, 1997). As well as having a deleterious effect on quality of life, CINV can also cause physiological impairment, loss of functional ability and a decline in performance status (National Comprehensive Cancer Network, 2010). When CINV is severe, it may lead to a clinical decision to cease chemotherapy or to implement dose delays or reductions (Vidall et al., 2011). The risk of chemotherapy dose delay, reduction or cessation is a serious cause for concern, particularly when a course of chemotherapy has been prescribed with curative intent. Patient perceptions of the most severe side effects of chemotherapy can be seen in Table 12.6, with CINV featuring consistently highly.

A recent study examining patient-reported chemotherapy indicators of symptoms and experience outcomes found that CINV remains a significant problem. Findings from ten UK treatment centres indicated that between 23% and 66% of patients reported moderate to severe nausea and that 3–49% reported vomiting as moderate to severe (Armes et al., 2013). Chemotherapy regimens vary in their **emetogenicity**, depending on the agent(s) used and their dosage. A widely used classification system is based on the frequency of emesis associated with a given agent when used without effective CINV prophylaxis. For example, highly emetogenic chemotherapy (HEC) denotes a CINV risk of >90% and moderately emetogenic chemotherapy (MEC) denotes a CINV risk of 31–90% (National Comprehensive Cancer Network, 2010; Hesketh, 2008). Other risk factors include a history of motion sickness, being female, high alcohol consumption and previous experience of CINV.

CINV is categorized according to the timing of its occurrence relative to the administration of chemotherapy:

- **Acute** CINV describes nausea or vomiting that occurs during the 24 hours following a dose of chemotherapy; it generally reaches a peak of intensity after 5–6 hours (National Comprehensive Cancer Network, 2010).

Table 12.6   Patient perceptions of the most severe side effects of chemotherapy

Rank	1983	1993	1995	1999
1	Vomiting	Nausea	Nausea	Nausea
2	Nausea	Constantly tired	Loss of hair	Loss of hair
3	Loss of hair	Loss of hair	Vomiting	Constantly tired
4	Thought of coming for	Effect on family	Constantly tired	Vomiting
5	Length of time treatment takes	Vomiting	Having to have an injection	Changes in the way things taste

Source: Middleton and Lennan (2011).

- **Delayed** CINV refers to nausea or vomiting that begins at least 24 hours following the dose of chemotherapy.
- Anticipatory nausea and vomiting occurs before chemotherapy is administered in approximately 10–44% of patients (Tipton, 2013), and is difficult to control. Triggers for anticipatory nausea and vomiting include previous unsuccessful control of emesis, and sights and smells associated with previous chemotherapy administration such as the hospital, chemotherapy nurse, perfume, etc.

Prevention of CINV is the optimal approach, with prescription of appropriate **anti-emetics** relevant to the emetogenicty of the chemotherapy drugs (Middleton and Lennan, 2011). It remains important to use evidence-based guidelines, such as UK Oncology Nursing Society Anti-Emetic Guidance (2013b) to ensure adequate emesis control. **NK1 receptor antagonists** (such as aprepitant) and **5ht3 antagonists** (including granisetron, ondansetron and palonosetron) are effective anti-emetics and act by blocking transmission of vomiting impulses to the vomiting centre in the **medulla oblongata**. Older compounds are still used, such as metoclopramide, domperidone, stemetil and the steroid dexamethasone (Tipton, 2013). Lorazepam is excellent for anticipatory nausea (British National Formulary, 2012).

Helpful advice to give patients on chemotherapy may include to eat little and often, to avoid strong smells and to explain that temporarily abstaining from food for 24 hours may be acceptable, as long as fluid intake is good. Non-pharmacological interventions have also been used (including acupressure, acupuncture, ginger) with some effect (Tipton, 2013; Dibble et al., 2000; Molassiotis et al., 2006; Ezzo et al., 2006; Ernst and Pittler, 2006). Nausea and vomiting is not only an unpleasant physical experience, but can also pose additional pressures such as lengthened periods of hospitalization, missed work and inability to undertake usual daily activities.

Effects on skin and nails

Some chemotherapy causes changes to the skin and nail beds (Morse, 2013), and several drugs are associated with altered skin pigmentation, a purely cosmetic reaction of which the aetiology is poorly understood. It is unclear why some drugs are associated with widespread pigmentation and others are confined to darkening of specific areas, such as the nails and tongue. **Hyperpigmentation** occurs more commonly in dark-skinned individuals. **Palmar-plantar** erythrodysesthesia (PPE), sometimes known as hand–foot syndrome, is an unpleasant effect of the drug capecitabine, where the patient first experiences tingling and/or numbness in the palms of the hands and soles of the feet that evolves into painful, symmetric and well-demarcated swellings and red plaques. This is followed by peeling of the skin before symptom resolution (Morse, 2013). The occurrence of PPE may result in discontinuation of capecitabine until resolved and then subsequent dose reduction. The use of pyridoxine is also commonly used in the treatment of PPE, along with measures to promote optimal skin comfort (Morse, 2013).

More severe nail toxicity is seen in taxane therapy. This can be a simple **erythema** or result in **desquamation** of the nails and separation of the nail plate from the nail bed. The incidence is more common in weekly regimens than three-weekly regimens but can have a devastating psychological effect on the patient. Cold gloves using the same technology as head cooling have been trialled in this situation, but although effective, the tolerability of the glove has been poor (Scotte et al., 2005).

Peripheral neuropathy

The symptoms of **peripheral neuropathy** vary depending on which nerves are affected, but the most commonly affected are the hands, feet and lower legs. This is because the longer the nerve, the more vulnerable it is to injury. Symptoms may be mild but progress with further treatment and so patients need careful assessment with each cycle of chemotherapy. It is often caused by drugs, such as vinorelbine, carboplatin, eribulin, oxaliplatin and the taxanes docetaxel and paclitaxol. As there is no treatment for the peripheral neuropathy itself, the causative agent would be discontinued, although withdrawing from chemotherapy may be a difficult choice for many (Argyriou et al., 2008).

Fatigue

Fatigue is a prevalent and common subjective complaint associated with chemotherapy, characterized by symptoms such as total body tiredness, diminished energy, reduced ability to concentrate, forgetfulness and an overwhelming desire to rest (Mitchell, 2013). Therapeutic approaches include assessing the impact on the patient's daily life and exploring management strategies tailored to the patient's individual wishes and circumstances. There are many different fatigue assessment tools available, but commonly used measures are the Piper Fatigue Scale (Piper et al., 1998) and the FACT-F (Functional Assessment of Cancer Therapy Fatigue; Yellen et al., 1997). Strategies to help patients cope with this side effect may include correcting physical causes (such as anaemia), encouraging a well-balanced diet and balancing periods of rest and activity (Mitchell, 2013).

Reflective activity

- List 10 activities you undertake every day that are important to you (this may range, for example, from cleaning your own teeth to going to work).
- Now reduce this list to five.
- Now select the one that is most important to you.

How easy or difficult was it to make these choices?

How may a patient with limited energy be helped to explore what is important to them so that their day can be adapted to make use of their available energy?

Mucositis

Mucositis, sometimes used interchangeably with the term **stomatitis**, refers to inflammation of the **mucosa**. The oral mucosa is a common site of injury for a patient on chemotherapy because the rapid proliferation (turnover) of cells in the mouth makes them particularly susceptible to damage. Neutropenia can lead to local infective complications or systemic infection through damaged mucosa, which can, in turn, lead to life-threatening **septicaemia**. Mucositis, particularly when severe, is a very painful condition, which can lead to significant adverse effects on quality of life, such as inability to eat or drink or communicate (Wujcik, 2013). The severity of mucositis can be undertaken using an assessment tool such as the Oral Assessment Guide (Eilers et al., 1988). Prevention in the form of good oral hygiene and mouthwashes can help to minimize the effects of mucositis and interventions such as analgesia (systemic or local), mouthwashes and promoting hydration can help to manage symptoms.

Diarrhoea and constipation

The gut also has a high proliferation rate and so diarrhoea is common because the bowel becomes inflamed. Any chemotherapy can cause diarrhoea, but it is significantly seen in 5Fu, capecitabine and irinotecan therapies. Some literature reports incidences of up to 16% of grade 3 or 4 diarrhoea (Chau et al., 2005; Saltz et al., 2001; O'Shaughnessy et al., 2002; Tveit et al., 2012).

If the bowels are opening four to five times a day, an anti-diarrhoeal should be commenced and the individual should contact the hospital for further advice. If diarrhoea is sufficiently severe, treatment may have to be discontinued. Prolonged inflammation of the bowel at best is debilitating – at worst can lead to perforation and death (Andreyev, 2010).

Constipation is often multifactoral and can be due to loss of appetite, anti-emetic therapy, inactivity, analgesia and chemotherapy agents. One particular group of chemotherapy drugs – the vinca alkaloids – are known to cause constipation due to neurotoxicity of nerves that affect the bowel. A clear aperient schedule should be discussed with patients receiving these drugs.

Fertility

Chemotherapy can produce significant effects upon a patient's fertility, but these depend on gender, age and the specific drugs prescribed (Lamb, 1995; Keen and Lennan, 2011): the more drugs a person receives at the same time, the greater the likelihood that fertility will be affected. Although female patients under 40 are more likely to resume normal function, premenopausal women who receive chemotherapy should be clearly informed of the risk of temporary or permanent ovarian failure. Permanent menopause is likely in perimenopausal women (Larsen–Disney, 2007; Chapman, 1982; Royal College of Physicians et al., 2007; Goodman, 2006) leading to menopausal symptoms such as hot flushes, night sweats, vaginal dryness and irregular menses. The Royal College of Physicians (2007) provide comprehensive guidance on the management of the effects of cancer treatment on reproductive function.

For women who wish to preserve their reproductive ability, there are two main options:

- Fertility preservation
- Embryo storage

Although the action is not clearly understood, fertility preservation may involve the use of hormones during chemotherapy to suppress ovarian cycling and induce a temporary **medical menopause**. It is also sometimes possible to store oocytes and ovarian tissue for future *in vitro* **fertilization** (IVF), although success rates are low. In general, delays in cancer treatment are not recommended; however, embryo storage is an established technique where it may be possible to delay cancer treatment for a few weeks in order to stimulate the ovarian cycle using fertility drugs and then to retrieve eggs. IVF with the partner or donor sperm can then be carried out, followed by cryopreservation of embryos.

Emotional distress due to loss of fertility function can be devastating (Partridge et al., 2004). The loss of a future family cannot be mourned quickly and it should be noted that even if the patient already has children, infertility or a premature menopause can be overwhelming. In addition, for those who retain a degree of fertility function, anxiety about future pregnancies due to chemotherapy cannot be underestimated (Beaumount, 2007). In fact, pregnancies are not recommended until at least two years post-completion of all treatment. This is not necessarily due to toxic effects of treatment but because patients are more likely to relapse within this initial two-year period, making overall management difficult and subsequently raising concerns for the future of the child.

For men, sperm banking (freezing sperm or sperm cryopreservation) prior to treatment is a simpler process and widely available. Providing a semen sample for freezing is a relatively straightforward procedure and can be quickly arranged, but the decision to bank sperm and the process for obtaining a sample is still likely to promote anxieties and concerns. Imagine a young man, for example, who is suddenly faced with a diagnosis of cancer, which requires treatments that are potentially unpleasant. In addition, he is confronted with having to make a decision prior to treatment about his potential for future fertility, a life event that he has not yet considered. If he then decides to bank sperm, the process of ejaculating into a container in a private room, and then handing it to a nurse may be simple, but also embarrassing. In general, it is recommended that at least two semen samples are collected over a period of one week and stored before treatment for cancer. Males should be sexually abstinent where possible for at least two days before each collection. The Human Fertility and Embryology Authority (HFEA) recommends that semen samples be produced onsite wherever possible. In exceptional circumstances, they can be produced at home, if delivered to the laboratory within 30–45 minutes of production. Success rates following this procedure are variable (Royal College of Physicians et al., 2007).

Reflective activity

Consider one or two of the common toxicities described previously. How were they managed in your own practice? What was the impact on the individual and their family?

CHAPTER SUMMARY

Although many of the side effects of treatment are manageable with prompt interventions supported by good patient information, the overall impact on an individual can be significant. A cancer diagnosis poses its own challenges but the consequences of treatment may inflict additional debilitating physical and psychological effects that challenge the individual's perception of self (Hewitt et al., 2005). Body image changes due to weight loss/gain, hair loss, skin texture and nail changes, for example, in addition to other side effects such as fatigue or nausea can confound problems. Added to this, the uncertainty of treatment success or failure makes the whole experience of cancer and its treatment a tremendous challenge for the patient and their family (Ream et al., 2013).

Chemotherapy is likely to remain the mainstay of treatment for the foreseeable future, but the development of targeted therapies associated with reduced risk of side effects are likely to increase (see also Chapter 15). In addition, with improved knowledge of cancer cell biology and genomics, approaches to individualized treatments are closer to becoming a reality.

Key learning points

- Cytotoxic chemotherapy predominantly kills cells by interfering with cell replication. It may be phase-specific or cycle-specific.
- Chemotherapy usually involves a course of treatment comprising cycles of chemotherapy, with intervals between to facilitate repair of normal cells and maximize damage to cancer cells.
- The four main approaches to chemotherapy are neoadjuvant, primary, adjuvant and palliative.
- Cytotoxic chemotherapy is usually given intravenously but may also be given orally, topically, intrathecally, subcutaneously or into a body cavity.
- Cytotoxic chemotherapy kills both normal and cancer cells, but is most effective on cells that divide rapidly. Administering combinations of chemotherapy increases cell kill.
- Treatment can result in physical, psychological and social consequences, which range from a significant threat to life to severe psychological distress.

Recommended further reading

- Yarbro, C.H., Wujcik, D. and Holmes Gobel, B. (2014) (eds) *Cancer Symptom Management.* 4th edn. Burlington, NJ: Jones and Bartlett Learning.

The following websites may also be helpful:

- www.skillsforhealth.org
- www.mynewhair.org
- www.hairlosssupport.me.uk/Head_Strong/
- The National Extravasation Information Service (www.extravasation.org.uk)

13 RADIOTHERAPY

KATE PARKER, ANN MALONEY AND DEBBIE WYATT

Chapter outline

- What is radiotherapy?
- How does radiotherapy work?
- Treatment intent and methods of delivery
- Treatment planning

- Side effects of radiotherapy and their management
- Psychosocial impact of radiotherapy treatment
- Support for patients receiving radiotherapy treatment

INTRODUCTION

This chapter explores the principles of radiotherapy and how this highly technical and specialized cancer treatment impacts on the lives of patients who need it. Radiotherapy continues to be the main non-surgical treatment for cancer, with over 50% of patients receiving radiotherapy at some stage of their illness (Hoskin, 2006). Radiotherapy is considered to be the second most effective treatment after surgery; 16% of people are cured of their cancer purely as a result of their radiotherapy and 40% are cured when radiotherapy is given in combination with other curative treatments (Department of Health Cancer Policy Team, 2012). The psychosocial consequences of radiotherapy treatment for each individual are varied, ranging from a sense of loneliness to the inconvenience of daily visits to a cancer centre, in addition to physical side effects of treatment. Understanding these experiences can help healthcare professionals to develop approaches to supporting patients through what can sometimes be a very difficult time of their lives.

WHAT IS RADIOTHERAPY?

Radiotherapy is the use of **high-energy X-rays** and similar rays (such as electrons) to kill cancer and treat some benign tumours (Glover and Harmer, 2014). Radiographs were discovered in 1895 by Roentgen, but it was Marie and Pierre Curie upon their discovery of radium in 1898 who made radiation therapy a recognized medical specialty and an effective alternative to surgery (Fröman, 2014). Treatment initially involved the use of **radioactive sources** but technological advances led to the development of **linear accelerator (linacs)** machines, which could generate a variety of radiation types in a much more controlled manner.

The initial discovery that radioactive sources could treat and even cure cancer heralded a new era in cancer treatment, but not much was known of the hazardous properties of radiation at that time. At first, radioactive sources such as **radium** and **cobalt** were used to deliver treatments, and then others such as **caesium, iodine and palladium** were included for internal treatment known as **brachytherapy.** An understanding of hazardous radiation properties means that radiotherapy treatment is governed by strict health and safety regulations (Ionising Radiation [Medical Exposure] Regulations 2000 [amended in 2006 and 2011]) and is subject to quality measures in the cancer peer review measures for radiotherapy in England (National Cancer Peer Review-National Cancer Action Team, 2013).

How does radiotherapy work?

In order to understand how radiotherapy works it is useful to have knowledge of the structure of atoms, which are the fundamental building blocks of all matter, including cells.

Atoms consist of protons (which have a positive charge), electrons (which have a negative charge) and neutrons (which have no electrical charge). Protons and neutrons are found in the centre, or nucleus of an atom, with electrons revolving around the nucleus in electron shells (see Figure 13.1). All atoms, except hydrogen, contain both protons and neutrons; the number of protons and electrons is equal in a stable atom, resulting in a neutral overall electrical charge (Baker, 2012a). If an atom gains an electron however, it becomes negatively charged (a negative ion), and if it loses one, it becomes positively charged (a positive ion). **Ionizing radiation** used in radiotherapy carries enough energy to cause atoms to gain or lose electrons by forcing electrons to leave their orbits around the nucleus. This, in turn, causes DNA damage and other cellular changes that result in cell death. (Morgan et al., 2011)

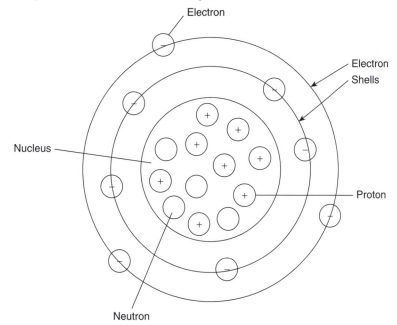

Figure 13.1   The structure of an atom

IONIZING RADIATION AND RADIOTHERAPY

Ionizing radiation can be electrically generated as X-rays or produced from naturally occurring or manufactured radioactive isotopes (Faithfull, 2008). **Isotopes**, which can be either stable or unstable, are atoms that have the same number of protons and electrons but a different number of neutrons. Unstable isotopes are called **radioisotopes** (radioactive isotopes) and these emit radiation as they disintegrate, shedding charged particles such as positrons, neutrons, alpha or beta particles and gamma ray photons in their attempt to become stable. In order to become stable they may exchange protons for neutrons or vice versa and can release or absorb particles (Baker, 2012a) that can lead to ionization of surrounding atoms. The **beta particles** released during this process have a limited range in tissue (i.e. they are only able to penetrate a small distance) but can be suitable for specific radiotherapy treatments. The radioisotope iodine-131(^{131}I), for example, is delivered orally as a liquid or a capsule to patients with benign or malignant thyroid disease. The ^{131}I is absorbed into the bloodstream from the stomach and is then taken up in the tissues of the thyroid. Due to the limited range of the beta particles emitted (3 mm in tissue), a high dose can be delivered to the thyroid whilst the dose to the body as a whole is limited (Rose et al., 2012). Despite the usefulness of beta particles in this instance, isotopes that emit **gamma ray photons** are more commonly used in radiotherapy. Gamma ray beams have a greater range in tissue, and these can be employed in external beam radiotherapy and brachytherapy. Cobalt-60 (^{60}Co) can be used as a source of radiation in external beam treatment machines (Mills et al., 2012) and iridium-192 (^{192}Ir) is commonly used as a source in brachytherapy (Symonds and Deehan, 2012).

Electrically generated radiation includes X-rays, electrons and protons. **X-rays**, which are high-energy photons, are the most commonly used form of radiation delivery and are often thought of as packets of energy. The higher the energy of the X-ray, the deeper the photons can penetrate. Different X-ray energies can be used therefore to treat a range of cancers at different depths within the body. When producing X-rays using electricity, a stream of electrons is emitted from a heated filament or an electron gun and these electrons are accelerated before bombarding a target made of a material such as tungsten. Due to interactions between the electrons and the atoms within the target, photons are emitted that deliver energy, which in turn damages DNA and kills cells. The energy of the resultant photons is dependent on the degree of acceleration of the emitted electrons and in clinical use can vary from 20 keV (kilovolts or thousands of volts) to 25 MeV (megavolts or millions of volts). It is worth noting that the photons produced will range in energy, in a spectrum, up to a maximum that is related to the energy the electrons have acquired when accelerated (Baker, 2012b). In contrast, gamma rays of specific energies are released from radioactive isotopes due to the decay of radioactive sources, for example Cobalt-60 source will emit gamma rays at 1.17 MeV and 1.33 MeV (Venables, 2006).

Prior to the introduction of ^{60}Co **external beam therapy** (EBT) machines and linear accelerators, which were developed after the Second World War, **kilovoltage X-rays** up to 300 kV were used to treat a wide range of tumour sites, including those in deep tissues within the body (Venables, 2006). Although kilovoltage X-rays are capable of penetrating into deeper tissues, they also deliver a substantial proportion of prescribed dose to the surface of the treated area. For a 10 x 10 cm area treated at 100 kV, the maximum dose is delivered on the skin surface and only 10% of the given dose reaches a point 10 cm within the patient. The same treatment beam at 220 kV would again deliver maximum dose on the skin surface with 29% of the given dose reaching a depth in tissue of 10 cm (Childs and Bidmead, 2012). Therefore, the use of kilovolt beams in a modern radiotherapy department would generally be limited to treating superficial skin lesions such as basal cell carcinomas (BCC) and bony metastases in superficial bones.

Megavoltage X-rays are vastly more energetic than the kilovoltage X-rays. When radiotherapy treatment is planned, the volume of tissue to be treated is considered, including the depth the maximum dose should be delivered at and the distance from entry to exit point (this is called the separation). In the megavoltage energy range, beams of 4–6 MV are considered to be low energy and are useful for treating areas with small separations, such as volumes in the head and neck. Higher energy beams, for example 10 MV and above, are useful for treating volumes situated more deeply in areas with larger separations, such as the pelvis, and would include prostate and gynaecological tumours. Considering the 10 x 10 cm beam discussed earlier at 4 MV, the maximum dose is delivered at a depth of 1 cm and 64% of the given dose will reach a point at a depth of 10 cm in tissue. A 15 MV beam would deliver the maximum dose 2.9 cm inside the patient and 77% of the dose would reach the point at 10 cm depth (Childs and Bidmead, 2012). Megavoltage beams therefore have a 'skin sparing effect' in that a smaller dose is delivered onto the skin surface than to the tissues beyond. This can lead to reduced skin reactions when compared to treatment with lower energies. Most radiotherapy in the Western world is in the form of megavoltage X-rays produced and delivered by **linacs** that can produce a range of energies.

Radiation can also be delivered by **electron particles** rather than photons. As electrons are negatively charged they interact with other charged particles in the material they pass through. Small amounts of energy are lost in multiple interactions (Baker, 2012b), which means that in clinical use an electron beam is less penetrating than a photon beam and is therefore used to treat more superficial structures. Electron beams at energies ranging from 4 to 20 MeV are commonly used in clinical practice (Mills et al., 2012).

The energy from a **proton beam** is deposited very differently to that of a photon beam. The energy deposited by a beam of protons increases as the speed of the protons decreases. When the protons come to a halt, they give up their remaining energy in a surge known as the Bragg peak (Baker, 2012b). This means that the point where the bulk of the dose will be delivered can be predicted based on the energy of the proton beam. In the clinical setting, this characteristic can be used to reduce dose to the tissue the beam travels to, until the point where dose delivery is required within the tumour (Jones and Symonds, 2012). The use of protons is increasing worldwide (Mills et al., 2012), with particular interest in their use in the treatment of paediatric tumours. This is due to the possibility of reduced long-term side effects as a result of the low dose delivered to normal tissue (Taylor, 2006).

Aim of radiotherapy

The aim of radiotherapy treatment is to deliver a specific dose of ionizing radiation to a target area (the cancer) whilst minimizing damage to normal cells in the surrounding tissues (Faithfull, 2008). One way of minimizing harm to normal tissues is through **fractionation** in which the patient is prescribed a total dose of radiation that is then divided into fractions (#) (i.e. the number of times the treatment is to be given). Radiation treatment is prescribed in units of measurement called **grays (Gy)**, although treatment machines (linacs) deliver the radiation in **monitor units** (MU). A prescription of 20 Gy of radiotherapy in 5#, for example, means a total of 20 Gy is delivered in 5 treatment sessions at 4 Gy per fraction. The number of fractions varies depending on the anatomical site being treated and the overall intent, although curative doses tend to range from 55 to 65 Gy over a period of 4–6 weeks (Faithfull, 2008).

Different tissues have different dose tolerances, which partially explains why skin reaction severity and tumour response are not predictable for an individual. Cells that divide rapidly are more susceptible to radiation than those that divide more slowly because they repeat the sensitive stages of the cell cycle more frequently. The term used to describe the speed and response of a tumour to radiation is called **radiosensitivity** and different tissues can be described as having high, medium or low sensitivity. Tissues with high sensitivity, such as the epidermis of the skin, react quickly to even small doses of radiation (Morgan et al., 2011), whereas those with low sensitivity, such as bone, are able to tolerate higher doses with less effect. The tolerance of normal tissues to radiation limits the dose that can be prescribed. For example, in the UK the tolerance dose for the spinal cord is considered to be 48 Gy in fractions of 2 Gy. Giving any part of the spinal cord a dose greater than this carries a 0.5–1% risk of causing radiation-induced paralysis (The Royal College of Radiologists, 2006) and should be avoided unless the aim is palliation. Some cancers are radio-resistant and therefore would not benefit from radiotherapy.

The effects of fractionated radiotherapy on both normal and malignant cells are governed by biological factors. Fractionation aims to take into account the four Rs of radiobiology, as described by Morgan et al. (2011).

The four Rs of radiobiology

- **Repair:** Each dose (fraction) of radiation aims to irreparably damage cancer cells but allow normal cells to recover before the next fraction is given. The ability of cells to recover from sub-lethal radiation damage normally occurs within 4–24 hours. Cellular repair mechanisms promote the recovery of both normal and cancer cells exposed to radiation, but with repeated exposure the ability of cancer cells to repair themselves decreases.
- **Reassortment/redistribution:** A cell's sensitivity to radiation varies as it undergoes different phases of the cell cycle, with cells in S phase most resistant to treatment and those in mitosis most sensitive. During treatment, more of the radiosensitive cells will be destroyed but less of the resistant ones. As the surviving cells continue to move through the cell cycle, some will have moved into the more sensitive phases of the cell cycle by the time the next fraction of radiation is given and so the chances of catching cells in these sensitive phases increases with each subsequent fraction of treatment (for further information on the cell cycle, see Chapter 4).
- **Repopulation:** An increase in cell division is seen in both normal and malignant cells following radiotherapy treatment. This enables damaged normal cells to regenerate, usually over a period of 5–7 weeks. Cancer cells may also proliferate over a course of radiotherapy, particularly in tumours that respond to treatment early. The total amount of malignant cells to be killed may therefore increase. Planned treatments aim to reduce the ability of cancer cells to repair themselves, but unplanned breaks in therapy should be avoided because interruptions to radiotherapy treatment may increase risk of local recurrence and reduce cure (The Royal College of Radiologists, 2008).

- **Reoxygenation:** Well-oxygenated cells respond better to radiotherapy (i.e. they are more radiosensitive). Small tumours and cells on the periphery of tumours tend to be well oxygenated and are therefore more sensitive to treatment; however, poorly oxygenated cells confer resistance to radiation. Early fractions tend to selectively kill oxygenated cells, but as these cells die, more oxygen becomes available to the remaining cells. Fractionated treatment allows time for poorly oxygenated parts of the tumour to reoxygenate, thus making the newly oxygenated cells more sensitive to radiation.

TREATMENT INTENT

Radiotherapy treatment can have a variety of different aims. For some people, it is used to help control their cancer symptoms, such as pain, whereas for others it is used to control their local disease.

Table 13.1   Approaches to treatment

Treatment approach	Treatment intent	Examples of treatment site, dose and number of fractions (#)
Curative	• Cure • Long-term control	• Prostate – 74 Gy/37#/ 51 days (Department of Health Cancer Policy Team, 2012)
Palliative	• Control growth of tumour • Prevent tumour invading other important structures, for example spinal bone metastasis invading the spinal cord • Symptom control, for example stop bleeding, reduce/relieve pain	• Cervix – 20 Gy/5#/ 1 week (Taylor and Powell, 2006) • Bone – 20 Gy/5#/ 1 week or 8gy/1# • Spine – 30 Gy/10#/ 2 weeks, 20 Gy/5#/ 1 week or 8 Gy/1# (Hoskin, 2006)
Adjuvant given after, or with other treatment(s), usually surgery	• Cure • Destroy microscopic cancer cells that are localized in the tumour bed • Maximum chance of longer-term control compared to a single treatment modality	• Breast – 40 Gy/15#/ 3 weeks (Haviland et al., 2013)
Neoadjuvant given (with or without chemotherapy) before surgery	• Cure • Shrink the tumour prior to surgery • Maximum chance of longer-term control compared to a single treatment modality	• Preoperative rectum – 25 Gy/5#/ 5 days (Royal College of Radiologists, 2006)
Consolidation given with other systemic modality, but not post-surgery	• Cure • Systemic treatment, such as chemotherapy, shrinks the tumour thus reducing the radiotherapy target • Maximum chance of longer-term control compared to a single treatment modality	• Small-cell lung cancer 50 Gy/25#/5 weeks (Royal College of Radiologists, 2006)

There are many influencing factors that contribute to the overall management plan of every patient with a cancer diagnosis. What determines the type of radiotherapy treatment they receive is also multi-stranded and includes patient factors and treatment intent (Department of Health Cancer Policy Team, 2012).

The clinical oncologist is responsible for prescribing the most appropriate radiation treatment based on a number of factors, such as diagnostic test results, histological information and the patient's general health. The possible benefits and expected side effects of each option are discussed with the patient, who ultimately decides which treatment option they would prefer to receive. It is only when all of this information is gathered that a treatment plan and its intent can be identified (see Table 13.1 for examples of approaches to treatment).

Radiotherapy and chemotherapy are often given concurrently and this is referred to as **chemo-radiation**. Some types of chemotherapy have radio-sensitising effects, which enhance the efficacy of radiotherapy to kill cells. Some regimes require the chemotherapy to be delivered before the radiation starts (neoadjuvant), during the radiotherapy (concurrent) or once the radiotherapy has finished (adjuvant) (Symonds and Meredith, 2012).

Unfortunately, patients cured of their primary cancer as a result of radiotherapy are at increased risk of developing subsequent **radiation-induced malignancies** (Brenner et al., 2000; Sigurdson and Jones, 2003; Health Protection Agency, 2011). These are malignancies that develop as a direct result of being exposed to ionizing radiation. This risk is taken into consideration by clinicians when weighing up the best treatment option.

METHODS OF DELIVERY

There are many different treatment techniques used in radiotherapy but they all fall into two main areas:

- **External radiotherapy**: delivered by using radiation sources from outside the body.
- **Internal radiotherapy**: delivered by placing a radioactive substance inside the body.

External radiotherapy, the most common type of radiotherapy treatment, is also referred to as **external beam therapy (EBT)**. It is most commonly delivered using high-energy electrically generated X-rays via a linear accelerator (linac) as discussed earlier in the chapter. There are several types of machines that produce these X-rays, but the main difference is that they can produce varying strengths of X-rays, which penetrate to different depths. Stronger beams are needed to reach deeper cancers because they have to pass through more tissue before reaching their target area.

Linacs stand alone within a treatment 'set' with the treatment couch sitting directly underneath the head of the machine, known as the gantry. The strict safety building regulations require the room (bunker) in which the linac is situated to have thick walls that cannot be penetrated by the exit beams once they have passed through the patient. During treatment, staff sit in a control area outside the room and monitor the patient on multiple CCTV systems.

Whilst the patient lies on the treatment couch, the gantry can rotate 360 degrees around them to allow any tumour in any position to be irradiated. The radiographers use green laser lights that intersect on the patient to help recreate the same position of the initial planning session and the invisible beam is projected out of the gantry. The linac makes a quiet beeping sound when the X-rays are switched on, but the patient does not see or feel anything.

Orthovoltage units are used to treat more superficial regions such as skin lesions. Apart from the energy, the main difference between orthovoltage and megavoltage is that the machine applicator (collimator) physically touches the target area.

Brachytherapy is the term used to describe radiation treatment in which the radiation source is in contact with the tumour (Faithfull, 2008). Sources in the form of pellets or seeds may be implanted directly into the tumour (interstitial therapy) or through hollow tubes, such as needles, or applicators (intracavity therapy) that have previously been inserted and positioned into the patient's tissues in theatre (Symonds and Deehan, 2012). Most implants can be removed once treatment has been delivered; however, some implants, such as radioactive seeds to treat prostate cancer, are left *in situ* (Symonds and Deehan, 2012). Removable sources are inserted temporarily into the needles or applicators through a process called **remote after loading** where radioactive sources stored in protective containers are moved by remote control to the target area (Colyer, 2003). Three types of remote after loading include **high dose rate (HDR), medium dose rate (MDR)** and, rarely, **low dose rate (LDR)** brachytherapy. HDR is the most frequent method of brachytherapy treatment in the UK, although MDR and LDR are sometimes used (Symonds and Deehan, 2012). HDR is most commonly used to treat the vaginal apex, oesophagus, lungs, breast and prostate, and it delivers treatment in a matter of minutes, which enables patients to attend on an outpatient basis. MDR treatment is most commonly used to treat gynaecological cancers. Once the applicator has been positioned, the patient is taken to a specially designated room where the after loading takes place to provide continuous radiation for 24–48 hours. Sources can be temporarily returned to their protective containers should anyone need to enter the patient's room (Colyer, 2003). **Unsealed sources** are radioactive isotopes that can be administered to the patient as a drink or injection. A main advantage of brachytherapy over external beam radiotherapy is that the dose can be delivered directly to the tumour whilst reducing exposure to normal tissues.

Treatment planning

The ideal **dose** and number of **fractions** are calculated to maximize damage to cancer cells and minimize damage to normal tissue; however, a number of other factors also need to be considered to translate the prescription into the optimum radiotherapy technique for each individual patient (Childs and Bidmead, 2012). This requires meticulous planning.

There are three main target volumes to consider in planning radiotherapy (Burnet et al., 2004):

- Gross tumour volume
- Clinical target volume
- Planning target volume.

Gross tumour volume (GTV) refers to the position and extent of the gross tumour and is derived from a diagnostic CT (computerized tomography) scan undertaken prior to treatment. The **clinical target volume (CTV)** includes the GTV plus a margin of surrounding tissue. Whenever planning radiotherapy treatment, a margin of tissue around the tumour is included to ensure that any microscopic disease is also exposed to radiation because every tumour cell must be eradicated if cure is to be achieved (Munro and Gilbert (1961) cited by The Royal College of Radiologists (2008b)). Over time, treatment techniques have become more complex and sophisticated with an emphasis on treating the visible tumour whilst sparing adjacent healthy tissue and critical structures. This helps to minimize short-term toxicities and damage caused by long-term side effects. Tumours in different parts of the body require different margining, for example a lung tumour may need a larger margin than a tumour in the pelvis because treatment has to account for the natural motion of the heart and breathing. The **planning target volume (PTV)** involves radiotherapy planning to ensure that the prescribed dose of radiotherapy is delivered to the clinical target volume (Conway and Johnson, 2012).

The dose of radiation emitted from the head of the linear accelerator does not remain constant as it passes through the patients' tissues towards the target volume. Instead, as the beam enters the body (or any solid matter placed in the path of the beam) some of that radiation is absorbed, and some interactions at the point of impact can actually create more radiation, known as **scatter**. As the beam of energy hits a surface such as the skin, it deposits some energy and then continues losing energy as it passes along its path. The highest amount of radiation is delivered just below the skin and is known as the region of **dose build up**. 'Fall off' refers to the gradual decrease in radiation dose as it passes through tissues. The denser the tissues, the more radiation that is deposited, and the lower the dose that passes through to remaining tissues. The dose distribution therefore varies throughout the radiation field and is referred to as the **isodose**. This change in dose can be displayed as percentage **isodose lines** or as a colourwash display showing dose gradients within the treated volume. An isodose of 100% is where the radiation dose will be at its highest and can be plotted at decreasing 10% intervals as the amount of radiation delivered to surrounding tissues falls off (Faithfull, 2008; see Figure 13.2).

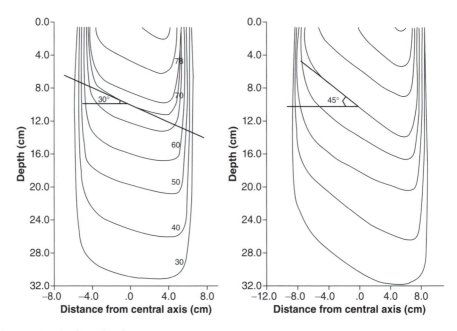

Figure 13.2 Isodose distribution

Source: Available from www.jacmp.org/index.php/jacmp/article/view/2060/1216

A margin, the size of which depends on the tumour and its location, is drawn around the gross tumour area, which accounts for any movement. This forms the PTV. Once the clinical oncologist defines the treatment field, the computer planning radiographers and physicists determine which beam arrangements and dose distributions will achieve the pre-scribed dose to the treatment field whilst minimizing the dose to **organs at risk** (i.e. how the dose of radiation will be distributed in the tissues). Each critical organ (e.g. spinal cord, lungs, heart, kidneys, small bowel) has a different sensitivity to radiation, which planners take into account when manipulating beams in order to minimize damage (Childs and Bidmead, 2012).

The number and arrangement of beams of radiation can be manipulated to achieve maxi-mum therapeutic effect. The size, shape and location of the CTV determine how many beams are needed to adequately distribute the radiation dose.

Treatment can be given from a number of different directions and angles, each of which is referred to as a **treatment field**. **Simple beam arrangements** involve delivery of radiation by one beam from a single direction (one treatment field) or multiple directions (up to five or six treatment fields). The maximum amount of radiation is delivered where the beams converge, thus minimizing damage to normal tissues (see Figure 13.3).

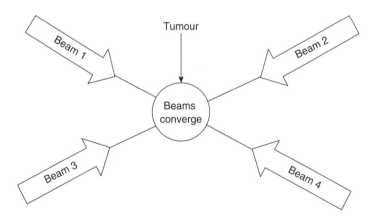

Figure 13.3   Beam convergence in multiple treatment fields

There are a variety of ways that planners can modify the beams to reflect the shape of the tumour and to homogenize the dose distribution whilst also sparing other tissue. The dose distribution can be modified to account for convergence of beams or tissue obliquity by using 'wedges' (Childs and Bidmead, 2012). Traditionally, these were wedge-shaped pieces of metal in the path of the treatment beam, but in some modern linacs, this effect is created by the primary collimator moving across the treatment beam. To minimize the dose to areas outside the PTV, it is also possible to shield these areas by using shielding materials. In most linacs currently in use in the UK, multi-leaf collimators are used to introduce shaped shielding. Multi-leaf collimators are individual 'fingers' of lead (0.5 or 1 cm wide and approximately 7–8 cm deep) that can be driven into a range of positions to shield areas which do not need to be treated.

A number of complex beam arrangements have also been developed, including:

- *Conformal radiation therapy*: the area (field) to be treated reflects the shape of the tumour and surrounding tissue.
- *Image guided radiotherapy (IGRT)*: localizing the beam to deposit the dose of radiation as accurately as possible into the target volume is of key importance. IGRT involves comparing a CT scan from planning with a CT scan taken whilst the patient is on the planning couch to establish if the patient's position needs to be adjusted (Society of Radiographers, 2013).
- *Intensity-modulated radiation therapy (IMRT)*: an extension of conformal therapy, which enables treatment beams to be shaped in 3D to match the shape of the tumour and surrounding margin. This is an important improvement, especially when the target is not well separated from normal tissues (Society of Radiographers, 2013). Current evidence suggests that in order to minimize the long-term effects of treatment, between a third and half of all radical radiotherapy treatment should be delivered as IMRT (Department of Health Cancer Policy Team, 2012).
- *Tomotherapy*: an enhancement of IMRT. With IMRT the gantry moves to a fixed position and stays stationary to deliver a beam to the specific shape of the tumour from that direction. It then moves to the next determined position, and so on, to deliver the beam to the tumour shape from multiple directions. Tomotherapy delivers the beam from many more angles through a complete 360-degree rotation known as an 'arc'.
- *Stereotactic ablative radiotherapy (SABR)*: a 3D technique using specially designed collimators attached to a linear accelerator, which delivers a high dose (five times larger than normal radiotherapy treatment) of radiation to a small volume, usually about 3 cm in diameter in one fraction (Society of Radiographers, 2013). Several stationary beams or multiple arc rotations concentrate the radiation dose to the lesion whilst sparing surrounding normal tissue. Surgical excision is the standard treatment of choice for operable lesions, but stereotactic radiosurgery has become a viable option for inoperable malformations (NHS England, 2013). More trials are needed to compare SABR against surgery and other forms of treatment (Department of Health Cancer Policy Team, 2012).

TREATMENT PLANNING

All radiotherapy treatment requires precise forward planning in order to ensure that the prescribed dose of radiation is delivered in the optimum way to the exact target area on every occasion. Therapy radiographers must immobilize and accurately position the patient in a 3D space each time the patient attends for treatment. It is imperative that the patient has a positive appointment at this stage because their first impression will enhance their overall experience.

Patients usually have a CT scan, which takes place in a pre-treatment planning suite, although MRI (magnetic resonance imaging) or PET (positron emission tomography) scans are also sometimes used. The scan information from these increasingly complex computer planning systems is fed into a planning computer to provide a detailed 3D dataset, which outlines the shape of the gross tumour area. These advances have led to a significant improvement in accuracy and patient outcomes (Department of Health Cancer Policy Team, 2012). Image enhancing aids such as contrast agents may also be given to help the clinician identify internal anatomy and accurately identify the treatment area. Pen marks and tattoos are then made on the patient's skin or specially made masks that are used to position the patient during subsequent treatments.

There are two specialist areas that are responsible for planning accurate radiotherapy positioning and immobilization: **mould room** specializes in techniques related to treatments of the head and neck, and **CT planning** specializes in all other anatomical areas of the body. Treatment for patients requiring radiotherapy to the head and neck involves making an individualized Perspex or thermoplastic mould of the patient's face and neck with holes cut out for the eyes, nose and mouth, which fits closely to the patient's skin. Planning marks can then be drawn onto the mask rather than onto the patient's skin. The mask will be worn and fixed to the couch each time the patient attends treatment in order to immobilize the head and neck and keep the patient in exactly the same position for each treatment. Although the patient is only required to wear the mask for short periods of time, a sensitive and supportive approach is required because people can find the experience claustrophobic (Wells, 2003).

The planning appointment usually takes place about a week after diagnosis once the planned management has been discussed with the patient (see the following example of a planning process).

Example of planning process for a patient with lung cancer

- Information given about what to expect at the pre-treatment appointment.
- Baseline assessments made: clinical history, height, weight, general health since last seen by the clinician and psychosocial assessment.
- Blood sample taken to check that kidney function is sufficient to tolerate the intravenous contrast agent, which is used to enhance the clarity of the CT scan of the chest.
- CT scan of the chest acquired with the patient in the treatment position. This is used to localize the area to be treated.
- Pin-head sized permanent reference marks with tattooing ink are made and used as external aids to treatment set up.
- The radiotherapy treatment booked and a schedule of appointments made, including appointments with other healthcare professionals, for example doctor or specialist nurse.
- Consent discussed and obtained by the doctor.
- Target area and critical structures outlined, followed by computer planning.
- Questions answered and other relevant information leaflets given.

Reflective activity

What misperceptions about radiotherapy treatment have you encountered?
Consider whether these five statements are true or false:

1. Patients receiving any type of radiotherapy become radioactive
2. Radiotherapy always causes severe skin burns

(Continued)

(Continued)

3. Radiotherapy always causes nausea and vomiting
4. Radiotherapy always causes hair to fall out
5. Radiotherapy always leads to infertility.

All five statements are false.

- Internal sources of radiotherapy emit radiation, but patients receiving external beam radiotherapy are not radioactive.
- Although the majority of patients will experience skin reactions at the treatment site, only 10–15% will be severe (Wells and MacBride, 2003).
- Side effects of radiotherapy are specific to the part of the body that has been irradiated, therefore:

  - nausea and vomiting may occur if parts of the gastrointestinal tract lie within the treatment field;
  - hair loss may occur if the skin or scalp lie within the treatment field; and
  - infertility may arise if the ovaries or testes lie within the treatment field.

SIDE EFFECTS AND THEIR MANAGEMENT

Radiation damages all cells that it passes through and patients can experience side effects as a result of their treatment. Increased side effects are associated with increased distress and decreased quality of life (Wengstrom et al., 1999) and patients can experience a range of psychosocial stressors specific to their radiotherapy such as anxiety and depression before, during and/or after treatment (Mitchell and Lozano, 2012), though this is not inevitable, and often not without challenges, as will be discussed in Chapter 18 of this book. Side effects are influenced by the anatomical structures being treated, the total radiation dose, number and frequency of treatments, the amount of tissue being irradiated and the physical and psychological state of the patient. Smaller treatment fields and lower doses of radiation, for example, are associated with fewer and less severe side effects (Faithfull, 2008), and a patient who is generally well may be able to tolerate treatment more readily than someone with co-morbidities. Any presenting symptoms that the patient may have are quite often exacerbated during treatment.

Radiotherapy side effects are local to the area being irradiated, but two common side effects occur regardless of treatment site: **skin reactions** and **fatigue**.

Radiotherapy induced skin reactions

Many patients have fears and worries about radiation skin reactions (Society of Radiographers, 2011a). Even with the most up-to-date radiotherapy techniques, up to 90% of patients will experience a dose-dependent skin reaction at the treatment site (MacBride et al., 2008); however, only 10–15% will be severe (Wells and MacBride, 2003). Skin reactions occur where the beam both enters and leaves the body and although some research suggests that people with dark and black skin report more severe reactions than people with fair skin (Ryan et al., 2007), others argue that there is insufficient evidence and that it is more dependent on the individual's response than their skin type (NHS Quality Improvement Scotland, 2010). Skin reactions vary considerably between patients (Morse, 2013), although they can be influenced by both intrinsic (related to the patient) and extrinsic factors (related to the treatment or external factors) (Kedge, 2009). A summary of factors influencing radiation-induced skin reactions can be seen in Table 13.2. These factors can either increase skin damage or delay healing.

Table 13.2 Predisposing factors for radiation-induced skin reactions

Intrinsic factors	Extrinsic factors
Older age	Higher doses of radiation
Co-existing disease	Increased volume treated
Infection	Smaller number of fractions
Reduced nutritional status	Radiosensitizers, e.g. some types of chemotherapy
Obesity	Site of treatment, e.g. where folds of skin come together
Previously irradiated areas	(e.g. infra-mammary fold, axilla) or where the epidermis is
Smoking	thin and smooth (e.g. perineum, groin, face, axilla).
Long-term UV exposure	Lower types of energy (less than 1 MV)
Genetic predisposition for less	Chemical irritants, for example perfume, aftershave
effective healing	Mechanical irritants, e.g. friction from clothes, shaving, etc.
Recent trauma, such as surgery	Extremes of temperature
Increased skin sensitivity to radiation	

Sources: Society of Radiographers (2011a)'; The Princess Royal Radiotherapy Review Team (2011); Morse (2013).

'These guidelines are currently being updated.

The maximum dose of megavoltage beams (energies above 1 MV) is deposited just below the surface of the skin (unlike kilovoltage beams under 1 MV that deliver maximum dose to the skin itself), but patients will experience skin reactions of varying severity from both high and low dose energies.

The Princess Royal Radiotherapy Review Team (2011) describes the three main levels of reaction as erythema, dry desquamation and moist desquamation. Although the inflammatory response is activated when radiotherapy commences, **erythema** tends to develop 10–14 days later, which is the time it takes damaged basal cells in the epidermis to migrate to the skin surface. Patients quite often describe an itching sensation prior to any visible colour change, but the skin becomes warm, dry, red and tight and has an appearance similar to the redness seen after sitting in the sun (Society of Radiographers, 2011b). The skin loses hair and may appear hyperpigmented as melanin cells in the skin migrate to the surface (Morse, 2013). Damage to the skin is minimal and may increase for 7–10 days after completion of treatment, but subsides after about 2–3 weeks. The mechanism is very different to a skin burn resulting from heat or strong chemicals, and changes due to radiotherapy should be described as skin reactions rather than burns. **Dry desquamation** occurs when an increased number of new cells are produced in the basal cell layer of the epidermis in an attempt to compensate for cells that have died. This occurs before dead cells have shed from the surface, which results in the irradiated skin becoming dry, itchy and scaly. It is not a permanent condition, however, and treatment can continue. With continued skin damage, the basal layer is unable to produce enough new cells to replace the ones that have died and skin appears blistered, moist and sloughs off as the broken epidermal layer exudes serum and causes pain and discomfort. This is known as **moist desquamation**. The exudate promotes healing, however, and the damage is reversible. Treatment may need to be suspended for a short time until healing has taken place, but can then be resumed. The final stage of skin necrosis, which involves damage to blood vessels, is now rarely seen due to advances in treatment technique (NHS Quality Improvement Scotland, 2010).

Reactions become apparent within 1–4 weeks of the start of treatment, but peak about 7–10 days after finishing treatment. The skin should be healing or have fully healed within 2–3 weeks of treatment completion (Glover and Harmer, 2014).

It is important to assess skin reactions in order to match interventions with the severity of the reaction. Consistency in grading skin reactions can be achieved by using tools such as the National Cancer Institute's Common Terminology Criteria for Adverse Events (CTCAE): radiation toxicities: dermatitis radiation (US Department for Health and Human Services, 2009) (see Table 13.3) or the Radiotherapy Oncology Group (RTOG) and the European Organisation for Research and Treatment of Cancer (EORTC) assessment tool (Cox et al., 1995), which is recommended by The Royal College of Radiographers (see Table 13.4). A UK survey of radiotherapy skin care by The Society and College of Radiographers (Society of Radiographers, 2011b) found RTOG to be the most commonly used tool. Observer-rated tools are limited, however, and a more holistic picture can be established using a tool that also assesses patient-rated symptoms, such as the Radiation-Induced Skin Reaction Assessment Scale (RISRAS) developed by Noble-Adams (1999) and the Skin Toxicity Assessment Tool (STAT) (Harris et al., 2012).

Table 13.3 National Cancer Institute's Common Terminology Criteria for Adverse Events (CTCAE): radiation toxicities: dermatitis radiation

Grade 1	Faint erythema or dry desquamation
Grade 2	Moderate to brisk erythema; patchy moist desquamation, mostly confined to skin folds and creases; moderate oedema
Grade 3	Moist desquamation in areas other than skin folds and creases; bleeding induced by minor trauma or abrasion
Grade 4	Life-threatening consequences; skin necrosis or ulceration of full thickness dermis; spontaneous bleeding from involved site; skin graft indicated
Grade 5	Death

Source: US Department for Health and Human Services (2009)

Table 13.4 Toxicity criteria of the Radiotherapy Oncology Group (RTOG) and the European Organisation for Research and Treatment of Cancer (EORTC)

Grade 0	No visible skin change
Grade 1	Follicular, faint or dull erythema/epilation/dry desquamation/decreased sweating
Grade 2	Tender or bright erythema; patchy moist desquamation/moderate oedema
Grade 3	Confluent, moist desquamation other than skin folds; pitting oedema
Grade 4	Ulceration; haemorrhage; necrosis

Source: Cox et al. (1995)

Skin care management commences prior to treatment in the form of patient education and advice on how to manage radiotherapy reactions when they occur. Skin care instructions only apply to the area directly affected by the radiation and should be tailored to the treatment area. For example, when skin folds and thin skin around the genitalia are within the treatment field, patients may need particular advice on keeping skin clean and dry (see the following for general patient advice).

General guidelines for managing radiotherapy skin reactions

- Washing: wash/bath as usual using warm water and soap. Pat dry to avoid friction.
- Skin care products: avoid perfumed products/aftershaves, talcum powder or creams. Unperfumed moisturisers, such as aqueous cream, may be used to promote comfort but only deodorants/products advocated by staff in the cancer centre should be used.
- Hair removal: can electric shave with care but avoid wet shaving in treatment area, no wax or hair removal creams.
- Clothing: wear loose fitting clothing.
- Swimming pools: fresh water is fine but avoid chlorinated pools because it has a drying effect on the skin. Be aware of shower temperature control.
- Irritants: avoid extremes of temperature, clothing that rubs, scratching/rubbing/massaging the area.
- Sun exposure: avoid direct sun exposure during treatment and afterwards until the skin has healed. Thereafter use high factor suncream of SPF30 or above because the area is at higher risk of harm from the sun.

Sources: The Princess Royal Radiotherapy Review Team (2011); Morse (2013)

There is no consensus regarding the best way to manage skin reactions, and approaches to managing dry and moist desquamation are not consistently evidence-based (Harris et al., 2012). Further research into best practice is needed (Society of Radiographers, 2011a), but skin care aims to prevent infection and further damage, maximize comfort, minimize pain and, where necessary, promote a moist environment for wound healing.

Where there are no visible skin changes, patients are advised to continue with their own skin care regime (Society of Radiographers, 2011a[2]). Tsang and Guy (2010) found that prophylactic use of aqueous cream was associated with reduced stratum corneum thickness and argue that more research is needed into the ingredient sodium laurel sulphate, which is a skin irritant. There is insufficient evidence to support the use of aqueous cream (Wells et al., 2004; Harris et al., 2012), although patients may find it soothing (Morse, 2013).

The now outdated approaches to erythema and dry desquamation included increased application of aqueous cream with hydrocortisone 1% and analgesia if needed, but there is contradictory evidence to support the use of hydrocortisone (Harris et al., 2012). If moist

---

[2]These guidelines are currently being updated.

desquamation develops, aqueous cream can be used on unbroken skin, but hydrocortisone and aqueous cream should not be applied where skin integrity has been lost. A swab should be taken if the skin shows signs of infection and the tissue viability nurse can advise on an appropriate dressing that is atraumatic, non-adhesive, absorbent and comfortable (Society of Radiographers, 2011a[3]; The Princess Royal Radiotherapy Review Team, 2011). Specific products such as petroleum jelly, steroids and gentian violet should not be used (Naylor and Mallett, 2001; Harris et al., 2012). For serious injury, which involves bleeding and necrosis, specialist advice should be sought.

Fatigue

Fatigue is a common side effect of radiotherapy that can be quite debilitating for patients (Fransson, 2011; Sawada et al., 2012; Alcântara-Silva et al., 2013; Langston et al., 2013; Guo et al., 2013). It usually begins in the first week of treatment, peaks about two weeks after treatment and gradually disappears during the following few weeks. The body has to expend a huge amount of energy to remove waste products in the blood from cells that have been killed as a result of radiation damage, and to generate new cells. Radiation to specific anatomical sites may also increase fatigue, for example if the lungs are in the treatment field, lung tissue may be damaged resulting in reduced oxygenation of the blood (oxygen is a key component in the production of energy).

Other factors may contribute to fatigue, such as co-morbidities, other cancer and non-cancer treatments, anaemia, infection, compromised nutrition, concurrent symptoms such as pain, insomnia, and anxiety and depression (Mitchell, S., 2013). It can therefore be difficult to establish the cause, and management is often challenging. Management of fatigue involves treating known contributory factors such as anaemia, pain and depression and assessing the severity of fatigue and its impact on patients' lives using a recognized assessment tool, such as the Piper Fatigue Scale (Piper et al., 1998) or the FACT-F (Functional Assessment of Cancer Therapy Fatigue; Yellen et al., 1997).

Traditionally, patients have been advised to rest if they feel tired; however, research has found that if patients maintain their 'usual' activities, they cope better physically and psychologically (Hickok et al., 2005; Janaki et al., 2010; Poirier, 2011; Kuchinski et al., 2009; Erickson et al., 2013). This may not necessarily be easy to achieve, especially because patients often feel worse during the two weeks after treatment when they are at home alone. Assessment of each patient's fatigue enables healthcare professionals to tailor evidence-based interventions to meet their individual needs (Erickson et al., 2013), for example psychosocial support (Kirchheiner et al., 2013) or education about exercise (Carayol et al., 2013). Macmillan Cancer Support (2014) is working in partnership with the Department of Health and Age UK on pilot projects aimed at coordinating and delivering short-term support packages for older people undergoing cancer treatment. One is exploring the benefit of providing practical support during treatment for those patients aged over 70 who may struggle with their daily activities during their treatment phase. Another is a home-from-hospital programme looking at supporting patients during their first week to 10 days post-treatment, which is the period of time when the treatment side effects are at their worst.

---

[3]These guidelines are currently being updated.

Table 13.5 Localized acute effects of radiotherapy

Area treated with radiotherapy	Examples of side effects
Scalp/brain	**Alopecia** results from damage to the hair follicles, which prevents replication of cells and can either be temporary or permanent. The extent and pattern of hair loss is dependent on the area irradiated and the dose of radiotherapy (Callaghan and Cooper, 2013). The likelihood of permanent hair loss increases with higher doses of radiotherapy, although temporary alopecia tends to resolve within 2–3 months of completing treatment (Lawenda et al., 2004). This can be distressing for patients and lead to an altered body image (for further information on altered body image, see Chapter 21). **Cerebral oedema**, the swelling of the brain, can occur as a result of radiation injury. This can lead to intracranial pressure, which can alter brain function by compressing brain tissue and leading to signs and symptoms such as changes in mental state, headache, increase in blood pressure, decrease in pulse and respiration, and nausea (Fields, 2013).
Head and neck area	**Oral mucositis** is the inflammation of the mucosa and almost always occurs in patients receiving treatment to the head and neck (Lalla et al., 2008) and can have a major negative impact on patients' quality of life due to, for example, pain and inability to eat, drink or talk, which can necessitate dose reduction and delay in treatment (Scully et al., 2003; Wujcik, 2013). It can be graded from mild to severe using a recognized scale such as the National Cancer Institute's CTCAE (US Department for Health and Human Services, 2009), and the RTOG and EORTC Radiation Toxicity Grading (Cox et al., 1995). It tends to develop and then worsen from the second week of treatment (Wujcik, 2013). Other structures in the treatment field can also be affected leading to **pharyngitis**, **oesophagitis** and alterations in taste. **Xerastomia**, or dry mouth, can develop when the production of saliva is reduced due to damaged salivary glands. It can cause physical and emotional distress by interfering with eating, drinking, tasting, swallowing and speaking (Dalton and Gosselin, 2013). Salivary changes also occur, mainly involving the saliva becoming extremely thick and sticky.
Chest and/or upper back	Gastrointestinal symptoms can include **oesophagitis**, **indigestion** (due to inflammation of the oesophagus) **nausea** and **dysphagia**. Respiratory problems can include **dyspnoea** due to **pneumonitis** from damaged airways, which compromises gaseous exchange, and **radiation fibrosis**, which makes the lungs less elastic (Joyce, 2013).
Abdomen/lower back	Damage to epithelial tissue that lines the gastrointestinal and genito-urinary systems can lead to **nausea** and **vomiting, diarrhoea, cystitis** and **sexual dysfunction**. The negative impact on sexual functioning for both men and women is multidimensional as a result of physical, psychological and social factors (Incrocci and Jensen, 2013). Men may experience impotence and women may experience vaginal stenosis (narrowing of the vagina) and vaginal dryness, which leads to painful intercourse. Both men and women may become infertile.
Red bone marrow	Red bone marrow produces all blood cells and is highly sensitive to radiation so the production of blood cells decreases. White blood cells are affected first, which may lead to infection and impaired healing. A reduction in red blood cells leads to anaemia and increased lethargy. Low numbers of platelets leads to bruising and bleeding.

concerns at the start of treatment would help to ensure that patients receive support tailored to their needs.

Physical side effects of treatment can also lead to considerable distress and have a negative impact on interactions and relationships. For example, mucositis can be so painful that it prevents the person from being able to eat or drink, skin reactions may lead to an altered body image and uncontrollable diarrhoea can cause embarrassment (Donovan and Glackin, 2012). Patients receiving radiotherapy for specific cancers have been found to experience particular distress, for example those with lung cancer have been found to have a higher degree of emotional distress than those with other types of cancers. Their quality of life changes over time as the disease progresses due to increasing physical symptoms such as fatigue (Ekfors and Petersson, 2004).

Other patients, for example those receiving treatment for prostate cancer, have well documented problems with sexual functions and urinary-related side effects (Queenan et al., 2010). A study of patients with breast cancer receiving adjuvant radiotherapy following surgery found fatigue to be the most troublesome side effect, followed by pain associated with skin reactions. Psychosocial symptoms happened over time, however, and the greatest need for support was following completion of treatment. For some women, the added loss of social roles within the family, at work and with friends and colleagues added further anxiety and depression (Sjovall et al., 2010). For the majority of patients, treatment is given as an outpatient and requires daily travel to the hospital. This in itself is time-consuming and disrupts a person's usual routines, such as work or caring responsibilities.

Support

There are a number of ways in which patients receiving radiotherapy can be supported prior to, during and following their treatment. Patients should be given quality information regarding their radiotherapy treatment and how it is to be delivered and also potential side effects and their management (Department of Health Cancer Policy Team, 2012). Patient-centred information is important (Bergenmar et al., 2014; Güleser et al., 2012). The Radiotherapy Patient Experience Survey, undertaken in 2013 by Quality Health for the Department of Health and the National Cancer Action Team, examined treatment-specific information given to patients receiving radiotherapy (Quality Health, 2013b). Patients reported that their information needs were largely met, with 30 of the 42 questions receiving ratings of 80% or over. Some aspects were covered well, such as clear explanation of treatment plans (90%), but others, such as information about how to manage side effects (72%), were less well addressed.

Some patients receive information prior to treatment by clinical nurse specialists, but all should have opportunities to discuss their treatment with therapy radiographers during radiotherapy treatment planning and assessment, and information given prior to the first fraction of treatment. Appropriate use of terminology and checking patients' understanding can play a large part in relieving anxiety and a skilled psychosomatic consultation in radiotherapy would help towards meeting patients' emotional needs whilst receiving treatment (Voigtmann et al., 2010; Kirchheiner et al., 2013). The use of a Distress thermometer can also provide a useful tool (Mann and Ford, 2011), but giving empathetic, honest and spontaneous attention is also important (Sjovall et al., 2010; Nijman et al., 2011). Nurses can also help by empowering patients; keeping them well informed; helping them to manage side effects, such as skin reactions and pain; and advising on fatigue because addressing symptoms increases patients' wellbeing (Sjovall et al., 2010).

Patients also derive support from family and friends (David et al., 2012; Queenan et al., 2010) and supporting carers during this time is therefore also important.

Key indicators to ensure good practice in the psychosocial assessment and support of patients receiving radiotherapy treatment include:

1. Individualized holistic patient assessment aimed at identifying patients at risk for anxiety and distress, pre-treatment, during treatment and after treatment (Macmillan Cancer Support, 2012b) (see Chapter 17 for further information on effective communication).

2. Screening tools that are used to help identify patients at risk of anxiety and depression (National Institute for Health and Clinical Excellence (NICE), 2009b). NICE recommends that any patient who may have depression (especially those with a past history of depression or who suffer from a chronic physical illness associated with functional impairment) should be asked the following two questions:

    a. During the last month have you been feeling down, depressed or hopeless?
    b. During the last month have you often been bothered by having little interest or pleasure in doing things?

3. Radiation therapists who are educated to recognize symptoms of distress. The Health and Care Professions Council (HCPC) (2013:8) *Standards of proficiency: radiographers 5.2* states that radiographers must 'understand the emotions, behaviours and psychosocial needs of people undergoing radiotherapy or diagnostic imaging, as well as that of their families and carers'.

4. Ensuring that the patient receives treatment from the same radiotherapy treatment team for the duration of treatment where possible.

5. Ensuring that the patient has access to a key worker (a relevant healthcare professional) for ongoing support and information.

6. Ensuring that the radiotherapy environment is uncluttered and organized, and that it provides a calm and comforting atmosphere (Jarvis, 2003).

7. Providing information that is individualized and tailored to promote patient understanding (Nijman et al., 2011) (for further information on information giving, see Chapter 17).

8. Empowering patients through patient education to promote early recognition of side effects and their management and by giving them the opportunity to choose treatment times to suit their individual lifestyles.

9. Helping carers and friends to support patients more effectively (Queenan et al., 2010).

10. Identifying and utilizing patients' own management strategies (Donovan and Glackin, 2012; Nijman et al., 2011).

11. Improving signposting of resources to support groups.

12. Establishing the patient's level of activity prior to starting treatment and tailoring advice accordingly. (Reduction of level of physical activity may contribute to increased fatigue (Kuchinski et al., 2009).)

13. Appropriately referring to other members of the multiprofessional team, e.g. site-specific cancer nurse specialists, dieticians, physiotherapists, occupational therapists, oncology social workers, benefits and welfare advisor, palliative care team, lymphoedema specialists, holistic therapists and clinical psychologists.

14. Promoting supported rehabilitation and self-management.

CONCLUSIONS

Radiotherapy is an effective curative and palliative treatment for cancer; however, it can be associated with unpleasant consequences, such as physical side effects and psychological distress. Recognizing the multidimensional impact of treatment on patients is central to achieving excellent care that is tailored to each individual's need. This should involve thorough assessment, meeting information needs, managing side effects and providing psychosocial support to reflect current evidence-based practice.

Key learning points

- Radiotherapy is the main non-surgical treatment for cancer.
- Ionizing radiation is used to kill cells by forcing electrons to leave their orbit around the nucleus of an atom.
- Ionizing radiation can be electrically generated or produced from naturally occurring radioisotopes.
- The aim of radiotherapy is to maximize damage to cancerous cells whilst minimizing damage to surrounding tissues.
- One way of minimizing harm to normal tissues is through fractionation.
- Radiotherapy can be given with curative or palliative intent, alone or in combination with other therapies.
- Radiotherapy can be delivered externally (external beam radiotherapy) or internally (brachytherapy).
- Meticulous planning is required to ensure that the prescribed dose of radiation is delivered in the optimum way to the exact target area on every occasion.
- A variety of radiotherapy techniques can be used to minimize damage to normal tissues and maximize harm to cancer cells.
- Patients will experience side effects local to the area of irradiation because radiation damages both normal and malignant cells.
- Most patients will experience skin reactions and fatigue.
- Radiation reactions should be assessed using a recognized assessment tool.
- Patients can experience physical, psychological and social distress as a result of radiotherapy.
- Management aims to establish patient concerns through effective communication and to tailor support to individual need.

Recommended reading

- Faithfull, S. and Wells, M. (eds.) (2003) *Supportive Care in Radiotherapy*. Edinburgh: Churchill Livingstone.
- Symonds, P., Deehan, C., Mills, J.A. and Meredith, C. (eds) (2012) *Walter and Miller's Textbook of Radiotherapy*. 7th edn. London: Elsevier Churchill Livingstone.
- Yarbro, C.H., Wujcik, D and Holmes Gobel, B. (eds) (2013) *Cancer Symptom Management*. 4th edn. Burlington, VT: Jones and Bartlett Learning.

14 HAEMATOPOIETIC STEM CELL TRANSPLANTATION

COLIN THAIN AND JACQUELINE BLOOMFIELD

Chapter outline

- The main indications for haematopoietic stem cell transplant (HSCT)
- Key biological factors in HSCT, sources of stem cells and stem cell donation
- The common short-term and long-term side effects of HSCT
- Psychological aspects of HSCT

INTRODUCTION

Haematopoietic stem cell transplantation (HSCT) is a procedure involving the infusion of haematopoietic **stem cells** to a recipient following chemotherapy, radiotherapy and, in some cases, other **immune suppressive therapy.** The procedure is undertaken for a range of malignant and non-malignant conditions and aims to repopulate and/or replace the existing **haematopoietic system** in the patient on which the procedure is being performed (Ljungman et al., 2010). The general term 'haematopoietic stem cell transplantation' has now replaced **'bone marrow transplantation'**, reflecting the various sources from which stem cells can be derived. It is now possible to harvest HSCs from peripheral blood, following mobilization of the stem cells using colony stimulating factors or chemotherapy, or from umbilical cord blood, as well as from bone marrow. HSCT is typically an intensive form of treatment, with significant morbidity and, in some cases, mortality, but it is potentially curative for some illnesses, and can result in long-term remission in others (Brown, 2010). This chapter provides a discussion of key issues related to HSCT, including biological aspects, types of transplant and phases in the transplant process. In addition, the implications of HSCT are addressed from both a physical and psychosocial perspective, including discussion of late effects.

HISTORY

Attempts to transplant bone marrow can be traced back to the nineteenthth century; however, the first use of the technique to treat end-stage **leukaemia** was reported in 1959. This involved the administration of bone marrow from an identical twin to his sister, who had received high-dose radiation therapy, and resulted in a three-month remission from the disease (Copelan, 2006). This event was instrumental in providing support to the concept that infusing marrow could provide haematological reconstitution in lethally irradiated patients with acute leukaemia (Appelbaum, 2007). However, subsequent attempts at transplantation were met with limited success, largely because many of the mechanisms involved in successful engraftment, and factors guiding optimal treatment and supportive care, were not well understood or readily available at the time (Ezzone, 2010).

As knowledge developed throughout the 1960s and 1970s, further incremental successes were reported. These included the successful transplant of bone marrow from a non-identical sibling to a patient with an immune deficiency and the use of the procedure for the treatment of aplastic anaemia and acute leukaemia (Appelbaum, 2007). Ongoing research also led to a better understanding of key issues such as pre-transplant treatment (conditioning regimes), the need to match donors and recipients, different sources of stem cells, and the importance of supportive care, particularly in the post-transplant period. These developments have contributed to improving the success of transplantation and to widening its application to include a range of illnesses (Gratwohl et al., 2010). HSCT is now considered the standard treatment for a variety of malignant and non-malignant illnesses, and long-term survivorship is increasing (Wingard et al., 2011). In 2006, there were over 50,000 transplants worldwide (Gratwohl et al., 2010), with over 31,000 procedures conducted in Europe in 2010 (Baldomero et al., 2011).

BIOLOGICAL ASPECTS OF HSCT

Haematopoiesis, the production of blood cells, takes place in the bone marrow, which in adults is found mainly in the bones of the pelvis and axial skeleton, and in the proximal **epiphyses** of long bones (Hoffbrand and Moss, 2011). The **pluripotent** or **haematopoietic stem cell** (HSC) can give rise to all types of blood cell, and is also capable of self-renewal. Figure 14.1 illustrates how, through a series of steps, HSCs give rise to the multiple blood cell lines. Each step represents a degree of differentiation, which also means that the cells are restricted in their developmental potential and lose the capacity for self-renewal (Hoffbrand and Moss, 2011). Although there are relatively few stem cells in the bone marrow (about 1 in 20 million nucleated cells in the marrow, according to Hoffbrand and Moss (2011)), they can be identified by the presence of the **CD34 protein** on the cell surface. This enables these cells to be collected ('harvested') in sufficient quantities to allow for transplantation (Ezzone, 2010). The transplanted cells are able to repopulate the bone marrow of the recipient.

It is essential that HSCs have the capacity for self-renewal because this allows the body to maintain a readily available supply of stem cells, enabling a quick response to demand for blood cells caused by events such as infection or blood loss by increasing production of particular cell lines. When a stem cell divides, it forms one replacement stem cell and one cell committed to **differentiation**. This occurs either along the **myeloid** cell line, giving rise to **granulocytes**, **myelocytes**, **erythrocytes** and **megakaryocytes** (and ultimately platelets), or

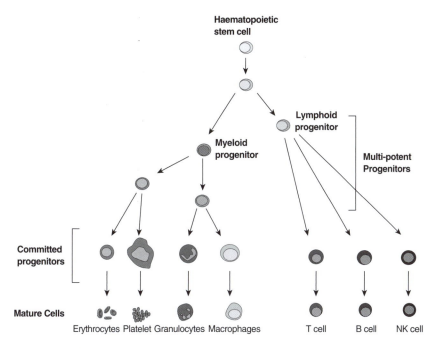

Figure 14.1 Haematopoiesis

along the **lymphoid cell line**, giving rise to **T-** and **B- lymphocytes and Natural Killer** (NK) cells (Hoffbrand and Moss, 2011; Brown, 2012). The question of which differentiation pathway a cell follows is complex and determined partly by chance and partly by the signals received by the **progenitor** cells in the form of transcription factors and haemopoietic growth factors. These in turn are produced according to the demands on the body at the time. Clearly, the presence of HSCs is essential to maintaining a healthy functioning **immune system**.

HSCT involves the replacement of the haematopoietic system or the restoration/'rescue' of immune and haematopoietic function following intensive chemotherapy, radiotherapy and/ or other forms of **immunosuppressive therapy**, which typically result in profound immuno-suppression and severe **pancytopenia**. This means that people undergoing HSCT are at high risk of infections, which are a major cause of morbidity and mortality (Anderson-Reitz, 2011). Although the immune system usually starts to recover within 1–3 weeks of receiving a trans-plant, this is a slow and gradual process. It may take several weeks for a normal **neutrophil** count (4–11 × 10^9/L) to be reached, and **immunodeficiency** (e.g. low helper T-cell count) may persist for many months following transplantation (Hoffbrand and Moss, 2011). Recipients will also experience **anaemia** and **thrombocytopenia** as a result of the effects of treatment on the stem cell population, placing them at further risk of complications.

Human leukocyte antigen (HLA) compatibility must also be considered in the context of HSCT. This is crucial when a patient is to receive a transplant from another person (**allo-geneic** transplantation). The HLA antigens are proteins encoded by a cluster of genes located on the short arm of chromosome 6 (Hoffbrand and Moss, 2011). The role of these proteins is to present antigenic material to T cells for recognition, with 'foreign' antigens provoking an immune response. Importantly, in the context of stem cell transplant from one person to another, there is a risk that the host's immune system will mount an immune response against the transplanted stem cells, or that the transplanted stem cells will recognize the host's cells as 'foreign' and mount an immune response against them. For these reasons, it is vital that donor and recipient are closely matched according to their HLA antigens through a process known as **tissue typing** (Hoffbrand and Moss, 2011).

The HLA proteins are divided into two classes. Class I antigens are termed HLA- A, -B and -C and are present on most nucleated cells. Class II antigens (HLA-DR, -DQ and -DP) are less widely distributed, but found on macrophages and B-lymphocytes (Hoffbrand and Moss, 2011; DeMeyer, 2009). An individual's HLA-type is inherited from his or her parents, 50% from each, so two siblings have a 1 in 4 chance of being identical. It is important that donor and recipient are HLA-matched because differences, especially in HLA-A, -B or -DR, will result in immune responses between donor and recipient, potentially leading to rejection (see later). A number of other HLA antigens also exist, but their significance is unclear in the context of SCT (DeMeyer, 2009). For patients without an HLA-matched donor, treatment options now include HLA-mismatched unrelated donors, umbilical cord blood, where mismatches are better tolerated and HLA-haploidentical family donors. However, T-cell depletion of the allograft is required to minimize potential graft rejection, although this increases the risk of disease relapse (Passweg et al., 2012b).

TYPES OF HAEMATOPOIETIC STEM CELL TRANSPLANT

There are three main types of HSCT – **autologous, allogeneic** and **syngeneic**. The first type of HSCT, autologous transplantation, uses the patient as the donor (Richardson and Atkinson, 2006). The patient is initially treated for their disease with an appropriate regime, which typically comprises cytotoxic chemotherapy. Stem cells are then harvested and stored whilst the patient is in remission. The patient is subsequently treated with high-dose chemotherapy (and possibly radiotherapy) and the stem cells are then re-infused to 'rescue' the patient from the subsequent profound pancytopenia (Hoffbrand and Moss, 2011). Autologous SCT is the most widely used type of HSCT (Gratwohl et al., 2010; Baldomero et al., 2011) with more than 20,000 of this type of transplant occurring in transplant centres throughout Europe in 2010 (Passweg et al., 2012a). Richardson and Atkinson (2006) note that the reduced toxicity and fewer side effects associated with autologous transplantation mean that it can be used in older adults and people who are unable to tolerate the more aggressive treatment associated with allogeneic HSCT; however, despite the reduced toxicity, the difficulty of the procedure should not be underestimated and expert care and support are still essential. Notably, there is also a greater risk of relapse associated with autologous HSCT. This is because tumour cells may contaminate the stem cell harvest and be reintroduced to the patient during the infusion (Hoffbrand and Moss, 2011).

The second type of transplant, allogeneic HSCT, involves the infusion of donated stem cells to a patient from either a related or unrelated donor. The first group to be considered as potential donors will be the patient's siblings due to the greatest likelihood of them being a compatible HLA tissue match. This is determined using a process called tissue typing. However, donors may also be found via unrelated donor registries. In the UK, these include organizations such as the Anthony Nolan Foundation and the British Bone Marrow Registry (see end of chapter). Similar organizations also exist in a number of other countries (UK Stem Cell Strategic Forum, 2010).

Since ethnic minority groups tend to be under-represented on these registers (Brown, 2010), for some patients, finding compatible donors can be very problematic.

Due to the fact that allogeneic HSCT uses stem cells from another person, it is a more complex procedure than that required for autologous HSCT, necessitating further immunosuppressive therapy in addition to treatment for the disease itself. Notably, one of the most serious risks associated with allogeneic HSCT is a condition known as **Graft-versus-Host Disease (GvHD)**, which occurs when the transplanted donor T (graft) cells mount immune responses to host antigens (Passweg et al., 2012b).

Ezzone (2010) notes that allogeneic HSCT has traditionally employed **myeloablative approaches**, which destroy the patient's bone marrow, resulting in severe myelosuppression, and placing the patient at risk of a number of other life-threatening organ toxicities. More recently, however, reduced-intensity non-myeloablative regimens (**'minigrafts'**) have been employed, which utilize lower dose conditioning treatments. The advantage of this is reduced toxicity, meaning that the treatment can be used for older patients, and for a wider range of conditions (Hoffbrand and Moss, 2011).

The third and least common type of transplant, syngeneic HSCT, involves transplanting stem cells from an identical twin. The advantage is that the twin is a perfect genetic match for the patient, so there is less likelihood of immunological response and graft rejection. As Richardson and Atkinson (2006) note, this makes syngeneic HSCT somewhat akin to an autologous transplant and for this reason, further immunosuppressive therapy is not required (Ezzone, 2010).

HSCT may also be categorized according to the source of stem cells, which can be harvested from the bone marrow, peripheral blood or umbilical cord blood.

Reflective activity

Consider the issue of donating stem cells. What do you think a potential donor needs to know in order to make a decision? Do you think there is a difference in the information required for sibling donor and unrelated donor transplants? Provide a rationale for your answer.

Find out the details of your country's HSCT register and arrangements for volunteering to donate.

STAGES OF HAEMATOPOIETIC STEM CELL TRANSPLANT

In terms of the treatment itself, Richardson and Atkinson (2006) assert that there are three key phases – pre-transplant, transplant and post-transplant.

Pre-transplant phase

In the pre-transplant phase, a range of physical and psychological assessments are performed to ensure that the patient is fit for the proposed treatment, and understands what the course of treatment involves. Ezzone (2010) notes that many of the procedures required during the pre-transplant phase are the same for all patients, regardless of type of transplant. Physical parameters assessed will include organ function (lung, kidney, liver and heart), infectious disease titres and disease staging. Fertility issues will also be discussed because HSCT will almost certainly impact on the patient's fertility. Where relevant, male patients should be offered the opportunity to bank sperm if this has not already been done prior to previous treatment. **Cryopreservation** of ova may also be possible for younger female patients, but this is only likely to be offered by specialist centres to certain groups of women, and the long-term success of this is currently unclear (Anderson-Reitz, 2011; Porcu et al., 2013). In the pre-transplant phase, allogeneic transplant patients will also undergo tissue typing to identify potential donors.

Assessment of potential donors is also essential at this stage. Additional to HLA-typing to determine compatibility between donor and recipient, the donor must be assessed for physical fitness to undergo donation, as well as being screened for infectious diseases that may be transmitted at transplantation. Of particular importance will be HIV and CMV (**cytomegalovirus**) status because transmission of either of these viruses to the donor during transplantation could be life threatening. The donor will also need to have full explanation of the potential risks involved, and be provided with the opportunity to ask questions and to discuss any concerns prior to giving consent (Thain, 2006).

Psychological assessment is of utmost importance, especially during the pre-transplant phase because it is known that a significant proportion of patients undergoing HSCT experience issues of a psychological nature. Recent longitudinal studies have indicated that between 14–90% of SCT survivors report psychological distress (Sun et al., 2011), and other issues such as mood disturbances, anxiety and depression may also negatively impact their recovery and long-term outcomes (DeMarinis et al., 2009). Patients, who are **immunosuppressed** as a result of conditioning treatments, may be required to be isolated in a single hospital room for up to four weeks to protect them from infection. Typical reactions during this period may include feelings of sadness, loneliness, depression, frustration, anxiety and hostility (Pulgar et al., 2012). The transplant procedure itself is complex and intense, associated with a range of life-threatening side effects and has the potential to cause prolonged psychological distress and emotional issues (Cooke et al., 2009). It has been postulated that the strongest predictor of long-term emotional health post-transplantation is emotional health prior to and during transplant (Jim et al., 2012). Pre-transplant assessment is, therefore, important in order to screen for emotional distress, identify existing or potential psychological issues, determine the effectiveness of coping strategies and to ascertain patient support needs (Trask et al., 2002; Cooke et al., 2009). Horne et al. (2013), in a qualitative study amongst staff in three UK transplant centres, suggest that, in the UK at least, this is rarely performed and is an area of transplant practice that could be developed.

Prior to transplantation, it is also essential that potential donors undergo psychological assessment in addition to the necessary physical investigations. Issues such as anxiety, uncertainty and feelings of guilt or pressure to donate may be evident (Munzenberger et al., 1999) and it is important that these are detected and addressed as early as possible to prevent negative psychological reactions to the experience of donation. Such reactions may include depression, withdrawal, lowered self-esteem, identity problems, guilt, resentment and anger (Weiner et al., 2007) and may be particularly prevalent if complications or disease relapse occurs.

Conditioning is the term used to denote the treatment given to the patient immediately prior to transplant. The exact form of this treatment varies according to the patient's illness and the type of transplant (Quinn and Stephens, 2006), and may include high-dose chemotherapy, **total body irradiation** (TBI) and **biological therapies**. Both Richardson and Atkinson (2006) and Ezzone (2010) detail a number of conditioning regimes and their indications. For example, a combination of high-dose **cyclophosphamide** and TBI is a common conditioning regime in haematological malignancy. HSCT is also used for solid tumour treatment, as noted in Table 14.1. This is most likely to be autologous HSCT, and the conditioning regime will typically comprise high doses of multi-agent chemotherapy.

The purpose of the conditioning regime is three-fold: (1) eradication of malignant cells; (2) immunosuppression to prevent rejection; and (3) to create marrow space for the transplanted stem cells (Richardson and Atkinson, 2006). Due to the intensive nature of traditional conditioning regimens, a wide range of acute side effects may be experienced by patients, including profound bone marrow depression, nausea, vomiting, **tumour lysis syndrome** and mucositis. Table 14.2 summarizes the main side effects and complications of HSCT, both early and late. Ultimately, most of the patient's organs and body systems can be affected, but during conditioning itself, it is the side effects of the drugs and radiotherapy (if used) that are the main concerns. Supporting the patient at this time can be challenging. It is not only the physical effects of the conditioning regime that may impact on the patient; it is also a very demanding time psychologically. Severe physical side effects can lead patients to question whether they have made the right choice, and research suggests that at this time, patients may experience psychological and emotional distress, anxiety and fears for

Table 14.1 Indications for HSCT

	Malignant	Non-malignant
Autologous	Multiple myeloma/plasma cell disorders	Autoimmune diseases
	Relapsed non-Hodgkin lymphoma	
	Relapsed Hodgkin lymphoma	
	Acute myeloid leukaemia (poor risk first, or second, complete remission – no donor)	
	Relapsed germ cell tumours	
	Neuroblastoma	
	Ewing's sarcoma	
Allogeneic	Acute myeloid leukaemia (poor risk first, or second, complete remission)	Bone marrow failure (e.g. severe aplastic anaemia)
	Acute lymphoblastic leukaemia (poor risk first, or second, complete remission)	Haemoglobinopathies
	Myelodysplastic syndromes	Immune deficiencies
	Relapsed non-Hodgkin lymphoma	Inborn errors of metabolism
	Chronic myeloid leukaemia (not chronic phase 1, unless poor response to tyrosine kinase inhibitors)	
	Multiple myeloma/plasma cell disorders	
	Chronic lymphocytic leukaemia	
	Relapsed Hodgkin disease	

Source: Based on Gratwohl et al. (2010); Baldomero et al (2011); Cutler (2012)

Table 14.2   Early and late complications of HSCT

Early complications	Infections – bacterial, viral, fungal, protozoal
	Gastrointestinal – nausea, vomiting, diarrhoea, mucositis
	Haemorrhage and haemorrhagic cystitis (high-dose cyclophosphamide)
	Fluid, electrolyte and nutritional imbalance
	Anaemia
	Pulmonary complications – infection, interstitial pneumonitis
	Renal toxicity
	Hepatic toxicity – veno-occlusive disease
	Acute Graft-versus-Host Disease (GvHD)
	Graft failure
	Psychological issues, including the protective isolation experience, anxiety
Late complications	Infections – cytomegalovirus (CMV) and *Pneumocystis carinii* pneumonia
	Chronic GvHD
	Infertility
	Relapse
	Psychological issues
	Haemostatic problems, including venous thromboembolism, bleeding complications, arterial thrombosis, premature atherosclerosis
	Ocular disturbances, including microvascular retinopathy, optic disk oedema, haemorrhagic complications, infectious retinitis
	Pulmonary effects, including restrictive lung disease, chronic obstructive lung disease
	Hepatic complications, including Hepatitis B and C, iron overload
	Complications of bones and joints, including avascular necrosis of bone
	Endocrine dysfunction, including hypothyroidism, autoimmune disease, gonadal failure

Source: Based on Richardson and Atkinson (2006); Anderson-Reitz (2011); Stussi and Tsakiris (2012) and Socie et al. (2003)

the future. It is imperative that nurses and other professionals take the time to explain the processes involved and potential side effects of the conditioning regimen and transplantation process and to listen to patients' concerns and answer questions (Quinn and Stephens, 2006). This will also allow for the timely identification of needs and the implementation of appropriate interventions aimed at preventing or minimizing complications.

The relatively recent advent of **reduced-intensity conditioning regimes** (RIC) has lessened the risks associated with toxicities for some transplant patients, which in turn has enabled allogeneic HSCT to be offered to patients who previously would not have been considered appropriate candidates for such treatments. These patients traditionally included those aged over 60, or those with co-morbidities who were considered to be at high risk of transplant-related mortality. HSCTs involving reduced-intensity conditioning regimens rely on an immune response from donor cells against residual disease, rather than amelioration of the diseased marrow, and are associated with less severe side effects and reduced risk of organ toxicities and related complications (Copelan, 2006). The outcomes of this type of transplant are still being studied, and standard SCT remains the treatment of choice in younger patients (Shelburne and Bevans, 2009; Ljungman et al., 2010).

Transplant phase

The actual transplant itself is often uneventful, and patients may experience a sense of anticlimax following the procedure (Brown, 2010; Richardson and Atkinson, 2006). Cells are administered by intravenous infusion, and the patient is likely to be pre-medicated with a steroid and antihistamine to prevent or minimize any reaction to the donor cells or **cryopreservative** (dimethylsulfoxide DMSO) in which the cells may have been stored. Cells that have been cryopreserved, as is always the case with autologous HSCT, are slowly thawed in a water bath at approximately 37°C immediately prior to infusion. Patients receiving stem cells for an allogeneic transplant are more likely to receive fresh cells, particularly if they are harvested from bone marrow. Infusion of stem cells normally occurs over a 60–90 minute period, during which a nurse will stay with the patient, closely monitoring vital observations and for any sign of allergic reaction (Sauer-Heilborn et al., 2004).

Following the stem cell infusions is a period of waiting for the cells to migrate to the cavities of the bone marrow and to start the process of haematopoiesis (**engraftment**). This can take between 10 and 21 days, although this is sometimes even longer in unrelated donor HSCT due to the greater immunosuppression necessary. This period may be difficult and challenging for both patients and their family. Understandably, they will be eager to know if the transplant has worked but until there are indications that engraftment has occurred, there is no way of knowing this, which can be very stressful. Monitoring of blood counts assumes high importance for the majority of transplant recipients as they search for tell-tale signs, such as increased white cell counts, especially **neutrophils** (Quinn and Stephens, 2006). The key issues for healthcare staff involved in the care of patients in the post-transplant period focus on ongoing assessment, as well as physical and psychological support of the patient and their family.

Reflective activity

You may be involved in caring for a patient who will have a HSCT in the future. How would you explain to that person what the process will involve and what they should expect? What strategies can you use to support the patient and their family during the transplant phase?

Post-transplant phase

The physical aspects of care in the post-transplant period relate mainly to preventing, recognizing and managing complications resulting from the conditioning treatment (Quinn and Stephens, 2006). The main potential complications are listed in Table 14.2, although this list is not exhaustive.

The intensity of the conditioning regime results in profound bone marrow suppression and subsequent anaemia, neutropenia and thrombocytopenia. How long this pancytopenia lasts depends on a number of factors, including the conditioning treatment itself, the origin of the stem cells and type of transplant, and whether haematopoietic growth factors are used to stimulate recovery. Patients undergoing allogeneic HSCT will receive other immunosuppressive therapy, such as ciclosporin, further delaying that recovery.

Despite advances in treatments, infections remain major causes of morbidity and mortality in patients undergoing HSCT (Anderson-Reitz, 2011). During the post-transplant phase, patients are susceptible to all forms of infective organisms, including gram-positive and gram-negative bacteria, viruses, fungi and protozoa. This susceptibility means that protective isolation is usually considered necessary. In most transplant centres, the patient is nursed in a single room with high-efficiency particulate air (HEPA) filtration or laminar airflow to reduce entry of airborne organisms. However, procedures vary quite widely, and the value of isolation has been questioned due to the lack of robust research evidence (National Institute for Health and Care Excellence, 2003).

Patients need to be monitored carefully for signs of infection, and treatment must be initiated promptly if **pyrexia** occurs. Typically, this is two temperature readings >38°C one hour apart, or one reading >38.5°C and represents a medical emergency. Initially, treatment will be with broad-spectrum antibiotics according to local protocols, with changes made if a specific organism is isolated or the pyrexia fails to respond. Further information about the management of infection in neutropenic patients can be found in Chapter 12. Other procedures required to minimize infection include scrupulous oral and general hygiene for the patient and vigilant attention to hand hygiene by all healthcare professionals involved in the patient's care, as well as visiting family members and friends. Protective isolation (reverse-barrier nursing) procedures, such as wearing protective clothing, on the part of visitors and staff are also commonly implemented during this phase. Patients are given prophylactic antiviral and antifungal drugs and, in some centres, will also receive prophylactic antibiotics (Brown, 2010).

In spite of all these procedures, it is probable that most patients will experience some type of infection during the post-transplant period, despite protective isolation. As noted by Quinn and Stephens (2006), many of these will be due to endogenous organisms. Of particular concern to HSCT patients are opportunistic infections such as *Pneumocystis carinii*, *Aspergillus* and *Cytomegalovirus* (CMV) (Hoffbrand and Moss, 2011). All these can cause **pneumonia**, which may be very difficult to treat and may lead to death. **Interstitial pneumonitis** caused by CMV is a frequent cause of death in HSCT patients. In allogeneic HSCT, if both patient and donor are CMV-seronegative, all blood products administered should be CMV-negative, such is the seriousness of the threat of transmission.

In addition to neutropenia, patients will also experience anaemia and thrombocytopenia during the post-transplant phase due to bone marrow depression. These effects are typically managed through regular blood product transfusions. Red cell transfusions need only be given once or twice a week, depending on haemoglobin levels and symptoms, whereas platelet transfusions may be required daily during the nadir in platelet count, until the count reaches $>20 \times 10^9$/L. It should be noted that there is a greater risk of major haemorrhage if the platelet count falls below 20×10^9/L. Patients should also be monitored for **petechiae**, bruising and other signs of spontaneous bleeding, and female patients will have their menstruation suppressed (e.g. using norethisterone), to further prevent the risk of haemorrhage.

Nausea and vomiting are well-recognized problems associated with chemotherapy and/or radiotherapy (Coates et al., 1983; Molassiotis and Borjeson, 2006), which can be adequately controlled for many patients with the timely administration of anti-emetics. However, the intensity of many conditioning regimes means that there is a very high risk of nausea and vomiting for patients undergoing HSCT (Einhorn et al., 2005; see also Chapter 12), but it is imperative that these conditions are monitored closely in HSCT patients and managed aggressively. Vomiting can become a serious problem if it cannot be brought under control, leading to **electrolyte disturbance** and nutritional deficits. Patients often require supportive interventions, such as electrolyte replacement, hydration therapy and/or total parenteral nutrition (TPN). The range of anti-emetics now available is wider than ever, but nausea and vomiting continue to be a challenge in this patient population (Navari, 2013).

The problem of **oropharyngeal mucositis** also represents a considerable challenge for many HSCT recipients. This is directly related to the impact of the conditioning treatment on the reproduction of mucosa and of the administration of cytotoxic drugs such as busulphan and melphalan, and TBI, which are particularly toxic to the oral mucosa. This damage can be exacerbated by super-imposed infections, such as **candidiasis**, which are associated with immunosuppression and the use of antibiotics. Mucositis is very painful, and can result in the patient being unable to swallow, aggravating dehydration and nutritional imbalances. A strict oral hygiene regime involving regular assessment and the use of mouthwashes can help to reduce the risk of super-imposed infection, but the mucositis may be so painful that performing this becomes impossible for patients (Quinn and Stephens, 2006). Local anaesthetic mouthwashes may help to alleviate the pain, but many patients require parenteral opiate infusions to control the pain (Richardson and Atkinson, 2006).

GvHD is a problem unique to allogeneic HSCT that occurs in the post-transplant phase. Caused by an immunologic reaction of the transplanted stem cells towards the host's tissues, GvHD is classed in relation to when it manifests, with acute GvHD emerging before 100 days post-transplant, and chronic GvHD occurring more than 100 days post-transplant (Hoffbrand and Moss, 2011). The patterns of occurrence are different and Hoffbrand and Moss (2011) note that acute GvHD affects the skin, GI tract and liver, with skin rashes most commonly apparent on the palms, soles, face and ears, whereas chronic GvHD typically affects joints, the oral mucosa and lacrimal glands. Liver involvement in acute GvHD manifests in raised bilirubin and liver enzymes, and gastrointestinal involvement is characterized by green, offensive-smelling diarrhoea.

Mild (grade 1) acute GvHD has a good outcome and requires little or no treatment. Indeed, this is often viewed as a positive sign because it is also associated with lower risk of relapse through the graft-versus-disease effect. This occurs when the donor T-cells recognize remaining malignant cells as 'foreign' and mount an immune response. Moderate (grade 2) GvHD does require treatment to prevent progression to grade 3 (severe) or grade 4 (life-threatening) (see Table 14.3). GvHD is a difficult problem to manage and can be challenging for healthcare professionals. Preventative measures include immunosuppressive therapy with ciclosporin, with or without methotrexate, commenced immediately prior to transplant. T-cell depletion of donor stem cells can also decrease the risk of GvHD, but this is associated with increased risk of relapse. As Richardson and Atkinson (2006) note, there is a fine balance between prevention of GvHD and reducing the incidence of relapse. If treatment of acute GvHD is required, this will usually be with high-dose steroids (1–2 mg/kg/day IV). Other options include anti-thymocyte globulin, monoclonal antibodies and thalidomide. Patients who experience acute GvHD are also at increased risk of infection due to the disruption of natural barriers and immunosuppression, and of malnutrition due to malabsorption.

Another serious acute side effect of HSCT is a syndrome of painful **hepatomegaly, jaundice** and fluid retention known as **sinusoidal obstruction syndrome**. This potentially fatal

Table 14.3   Acute Graft-versus-Host Disease

Grade	Skin	Liver (bilirubin, μmol/L)	Gut (diarrhoea)
1	Rash <25% body surface	20–35	500–1000ml/day
2	Rash 25–50% body surface	35–80	1000–1500ml/day
3	Erythroderma >50% body surface	80–150	1500–2500ml/day
4	Bullae, moist desquamation	>150	>2500ml/day; severe pain +/– fistula formation

Source: From Hoffbrand and Moss (2011) and Anderson-Reitz (2011)

condition is caused when damaged sinusoidal endothelium sloughs and then obstructs the hepatic circulation. In severe sinusoidal obstruction syndrome, renal and respiratory failure may occur. Total body irradiation, busulphan, cyclophosphamide and many other preparative agents cause sinusoidal obstruction syndrome, which limits maximal doses. Because there is no effective treatment for the syndrome, its prevention is critical and the patient should undergo vigilant monitoring for signs and symptoms. Replacing cyclophosphamide with fludarabine appears to reduce the risk of sinusoidal obstruction syndrome (Copelan, 2006).

The immediate post-transplant period, therefore, poses many challenges for patients, carers and staff. The patient is acutely ill and vulnerable, and needs a great deal of supportive care from the multidisciplinary team. There is high morbidity and significant mortality associated with the procedure, especially in unrelated donor transplantation. The most common causes of death in the early post-transplant period are infection, acute GvHD and graft failure.

The post-transplant period is characterized by uncertainty and waiting whilst the team monitor and treat the effects of the conditioning treatment and support the patient and family members through to discharge. From a psychological perspective, transplant recipients often require intensive support at this time. Not only is the patient faced with considerable changes to their appearance and body image, but they may also experience significant levels of stress, anxiety and uncertainty for their future (Sun et al., 2011). These issues may be further compounded by the effects of fatigue, pain and other physical symptoms. Health professionals must therefore work to maintain a therapeutic relationship with the patient and their family. The provision of adequate psychological and emotional support is essential at this time. This will require the appropriate use of reassurance, encouragement and motivation, as well as input from specialist psychologists, counsellors and patient and carer support networks (see also Chapter 22).

LATE EFFECTS

Discharge from hospital following HSCT is often greatly anticipated by the patient and their family; however, it is important to recognize that this does not mean that the patient can immediately return to normal life. During the immediate post-transplant phase, there are still a great many challenges facing the patient and potential complications that can occur during immune reconstitution, which may take up to two years to be established (Passweg et al., 2012b). As such, the patient is often required to return to hospital as an outpatient for several weeks or months for monitoring and supportive interventions, such as medications, immunosuppressive therapy and blood transfusions.

While many long-term transplant survivors enjoy general good health, for others, complete restoration of health status is not achieved in the long term and the deleterious impact of late effects on physical and psychological function may be considerable (Mohty and Mohty, 2011). Aside from the infective complications such as CMV and *Pneumocystis carinii* discussed previously, the main complications occurring late in the post-transplant period are disease relapse, **graft failure**, infertility and chronic GvHD (allogeneic transplants).

Disease relapse is a risk in the post-transplant period and the most common cause of death in the first year following both autologous and allogeneic transplant (Nivison-Smith et al., 2000). This may be attributed to a number of factors, including the reinfusion of malignant cells contained in autologous stem cell infusions, or residual malignant cells not being eradicated by the conditioning regimens or a lack of graft-versus-disease effect. Graft failure also represents a considerable risk at this time.

Chronic GvHD may evolve from acute GvHD, or may develop independently (Hoffbrand and Moss, 2011), and is the main cause of mortality following allogeneic HSCT (Wingard, 2002). This can be a complex and debilitating condition that patients may struggle with for prolonged periods (Anderson-Reitz, 2011). It can often lead to considerable psychological distress, due to its impact on appearance, body image and activities of daily living and has the potential to impact markedly on quality of life.

Most patient who receive TBI as part of conditioning will be rendered infertile, and many patients who receive high doses of chemotherapy will experience transient or permanent fertility problems. As discussed previously, males should be offered sperm banking prior to commencing treatment, and should be encouraged to take this up (Quinn and Stephens, 2006). For females, the options are less straightforward, but may include embryo cryopreservation, or oocyte or ovarian cryopreservation. Dannie (2006) discusses the options in more depth, but it should be noted that oocyte and ovarian cryopreservation are not widely available.

Other late effects may also include ocular conditions such as **microvascular retinopathy**, **optic disk oedema** and **infectious retinitis**, pulmonary complications such as **restrictive lung disease** and **chronic obstructive lung disease**, liver abnormalities, haemostatic problems and complications of the bones and joints (Socie et al., 2003). The onset, severity, treatment options and response to treatment are influenced by a variety of factors, including patient age, gender and co-morbidities, disease stage, conditioning regime and graft source (Mohty and Mohty, 2011).

In addition to physical effects, many transplant recipients will also experience the continuing psychological effects of the illness and treatment, such as fear of relapse, loss of control and continuing uncertainty of outcome. This may result in depression and have a lasting impact on quality of life.

Potential psychological effects of HSCT

- Alteration in body image
- Anxiety
- Fear of recurrence
- Sleep disturbances

(Continued)

(Continued)

- Depression
- Loss of control
- Altered quality of life
- Decrease in social function
- Post-traumatic stress disorder
- Loss of identity
- Alteration in family roles

Source: Cooke et al. (2009)

Furthermore, there are increased reports of fatigue, lack of energy, sleep disturbances, cognitive difficulties and problems with sexuality and intimacy among patients post-HSCT (Socie et al., 2003; Yi and Syrjala, 2009; Packman et al., 2010). These issues have the potential to impact on family and social relationships, self-esteem and impede the ability to return to work or school, further decreasing quality of life. Interventions aimed at improving psychosocial function are therefore crucial at this time and will include strategies to prevent and minimize emotional distress, promote sleep and to restore social functioning (Rischer et al., 2009; Packman et al., 2010). A summary of interventions that may be used to address the psychological effects of HSCT is presented next.

Strategies that can be used to address the psychological effects of HSCT

- Assessment and ongoing monitoring
- Anti-depressant medication
- Psycho-educational sessions
- Support groups
- Social support
- Cognitive–behavioural therapy
- Complementary and alternative therapies

Source: Cooke et al. (2009)

CHAPTER SUMMARY

Haematopoietic stem cell transplantation (HSCT) is an established curative option for a wide range of malignant and non-malignant conditions. Despite advances in treatment and supportive care, HSCT remains an intense treatment associated with high rates of morbidity and mortality. Patients undergoing HSCT and their families have comprehensive needs and will require considerable physiological, psychological and emotional support during all phases of the transplant process. This care must be provided by skilled healthcare professionals who understand the complexities of the treatment and its potential implications and effect on survivorship and quality of life issues.

Reflective activity

Identify your local SCT unit and arrange a visit. Write some learning objectives before you visit and reflect on what you learned. What did the staff see as the biggest challenges in working in SCT?

Key learning points

- The pluripotent or haematopoietic stem cell (HSC) gives rise to all types of blood cell, and is also capable of self-renewal.
- HSCT involves the replacement or rescue of the haematopoietic system following intensive chemotherapy, radiotherapy and/or other forms of immunosuppressive therapy.
- The three main types of HSCT are autologous (patient is donor), allogeneic (from a related or unrelated donor) and syngeneic (identical twin is donor).
- The three key phases to treatment are pre-transplant, transplant and post-transplant. Conditioning is the term used to denote the treatment given immediately prior to transplant, such as high-dose chemotherapy or total body irradiation (TBI) in order to:

  - Eradicate malignant cells,
  - Cause immunosuppression to prevent rejection, and
  - Create marrow space for the transplanted stem cells.

- Acute side effects include profound bone marrow depression, nausea, vomiting, tumour lysis syndrome and mucositis. Late effects include infertility, microvascular retinopathy, pulmonary complications, liver abnormalities, haemostatic problems and complications of the bones and joints.
- Graft-versus-Host Disease (GvHD) is caused by an immunologic reaction of the transplanted stem cells towards the host's tissues in allogeneic HSCT.
- Physical management relates mainly to preventing, recognizing and managing complications resulting from the conditioning treatment.
- The psychological effects of the illness and treatment, such as fear of relapse, loss of control and continuing uncertainty of outcome should not be underestimated.

Recommended further reading

- Hoffbrand, A.V. and Moss, P.A.H. (2011) *Essential Haematology*, 6th edn. Chichester, UK: Wiley-Blackwell.
- Mohty, B., and Mohty, M. (2011) 'Long-term complications and side effects after allogeneic hematopoietic stem cell transplantation: an update', *Blood Cancer Journal*, 1(16): 1–5.

(Continued)

(Continued)

- Sun, C.L., Francisco, L., Baker, K., Weisdorf, D.J., Forman, S.J. and Bhatia, S. (2011) 'Adverse psychological outcomes in long-term survivors of hematopoietic cell transplantation: a report from the Bone Marrow Transplant Survivor Study (BMTSS)', *Blood*, 118(17): 4723-31.

The following websites may also be of interest:

- Anthony Nolan www.anthonynolan.org/
- British Bone Marrow Registry www.nhsbt.nhs.uk/bonemarrow/
- Center for International Bone Marrow Transplant Research www.cibmtr.org/pages/index.aspx

15 BIOLOGICAL THERAPY

ANOOP HARIDASS AND HELEN NEVILLE-WEBBE

Chapter outline

- Small molecule tyrosine kinase inhibitors (TKIs) and similar drugs
- Monoclonal antibodies
- Cancer vaccines
- Biological response modifiers
- Colony stimulating factors (CSF)/ growth factors
- Psychosocial aspects of treatment

INTRODUCTION

The immune system consists of specialized cells that can sense, adapt and respond to a variety of challenges that the body is exposed to. Cancer cells negotiate this sophisticated detection system and escape destruction by it. This is emerging as one of the newer hallmarks of cancer (Hanahan and Weinberg, 2011). Therapies that can turn this system into an ally, so-called **biological therapies**, have huge potential in the management of cancer, and have been investigated in depth over the last few decades, with promising early results.

Biological therapies are drugs that use the body's immune system to fight cancer or lessen the effect of other anticancer treatments. Targeted cancer therapies are drugs or other substances that block the growth and spread of cancer by interfering with specific molecules involved in tumour growth and progression. These therapies, therefore, aim to destroy cancer cells (which contain a specific molecule) but not normal cells (which contain few or none of the specific molecules). Normal cells are less affected by the treatment and less likely to result in side effects for the patient. The first targeted treatment used was tamoxifen (Cole et al., 1971), which targeted the **oestrogen hormone receptor** (ER) in patients with breast cancer. Biological therapies are used as umbrella terms to include a wide variety of anticancer agents, which include:

1. Small molecule tyrosine kinase inhibitors (TKIs) and similar drugs
2. Monoclonal antibodies
3. Cancer vaccines
4. Biological response modifiers
5. Colony stimulating factors (CSF)/growth factors

Treatments are designed to target either **signalling pathways** inside a cell or **receptors** on a cell wall. An overview of the underlying principles behind each of the groups of drugs and examples of commonly used drugs in each of these groups will be addressed in this chapter, in addition to the impact on patients.

Small molecule tyrosine kinase inhibitors and similar drugs

Cancer cells have complex mechanisms to promote growth and proliferation. These include utilization of normal substances in the body as triggers for growth (growth factors). The signals from these substances are translated to actual growth triggers via signalling chains in the cancer cell. A better understanding of the molecular basis of cancer through research has led to the development of several new small molecules, which are capable of blocking these signals at various levels in the chain, thereby preventing growth. A vital link in the signalling chain is a group of enzymes called **receptor tyrosine kinases** (RTK) and inhibitors of this group of enzymes are called **tyrosine kinase inhibitors** (TKI). Several drugs that belong to this group are in regular clinical use for different types of cancers, ranging from leukaemia to lung cancer. Due to their small size they can penetrate far and wide into the tissues and reach protected areas of the body like the brain, which other anticancer agents like chemotherapy may not.

As these drugs are targeted against a specific molecule in the cancer cell, testing the cancer tissue (usually a **biopsy** specimen) for the presence of these targets is usually necessary; they are likely to be ineffective in the absence of the target. As a result of this, these drugs will only be useful in a smaller subgroup of cancers that express these targets. The subgroup can range from as low as 5%, for example in the case of epidermal growth factor receptor (EGFR) mutations in lung cancers (Riely et al., 2006) to as high as 80%, as in the case of bcr-abL in Chronic Myeloid Leukaemia (CML) (Druker et al., 2006). These drugs are usually available in oral form (tablets), which are taken daily. The schedules may range over several days to weeks with intermittent gaps. At present, most of these drugs are used in isolation, but there are studies in progress that are testing to see if combining these drugs with other biological agents or chemotherapy can be more effective.

Although the effects of targeted therapies on normal cells are likely to be minimal, some can cause significant physical side effects (see Table 15.1) such as fatigue, skin rashes and diarrhoea which can also lead to psychosocial problems such as distress and embarrassment, or a reluctance to go out or be with others.

EGFR TK targeting agents

Epidermal growth factor receptors (EGFR) are over-expressed, that is, present in increased numbers, in a broad range of cancers and serve as drivers for growth of the cancer cells. Drugs that can block this receptor pathway have proven to be important weapons in the fight against cancer. Some of the small molecule inhibitors that belong to this group are:

Erlotinib (Tarceva®): Erlotinib belongs to a family of drugs that inhibit the EGFR. Certain types of lung cancer, like adenocarcinoma, have mutations in the EGFR pathway that make

Table 15.1 Small molecule tyrosine kinase inhibitors and similar drugs

	Target	Cancers treated	Posology	Common side effects	Similar agents
EGFR TK targeting agents					
Erlotinib	EGF (erbB1 or HER1) RTK	Metastatic non-small-cell lung cancer with EGFR activating mutations	Oral tablet 150 mg daily	Skin rash, diarrhoea, fatigue, shortness of breath, liver function (blood) test abnormalities	Gefitinib (Iressa®)
Lapatinib	HER2-neu (EGFR2 or erb B2) RTK	Metastatic Her2+ breast cancer	Oral tablet 1250–1500 mg daily	Diarrhoea, redness and soreness of palms and soles, nausea, heart muscle weakening, liver function (blood) test abnormalities	None
VEGF RTK targeting agents					
Sunitinib	VEGF RTK, C-kit (CD117), PDGF RTK	Metastatic kidney cancer Early and advanced GIST Advanced gastrointestinal neuroendocrine cancer	Tablet 37.5–50 mg oral daily either 4 weeks on and 2 weeks off, or continuous	High blood pressure, fatigue, diarrhoea, hand–foot syndrome and rashes	Sorafenib (Nexavar®), Pazopanib (Votrient®)

(Continued)

Table 15.1 (Continued)

Other TK targeting agents	Target	Cancers treated	Posology	Common side effects	Similar agents
Imatinib	bcr-abl TK, C-kit (CD117), PDGFRα TK	CML Advanced GIST	Oral tablet 400–800 mg daily	Fluid retention – ankle swelling/puffy eyes, nausea, diarrhoea, fatigue, muscle cramps and rashes	Dasatinib (Sprycel®), Nilotinib (Tasigna®)
Vemurafenib	V600E mutated B-raf	Metastatic melanoma	Tablet 960 mg twice daily oral	Joint pain, skin rash, fatigue, light sensitivity, nausea, hair thinning, squamous skin tumours, heart rhythm abnormalities	None
Temsirolimus	mTOR (mammalian target of rapamycin)	Advanced kidney cancer	IV infusion 25 mg/week	Fatigue, drop in blood counts, rash, mouth ulcers, nausea, change in blood biochemistry (phosphate, glucose, creatine, cholesterol), liver function abnormalities. Most of the side effects when they occur tend to be tolerable and reversible. Regular monitoring of blood chemistry and counts is advisable.	Everolimus (Afinitor®)

this an attractive option in treating patients with advanced disease. Clinically, patients with no smoking history, who are female, of Asian ethnicity and have adenocarcinoma type of lung cancer, appear to benefit more from this treatment (Shepard et al., 2005).

Lapatinib (Tyverb®): This drug is used in conjunction with chemotherapy to treat advanced breast cancer (Geyer et al., 2006). It blocks the RTK for a growth factor receptor called HER2 that is over-expressed in 15–20% of breast cancers. The smaller size of the lapatinib molecule allows it to penetrate into protected tissue areas, specifically the brain, unlike other HER2 targeted drugs and this is an increasing area of use for this agent.

VEGF RTK targeting agents

The ability to induce the growth of new blood vessels to act as conduits for nutrition and oxygen to the cancer cell (a process called **angiogenesis**) is considered one of the hallmarks of cancer (Hanahan and Weinberg, 2011). A group of growth factors called VEGF (**vascular endothelial growth factor**) are the main agents that trigger the process of new blood vessel formation in the tissues. Blocking the VEGF pathway can be an efficient way of curtailing the growth of the cancer by depriving the cancer cell of new nutrients and oxygen that the blood vessels can supply.

Sunitinib (Sutent®) was developed as a TKI that targeted multiple RTKs, including VEGF RTK, a growth factor involved in the generation of new blood vessels that certain cancer cells use to create new sources of nutrition and oxygen to fuel their growth. It is mostly used in the management of advanced kidney cancer (Motzer et al., 2009), a disease that is resistant to conventional chemotherapy treatment options. It has also been found to be useful in the treatment of GIST (gastrointestinal and stomach tumours), which become resistant to imatinib (Demetri et al., 2006).

Other TK targeting agents

Imatinib (Gleevec®): Imatinib was one of the earliest biological therapy drugs to be discovered. Imatinib is a TKI that inhibits the bcr-abl TK found in 80% of chronic myeloid leukaemia (CML) cells. The drug has had a significant impact in controlling the disease, improving survival, and has very low toxicity. It has also been found to be effective in treating rare types of advanced sarcoma that arise in the gastrointestinal tract called GIST, which are unresponsive to any other type of systemic treatment.

Vemurafenib (Zelboraf®): This is a new oral drug used in the treatment of advanced melanoma, the most lethal form of skin cancer, that blocks an important signalling pathway (V600E mutated B-raf) and improves survival in patients with this cancer (Flaherty et al., 2010). It is hoped that drugs of this type will provide better outcomes for this form of cancer, which has quite a dismal outlook once it has spread from its site of origin.

Temsirolimus (Torisel®): mTOR (mammalian target of rapamycin) is an important intracellular enzyme (kinase) which can coordinate and interpret several signals from other pathways inside the cell, which deal with growth, proliferation, angiogenesis and cell survival. It is over-activated in a large number of cancers. Inhibition of mTOR can have a knock-on effect on several signalling pathways, leading to programmed cell death (apoptosis). Several agents have been developed that can block this kinase and after early success in treating advanced renal cancer (Hudes et al., 2007), trials in several other tumour types, including breast, brain and pancreatic cancer are ongoing.

MONOCLONAL ANTIBODIES (MOAB)

Antibodies are proteins produced by the immune system to help fight infections. They can be synthesized in the laboratory and targeted to specific molecules in the cancer cell, resulting in prevention of cancer cell growth and replication, and prevention of angiogenesis. **Monoclonal antibodies** can also be considered as targeted treatment because they are very specific to the molecule against which they are targeted. This means that a similar method of testing for targets in the cancer cells is required for this group of drugs as well. Some of the most effective anticancer drugs to be discovered recently belong to this group. Unlike the small molecules, the MoAbs work by binding to the target molecule on the cancer cell surface and initiating an immune reaction that destroys the cell or by blocking the molecule (usually a growth factor or its receptor) and preventing the effects of growth factors on the cancer cell.

As these are proteins, they can only be given in intravenous (IV) form as a drip or **subcutaneous infusion** over a short period of time. Trials indicate that the subcutaneous route is welcomed by patients (Pivot et al., 2013). MoAbs are relatively large molecules that can be inhibited by normal barriers, like the barrier between the brain and the blood where they may be unable to penetrate the tissue. The protein nature of these drugs also means that they can trigger severe allergic reactions in a very small proportion of patients, which makes monitoring during administration necessary. Other side effects may include fatigue, flu-like symptoms and diarrhoea, depending on the specific treatment administered. MoAbs can also act as couriers to carry either chemotherapy agents or a radioactive isotope (called radio-immunotherapy) to specific targets on the cancer cell by chemically tagging such agents onto the antibody molecule itself. Agents such as ibritumomab tiuxetan (Zinzani et al., 2010) are used for **radio-immunotherapy** of B-cell non-Hodgkin lymphoma that is no longer responsive to standard therapies. Some of the commonly used MoAbs are listed and also in Table 15.2.

Trastuzumab (Herceptin®): Trastuzumab is a humanized MoAb, which is used in the treatment of both early (Piccart-Gebhart et al., 2005) and advanced breast cancer. This drug was instrumental in instigating a widespread interest in developing similar drugs due to its efficacy in controlling HER2+ breast cancer, a disease which only makes up 15–20% of all breast cancer but has a disproportionately high mortality due to its aggressive biological behaviour. Conjugate drugs with a chemotherapy molecule attached to the trastuzumab antibody (called TDM-1) (Mathew and Perez, 2011) are under investigation for the treatment of advanced HER2+ breast cancer.

Cetuximab (Erbitux®): Cetuximab is a **chimeric** (that is, composed of parts from different sources) MoAb, which has been found to be effective in delaying disease progression when used in combination with chemotherapy to treat metastatic colorectal cancers (Van Cutsem et al., 2009). Subsequently, a smaller subset of patients with colorectal cancer, in whom KRAS (a protein involved in the downstream signalling of EGFR) was not mutated, were identified as patients who benefited from this targeted treatment. EGFR is also over-expressed in head and neck cancers, and inhibition of this receptor is beneficial in the treatment of these cancers (Bonner et al., 2010).

Table 15.2 Monoclonal antibodies

	Target	Cancers treated	Posology	Common side effects	Similar agents
EGFR TK targeting agents					
Trastuzumab (Herceptin®)	HER2-neu (EGFR2 or erb B2) receptor	Her 2+ breast cancer Her 2+ stomach cancer	IV infusion 2mg/Kg weekly or 6mg/Kg three weekly SC	Flu-like symptoms, weakening of heart muscle (usually reversible). These are usually tolerable but regular monitoring of heart muscle function is advisable. Risk of severe allergic reactions	Pertuzumab (Omnitarg®)
Cetuximab (Erbitux®)	EGFR1 or erb B1 receptor	Advanced head and neck cancer Metastatic colorectal cancer with wild type KRAS	IV infusion 400mg/m² followed by 250mg/m² weekly	Acneiform skin rash, nausea, diarrhoea, sore eyes, hair changes, fatigue. Risk of severe allergic reactions	Panitumumab (Vectibix®)
VEGF RTK targeting agents					
Bevacizumab (Avastin®)	VEGF-A	Colon cancer Lung cancer Breast cancer Brain cancer	IV infusion 5-15mg/kg 2-3weekly.	High blood pressure, bleeding, bowel perforation, fatigue. Risk of severe allergic reactions	-none-
Other anticancer monoclonal antibodies					
Rituximab (MabThera®)	CD20	CD20+ Non Hodgkin lymphomas	IV infusion 375mg/m2 weekly to 6 monthly depending on type of lymphoma.	Risk of severe allergic reactions, fall in blood counts, risk of viral infections, fatigue	Ofatumumab (Arzerra®)

VEGF targeting agents

Angiogenesis is the ability of a cancer to induce the growth of new blood vessels, which then act as conduit for nutrition and oxygen to the cancer cell. This is considered to be one of the hallmarks of cancer (Hanahan and Weinberg, 2011). A group of growth factors called VEGF (**vascular endothelial growth factor**) are the main agents that trigger the process of new blood vessel formation in the tissues. Blocking the VEGF can be an efficient way of curtailing the growth of the cancer by depriving the cancer cell of new nutrients and oxygen that the blood vessels supply.

> **Bevacizumab** (**Avastin®**): Bevacizumab was the first drug to target angiogenesis by blocking the VEGF-A **ligand**, or 'binding site'. It showed early promise in colon and lung cancer in conjunction with chemotherapy. Its use in breast cancer is still only done in the context of a clinical trial (outside the USA) because the drug has not shown a clear survival improvement. Its use in brain cancer is being investigated as part of a multinational clinical trial (Chinot et al., 2011).

> **Other anticancer monoclonal antibodies**

> **Rituximab** (**MabThera®**): Rituximab was found to be one of the earliest chimeric antibodies targeted against CD20 (a protein found on the surface of most B-lymphocytes, which is a type of immune cell). Addition of this drug to standard chemotherapy for lymphomas revolutionized the management of this illness due to the large gains in efficacy of the combined treatment (Coiffier et al., 2002). Rituximab has now become the standard of care in the treatment of B-cell lymphomas.

CANCER VACCINES

Vaccines are weakened versions or parts of infectious organisms like viruses and bacteria that, when injected into the body, provoke a subsequent **protective immune response** towards that particular virus or bacteria. Vaccines have played a major role in preventing severe infectious diseases, such as small pox, meningitis and polio. **Cancer vaccines** work in a similar manner by stimulating an immune response to molecules (antigens) found in the cancer cell. By isolating specific proteins on the surface of the cancer cell and exposing immune response-generating cells to these proteins, researchers hope to generate a widespread immune response against the cancer cells.

Although early results in cancers like melanoma and kidney cancer have shown some hope, these vaccines are not in regular use due to a general lack of efficacy.

BIOLOGICAL RESPONSE MODIFIERS

Biological response modifiers include naturally occurring substances like **interferons** and **interleukins**, called **cytokines**, which work by enhancing the efficacy of the immune system in a non-specific manner in dealing with cancer cells.

Interleukin-2 (IL-2): IL-2 is used in the treatment of kidney cancer and melanoma. It works by activating the immune cells against the cancer cells and making them more effective in destroying the cell. This can be a double-edged sword because the activation of the immune cell is non-specific and can lead to a runaway inflammatory reaction that can be fatal without intensive medical support. Side effects of the treatment depend on the amount/dose of the IL-2 given. Low dose IL-2 is given as an injection under the skin and has the side effects of fatigue, weight loss, flu-like symptoms, flushing, nausea, confusion and low blood pressure. High dose IL-2 is given as an intravenous infusion and requires intensive medical monitoring because it can cause all the symptoms of low dose IL-2 to a greater degree, in addition to heart rhythm abnormalities, drowsiness and respiratory failure. Due to this, it is usually administered in an intensive care setting.

Interferon alpha: This is another cytokine, which is used in the treatment of kidney cancer and melanoma. Similar to IL-2, it works by making the immune system more effective at destroying the cancer cells. It is usually given as an injection under the skin and has similar side effects to low dose IL-2. In addition, it can have an effect on the mental state of the patient, causing depression, confusion, anxiety and irritability.

Cytokines are now rarely used in routine practice, having been supplanted by more targeted agents, as discussed elsewhere in this chapter.

COLONY STIMULATING FACTORS (CSF)/GROWTH FACTORS

These are substances that can be naturally produced in the body but do not have a direct anticancer effect; however, they are very helpful in supporting a patient undergoing other anticancer treatments like chemotherapy.

Recombinant granulocyte-CSF (Filgrastim): This treatment is used to increase the rate of recovery of infection-fighting white blood cells in the body. Patients on chemotherapy treatment often have a temporary drop in the number of infection-fighting white cells, leaving them in an immune compromised state vulnerable to opportunistic infections, which can be fatal. Injections of filgrastim can help boost the levels of white blood cells (the neutrophil component), helping to return the patient's immune system to a level capable of fighting infections. Return of white blood cell counts to normal levels also prevents delays of future chemotherapy cycles, which in turn preserves the efficacy of the chemotherapy treatment. The drug is usually given as an injection under the skin, either daily until there is recovery of the white blood cell count, or every 2–3 weeks at the completion of each chemotherapy cycle, in the case of the long-acting preparation. The main side effects of this drug include injection site reactions, flu-like symptoms and bone aches.

Erythropoietin: This is a **glycoprotein** normally produced in the body to increase the production of the oxygen-carrying component of the blood, the red blood cells. Apart from various non-cancer related uses, for example the prevention of anaemia in kidney failure patients, this drug (or its synthetic variants) can be used to prevent chemotherapy-induced anaemia in people with cancer as an alternative to blood transfusions. Although its early use was effective in improving red blood cell levels and preventing anaemia, concerns regarding the stimulation of cancer cell growth and worsening cancer cure rates were raised (Bohlius et al., 2009); its use in this setting remains controversial. This drug is given as an injection under the skin and dosage and duration of therapy vary depending on the type of preparation. The main side effects of this drug are high blood pressure and risk of heart failure in patients with predisposing heart conditions.

PSYCHOSOCIAL ASPECTS

Biological therapies are a rapidly developing and expanding aspect of cancer care and are likely to be the leading treatments in the near future, when individualization of treatment is the ultimate aim of cancer treatment; however, the psychological impact of cancer and its treatment are only beginning to be realized. In such a rapidly changing field as cancer medicine, it is important not to lose sight of the fact that long-term losses can be eclipsed by short-term gains. Although the side effects of most of the targeted agents may not be as severe as conventional chemotherapy or radiotherapy, the effect on the quality of life can be just as significant. Seemingly minor medical issues, such as having an itchy rash, which makes it difficult to go out in the sun on a warm day, can actually have a profound negative impact on the psychological state of the patient. It is also important to highlight that most of these drugs are not used in a curative setting and most are given on a regular basis until the cancer no longer responds to the treatment. Whilst there is a real possibility of converting cancer into a chronic disease, with potential for a corresponding increased survival, it does mean a patient is living with the burden of chronic disease and the ongoing effects of cancer treatments. As the effects of any treatment will vary between individuals and their specific treatments, assessment and monitoring by nurses and other healthcare professionals are key to reducing and/or minimizing negative consequences. Failure to do so can have a serious detrimental impact (Macmillan Cancer Support, 2013c).

Furthermore, treatments such as surgery provide a clearer answer to the question of whether the tumour has been removed. Assessing responses to treatment with biological agents can be quite difficult because imaging to measure response of the cancer (a standard approach when using chemotherapy agents) is not so clear cut for these therapies. This adds an ongoing stress to the person with cancer and to their families and carers. To minimize the psychosocial impact of such agents, the following approach is suggested as elements of good practice.

Give clear information regarding:

- What the drug is being given for;
- How it is to be given;
- How it is to be taken;
- The aim of the treatment;
- Common side effects and how to manage them; and
- The risk of potential serious side effects and whom to call if there are problems.

For further information on approaches to effective communication, see Chapter 17.

The point of contact for adverse events, such as serious side effects, will usually be the designated cancer nurse specialist and/or a 24-hour nursing helpline, allowing potentially serious adverse effects to be managed as early as possible. As treatment will be long-term, it is possible in certain cases to allow necessary planned treatment breaks or 'drug holidays', particularly to enable family holidays. It is important to maintain a clear line of communication with all other teams involved in the care of the patient, such as the GP, palliative care teams, district nurses and other medical teams. Some patients find patient-centred support groups helpful because it allows sharing of common experiences and reinforcement of coping strategies (see also Chapter 22). Early on in the disease process, it is also helpful to refer the patient to a benefits advisor to discuss financial help and aid for travel to hospital, accommodation, disability allowances, issues surrounding time off from work for patients in employment and travel insurance, which becomes difficult once a diagnosis of 'cancer' has been made.

Reflective activity

- Choose one drug from Table 15.1 and one drug from Table 15.2.
- Reflect on how you would explain the potential side effects of each treatment to the patient.
- What may be the psychosocial impact of each treatment on the patient and how would you support them through this aspect of their care?

CHAPTER SUMMARY

Biological and targeted anticancer therapies are a promising part of current therapy and increasingly the solid foundation for the development of truly personalized cancer management. With more research into identification of newer targets for therapy and development of newer drugs, their use is likely to increase significantly. As they differ considerably from conventional anticancer therapy, and are used for longer periods, it is imperative that any healthcare professional involved in the care of such patients has a clear understanding of their mechanism of action, clinical uses and side effects.

Key learning points

- Biological therapies are drugs that use the body's immune system to fight cancer or lessen the effect of other anticancer treatments.
- Targeted cancer therapies are drugs or other substances that block the growth and spread of cancer by interfering with specific molecules involved in tumour growth and progression.
- The effects and side effects can be very different from conventional chemotherapy and radiotherapy and are dependent on the target of the individual drug.
- Patients may experience psychosocial problems resulting from their cancer and treatment that require sensitive assessment and tailored interventions.
- Most of these drugs are used in a continuous fashion and, in the future, may have the ability to convert cancer into a chronic disease with the subsequent impact on long-term and continuing care.

to the cell. Other mutations called **translocations** involve the breakage and movement of **chromosome fragments**. Breakage and rejoining may occur within a gene, leading to its inactivation, and movement of a gene in this manner can lead to an increase or decrease in the level of protein production, resulting in the deregulation of normal cell growth. An example would be an exchange between chromosomes 9 and 22, observed in over 90% of patients with chronic myelogenous leukaemia (CML). Translocations are common in leukaemias and lymphomas and are less commonly identified in cancers of solid tissues.

In the human genome, many genes are responsible for controlling cell growth in a precise way. Generally, a single mutation in one of these genes is not sufficient to cause cancer. An accumulation of additional mutations in key regulatory genes is required to cause malignancy. Different tissues and types of cells will require different combinations of genes to be mutated in order to become cancerous.

GENES THAT PLAY A ROLE IN CANCER

The development of cancer is a multistep process involving the interaction between genes and their environment, during which cells acquire a series of mutations that lead to unrestrained cell growth and evasion of cell death. Alterations in three types of genes lead to cancer: **tumour suppressor genes**, whose normal function is to act like 'a brake' to inhibit cell growth and division, **proto-oncogenes**, which normally act like 'an accelerator' to increase cell growth and division, and **DNA repair genes**, the products of which are involved in the processes where a cell identifies and corrects damage to the DNA.

The normal function of tumour suppressor genes is to suppress tumour development by regulating the processes of cell growth and cell death (**apoptosis**). However, when tumour suppressor genes become altered or inactivated (due to inherited or environmental mutations) they lose the ability to inhibit cell growth, allowing cells to grow uncontrolled and develop into a cancer. *p53, BRCA1* and *BRCA2* are all examples of tumour suppressor genes (Hollstein et al., 1991; Roy et al., 2011).

The *p53* gene plays a central role in the cell's response to DNA damage and more than 50% of human tumours contain a mutation or deletion of the *p53* gene. When DNA damage is detected in a cell, *p53* stops the cell from dividing, preventing cells from passing on the DNA damage to the daughter cells. Also, *p53* can stimulate cells with damaged DNA to commit 'cell suicide' if repair cannot be performed. When the *p53* gene cannot function correctly because of mutation in itself, the cells with DNA damage continue to divide and accumulate further DNA damage that can eventually lead to the formation of cancer. A defective *p53* gene deprives the cells of crucial signals that normally put the 'brakes' on inappropriate cell division and tumour development. People who inherit a mutated copy of *p53* often develop tumours in early adulthood, a disease known as **Li-Fraumeni syndrome**.

Oncogenes are altered forms of normal genes called proto-oncogenes. Proto-oncogenes code for proteins responsible for promoting cell growth, and are important for normal development and maintenance of human tissues and organs. However, if a mutation occurs in a proto-oncogene, the products contribute to unregulated cell division and can cause normal cells to become cancerous. The mutant proteins are no longer sensitive to the controls that regulate the normal form of the protein and cells divide continuously, even in the absence of any signals telling them to divide. The action of the mutant protein confers a growth advantage or increased survival of cells. Examples of proto-oncogenes include *RAS, WNT, MYC, ERK*, and *TRK* (Chow, 2010).

DNA repair genes code for proteins involved in the mechanisms that attempt to correct errors arising in DNA, thereby minimizing alterations in the cell. However, when a DNA repair gene is mutated, its product may no longer be functional, leading to failure in repair and allowing further mutations to accumulate in the cell. These mutations can increase the frequency of cancerous changes in a cell.

Many oncogenes, tumour suppressor genes and DNA repair genes have been identified and shown to influence aspects of tumour development or behaviour. The accumulation and interactions of genetic lesions during tumour initiation and progression is well characterized for many human tumour types, and such information is proving to be tremendously valuable in diagnosis and treatment options.

PRINCIPLES OF GENE THERAPY

The enhanced understanding of the genetic basis of cancer has facilitated the development of new molecular therapeutic approaches to fighting the disease. Advances in understanding and manipulating genes provide the opportunity for scientists to transfer functional genes into cells of a target tissue in order to correct defective genes or to replace absent genes in a cancer cell.

Gene therapy is an experimental technique that attempts to treat diseases, including cancer, by means of genetic manipulation and is designed to insert genetic material directly into cells to restore the normal function of a faulty gene. Researchers are testing several approaches to gene therapy, including:

- Replacing a mutated gene that causes disease with a normal copy of the gene.
- Inactivating a mutated gene that is causing disease.
- Introducing a new gene into the body to help fight a disease.
- Inserting genes into cancer cells to make them more susceptible to or prevent resistance to chemotherapy, radiation therapy or hormone therapy.
- Creating 'suicide genes' that can enter cancer cells and cause them to self-destruct.

ADMINISTRATION ROUTE FOR GENE THERAPY

Gene therapy involves one of two routes of administration, *ex vivo* gene therapy or *in vivo* gene therapy.

In *ex vivo* gene therapy, cells are removed from the patient and grown in the laboratory. During this time, the genetic material is transferred and the cells are returned to the patient by injection into a vein. An advantage of this approach is that only those cells where gene transfer has occurred are selected. However, *ex vivo* gene therapy is more demanding and expensive than *in vivo* gene transfer, and needs to be personalized for each patient. In contrast, *in vivo* gene therapy, where the therapeutic DNA is directly administered to the patient, can be applied once optimized to a number of patients with the same disease. However, some tissues such as brain, cartilage and connective tissue are difficult to reach *in vivo*. Also, once administered *in vivo*, the gene might enter cells other than the desired targets, causing unwanted effects. It is also possible that the vehicle used for gene delivery might elicit an immune response.

DELIVERY SYSTEMS FOR GENE THERAPY

For both *in vivo* and *ex vivo* gene therapy, the success of gene replacement relies on an effective delivery system to transport the genetic material to the intended target cell at adequate levels to produce the desired effect without toxicity. In addition, a good gene delivery system should be able to protect the gene against degradation. Researchers need to be able to deliver genes consistently to a precise location in the patient's DNA, and ensure that new genes are precisely controlled by the body's normal physiologic signals.

Gene delivery systems (**vectors**) can be divided into two broad categories: **viral vectors** and **non-viral** (physical and chemical) **vectors** (Table 16. 1).

Viral vectors

All viruses have evolved a way of introducing their genes into human cells as part of their replication cycle, and this ability to invade cells as part of their natural infection process has been recognized as a potential strategy for gene therapy. Scientists have exploited this capability and manipulated the virus genome to remove the disease-causing genes and use the virus as a vehicle to deliver the therapeutic genes. Viruses have the potential to be excellent vectors because they have a specific relationship with the host in that they colonize certain cell types and tissues in specific organs.

A number of viruses have been used for human gene therapy, including retrovirus, adenovirus, adeno-associated virus, herpes simplex virus, lentivirus and vaccinia virus (Table 16.1).

Many clinical trials conducted in the 1990s took advantage of the properties of viral vectors based on retroviruses because of their relative genetic simplicity, their efficiency in infecting many different cell types, and their ability to integrate their genetic material into the genome of the host cell (Barquinero et al., 2004). However, the genetic material of a retrovirus can be inserted in any position in the genome of the host and if the genetic material is inserted in the middle of an important regulatory gene of the host cell, the gene will be disrupted causing more harm than good. This problem has recently begun to be addressed by using **recombinant technology** to try and direct the site of integration to specific sites within the host genome.

Adenoviral vectors, a common cause of upper respiratory tract infections, are an attractive alternative to retroviruses because they have many sought-after characteristics for use as a gene therapy vector (Kay et al., 2001). Adenoviruses can infect a large range of human cells, carry a large genetic payload, and its DNA can be easily manipulated by researchers using recombinant techniques. In addition, unlike the retrovirus, the genetic material of the adenoviruses is not incorporated into the genome of the host cell. However, this means that the genetic material introduced via an adenovirus is not replicated when cells divide, and so is not present in any daughter cells. As a result, treatment with a modified adenovirus may require administration of high doses for health benefits, which may cause toxic effects. Adenoviral vectors are an extremely common human pathogen and *in vivo* delivery may be hampered by an immune response to the virus. Also, these viruses live for several days in the body, and some concern surrounds the possibility of infecting others with the viruses through sneezing or coughing.

Despite some disadvantages, adenoviruses have shown real promise in treating cancer. In October 2003, China became the first country to approve the commercial production of a gene therapy, Adenovirus-p53 Injection (Gendicine®) for head and neck squamous-cell

Table 16.1 Gene delivery systems

	Description	Advantages	Challenges
Viral delivery methods			
Retrovirus	Enveloped single-stranded RNA virus, which has been widely used in gene transfer methods.	Stably integrates DNA into the target cell genome, which means that retroviral vectors can be used to permanently modify the host cell DNA.	Random insertion of DNA into the host genome with risk of malignancy. Limited packaging capacity. Inactivation by human complement.
Adenovirus	A non-enveloped, double-stranded DNA virus associated with mild human infections such as upper respiratory tract.	Efficiently infect and express their genes in a wide variety of cell types.	Immune response against the viral vector.
Adeno-associated virus (AAV)	Non-pathogenic human parvoviruses, dependent on a helper virus, usually adenovirus, to proliferate.	Non-immunogenic. Simple structure. AAV genome integrates into a specific location on human chromosome 19, although is unable to replicate without a helper virus.	Limited packaging capacity for therapeutic gene.
Herpex simplex virus (HSV)	A double-stranded, linear DNA virus belonging to the herpes viridae family.	HSV can infect a wide range of cell types. Large capacity for the insertion of foreign genes.	As most humans are infected with HSV, pre-existing neutralizing antibodies could reduce the efficiency of intravenous or intratumoral delivery of HSV vectors.
Lentivirus	Complex retroviruses, the most common of which is the human immunodeficiency virus (HIV).	Can target a broad range of cell types.	Genetically more complicated. Safety issues regarding the use of an HIV virus.
Vaccinia virus	A large, complex, enveloped virus belonging to the poxvirus family.	Replicates in the cytoplasm of the cell, thereby excluding the risk of integration of DNA into the host genome. Infects a broad range of cells. Has a high capacity to carry large genes.	Inefficient delivery to sufficient numbers of cancer cells.

(Continued)

Table 16.1 (Continued)

	Description	Advantages	Challenges
Physical delivery methods			
Naked DNA	Direct injection *in vivo* into skeletal or cardiac muscle.	Easy to mass produce and quality control. Low immunogenicity.	Gene delivery is highly inefficient and variable. Requires a large amount of DNA.
Electroporation	Injection of DNA into muscle tissue followed by controlled electrical pulses that makes the cell membrane temporarily permeable, allowing DNA to enter the cell.	Simple to set up for skeletal muscle and skin.	Low efficiency. Limited applications.
Pressurized vascular delivery	Use of pressure to achieve close contact with the desired cell type.	Relatively easy to set up.	Usually invasive. Low efficiency. Short transitionary effect.
Sonoporation	Application of ultrasound results in membrane permeabilization enhancing the delivery of DNA to cells.	Non-invasive and well tolerated.	Kinetics of sonoporation are complex. Low efficiency of transfer of DNA.
Gene gun	DNA is coated onto the surface of gold particles, which are then accelerated by pressurized gas and propelled into cells. The momentum allows the gold particles to penetrate the tissue and release DNA into cells.	Relatively easy to set up.	Limited for gene transfer to skin, mucosa, or surgically exposed tissues within a confined area.
Chemical delivery methods			
Liposomes/ cationic lipids (lipofection)	Therapeutic DNA is enclosed within a cationic vesicle, which fuses with the cell membrane and releases the therapeutic gene into the cell.	High efficiency *in vitro*. Lower immunogenicity. Easier to produce.	Low efficiency of gene transfer.
Cationic polymers	Synthetic or naturally occurring cationic polymers in linear or branched configuration facilitate DNA uptake through charge interactions with cell surface.	High efficiency *in vitro*.	Toxicity to cells.
Dendrimers	Synthetic branching molecules that are slightly positively charged. This allows them to be loaded with DNA (which is slightly negative charged) for insertion into a cell.	Potentially used for the delivery of long stretches of DNA. Low toxicity.	Low efficiency of gene delivery.
Nanoparticles	Use of nanoparticles coated in DNA to deliver genes into cells.	High efficiency *in vitro*	Scale-up of production may prove difficult.

carcinoma (HNSCC). Gendicine® uses an adenoviral vector to transfer p53 tumour suppressor genes directly into tumour cells to suppress tumour growth by inducing cell death (Peng, 2005). In phase II and phase III clinical trials, Gendicine® was shown to have synergistic effects with radiotherapy and chemotherapy. One hundred and thirty-five HNSCC patients (77% stage III or IV) were randomized to receive radiotherapy alone or in combination with Gendicine®. Those receiving the gene therapy in addition to radiotherapy had a 93% response rate with complete remission in 64% compared to 79% and 19%, respectively in the radiotherapy group (Peng, 2005).

Non-viral systems

Although viral vectors have the potential to transfer the therapeutic gene with high efficiency, the **acute immune response**, revealed in gene therapy clinical trials have raised safety concerns about some commonly used viral vectors. The limited capacity of the genetically modified viruses and issues related to the production of viral vectors present additional challenges in the use of these vectors. Methods of non-viral gene delivery, such as the application of physical and chemical approaches, have been explored as alternative methods for gene delivery (Wells, 2004; Park et al., 2006). Physical approaches, including needle injection of naked DNA, electroporation, gene gun, ultrasound and pressurized delivery, are carrier-free methods that employ a physical force to permeate the cell membrane and facilitate entry of DNA into the cells. Chemical approaches use synthetic or naturally occurring compounds as carriers to deliver the therapeutic gene into cells. Although non-viral systems have the advantage that they are safer, easier to produce, less immunogenic and have no limitation on the size of a transferred gene, the majority of non-viral approaches are still much less efficient than viral vectors, especially for *in vivo* gene delivery that hinders their use for *in vivo* therapeutic applications.

RISKS AND CHALLENGES FOR GENE THERAPY

Numerous challenges remain to be overcome before gene therapy becomes available as a widespread, safe and effective treatment option for cancer.

Any foreign object introduced into human tissues causes an immune response, and the risk of stimulating the immune system that reduces the effectiveness of gene therapy is always a potential risk. The immune system may not allow the repeated treatments of gene therapy required for some patients. Although viruses are the current delivery system of choice by researchers, they present a variety of potential problems to the patient, including toxicity, immune and inflammatory responses. In addition, there is always the fear that the viral vector, once inside the patient, may recover its ability to cause disease. Other concerns include the possibility that transferred genes could be 'over-produced', making so much of the missing protein as to be harmful, and that the virus could be transmitted from the patient to other individuals or into the environment.

In addition to safe and effective gene delivery systems for gene therapy, a major challenge for researchers is to define the best candidate genes. This is made more difficult by the multiple genetic changes that occur within a cancer cell. The more invasive the cancer, the more likely it is to utilize **multiple signalling pathways** involving many different aberrant genes. Sometimes the inhibition of the target gene and its pathway is not sufficient to inhibit the disease process because the cancer cells have redundant or alternative pathways. Therefore, in any gene therapy approach, targeting one or a limited number of these pathways might not be sufficient to stop uncontrolled cell growth.

As with all treatments for cancer, the psychosocial impact on the patient cannot be underestimated. A patient's anxieties about their cancer diagnosis, the effectiveness of treatment and potential side effects requires an holistic and supportive approach. As gene therapy is still only in the early stages of development, most gene-based treatments are tested through clinical trials and patients may experience additional concerns associated with this approach to treatment (for further information on clinical trials, see Chapter 32).

Reflective activity

- What concerns may patients receiving gene therapy experience?
- How can patients be supported through their treatment?

SOMATIC GENE THERAPY

Most of the current work in applying gene therapy involves **somatic gene therapy**. In this type of gene therapy, therapeutic genes are inserted into tissue or cells to produce a naturally occurring protein that is lacking or not functioning correctly in an individual patient. This type of gene therapy affects only the targeted cells in the patient, and is not passed on to future generations. Somatic gene therapy treats a consenting patient and the effects begin and end within the body of that patient.

Technology is available for gene therapy to target reproductive cells (**germ cells**), which would allow the inserted gene to be passed on to future generations. This approach is known as germ line gene therapy and is a topic of much debate. Successful germ line therapy could eliminate some genetic diseases from a particular family and spare future generations in a family from having a particular genetic disorder. However, the genetic change propagated by germ line gene therapy may actually be deleterious and harmful, with the potential for unforeseen problems. There is no guarantee that germ line gene therapy would not cause unknown damage to a foetus or that a child born having received germ line gene therapy would not develop any disorders during their lifetime as a result of the treatment.

CHAPTER SUMMARY

During the past two decades, there have been major advances in understanding the genetic basis of cancer and offering new opportunities for the molecular prevention and treatment of the disease. Despite delays during the last two decades in developing successful gene therapy for cancer, gene therapy could become a powerful method of safe and effective anticancer treatment (Brenner et al., 2013). One of the most promising approaches to emerge from this improved understanding is the possibility of using gene therapy to selectively target and destroy tumour cells. Our understanding of the genes involved in malignant pathways allows researchers to explore the possibility of correcting an abnormality in a tumour suppressor gene, such as *p53*, by inserting a copy of the wild-type gene. This has significant implications because *p53* alterations are the most common genetic abnormalities in human cancers. However, despite the promise of such approaches, a number of difficulties remain to be overcome, the most important of which is the need for more efficient systems of gene delivery.

There are many clinical trials for cancer gene therapy that have been approved in the USA and other countries. It is thought that this large number of projects about gene therapy for cancer will provide important information on the safety and efficiency of gene transfer and efficacy in humans so that in the future there will be many gene therapy-based drugs that will be safe and effective for the treatment of a range of cancers.

Key learning points

- The majority of cancers arise from random mutations that are acquired in a cell during a person's lifetime.
- Alterations in three types of genes lead to cancer: tumour suppressor genes, proto-oncogenes and DNA repair genes. Gene therapy attempts to treat cancer by inserting genetic material directly into cells to restore the normal function of a faulty gene.
- Gene therapy is either *ex vivo* (cells are removed from the patient and grown in the laboratory and then injected back into the patient) or *in vivo* (therapeutic DNA is directly administered to the patient).
- Genes are delivered into cells via viral and non-viral vectors.
- Repeated stimulation of the immune system can reduce the effectiveness of gene therapy.
- Psychosocial support for patients is important.

Recommended further reading

- Giacca, M. (2010) *Gene Therapy*. New York, NY: Springer.
- Hunt, K.K., Vorburger, S.A. and Swisher, S.G. (2007) *Gene Therapy for Cancer*. New York, NY: Humana Press Inc.

The following websites may also be of interest:

- www.cancer.net/patient/All+About+Cancer/Genetics/The+Genetics+of+Cancer
- www.nature.com/scitable/topicpage/cell-cycle-control-by-oncogenes-and-tumour-14191459
- www.cancerquest.org/cancer-genes-overview.html

17 EFFECTIVE COMMUNICATION IN CANCER CARE

CATHERINE HEAVEN AND CLAIRE GREEN

Chapter outline

- The importance of effective communication

  - Consequences of inadequate assessment and ineffective communication
  - Barriers to effective communication

- Global assessment

  - Context
  - When to conduct an assessment
  - Structuring a consultation effectively
  - Responding to cues

- Key communication skills

  - Facilitative skills and behaviours
  - Blocking behaviours

- Managing difficult communication situations

  - Handling anger
  - Handling strong emotions
  - Handling difficult questions
  - Breaking bad news

- Improving skills

INTRODUCTION

'Communication is the key to a high quality patient experience'. (Royal College of Nursing, 2012)

The way we **communicate** with patients and their families is potentially the single biggest factor in influencing their healthcare experience. Building on the report of Lord Darzi (DH 2008a) , the Department of Health and the NHS Institute commissioned a review to identify 'what matters to patients' (DH, 2008a; Robert et al., 2011). The findings identified that **relational aspects**, that is those things which make a person feel cared for (dignity, empathy, emotional support) were significantly more likely to affect people's overall experience of care when compared to the **functional aspects** of care (e.g. waiting times, noise, food, cleanliness). Four of the top five factors reported by the study were associated with how the healthcare staff related to patients rather than what they did for them (Robert et al., 2011).

Today's patients want to feel informed, supported and listened to so that they can make meaningful decisions and choices about their care; they want to be treated as a person not a number (Entwistle et al., 2012; Robert et al., 2011). Because of this, the UK Government has made it clear that the patient experience is a crucial part of quality healthcare provision and sets out its standards within the NHS Constitution, the Outcomes Framework 2011/12 and the NICE Quality Standards for Experience and Mental Health Experience (NICE, 2013a).

This chapter will focus on how we can build that quality of relationship with patients and their families. It will explore how communication affects the quality of patient services and reflect on the barriers to effective communication in today's healthcare system. The second part of the chapter will then give a detailed account of the types of skills and approaches that can facilitate effective global assessment and information transfer, as well as considering how we can ensure patients and their families feel listened to and are involved in conversations.

THE IMPORTANCE OF EFFECTIVE COMMUNICATION

There are many reasons to ensure that we communicate effectively with patients and their carers, not least the need to ensure that the care provided is appropriate to their needs. In relation to improving patient experience, the NHS Confederation recognized the need to assess people individually, and not make assumptions about their needs, wishes and preferences.

> Improving the experiences of all patients starts by treating each of them individually to ensure they receive the right care, at the right time, in the right way for them. (NHS Confederation, 2010)

Over recent decades a number of studies have looked at how well we assess cancer patients concerns and worries (Heaven and Maguire, 1997, Maguire, 2002; Farrell et al., 2005; Cocksedge and May, 2005; Jansen et al., 2010; Finset, 2011; Mulley et al., 2012; Heyn et al., 2012). All of these studies show how patients' concerns and worries were not fully identified during interactions, suggesting that up to half of patients' worries remain hidden in consultations, despite staff having adequate time, a good environment and a willingness on the part of the health professional to try to listen carefully to what they were being told (Heaven and Maguire, 1997; Farrell et al., 2005; Heyn et al., 2012). The studies highlight that health professionals often missed a great deal of information and occasionally overestimated patients' concerns based on their own assumptions rather than focusing on the cues being given by the patients they were talking to (Heaven and Maguire, 1997; Henderson, 2003; Lee et al., 2010).

The consequence of missing or misunderstanding patients' problems, needs, preferences and concerns are far ranging. An increasing amount of evidence highlights the impact of good or poor communication, including confusion and isolation; distress; non-compliance with treatment regimes leading to poor outcomes; longer hospital stays; higher levels of medication and poor symptom control; patients' dissatisfaction leading to complaints and possibly litigation; greater number of GP visits; and a requirement for more community and psychological support for problems such as anxiety, depression or adjustment disorder (Schofield et al., 2003; Little et al., 2001; Kim et al., 2004; Maguire, 1999; Cocksedge and May, 2005; Deadman et al., 2001; Charlton et al., 2008).

What is clear from the studies is that most professionals aspire to give holistic care and genuinely wish to ensure that they are listening to their patients' specific concerns. Lack of skills, lack of confidence and fear of the consequences of talking more openly often hold people back in busy clinical settings. These inhibitory factors are explored in the next section.

BARRIERS TO EFFECTIVE COMMUNICATION

Communication is a two-way process, requiring a sender and a receiver to be working together to ensure clear transmission of a message. When assessing or gathering information, the patient, family member or carer is in **sender mode** and the health professional is in **receiver mode**; however, when the health professional is giving information, these roles are reversed. It can be difficult to switch backwards and forwards between assessment (**listening**) and information giving (**telling**) modes during the course of an interview, and this is why most models of clinical interviewing focus on assessment first, followed by information giving (Maguire, 1999; Silverman et al., 2008). **Communication breakdowns** relate to both sender (in this case a patient, relative or carer) and recipient (in this case the healthcare worker/healthcare professional) factors, as described next.

Patient factors

Fears: Patients report concern about asking key questions or mentioning key side effects due to fear of hearing bad news, or fear of seeming ungrateful to the health professionals (Maguire, 1999). Patients also report feeling concerned about losing control if they are angry and upset (Maguire, 1999; Zimmerman et al., 2007; Mulley et al., 2012), and fear burdening or upsetting the health professionals. In a 1997 study, Heaven and Maguire report this as a common reason why hospice patients did not disclose their concerns and worries to the nurses who were caring for them. The patients reported 'liking' the staff too much and not wanting to upset and hurt them, nor to become a burden to them by sharing worries (Heaven and Maguire, 1997; Farrell, 2013).

Beliefs: Strong cultural or religious beliefs can also inhibit patients or family members from talking about their concerns (Mustafa et al., 2004). Beliefs about the health professionals being too busy are common, as are beliefs that other people have more important problems that the professionals should focus on, or worry about taking up too much of the professional's precious time (Booth et al., 1996; Maguire 1999). Sometimes patients report the misguided belief that 'nothing can be done about a particular problem, so why talk about it', meaning that symptom control medication, vital home care features or simple emotional support cannot be offered (Maguire, 1999).

Skills: If a patient or carer does not have the ability to express themselves because of language difficulties, general language skills or literacy, health literacy issues, or physical disabilities, communication is hampered (see also Chapters 9 and 10). In the UK in 2012, it was reported that 'one in five of the population are so poor at reading they struggle to read a medicine label or use a cheque book' (World Literacy Foundation, 2012). Health professionals often overestimate the literacy levels of the client group they are working with, and communicate and expect understanding at the level at which they themselves function.

Environment: A final factor affecting disclosure is the healthcare setting itself (Zimmerman et al., 2007; Janssen and MacLeod, 2010). Patients are aware of how busy staff are, and expect very short consultations with key facts only and little time for questions (Janssen and MacLeod, 2010). The environment can also offer little privacy, with multiple interruptions and many people present, for example students or large teams of professionals. Interestingly, Oguchi et al. (2011) showed a reduction in disclosure when family members were present during consultations, showing patients often protect their relatives from the reality of their problems. Alternatively, patients may be inhibited when key carers who they rely upon for support and help are not present in a consultation (Mellon et al., 2006).

Professional health worker factors

Fears: Health professionals also express fears about 'going too far', 'pushing people over the edge' or 'upsetting people uncontrollably' , all of which inhibit them in asking key questions, clarifying what somebody might mean or explaining something more graphically (Booth et al., 1996). Professionals also express fears about 'opening up a can of worms', which they don't then feel skilled or sufficiently supported to deal with, or 'making things worse for the person not better', both of which will further inhibit communication and potentially lead to poor decision making. Carrying these fears around in day-to-day practice is also highly stressful (Parle et al., 1997; Heaven et al., 2003).

Beliefs that certain problems are inevitable or can't be addressed, and therefore do not warrant discussion, have been shown to inhibit professionals, as well as the belief that 'we should not raise false expectation by talking about these things' (Booth et al., 1996). Henderson (2003) reported that many nurses hold the opinion that 'they know best', and that patients lacked relevant medical knowledge to make decisions (Henderson, 2003). For these reasons, professionals often stay in control of the conversation, but miss out on hearing about vital pieces of information, and run the risk of being seen as uncaring by the patient they are talking to (Henderson, 2003).

The **environment** also inhibits professionals starting open and frank conversations. Lack of privacy, lack of time and lack of space are all things mentioned as reasons for holding back, as well as frequent interruptions from both people and technical devices (Janssen and MacLeod, 2010). Community staff often talk about the difficulty of the home environment. A study of nursing staff showed that the less supported staff felt, or the more conflict there was in their working team, the more these health professionals avoided emotionally taxing situations with patients (Booth et al., 1996; Wilkinson, 1991). Many of these factors seem to relate to the organizations within which health professionals work. Another key inhibitory factor is the many standardized treatment or care plans and regimes. These are often written to ensure optimal practice, to avoid mistakes and to streamline services to create an efficient effective system. Unfortunately, they make it hard for the health professionals working in those systems to provide truly individualized care, tailored to each individual person's needs, wishes and preferences.

Communication skills: Many health professionals report they were not given adequate training in communication skills (Turner, M. et al., 2011; Jack et al., 2013; Langowitz et al., 2010), especially in giving complex information, breaking bad news and handling strong and difficult emotions (Zimmerman, 2007). They report not feeling comfortable in integrating the listening and giving parts of their consultation, not feeling confident in knowing how to keep focus whilst allowing the patient the reins, or knowing what questions to ask when emotional issues or anxiety or depression are mentioned. Professionals also acknowledge being concerned about closing interviews, which have been emotional. Lack of training in communication skills has been linked to burn out in both the nursing and medical profession (Ramirez et al., 1996; Berman et al., 2007).

HOLISTIC ASSESSMENT

Holistic assessment (or **global assessment** as it is sometimes called) appears in the literature to be used in an interchangeable way – the purpose is to attempt to ensure that all aspects of a patient or family's concerns, symptoms, problems, worries and needs are incorporated into the gathering of information, not just those aspects associated with the professional's scope of practice. In short, this is about treating the patient as an individual and not merely as a disease or set of symptoms. The aim is to elicit not just the facts of the situation, but also the patient's perception, all the illness-related concerns and needs of the patient, and to give information tailored to the patient's wishes and needs (Heaven and Maguire, 1993).

The domains of holistic assessment suggested by Richardson et al. (2007) are background information and assessment preferences, physical needs, social and occupational needs, psychological wellbeing and spiritual wellbeing. Other holistic assessments tools also cover informational, financial and religious aspects (Harrison et al., 1994; DH, 2012c). Department of Health guidance on assessment in medical and non-medical fields suggests that all patients should receive holistic assessment, especially in cancer and end-of-life care situations (DH, 2008c, 2012c).

In 2012, Professor Sir Mike Richards, the then English National Cancer Director stated that:

> Holistic needs assessment should be part of every cancer patient's care. It can make a huge difference to a patient's overall experience and has the potential to improve outcomes by identifying and resolving issues quickly.
>
> Undertaking an holistic needs assessment with the patient enables them to more fully engage in their care and facilitates choice. It enables the patient to take greater control of what happens to them and supports them to self-manage their condition. By helping patients identify their concerns teams will know where best to concentrate their effort and they will be able to develop a care plan that is tailored to an individual patient's needs. (DH, 2012c).

To be effective in conducting holistic global assessments, practitioners need to consider a number of things. These will be covered in five sections:

1. The context of the conversation
2. When the assessment should take place – the timing of the assessment
3. How the conversation is to be structured

4. Being responsive to the cues and concerns
5. Key communication behaviours and skills (facilitative and inhibitory)

Context

How a practitioner assesses a person's needs, preferences and concerns depends on a number of factors. These may include the **setting**, whether it is an emergency situation with a pressing physical need, whether the conversation is in the context of acute care where you may only have a single face-to-face meeting, or whether this is the first of many meetings in a chronic care setting, and **prior relationship** and **prior shared knowledge**. For example, clarifying the meaning of a phrase used by a patient may be vital if you have never met the patient before, whereas it may be entirely unnecessary if there is a prior relationship or prior meetings.

When to conduct an assessment

NICE Guidance recommends that assessment should be an ongoing process throughout the course of a cancer patient's illness (NICE, 2004b). Structured assessments should be undertaken at each of the following key points in the patient pathway:

- Around the time of diagnosis
- Commencement of treatment
- Completion of the primary treatment plan
- Each new episode of disease recurrence
- The point of recognition of incurability
- The beginning of end of life
- The point at which dying is diagnosed
- At any other time that the patient may request
- At any other time that a professional carer may judge necessary.

This guidance refers to a formal assessment process; however, assessment could be considered a much more fluid concept. For example, if assessment refers to the process by which a health professional weighs up and takes in information about their client and his or her family, it can be considered something which starts before individuals meet, through reading notes, listening to handovers and through seeing an environment. It continues every second the health professional is with the patient and family, and then continues after the meeting when the professional reflects and analyzes the information he or she has gathered in the encounter.

This chapter will limit itself to the formal or semi-formal process of talking to patient or family members, and will consider verbal and non-verbal cues that might be considered and how these can be picked up.

Structuring a consultation effectively

Evidence suggests that one of the simplest things we can do to facilitate disclosure is to structure our consultations effectively (Maguire et al., 1996; Silverman et al., 2008). This can help to maximize patient disclosure of concerns and help the patient's ability to recall any information given. Reviews of healthcare professional conversations show that information is given throughout the consultation (Heaven et al., 2006). This creates difficulties because it requires the patient to switch between receiver and sender of messages, as described earlier in the chapter. As a consequence, when the consultation has little structure, information obtained and recalled by the patient is suboptimal (Zimmerman et al., 2003, Jansen et al., 2010).

Throughout the literature, there are a number of models that consider the *content* of an assessment (Richardson et al., 2007), and the *process* of moving through an assessment interview (Silverman et al., 2008; Heaven and Maguire, 1993). Two models are considered here: The **Cambridge–Calgary Model**, which has been developed to help medical students learn medical assessment, but which is now commonly taught to nursing students (Silverman et al., 2008), and the **Maguire Model**, developed within cancer care for all types of professionals to incorporate into their assessment interviews (Heaven and Maguire, 1993) (see Table 17.1).

Both models consist of five sequential steps and can be used by healthcare professionals to direct the flow of the interview with the patient, thereby optimizing the flow and direction of information. Both models fully involve the patient at every step and can be defined as holistic. The Calgary–Cambridge model emphasizes the role of physical examination in the information gathering mode whilst the Maguire model does not mention physical examination specifically, but separates out the history-taking element and the assessment of the current concerns and situation.

Adopting the scene setting approach is a highly effective approach when meeting a patient for the first time, or when a number of things have happened since last meeting the patient because it gives a clear picture of the course of the illness from the patient's perspective and allows for a better understanding of the patient's experience. This will enable the practitioner to obtain a global understanding of the person's past and current reactions and expectations. However, on occasions, depending on the urgency or intensity of the problem, a full review of the patient's experience to date might not be possible. On these occasions, focusing on the immediate issues, the **current concerns approach**, may be more appropriate because it enables the professional to assess and manage the immediate problems. A concerns approach is also holistic, covering psychological, social and spiritual aspects of the particular concern or problem, not just the physical (Heaven and Maguire, 1993). Good-practice guidance drawn from these models for an interview process and structure is outlined next.

Table 17.1   Models of assessment

	Calgary–Cambridge Model	Maguire Model
Initiating	Preparation, establish rapport, reasons time	History of illness Plus concerns and impact
Information gathering	Exploration of problems (biomedical and patient perspective) Physical examination	Current concerns, impact, view of future
Giving	*Explanation and planning:* Providing the correct type and amount of information Aiding recall and understanding Achieving a shared understanding Shared decision-making	*Information giving and plan of action:* Tailor information Check understanding Share decision-making Negotiate a plan of action
Closing	Ensuring appropriate point of closure Forward planning	Summarize Screen for further concerns and questions

Introductions: This can set the tone of the interview. Clarity about role and purpose of the consultation are important and will aid disclosure. Healthcare professionals often make assumptions that patients and their families understand the purpose of the consultation, the different roles of professionals and what each person is trying to achieve in each conversation. However, if we consider the fact that most patients are seen by 8–10 different types of professional in any admission, it is not surprising that patients report confusion about role and purpose of the consultation, and frustration at being asked to repeat important details. Explaining our intentions, and the exact nature of our roles, can alleviate this frustration and empower the patients and their family to help and enable the healthcare professional to collect the information needed to best help the individual.

Introducing the concept of time may seem alien to those working in high intensity and emergency settings where speed in delivering care is essential and use of time is often dictated by physical need; however, it is important to consider creating a time boundary because it has been shown to aid disclosure by helping to focus the patient on important issues and creating a basis for the healthcare professional to manage the time more effectively. Negotiating a time boundary is important in shorter time-restricted consultations where efficient use of time is crucial; however, mentioning 'time' concerns many healthcare professionals who fear short-changing or insulting the patient by seeming to limit the conversation before it is started. When done in conjunction with an exploration of the purpose in an interview, and mentioned in a way that informs the patient and family of what to expect, a *negotiated* time frame works well; it gives the patient a sense of control, ensures that the patient and family have time for the conversation and maximizes the use of the time available. For example:

> 'Mrs Shield I would like to go through a number of things with you … would that be OK? … (Pause and wait for a response) …. We have about 20 minutes just now, but we could make more time if needed, so please don't feel there is a need to rush, I really need to get a good sense of how things are for you at home … would that be OK with you ? … (Pause) … Do you have 20 minutes to spare..? … (Wait for a response) … Thank you …'

Gathering the information: This involves actively eliciting and clarifying the 'story' and concerns. It is important to elicit the patients' perspective of the **facts** of the situation (what happened, what was done, who said what to whom – essentially, 'What have you been told');the person's **perceptions and understanding** of what was happening (what their interpretation was, what they understood about what was happening to them or what was said to them – essentially, 'What do you understand?'); and also the **feelings** that were associated with the perceptions (were they worried, upset, angry, fearful about things, at what stage and how they coped with these emotions – essentially, 'How did it leave you feeling?').

Integrating what happened with the person's perceptions and also their feelings during the 'story telling' can be highly effective in helping the individual remember things more accurately because it reconnects the individual with the emotions they experienced at the time. It also allows for the impact of previous information to be ascertained and concerns to be identified. It also shows the person (patient or family member) that the practitioner is interested in them as a whole person, holistically, not just in their symptoms.

Many practitioners worry about identifying a broad range of concerns that do not fall into their domain of practice or speciality, fearing that this will raise patient or family expectations in relation to the health professional finding some solution. This is not the case. Collecting information to get a full picture, no matter what the domain, is vital if the patient is to feel truly understood and valued as a complete individual. Research literature would suggest that the range of concerns experienced by people with cancer is broad. Most patients, when talking to professionals, discuss 3–4 major concerns (Anderson et al., 2001), but these range in nature and are dependent on gender, age and stage of illness. A study of over 800 cancer patients (Parle et al., 1996) suggested the most common concern of newly diagnosed cancer patients is the illness itself, whilst the most common concern of late-stage cancer patients and palliative care patients is either lack of independence or pain (Heaven and Maguire, 1997; Brown et al., 2000; Anderson et al., 2001).

The information gathering stage should end with a summary. This summary has two functions. It allows the health practitioner to capture what they have heard, collect their thoughts and check they have covered all aspects they intended to cover. It also helps the practitioner to ensure that further clarity is not needed on any aspect of what the patient or family member has said. For the patient or family member, the summary is also both helpful and important. The summary allows the patient to hear what the professional has taken on board and empowers them to correct misunderstandings and reiterate important things that may have been missed on first telling.

Giving information: There is evidence to suggest that patients retain less than half of the information given to them and understand less (Schofield et al., 2003); therefore, it is important to give information relevant to the patient's concerns and preferences, and to deliver it in a way that is tailored to the level of detail and understanding the individual requires. This can be achieved by relating the information given to the needs, concerns and worries identified in the information gathering stage of the interview. This will empower the individual to make well-informed treatment decisions and choices.

A common pitfall for health practitioners is the tendency to move quickly into information giving and to give as much information to the patient as possible, in order to fully inform the patient and reassure the patient that something can be done. Unfortunately, this can result in the patient feeling overwhelmed and struggling to keep up as he or she struggles to make sense of what has been said. This can lead to misunderstanding and misinterpretation and can result in the patient feeling that inadequate information or even no information has been provided (Hanoch et al 2007; Jansen et al., 2010).

Research has also shown that both worries and emotions can get in the way of patients hearing or taking in the information provided for them (Jansen et al., 2010). It is therefore important that practitioners ensure they have allowed sufficient time and space in their conversations for individuals to express these concerns and fears before starting to give information. Acknowledgement by the professional of the emotions expressed or even hinted at by patients have been shown to positively impact on the recall information; however, if the patient's emotions are ignored (see section on distancing and blocking), the amount of information recalled by the patient is significantly less (Jansen et al., 2010).

Information can always be backed up in written form. Many patients and families may never read the information they are given in paper form; however, others will find it a vital lifeline in helping them remember what has been said during a consultation. Given the literacy issues discussed earlier, health professionals need to ensure that written information is tailored to the particular person's needs. Tailoring written information has been shown to reduce the likelihood of patients becoming depressed over time (Schofield et al., 2003), and can be achieved by showing individuals sections of pamphlets, annotating booklets with words used by the patient themselves and highlighting particular sections in text to show what is particularly relevant. The key behaviours for giving information well are summarized in the following box.

Key behaviours when giving information

- Check you have fully understood the patient's perception and concerns
- Summarize (signpost) the areas to discuss
- Obtain permission to give appropriate information
- Use simple jargon-free language
- If jargon is used, explain
- Seek permission to give additional chunks of information
- Pause to allow the patient to assimilate the information or respond
- Check understanding
- Check impact on patient and acknowledge
- Obtain permission from patient before giving further information or clarifying details
- Notice any cues and acknowledge
- Use empathy especially if the information was unexpected or upsetting
- Check for new concerns or questions
- Summarize

Shared decision-making: Once information is received, shared decisions can be made. Well-informed choice is dependent on a good understanding of both the benefits and costs of available options, including the no treatment option. In 2010, the UK Government review of information giving in healthcare introduced the concept of 'No decision about me without me' (DH, 2010a). In reality, achieving this in all situations can be a challenge, especially because many decisions are often made at multidisciplinary team (MDT) level and are influenced by multiple variables. The Kings Fund reviewed medical decision-making and suggested that health professionals should follow a new model. They summed up current practice as being represented by the following equation, showing that treatment decisions (T) are most commonly a function of (f) medical diagnosis (Dm). They suggest in their review that, , it should be a function of patient preferences (Dp) and medical diagnosis (Dm):

Current treatment decision: $T= f (Dm)$

Recommended process: $T= f (Dm,Dp)$

Mulley et al. (2012:4).

There is also evidence that when healthcare professionals ignore patients' emotions and cues, patients have greater difficulty making decisions (Smith et al., 2011). It is important to note that patients' decisions may also change during the course of the illness and with any new information. Often, immediately after a diagnosis and especially if the diagnosis came as a shock, patients opt to have treatment decisions made for them, whilst later on they may choose to be more actively involved in care and treatment decisions. Decision preferences therefore need to be checked with the patient throughout the course of the illness (Vogel et al., 2008). A summary of key behaviours in enabling shared decision-making is given in the following box.

Keys skills for shared decisions and negotiated planning

- Offer treatment choices
- Summarize and signpost
- Requires prior global assessment of needs
- Describe risks and benefits
- Check understanding and new concerns
- Provide further information
- Elicit new concerns
- Provide further information
- Elicit preferences
- Summarize plan
- Screen for questions or concerns
- Check how patient feels

Negotiated plan of action: Once treatment decisions have been identified, a plan of action can be drawn together and checked with the patient, before further concerns and questions can be addressed. This process is similar to shared decision-making and involves the same skills.

Closing the session: Each consultation or global assessment needs an ending. The objectives in this part of the consultation are:

- To draw the consultation to a close
- To check that all the patient's concerns have been identified
- To confirm the negotiated treatment plan along with an agreed contingency plan
- To increase compliance and therefore patient wellbeing.

It is important when closing the consultation to recap what has been discussed. This would ideally include a summary of worries the patient came with, the information given to the patient, new concerns and the agreed plan of action. This summary should be checked with the patient. The healthcare professional should also screen for anything that is unclear and for questions or concerns left unanswered. Finally, it is important to check how the patient is left , especially if the consultation has been difficult.

RESPONDING TO CUES AND CONCERNS

To effectively optimize eliciting of needs, concerns, preferences and choices, and the giving of information, the healthcare professional needs to be attentive to the patient's cues and link the responses they give to those cues (Zimmerman et al., 2003). Patient cues are:

... verbal or non verbal hint which suggests an underlying unpleasant emotion and would need clarification from the health provider. (Del Piccolo et al., 2006:150).

Patients tend not to immediately and clearly disclose all their concerns; instead they tend to hint at worries and concerns to determine if the healthcare professional is interested (Heyn et al., 2012). The Verona Sequence Analysis Group defined seven categories of cues, which include hints of emotions, use of metaphor, profanity and mention of symptoms of distress (Del Piccolo et al., 2006).

Patients give a varying number of cues in every interview (Heaven et al., 2006, Zimmerman et al., 2003; Jansen et al., 2010), and so it is often difficult to determine which cue to explore. In this situation, it can help to reflect cues back to the patient and to allow them the opportunity to add or say more about those things that are creating most distress. Alternatively, the most relevant or biggest cue can be selected to work with. There is evidence that facilitating the first patient cue is of particular importance, especially in a patient-centred holistic assessment. There is a 20% decrease in the total number of cues in an interview when the first cue is not acknowledged appropriately (Fletcher, 2006), suggesting that if cues are ignored, patients make assumptions that this area of concern is not relevant to the healthcare professional's agenda. Working with cues is therefore essential for a patient-centred holistic consultation to be achieved.

Working with cues is also important when giving information and negotiating decisions with the patient. Patients often find it difficult to disagree openly with healthcare professionals, and therefore cues can be a useful way of gauging people's reactions to what is said. Patients and families often show us their preferences and their understanding through cues, many of which can be non-verbal, for example smiles and nods of affirmation, or frowns, quizzical looks, agitations, vacant expressions or reduced eye contact.

KEY COMMUNICATION SKILLS

Facilitative skills and behaviours

Facilitative skills are those used to gather information, listen to the patient, acknowledge what the patient says, and give appropriate information (see Table 17.2); however, these skills are significantly more powerful in relation to eliciting information and enabling patients to feel understood, when linked to cues (Zimmerman et al., 2007, Fletcher, 2006; Uitterhoeve et al., 2009).

Blocking behaviours

Blocking and distancing are terms used to describe those communication behaviours that inhibit and discourage the patient from saying anything further in relation to the cue/s they have just disclosed. It is frequently unconscious behaviour and is often used when the healthcare professional feels uncomfortable about exploring emotions. This behaviour can lead to some concerns being disclosed at the very end of the interview when time runs short (Beckman et al., 1985). Two main types of blocking behaviours occur: overt and distancing.

Overt blocking occurs when the healthcare professional consciously or unconsciously moves away from a cue by asking a completely unrelated question.

Table 17.2   Facilitative skills and behaviours

Facilitative skill or behaviour	Function
Open questions	Frequently start with 'how' or 'why'. Encourage the patient to talk freely. Can be vague and difficult for a patient to answer.
Open directive questions	More effective than true open questions because they direct the patient towards the topic in question. Asking psychological open focused questions allows worries and concerns to be disclosed. Example: 'How do you feel about the proposed treatment plan?'
Closed questions with a specific function (precision and directive questions)	Are often used to obtain details such as time, dates and duration. These questions can help the patient to refocus on events and to recall the associated feelings. Often result in a yes or no response, or a short answer and as a category are inhibitory. Example: 'When did you learn about your diagnosis?'
Screening questions (closed question)	Used to check for missing concerns or details. Normally 'anything else' is the phrase used but there is evidence that 'something else', which has a positive polarity, will elicit significantly more concerns (Heritage et al., 2007). Example: 'Is there something else about the chemotherapy that worries you?' as opposed to 'Is there anything else about the chemotherapy that worries you?'.
Educated guesses (closed question)	Tentative questions that are used to tentatively check out ideas about the patient's experiences, thoughts and feelings. Shows the professional is trying to understand the patient experience regardless of whether the guess is right or wrong. Note: guess will become an assumption if space isn't given to the patient to respond and patient disclosure will be inhibited. Example: 'It sounds like life has been a real struggle for you, would that be right?'
Negotiation	Demonstrates not only a willingness to listen, but respect. Example: 'Can you bear to tell me how you feel?'
Minimal prompts	Minimal verbal behaviours, such as 'Okay', 'Right', 'I see', 'Go on'. Encourage the patient to continue to talk and disclose.
Pauses	Essential when giving information. Allows the patient time to process what has been said and respond (Eide et al., 2004, Zimmerman et al., 2003).
Reflection	Repeating back the patient's own words. Acts as a form of acknowledgement and as an encouragement to continue.
Paraphrasing	Repeating back what the patient has said but in different words. Allows the healthcare professional to check their own understanding and allows the patient to feel heard.

Facilitative skill or behaviour	Function
Summarizing	Term used to describe paraphrasing back more than two items. Allows the patient to feel heard and the healthcare professional to check their own understanding.
Empathy	This is a brief phrase to show that the health professional has understood and appreciated the emotional impact of what the patient has experienced. Helps the patient to make clearer decisions and recall significantly more information (Smith et al., 2011; Jansen et al., 2010). Examples: 'How awful', 'I can see this information is really upsetting you'.
Exploration	This term is interchangeable with clarification but is more accurately used when exploring a new cue, feeling or concern. Example: 'Can you tell me why you feel so strongly?'.
Clarification	Refers to the use of questions to clarify the details of a cue or concern that is unclear or ambiguous. The term is interchangeable with exploration. Example: 'Can you tell me what you understand by the word tumour?'

Example: Patient: 'I was really worried when I woke up'

Interviewer: 'What family do you have?'

Distancing behaviour is the result of more subtle behaviours and normally takes the form of a question linked to the patient's statement, but not to the cue contained in that statement. Examples include:

Switching time frame: 'Are you worried now?'

Switching person: 'Was your partner worried?'

Switching topic/factual clarification: 'What time did you wake up?'

A more appropriate response would be: 'What was worrying you?'

There are also many other distancing/inhibitory behaviours that can act to reduce patient disclosure of concerns and these are described in Table 17.3.

MANAGING DIFFICULT COMMUNICATION SITUATIONS

There are many different types of situations that healthcare professionals struggle to handle. These include handling strong and difficult emotions; being asked difficult questions; breaking bad news under difficult circumstances; and relatives making inappropriate demands.

Table 17.3 Distancing and inhibitory behaviours

Other inhibitory behaviours	Description
Giving premature advice, reassurance or information	Information given before concerns have been elicited. May not, therefore, address the real issues. Giving information can signify moving to end of the consultation.
Minimizing	Phrases used by healthcare professionals to lessen the impact. Example: 'It is only a small cancer'.
Normalizing	Usually an attempt to reassure the patient. Can act to minimize the concern and inhibit future disclosure.
Closed questions	Restrict the response to generally one word or very short answer.
Multiple questions	Occur when more than one question is asked at the same time. The patient tends to answer the easier question, which is usually the last question and the more powerful first question is lost. Example: 'How did you feel about that or did you go to your GP?'

Managing strong emotions

Being presented with strong emotions, such as anger, is hard to handle and can be frightening. There is a tendency for the fearful professional to minimize or even ignore strong emotions in the hope that this will calm the situation or avoid a challenging confrontation. However, this is not effective. Emotion needs to be named, acknowledged, legitimized and explored, so that the patient may feel understood. This will then enable a discussion of underlying fears. Two helpful approaches developed by the Maguire Unit (2013; unpublished) for doing this – ANGER and RELEASE – are given below.

Handling and diffusing anger (ANGER)

Acknowledge: Acknowledge the emotion by naming the anger. Do not minimize.

Negotiate: Negotiate to obtain permission to explore the reasons: 'Could you tell me what is making you angry?'

Gather: Gather and acknowledge all the reasons (do not justify or explain) – summarize.

Empathize: Empathize and apologise if appropriate. Acknowledge and explore any new emotions.

Respect: Respect the person's reasons for being angry. Once the feelings have been validated and the underlying concerns explored, the patient will be more likely to hear advice or explanations.

Handling other strong emotions (RELEASE)

Reflect: Reflect back the actual emotion or behaviour you see or hear and pause: 'I can see you're upset'.

Explore: Explore the reasons driving the emotion: 'Can you bear to tell me why?'

Listen: Listen and acknowledge: 'So you're upset because ...'

Empathize: 'It sounds awful'.

Ask: Ask for other reasons: 'Is there something else upsetting you?'

Summarize: Summarize back all you have heard.

Empathize: Empathize throughout and before giving relevant information.

Handling difficult questions

Answering difficult questions may result in breaking bad news or giving uncertain information. Typical questions can be 'How long do I have?', 'I am going to die aren't I?' or 'It is cancer isn't it?'. The key principle is to acknowledge and explore the question before giving information that addresses the question (**explore before explain**). By exploring the question, the patient's perceptions, concerns and fears can be identified, which can then be addressed in one of the following ways: (1) the patient may already know the answer and, therefore, what is needed is an empathic confirmation whereby the associated fears and concerns can be addressed; or (2) the patient can be appropriately reassured due to unfounded fears and beliefs. Finally, the patient might not be fully expecting bad news and the news will have to be delivered slowly and sensitively (see breaking bad news).

A helpful strategy is:

- Acknowledge the importance of the question and say you will do your best to answer the question but that it would be helpful to understand what is making them ask the question.
- Once you have obtained the reasons, acknowledge them. Clarify anything that is unclear or ambiguous. Check for other reasons and concerns making them ask the question.
- Empathize with the patient's fears.
- Check the patient still wants the answer.
- Confirm their suspicion using a warning shot if necessary, to prepare the patient for the news.

Breaking bad news (delivering significant information)

Breaking potentially distressing news is difficult and receiving it can be devastating. Bad news is bad news however it is delivered, but the way it is delivered can affect how a person copes with the news. Often it is difficult to second guess what is going to be perceived as bad news by the patient, so the giving of any information, especially complex information, should be undertaken carefully (Fallowfield, 1993). Bad news needs to be given in a way that allows the person to understand and manage what is being said to them and also in a way that allows the person control over pace, and an opportunity to express their resulting fears and concerns before any information and advice is given. There are several models for the delivery of bad news and all have the same core components:

Start where the patient is: First, fully assess the patient's perception of what is wrong: 'What have you been told?', 'What did you understand?', or 'How did you feel?'.

Then, if the patient is not aware of what is wrong:

Give a warning shot: 'I'm afraid the results are not what we were hoping for',

Pause,

Deliver further information in small amounts (chunks) allowing each bit of information to sink in before checking if it's okay to continue,

Pause,

Empathize and elicit concerns before moving into giving information,

Give information and advice in response to concerns.

If the patient is aware of what may be wrong:

Deliver a compassionate warning shot,

Pause,

Confirm their understanding: 'I'm afraid you were right in your thinking, I'm so sorry',

Empathize and elicit all concerns before giving any information and advice: 'I can see how upset you are',

Pause: 'Can you bear to tell me what's going through your mind?',

Give information in response to patient's concerns.

IMPROVING SKILLS

Learning to communicate effectively through experience alone has been shown not to be effective (Cantwell and Ramirez, 1997), but communication is a skill that can be taught and there is evidence that workshops in communication skills are effective in changing behaviour. Although a sound knowledge base and observation of good practice can facilitate change, workshops give participants a chance to practice, optimize and maximize the ability to acquire and hone skills (Maguire et al., 1996, Wilkinson et al., 2008c, Fallowfield et al., 2003). Following the publication of NICE Guidance on supportive and palliative care (2004c), which recommended that accredited courses should be available to all staff working with cancer patients, and the increasing demand for training, the National Cancer Action Team commissioned the development of a national **Advanced Communication Skills Programme**, developed and evaluated by leaders in the field, and widely available across the NHS in England.

CHAPTER SUMMARY

An effective holistic assessment performed using facilitative skills and behaviours in the context of patient cues can be considered to be an assessment that is truly patient-centred and holistic. This type of assessment will allow not only the medical symptoms and diagnosis to be ascertained, but will importantly allow the patient to have their concerns addressed and their preferences taken into account. It will allow the patient to feel they have been treated as an individual with their wishes respected.

Key learning points

- Communication is the key to delivering high quality patient experience.
- Clinical outcomes can be affected when communication is not patient-centred. There are a number of reasons why open communication is not always easy to achieve – understanding both patients' and professionals' barriers can help overcome these hurdles.
- Structuring consultations not only improves patient disclosure and recall of information but may also help you know how to move through an interview more effectively.
- Always think about eliciting facts, perceptions and feelings.
- Ensure you have gathered all the information before you start giving any information.
- Negotiate before giving information and always tailor what you say to what is needed.
- Use facilitative skills and behaviours to both gather and give information.
- Linking your skills to the cues given by patients will make you a much more powerful and effective communicator.
- Be aware of the tendency to block and distance.
- Know your referral pathways.

Recommended further reading

- Heaven, C.M. and Maguire, P. (1993) *Assessing Patients with Cancer: the Content, Skills and Process of Assessment*. 2nd edn. London: Cancer Research UK.
- Kai, J. (ed.) (2005) *PROCEED: Professionals Responding to Ethnic Diversity and Cancer*. London: Cancer Research UK. Copyright: University of Nottingham.
- Silverman J., Kurtz S. and Draper J. (2008) *Skills for Communicating with Patients*. 2nd edn. Oxford, UK: Radcliffe Publishing.

18 PSYCHOSOCIAL ADJUSTMENT TO CANCER

NICHOLAS HULBERT-WILLIAMS AND GILL HUBBARD

Chapter outline

- Prevalence and causes of psychological distress and co-morbidity
- The process of psychosocial adjustment to illness
- Cognitive models of appraisal and coping
- The social context of adjustment
- A functional contextual approach to adjustment

CONTEXT SETTING – PREVALENCE AND CAUSES OF PSYCHOLOGICAL DISTRESS AND CO-MORBIDITY

In a review article published in 1994, Andersen et al. highlighted the importance of paying attention to the **psychological stress** of cancer as a potentially important influence on an individual's disease outcomes (via health and compliance behaviour pathways). They developed a theoretical framework – the **Biobehavioural Model** – that linked psychological response to physiological disease progression. Even though convincing and conclusive empirical evidence on a causal relationship between psychological and physical health has not been forthcoming, this was an important message and the following two decades bore witness to an exponential rise in published work that attempted to understand the broader impact that cancer has beyond the physiological aspects. **Psychosocial oncology** as a discipline works towards achieving greater recognition of this broader impact and the need to conduct research and develop services to address *all* important patient concerns: their psychological stress; experiences of **distress**, low mood and **depression**; and their fears and **anxieties**. Within this context the term '**adjustment**' is used to refer to the process of change and adaptation that occurs as the individual attempts to integrate cancer into their lives whilst at the same time maintaining some sense of normality and **psychosocial homeostasis**.

Through the course of cancer diagnosis and treatment, few individuals maintain pre-diagnosis levels of psychological health and wellbeing without some challenges. There is inconsistency in published literature, however, about how common psychological disorders, for example anxiety and depression, actually are, Maguire (2000) suggested that such clinical disorders are apparent in around one-third of all cancer patients, but distress, a term used to refer to subclinical symptoms of mental health, is far more common (Dunn et al., 2013). For some, this distress may emerge in the form of fear (of recurrence or of death); for others it may be a general feeling of stressed agitation, or a persistent low mood that doesn't meet clinical cut-off for depression.

In many cases, distress can be relatively easily resolved by addressing any **unmet psychosocial needs** that a person may have (Carey et al., 2012). Unmet needs can be defined as a 'desire or requirement for help or support that underlies [a person's] emotional and psychological wellbeing' (Swash et al., 2014: 1131), and many people with cancer report having at least one unmet need (Harrison et al., 2009). Unmet needs do not always relate to the physical care of the patient with cancer and thus it may not always be appropriate for the healthcare professional to meet them: unmet emotional support needs, for example, may be better met by provision of a support group or access to a psychological counselling service (see Chapter 22).

In the next chapter of this textbook, Alex Mitchell gives a thorough account of the definitions of some of these negative consequences and how they may be screened for in routine clinical practice. Within psychosocial oncology, however, we are often too focused on negative outcomes, when in fact the same predictive factors may also help us to understand who may respond to the challenge of cancer in a more **adaptive** way. Some cancer survivors often reflect more positively on ways that their life has improved since their cancer diagnosis; we refer to this as **benefit finding** or **post-traumatic growth**. Early reports suggested that benefit finding was reported by around 90% of cancer survivors (Collins et al., 1990), and that these range from a sense of appreciation for life, more tolerance of stressors, or improved social and personal relationships. It is important to note that benefit finding is not simply a return to pre-diagnosis psychosocial functioning, but clearly identifiable self-reported improvements.

Whether the impact of cancer is positive or negative, this has clearly observable consequences on overall **health-related quality of life**. Quality of life represents much more than a simple measure of physiological or health status, and is defined by the World Health Organization (WHO) as:

> … an individual's perception of their position in life in the context of the culture and value systems in which they live and in relation to their goals and expectations, standards, and concerns. It is a broad ranging concept affected in a complex way by a person's physical health, psychological state, level of independence and their relationships to salient features of the environment. (WHO, 1999: 3).

As such, quality of life is understood to be a multidimensional index of wellbeing and an extensive literature has related this construct to cancer outcomes. Montazeri, for example, reviewed 104 studies linking quality of life to cancer survival documenting numerous significant independent predictors of mortality from the various subcomponents of quality of life (Montazeri, 2009). Similar data from 30 randomized controlled trials from the European Organization for Research and Treatment of Cancer (EORTC) was reported by Quinten et al. (2009): parameters of physical functioning, pain and appetite loss provided small but significant prognostic information, in addition to traditional markers of age, gender and metastases.

In this chapter, we outline some of the theoretical frameworks linking both psychological and sociological perspectives that may help us to understand why such variation in non-physiological impact of cancer occurs, and how these perspectives have changed over time. This is of vital relevance to both the psychosocial oncology research community (who need a broad appreciation of the context in which their participants are functioning), but also, and perhaps more importantly, to the clinicians who are under pressure to deliver holistic and individually tailored care to people with cancer.

THE PROCESS OF PSYCHOSOCIAL ADJUSTMENT TO ILLNESS

Initial disruption and challenged identity

Early work into illness adjustment attempted to elucidate a temporal process of adaptation and adjustment to explain the differences in emotional and psychological behaviours observed within various patient groups. Although many such models were proposed, most are in agreement that the initial few days following diagnosis place the individual in a state of uncertainty, crisis, disarray and psychological bewilderment whilst the full implications of their illness are being processed. There is evidence that, in this initial phase, **cognitive processing** is slowed and these patients will often report emotional numbness (Holland and Gooen-Piels, 2000).

Moos and Schaefer's **crisis theory of illness adjustment** (1984) suggests that this state of distress occurs because the new diagnosis has challenged four important aspects of the patient's everyday life: their identity, their environment, their self-perceived 'role' and their relationships. This has parallels with the sociological theory of **biographical disruption** (Bury, 1982, 1991, 2001): cancer diagnosis fundamentally disrupts the expected life course, necessitating reorganization of self-identity and a sense of uncertainty about what the future might hold (Hubbard and Forbat, 2012). These disruptions arise because illness throws into the air people's taken-for-granted assumptions about their bodies, selves and the social world in which they live, bringing to the fore pain, suffering and death, which are normally only seen as distant or remote possibilities in one's life or are perceived as the plight of others (Bury, 1982).

These themes of identity and loss through illness have formed the focus of much of Charmaz's work (1983, 1994, 1995, 2002). Bury and Charmaz both situate their work within the tradition of **symbolic interactionism**, which is a sociological theory of human interaction (Blumer, 1969; Cooley, 1902; Mead, 1934). A symbolic interactionist framework conceives of identity as a means of defining and differentiating self from others and takes into account people's preferred identities and identity goals that they desire, hope and plan for in the future. Identity requires empirical validation in daily life; yet, with the onset of chronic illness, daily life upon which former identities have been built will also have changed. According to Charmaz (1983), **'loss of self'** is experienced by people with chronic illness because their former actions, lives and selves are now precluded (or at least perceived to be so) by illness.

She notes that whereas acute illness may cause only temporary disruptions of self, chronic conditions can lead to continued and repeated losses of self. Understanding cancer as a disease that interrupts sense of self is evident in much of the adjustment literature (Bellizzi and Blank, 2007; Meiklejohn et al., 2013).

Charmaz's later work examined how people repair loss of self brought about by chronic illness, noting that some people struggle against illness and engineer their lives in order to regain, restore and preserve a pre-illness sense of self and identity (Charmaz, 1995). Her analysis of men's experience of illness (Charmaz, 1994) for instance, illuminates some of the processes employed to preserve pre-illness identities: **bracketing** is a means of removing illness from the general flow of life or confining it to a separate place, whereas **viewing illness as an enemy** serves to objectify and externalize it in order to preserve a pre-illness identity. Other patients, however, may adapt to illness and establish a new identity in the process: 'Adapting implies that the individual acknowledges impairment and alters life and self in socially and personally acceptable ways' (Charmaz, 1995: 657). The extent to which adaption is possible and successful is dependent on context. She suggests that middle class and professional men, for example, are better able to alter their paid work to fit around their bodily needs. Hence, they are able to maintain an identity goal (their paid employment) by altering their daily activities to accommodate the impact of illness. Thus, her understanding of disruption takes cognizance of context.

The process of integrating illness into life

There are a number of models that attempt to describe and map the process of adjustment following this initial phase of crisis. According to Shontz (1975), this initial distress is followed by a stage of loss and **helplessness**; then **denial** and retreat; and then a stage of adjustment and **acceptance**. Morse and Johnson (1991) suggest that the initial uncertainty is necessary to understand the meaning and severity of the illness diagnosis, and is followed by two phases of **coping**: first, coping with the crisis and stress that has resulted from the diagnosis event, and second, coping to gain personal control over the situation. The final stage of their model, restoration of wellbeing, comes only when the individual has psychologically accepted the diagnosis and gained emotional equilibrium. In Holland and Gooen-Piels's (2000) model of adjustment, the phase of long-term adaptation can only be reached where the individual has acknowledged the reality of their situation (their 'dysphoria' phase), and it is at this stage that we see a distinction between those who respond negatively, with distress or anxiety, and those who take a more positive perspective, reporting feeling hopeful and **optimistic**.

Whilst there is certainly some evidence that those coping with illness may experience these varying emotional responses, less evidence is available to support the temporal nature proposed by these models. It is very rare, for example, for a person with cancer to progress through each of the stages in the specified order and in a logical process: adjustment is simply far more complex than that, and even those who are accepting and seem to be well adjusted may have setbacks and feel helpless or more emotional now and again. Furthermore, such attempts to model adjustment are primarily descriptive and thus they don't sufficiently explain the why, or process, underlying the psychological responses. For that, we may find some answers in psychological theories of **appraisal** and coping.

Cognitive models of appraisal and coping

Since the cognitive revolution of the mid-twentieth century, psychology as a discipline has focused on not only observable behaviour, but also understanding the 'unseen' psychological processes that occur within the mind (see Brysbaert and Rastle (2009) for an excellent introductory text on the history of psychology). Although these cognitive processes can't be objectively observed, measures have been developed to assess them, and research has demonstrated how such constructs may be predictive of subsequent illness behaviours, such as coping or outward symptoms of psychological distress.

Defined in psychological terms, coping refers to the cognitive and/or behavioural efforts made by an individual to manage a stressful situation. This can include an entire array of responses ranging from engaging with negative health behaviours (e.g. smoking, getting drunk) to seeking out information, seeking emotional support from family and friends, or seeking solace in religious or spiritual practice. Coping is a psychologically interesting concept because it is so subjective: a coping strategy perceived by one person to be psychologically adaptive may be perceived by another to be maladaptive. Indeed, that same person may appraise the same coping method in two very different ways, with respect to the same stressor, on two different occasions. It is even common for individuals to report using many different coping approaches to manage the various demands associated with a stressor, sometimes in turn, at other times concurrently (Lazarus, 1993).

Similarly, from the sociological literature, Bury (1991) introduces the concept of coping to refer to processes whereby individuals learn to tolerate their illness and suggests that it 'involves maintaining a sense of value and meaning in life, in spite of symptoms and their effects' (Bury, 1991: 461). Examples of coping include normalization and bracketing off the impact of illness so that the effects on identity are minimized. According to Bury (2001) there are two processes of normalization. People normalize in the sense of keeping their pre-illness lifestyle and identity intact by either maintaining as many pre-illness activities as possible and/or by disguising or minimizing symptoms. Other people find ways to incorporate their illness into an altered lifestyle so that normal life is re-designated as containing the illness. Recent qualitative studies draw on understanding illness as a process of normalization, suggesting that some patients with cancer make considerable attempts to regain normality (Molassiotis and Rogers, 2012).

There are numerous measures of coping and, quite confusingly, each one tends to use different labels and dichotomies for the resultant variables. Folkman and Lazarus's (1985) 'Ways of Coping Scale', for example, differentiates eight dimensions of problem-focused (e.g. planned problem solving) and emotion-focused (e.g. escape-avoidance) coping; Endler and Parker (1990) meanwhile differentiate between task (e.g. solving strategies), emotion (e.g. self-preoccupation) or avoidance-oriented (e.g. distraction) coping; and Carver et al.'s (1989) COPE measure categorizes 15 different strategies (e.g. seeking emotional support, turning to religion, acceptance, etc.) without making any overall thematic categories. Within the cancer literature specifically, one of the most commonly used measures of coping is Watson et al.'s Mental Adjustment to Cancer Scale (Watson et al., 1988). This framework categorizes coping into five themes (helplessness/hopelessness, anxious preoccupation, cognitive avoidance, fatalism and fighting spirit), and is predicated on the idea that each individual will vary in the extent that they adopt these different responses.

This lack of consistency in how coping is defined and measured can make it difficult to draw meaningful conclusions from the literature. What the evidence does seem to show is that although a denial or avoidance coping strategy may be productive for short-term coping, more active strategies may encourage better long term adaptation (Taylor, 2008) whilst emotion-focused strategies are more predictive of greater distress in the longer term (McCaul et al., 1999; Stanton et al., 2000). According to Cheng, Hui and Lam (2004), those who cope best with stress are those who are able to tap into a variety of different methods of coping in a flexible and ongoing reflective way. Coping not only has direct effects on illness-related behaviours and outcomes (e.g. perceived stress, anxiety), but also has indirect effects on other health-related behaviours (e.g. adherence, lifestyle), and may potentially act to blunt stress-related physiological changes (thus bringing us full-circle to Andersen et al.'s (1994) Biobehavioural Model). As such, coping is an important construct, and is especially relevant in the context of providing individually tailored care and support.

The seminal work of Richard Lazarus and Susan Folkman in the 1980s led to one of the most adopted frameworks for understanding an individual's coping responses: the **Transactional Model of Stress and Coping**. Lazarus and Folkman suggested that this model could be applied to any situation that has the potential to result in psychological stress for the individual, and it therefore has relevance to be applied to understanding response to both the overall cancer experience or to specific aspects of it (e.g. attending the first radiotherapy session, attending follow-up appointments). This model was the first to comprehensively draw together a framework to explain why individuals cope with and respond to stress differently: they did this by introducing the concept of cognitive appraisal (Lazarus and Folkman, 1984).

Appraisal can occur both consciously or unconsciously and is influenced by a range of variables, including situational, temporal and personal factors. For example, a patient receiving a cancer diagnosis may appraise it as a threat (e.g. to future goals), as a challenge (to overcome), or as a loss (e.g. of their role as primary wage-earner for the family). These appraisals can vary considerably dependent on clinical characteristics, past experience, and even patient demographic. For example, diagnosis of cancer recurrence will be appraised in a very different way to diagnosis of a primary tumour. These cognitive variations go on to determine both the emotional response and the type of coping adopted, which in turn affect psychosocial outcome. The underlying motivation behind this process is to retain (or return to) pre-illness equilibrium or normality in the same way already discussed in the context of sociological perspectives on illness. Compared with research on coping responses to cancer, fewer studies have explored variation in cognitive appraisal. Those that have, however, suggest it may be a more powerfully predictive factor of psychosocial outcome than direct measurement of the resultant coping strategies adopted (Rand et al., 2012; Hulbert-Williams et al., 2012a).

In later versions of the Transactional Model, the concept of appraisal was further developed, and a distinction drawn between primary appraisal (cognitive evaluation of implications of the event) and secondary appraisal (cognitive evaluations of the individual coping resources available) (Folkman et al., 1986). Although Lazarus suggested even more specific forms of appraisal in his later work (Lazarus, 1999), a recent theory test of this in a cancer population reported a failure to verify the associations between appraisals, emotions and coping responses in this specific way (Hulbert-Williams et al., 2013).

Leventhal and colleagues' (1980, 1992) **Self-Regulation Model** of illness and illness-related behaviour is based on similar themes of appraisal and coping; however, in this framework the psychological process is split up into aspects related to the physical health threat and the emotional reaction separately. These illness **representations** initially form at the point of symptom experience and are influenced by both personal history and the broader socio-cultural context. The Self-Regulation Model categorizes five areas that are related to illness adaptation: (1) illness identity, (2) consequences of illness, (3) perceived cause, (4) expected timeline, and (5) curability and control (Leventhal et al., 1980).

Oncology-specific models of adjustment have also been proposed, for example James Brennan's **Social-Cognitive Theory of Cancer Adjustment** (2001). This process model encompasses a broad range of psychosocial components primarily centred around the notion that distress results when diagnosis (and its sequalae) requires greatest reorganization of the patient's mental map (Brennan and Moynihan, 2004), a term used to refer to individual cognitive **schema** and experience of the world.

These models have common features: they each assume that illness is stressful and distressing because it results in disruption to normality and equilibrium. Furthermore, they all assume that adjustment to the stress of illness is something that happens at a very individualistic level, and that it is the result of complex cognitive and coping processes. There are many demographic and dispositional factors that are known to affect variation in cognitive appraisals and coping (albeit to differing levels of evidence), and most of the models cited account for the potential influence of these factors. Examples from the cancer literature of potentially **mediating** variables include gender and age (Schnoll et al., 1998; Compass et al., 1999; Fife et al., 1994), optimism (Epping-Jordan et al., 1999; Hulbert-Williams et al., 2012a), self-efficacy (Beckham et al., 1997; Lev, Paul and Owen, 1999), religious and spiritual engagement (Laubmeier et al., 2004; Kristeller et al., 2011), and many others besides.

More recent theory development literature, from both sociological and psychological disciplines, has begun to challenge the individualistic and cognitive focus in these models of adjustment. In the second half of this chapter, we outline two alternative ways of understanding adjustment that may lead to a better understanding of cancer adjustment, and more effective supportive care interventions for both patients and their families.

The social context of adjustment

One of the core critiques levelled against these models is that they focus too much on the individual process, paying little regard to the 'social' world in which each individual exists: this is an essential part of the puzzle if the goal is to fully understand the cancer experience from a truly **biopsychosocial** perspective. To explain, for example, why certain patients are anxious or distressed, it isn't enough to know how they are thinking about their cancer or what coping methods they are employing, it is important to also know about their **relational networks** and how their close family and friends are also adjusting and the dyadic nature of these parallel processes (Hubbard et al., 2013). The work described earlier on coping and cognitive appraisal research has examined individual stress and coping patterns. Whilst there are some rather dated examples of attempts to also expand this work to examine individual stress and coping patterns of partners of cancer patients (e.g. Klein et al., 1967), these often treat the patient and partner as separate entities. This well-established body of work has described the impact of illness on people as individuals but falls short of examining the connections between patient and partner psychosocial adjustment following cancer diagnosis.

More recent literature has instead focused on the connections between the patient and their partner. For example, studies report that increasing anxiety in patients closely correlates with increasing anxiety in partners as well (Dorros et al., 2010), and that the strategies one person uses to cope with illness also affect the strategies used by their partner. This literature suggests that although there may be concordant rates of psychological distress within a couple, there may also be a complementary pattern of distress with only one partner exhibiting distress at any one period in time. This work improves our understanding of the impact of cancer beyond the patient at an individualistic level by describing their social connections with other family members (see also Chapter 20), but it does not necessarily explain the nature of this interaction.

Work that has focused on couple relationship dynamics offers explanatory potential for understanding these connections better. This work has been described as a systemic approach to understanding psychosocial adjustment and explains the impact of illness as a shared experience impacting on the couple as an interactive unit. A key psychosocial adjustment concept within the systemic approach is **dyadic coping** (Bodenmann, 1997). Dyadic coping, as opposed to individual coping, describes couples' efforts to cope jointly with a common or shared stressor. Stress is conceptualized as dyadic if it affects both partners, and where the stress signals of one partner influences the coping reactions of the other partner to these stress signals. Dyadic coping acknowledges that couples cope both individually and collectively as a unit to shared stressors and it focuses more on this shared experience than the individual stressor response. A recent review article on the influence of relationship quality (**attachment**) on dyadic coping and adjustment drew together key research in this field, and suggests that the development and evaluation of supportive care interventions, which are tailored to attachment styles of couples or family units, should be a long-term goal within cancer care (Nicholls et al., 2014).

A functional contextual approach to distress

Despite a common (misplaced) perception that the cognitive revolution was a whole-discipline paradigm shift in psychology, the late 1980s and early 1990s witnessed a re-interest in much earlier models grounded in **radical behaviourism**. An applied arm of this work (focusing on psychological wellbeing) has given rise to **'third-wave'** psychological interventions (Hofmann and Asmundson, 2008) such as **Acceptance and Commitment Therapy** (ACT) and **Dialectical Behaviour Therapy** (DBT).

These alternative intervention approaches are rooted in a behaviourally based psychological framework: **Contextual Behavioural Science**. Perhaps the most pertinent difference between these approaches and the cognitive approaches discussed earlier is that mental events are considered as outcomes in their own right, not as the causes of other behaviours. They also have clear and demonstrable influences from the newer fields of **Positive Psychology** and **Buddhist Psychology**, and as such they have developed a framework of wellbeing and distress that is quite different from that with which readers may be familiar – it is this that may be suggested to better suited to understanding cancer-related adjustment (Hulbert-Williams et al., 2014). These models challenge the basic assumptions underlying other models of psychological wellbeing, whereby they position distress in medical terms and resulting from problematic, faulty or inappropriate cognitive responses. The inevitable consequence of these frameworks is that interventions should aim to challenge, change or fix these cognitive or coping responses. Contextual behavioural models of wellbeing instead suggest that feelings of distress and suffering are simply normal and expected responses to difficult situations (Hayes et al., 2011); the goal of these interventions, therefore, should be in helping individuals to accommodate suffering and distress into their lives, rather than avoiding or changing their perception of it. This is predicated on a good deal of experimental psychology research which concludes that attempts to suppress or challenge thoughts and cognitions is rarely an effective therapeutic technique and can, in fact, often lead to those thoughts becoming more problematic in the longer term (Longmore and Worrell, 2007; Hayes et al., 2011). Essentially, these models propose that distress arises because we try to control experiences and evade suffering, rather than finding ways to live with suffering and to build resilience against the negative effects of these experiences (Hayes et al., 2006).

Psychological flexibility has been introduced as a construct that rests at the centre of the ACT model (Wilson and DuFrene, 2009); proponents of this theory suggest that flexibility acts as a buffer to psychological distress, such that the higher an individual's level of flexibility, the less likely they are to experience negative consequences from stressor adaptation and may be more likely to find benefit or growth. Whilst there is not the space in this chapter to explain this model in great depth, a summary of what flexibility in this context represents may be helpful. From an ACT perspective, flexible individuals are characterized by:

- An awareness and acceptance of all experiences (not just positive or desirable ones), real and/or imagined, in an open, and non-judgemental way (these are the theoretical components of **mindfulness** and **acceptance**);
- An ability to be able to experience thoughts as merely passing thoughts, not something to be constantly held on to or ruminated about (this component is **cognitive defusion**), and not as something that defines self-identity (the component, **self as process and context**); and,
- A recognition of honest and individually defined values (the component, **valued living**) and a commitment to live in accordance with these self-defined values (the final component, **committed action**).

Although the evidence base for third-wave interventions in cancer is only small (see Chapter 22), Hulbert-Williams and Owen (2015) outline why this model may be so suitable for understanding the adjustment challenges that people with cancer face: distress-related responses to cancer are not unreasonable, and they are certainly not 'abnormal' from a psychological perspective. As such, attempts to challenge and change these responses are likely to be futile. Instead, a **transdiagnostic approach** (such as that offered by ACT) that advocates **resiliency** and psychological flexibility as a means of coping may be more effective. There is already a growing literature with cancer patients that demonstrates, for example, (1) the importance of living in accordance with values (Ciarrochi et al., 2011), and (2) varying levels of psychological flexibility (Hulbert-Williams and Storey, under review) as important correlates of psychosocial outcome in cancer patients.

Although this model is currently relatively unknown in psychosocial oncology, it incorporates some important features that we've covered elsewhere in this chapter, from both earlier psychological and sociological perspectives. For example, there is less focus on the micro-cognitive responses of the individual, and more appreciation of the challenge that cancer may present to self-identity, relationships and living according to one's values. In this way, it perhaps marks an important step towards developing a more integrative model of cancer adjustment.

CHAPTER SUMMARY

The importance of understanding the psychological and social impacts of cancer has been established for some time, and a substantial literature has emerged indicating that those who respond to cancer with distress have significantly poorer longer-term psychosocial outcomes (Lam et al., 2010), for example they may have comparatively poorer quality of life. Whilst attempts to model the process of emotional adaptation to cancer were useful in terms of population descriptions, more recent research has attempted to identify observable and measurable predictors of outcomes, such as cognitive appraisal and coping. Although there is some correlational evidence for the importance of these variables, they have also been critiqued for their individualistic framework of adaptation. We ended this chapter with a brief overview of two alternative frameworks – one from a sociological perspective, the other from a behavioural psychological perspective – that may offer new directions for research in psychosocial oncology. There is clearly much more work to be done in developing a sound and clinically useful model of psychological adjustment to cancer, but there is still an important take-home message: those providing care and support for people with cancer need to be aware of the prevalence of psychological distress and why this may occur if they are to provide holistic and individually tailored healthcare. Furthermore, every person with cancer exists in a social unit and so to not take this into account may undermine the support provided: cancer care may benefit from taking a more **systemic** perspective, enquiring about wider aspects of family functioning, such as how a couple affected by cancer communicate their own stress to each other, the degree to which both partners respond to each other's stress and the degree to which both partners work together to manage dyadic stress.

Key learning points

- Cancer has a broad and wide-reaching impact beyond the physical and functional level: psychological and social outcomes are also of importance.
- This psychosocial impact is evident not only on the patient, but also their family and wider support network.
- Various models of the process of psychological adjustment to cancer have been proposed, but these have limitations.
- Attempts to predict adjustment from psychological and sociological factors are limited by their individualistic nature.
- Models that take into account the wider family and social network around the patient may add an additional and important level of understanding.
- As an alternative, considering cancer adjustment within a functional contextual framework of psychological wellbeing may be more appropriate and lead to more acceptable and useful interventions.

Recommended further reading

- Lazarus, R. (1993) 'From psychological stress to the emotions: a history of changing out-looks', *Annual Review of Psychology*: 44: 22–39.
- Hulbert-Williams, N. and Owen, R. (2015) 'ACT: Acceptance and Commitment Therapy for Cancer Patients', in J. Holland, W.S. Breitbart, P.B., Jacobsen, et al. (eds), *Psycho-Oncology*, 3rd edn. New York, NY: Oxford University Press.
- *Sociology of Health and Illness and Psycho-Oncology* are two very relevant scientific journals that regularly include articles on the topic of adjustment to illness.

19 ASSESSMENT OF PSYCHOLOGICAL WELLBEING AND EMOTIONAL DISTRESS

ALEX J. MITCHELL

Chapter outline

- The importance of psychological wellbeing in cancer
- Screening tools for psychological wellbeing
- Implementation of screening in clinical practice

- Clinical case-finding of psychosocial wellbeing
- Challenges and benefits of screening for psychological co-morbidity

---

INTRODUCTION

Psychological wellbeing covers a wide area that may be described by broad concepts of **quality of life** (QoL) and **distress**, as well as traditional mental health diagnoses, such as **depression, bipolar disorder** and **anxiety**. There is a strong case for evaluating unmet needs when assessing psychological complications because these are often related to underlying disease burden. It is well documented that many cancer patients report that their psychological needs are not met (Harrison et al., 2009). Unmet needs closely correlate with distress. Addressing unmet unresolved concerns helps alleviate distress in most cases (Carey et al., 2012). Currently, there is no single acceptable tool that enables clinicians to assess all relevant aspects of psychological health. Fully structured and semi-structured interviews are available, but these are designed for research purposes as a criterion reference. The most popular is the **Structured Clinical Interview** for Diagnostic and Statistical Manual: Mental Disorders (DSM) (SCID) (Spitzer et al., 1992). Other examples include the **Composite International Diagnostic Interview** (CIDI) (Wittchen et al., 1991) and the

Mini-International Neuropsychiatric Interview (MINI) (Sheehan et al., 1998). Mental health problems are sometimes overlooked by busy cancer professionals in palliative and non-palliative settings because these clinicians do not have the time to use lengthy assessment tools and often prefer to use their own clinical judgement (Söllner et al., 2001; Jones and Doebbeling, 2007); yet all professional groups should look out for emotional complications and nurses are no less accurate than doctors (Mitchell and Kakkadasam, 2011). Less than a third of recorded consultations are found to contain discussions of emotional concerns (Rodriguez et al., 2010; Taylor C. et al., 2011). To address this, several organizations have recommended (but not mandated) screening for emotional complications of cancer (Institute of Medicine, 2007; National Comprehensive Cancer Network (NCCN), 2008; NICE, 2004b; Neuss, 2005). It is important to understand screening conceptually because this will influence later interpretation of results. **Screening** can be defined pragmatically as 'the application of a diagnostic test or clinical assessment in order to optimally rule-out those *without* the disorder with minimal false negatives (missed cases)' (Mitchell, 2010a; Mitchell and Malladi, 2010). Screening is often performed in a large population as the first of several diagnostic steps. The related procedure of case-finding can be defined as 'the application of a diagnostic test or clinical assessment in order to optimally identify those *with* the disorder with minimal false positives (misidentifications)' . **Case-finding** is often performed as a second step in a selected population at high risk for the condition following initial screening and, by implication, is a more thorough in-depth process. All tests (including clinical judgement) should be evaluated for suitability for purpose. In this context, that means not only accuracy, but also acceptability and effectiveness in clinical practice. In short, does the proposed test method bring added value to clinical practice when compared to routine care? Possible benefits of screening include prompt recognition, timely treatment and potentially earlier resolution of psychological complications. Potential hazards of screening include heightened anxiety, **false positives and negatives**, cost (including time) and diversion of precious resources.

Defining psychiatric complications

Depression is the most studied psychological complication of cancer and is itself one of the strongest determinants of QoL. Depression also influences receipt of medical care, participation in treatment and possibly mortality (Bui et al., 2005; Kennard et al., 2004; Skarstein, 2000; Satin, 2009). The **point prevalence** of major depression in the first two years following a cancer diagnosis is approximately 15%, with a gradual reduction in severity as patients transition to long-term survivors (Mitchell et al., 2011a). The most commonly applied criteria are those set out in *Diagnostic and Statistical Manual of Mental Disorders* (DSM-IV) (American Psychiatric Association, 1994), describing major depression, which has recently been updated (DSM-V) (American Psychiatric Association, 2013). Uncertainty exists regarding less common forms of depression. Diagnosis of major depression requires five out of nine qualifying symptoms, together with a minimum duration of two weeks and clinical significance defined by concomitant distress or impaired daily function. Other forms of depression include minor depression, **dysthymia**, **adjustment disorder** with predominant depression and a research category of **brief reactive depression**. Differences between depression subtypes can by found in the DSM source book (APA, 2013), but crucially all of these alternative categories include patients who do not fulfil criteria for major depression but have troubling symptoms nonetheless. Given the focus on depression, it may be surprising that anxiety is actually the most common patient-reported emotional complication of cancer (Mitchell et al., 2011). Self-reported anxiety is typically found in more than 40% of patients in the early stages of treatment, but like depression, anxiety is underestimated by clinicians (Mitchell et al., 2011). Anxiety and depression are frequently overlapping, but anxiety is independently associated with poorer QoL amongst cancer patients (Brown et al., 2010). Anxiety has many subtypes, but the main ones are **generalized anxiety disorder** (GAD), **panic disorder**, and **post-traumatic stress disorder** (PTSD). Unfortunately, the criteria for GAD may be too restrictive for medical settings because they require 'excessive anxiety' for at least six months. In addition, there is low agreement between ICD10 (WHO International Classification of Diseases, 10th edn) and DSM-IV criteria for GAD (Slade et al., 2001). It is well known that depression and anxiety are relatively narrow concepts with complex criteria: one broader category that may be of more use is **adjustment disorder**, which lacks specific symptom criteria but encompasses symptoms of depression and anxiety and occurs in about one in five cancer patients acutely (Mitchell et al., 2011). The term adjustment disorder was revised in DSM-III and again in DSM-IV to describe a reaction that occurs within three months (ICD10 uses once per month window) of an identifiable stressor and consists of mild symptoms of depression, anxiety or trauma stress.

A newer direction is to use simpler, patient-defined terms rather than psychopathological ones. Hence '**distress**' has been proposed as a simple user-friendly concept that could be considered as a sixth vital sign in medical settings (Holland and Bultz, 2007). Distress is 'the experience of significant emotional upset arising from various physical and psychiatric conditions' (Carlson et al., 2010: 271; Graves et al., 2007). Although not a specific category in DSM-IV or ICD10, it does appear as a qualifier or clinical significance criteria. Accumulating evidence suggests that the presence of distress is associated with reduced health-related quality of life (Shim et al., 2006), poor satisfaction with medical care (von Essen et al., 2002) and possibly reduced survival after cancer (Faller et al., 1999). It is not yet clear, however, to what extent distress adversely influences outcomes once psychiatric disorders are accounted for. Unfortunately, interventions for distress and related emotional disorders have failed to show any benefit on survival as a whole, implying distress is linked with mortality through confounding factors such as patients' self-awareness of deterioration (Chow et al., 2004; Smedslund and Ringdal, 2004). That said, distress and related emotional disorders are strongly linked with quality of life and, therefore, remain a valid target for intervention.

SCREENING TOOLS FOR PSYCHOLOGICAL WELLBEING

Details of how, and how often, to screen are disputed and subject to much local variation. According to the US NCCN, distress should be recognized and monitored through regular and repeated screening and treated promptly at all stages of disease (Holland et al., 2010). A 2002 US National Institutes of Health (NIH) conference statement called for the routine use of screening tools to identify untreated depression among patients with cancer (Patrick et al., 2003). The 2004c UK NICE guidelines recommended screening for psychological distress, including depression, in cancer patients at key stages through treatment and survivorship. Similarly, the Canadian

Partnership Against Cancer (CPAC; Howell et al., 2009) and the US Institute of Medicine (IOM) recommend routine distress screening in cancer settings (IOM, 2007). However, none of these important consensus statements were able to offer thorough evidence-based advice regarding which tool to use and its likely added value in clinical practice (see the following box for a summary of currently available screening tools). Such evidence has been accumulating rapidly and can be divided into **diagnostic validity studies** (how accurate is the screening tool) and **implementation studies** (how well does screening work in practice). The aim of screening is fundamentally to facilitate effective and efficient treatment by focusing on people who would most benefit from a proven intervention; however, to justify the time and effort required, screening must be more worthwhile than not screening (treatment-as-usual). Let us consider first availability and accuracy of tools before considering implementation studies.

Common tools for psychological wellbeing in cancer settings

Distress

- Profile of Mood States (POMS)
- Brief Symptom Inventory (BSI)
- General Health Questionnaire (GHQ)
- Symptom Checklist 90-R (SCL-90)
- Distress Thermometer

Anxiety

- State-Trait Anxiety Inventory (STAI)
- Hospital Anxiety and Depression Scale – Anxiety
- Impact of Events Scale (IES)
- Fear of Progression Scale (FoP12)
- Generalized Anxiety Disorder QQ (GAD7)

Depression

- Beck Depression Inventory (BDI-II)
- Center for Epidemiologic Studies Depression Scale (CES-D)
- Hospital Anxiety Depression Scale (HAD)
- Patient Health Questionnaire (PHQ-9)

Quality of life

- European Organization for Research and Treatment of Cancer Quality of Life Core Questionnaire (EORTC QLQ-C30)
- Functional Assessment of Cancer Therapy – General (FACT-G)

Bipolar disorder

- Mood Disorders Questionnaire (MDQ)

Screening for depression

Numerous tools have been developed to screen for depression, varying from 1 to 90 items in length (Vodermaier et al., 2009). Most are pencil and paper self-report tools but some examples include brief structured verbal questions and computerized stations in waiting areas (Zealley and Aitken, 1969). The best-known conventional self-report mood scale is the Hospital Anxiety and Depression Scale (HADS) (Zigmond and Snaith, 1983). Two recent reviews found that the HADS could not be recommended as a case-finding (diagnostic) instrument, but it may be suitable as an initial screening tool (Luckett et al., 2010; Mitchell et al., 2010b). In addition, the HADS is probably too long for routine use, at least in paper and pencil format, although it has been successfully implemented by touch screen in some well-resourced areas (Strong et al., 2008). According to the Depression in Cancer Consensus Group, as of 2012, there were 63 diagnostic validity studies involving 19 tools designed to help clinicians identify depression in cancer settings (Mitchell et al., 2012a). However, only eight tools had reasonable independent replication. These tools included the Beck Depression Inventory (BDI) (Beck et al., 1996), BDI fast screen (Beck et al., 1997), Distress Thermometer (DT) (applied to depression) (Morasso et al., 1996), Edinburgh Postnatal Depression Scale (EPDS) (Cox et al., 1987), Patient Health questionnaire (PHQ-9) (Spitzer et al., 1999), PHQ-2 (Kroenke et al., 2003), the structured two stem questions ('low mood' and 'loss of interest') (Whooley et al., 1997) and the Center for Epidemiological Studies Depression Scale (CES-D) (Radloff, 1977). After pooling the results for each scale for the purposes of depression screening, the Depression in Cancer Consensus Group concluded that two stem questions (e.g. 'Are you depressed?' and 'Have you lost interest?') had the highest level of evidence (with high acceptability) for identifying cases of depression; the BDI-II had intermediate evidence. In pragmatic terms, they estimated that for every 100 people screened for depression in a non-palliative setting, the BDI-II would accurately detect 17 cases, missing two and correctly reassuring 70, with 11 falsely identified as clinical cases (Mitchell et al., 2012a).

Screening for anxiety

Clinicians rarely use formal instruments when assessing anxiety, but typically rely on verbal and non-verbal cues (Frojd et al., 2007); however, recognition of anxiety appears to be significantly worse than recognition of depression (Mitchell, 2012). Several screening options could theoretically help. A single verbal item ('How anxious have you felt this week?') and a single Anxiety Thermometer rapidly screen for anxiety and can be quickly adopted into routine care, but may lack specificity (Mitchell, 2007). That said, a focused anxiety question is a more accurate way of gauging anxiety compared with the DT alone (Mitchell, 2010). A number of brief generic self-report questionnaires have been extensively studied in non-cancer settings but there are still limited data in cancer patients. These include the anxiety subscale of the HADS, the STAI and the GAD7. Several cancer-specific anxiety questionnaires have been proposed and validation is ongoing. A notable example is the Fear of Disease Progression Scale, which deserves further study (Herschbach et al., 2005).

Screening for distress

Given the difficulties in defining and identifying psychiatric disorders, an alternative approach is to look for broader distress. In the UK, this has been advocated by NICE and the National Cancer Survivorship Initiative (NCSI). In 1998, the NCCN released the Distress Thermometer (DT), a one-item, visual–analogue scale (VAS) (Roth et al., 1998; NCCN, 2004) which is now commonly used. One immediate difficulty, however, when evaluating distress tools, is that a gold standard measure of distress is itself undefined. A close approximation might be any psychiatric disorder using a full semi-structured interview, and a weaker approximation would be a screen for anxiety or depression. The latter is typically generated by studies relying on the HADS as a comparison tool. Bearing this limitation in mind, our group reviewed the tools proposed for distress against an interview-based gold standard (Mitchell, 2010). Very few studies had supportive evidence from independent replication. When studies were limited to those tested against distress defined by semi-structured interview, only six methods had been validated. These were the HADS (13 studies), the DT (four studies), a single verbal question (four studies), the Psychological Distress Inventory (one study), combined DT and Impact Thermometer (one study) and combined two-verbal questions (one study). Of the longer approaches, the Psychological Distress Inventory, a 13-item scale, was the first to measure distress in patients with breast cancer and a cut-off of 28 was proposed as clinically significant (Morasso et al., 1996). Validation data on several well-known generic distress scales such as the General Health Questionnaire (GHQ) are awaited. In our review (Mitchell et al., 2012), we concluded that all tools have approximately the same screening accuracy and therefore the choice of a short screening tool for distress can be based on acceptability or cost effectiveness. Best evidence supports use of the DT or single verbal question. We concluded that for case-finding, data were sparse and no method was satisfactory. From very limited evidence, the optimal short methods for identifying distress are possibly two verbal questions. All short methods may be augmented by repeated application, by an assessment of unmet needs (problem checklist) and by clarification regarding the need for professional help.

It is worth noting that following the success of the NCCN DT, several promising variants on the thermometer format have also been developed. Lees and Lloyd-Williams tested a visual–analogue scale anchored with a sad face and happy face (Lees and Lloyd-Williams, 1999) and reported a high correlation with the HADST, but they did not report sensitivity or specificity. Gil and colleagues conducted a multicentre European study to assess the value of both the DT and a Mood Thermometer, although the comparator was the HADS (Gil et al., 2005). Interestingly, the DT was more highly associated with HADS anxiety scores than depression scores, while the MT was related to both HADS anxiety and depression scores. Recently, our group developed a five-item, seven-item and a modular version of the Emotion Thermometer designed to measure multi-domain emotional complications of cancer (see www.emotionthermometers.com). It appears to have good validity against DSM-IV-defined depression and HADS total scores in early cancer, but studies are awaited regarding interview-defined distress (NCCN, 2007).

Screening for bipolar disorder

Screening for bipolar disorder is a relatively new area that has long been overlooked in cancer settings. Several problems interfere with an apparently simple detection task. First, patients with bipolar disorder spend at least three times as long with depressive rather than **manic/hypomanic** symptoms (Kupka et al., 2007). Second, patients may not recall past manic symptoms at all or may not recall them as problematic. Third, the disorder is relatively uncommon outside of psychiatric settings (Rouillon et al., 2011). In the landmark Derogatis prevalence study, only 1 out of 215 cancer patients had bipolar disorder (Derogatis et al., 1983). A more recent study found mania in a concerning 3.5% early after a diagnosis of breast cancer (Gandubert et al., 2009). Several screening tests and self-completed questionnaires have been developed to facilitate the early detection of bipolar disorder, including the Mood Disorders Questionnaire (MDQ) and the Bipolar Spectrum Disorders Scale (Picardi, 2009). Hirschfeld et al. (2000) introduced the MDQ, a single-page screener for a lifetime history of manic or hypomanic symptoms using 13 yes/no items. The MDQ initially demonstrated a sensitivity of 73% and a specificity of 90% when compared to a semi-structured telephone interview using the SCID in high-risk outpatient psychiatric clinics (Aaronson et al., 1993). Outside of psychiatric settings, use of the MDQ has proven more problematic. Dodd et al. (2009) compared the MDQ and SCID in a community-based sample of 1066 women. Only 24 women had bipolar disorder, demonstrating the issue of low prevalence outside the specialist settings. The sensitivity and specificity of the MDQ were 25% and 99%, respectively. No studies have yet been conducted in cancer settings, but given the high false–positive rates, several authors propose that screening for bipolar should be confined to those with current depression, focusing on the longitudinal history of bipolar disorder (Tafalla et al., 2009).

Screening for impaired QoL

Many generic QoL instruments are available and have been used in cancer settings. These include the Mental Health Inventory short form (MHI-5), the Brief Symptom Inventory (BSI), the Short Form health survey 36 (SF36) and the Nottingham Health Profile (NHP). Generic QoL instruments may omit important cancer-related complications and, therefore, several cancer-specific QoL instruments have been developed and validation performed. These include the EORTC QLQ-C30 (European Organization for Research and Treatment of Cancer Quality of Life Core Questionnaire) (Aaronson et al., 1993) and the FACT-G (Functional Assessment of Cancer Therapy – General) (Cella et al., 1993) and its various modules. The EORTC QLQ-C30 was originally validated in multiple European countries and published in 1993 and since used in almost 10,000 clinical studies. The EORTC QLQ-C30 comprises a global HRQoL scale (two items) and five functional scales: physical functioning (five items), role functioning (two items), emotional functioning (four items), cognitive functioning (two items) and social functioning (two items). There are three symptom scales (fatigue – three items), nausea and vomiting (two items) and pain (two items) and six single items relating to dyspnoea, insomnia, loss of appetite, constipation, diarrhoea and financial difficulties. Specific QoL instruments have been used in trials comparing different oncologic treatment regimens, but such instruments have rarely made the transition into clinical practice (Bezjak et al., 1997; Morris et al., 1998; Bezjak et al., 2001).

Given the early promise of QoL screening but disappointing uptake, a few noteworthy studies have looked at barriers to QoL screening. Carlson et al. (2001) asked 46 cancer patients from a pain and symptom control cancer clinic to complete a computerized EORTC QLQ-C30 along with a feedback questionnaire. Staff members also completed a satisfaction form. Only

39% of patients stated that a QoL report was 'very helpful' in guiding their interaction with staff, and about 70% of clinic staff found the instrument useful in promoting communication and in identifying patient concerns. Allenby et al. (2002) studied the acceptability of QoL screening in a randomized trial evaluating the use of self-reported psychosocial information. Patients completed the Cancer Needs Questionnaire (CNQ), EORTC QLQ-C30 and the Beck Depression Inventory-Short Form using touch screen. Of 450 patients, 244 (54%) were 60 years or older and nearly all found the touch screen simple to use. The average time to complete the CNQ was 9 minutes, EORTC QLQ-C30 4 minutes and BDI 3 minutes, hinting at a rather lengthy burden. Factors influencing time for completion were prior use of computers, physical condition, education and overall level of needs. More recently, Carter and colleagues in Australia (2008) asked 388 patients and 234 carers to complete the World Health Organization-Quality of Life-BREF (WHOQOL-BREF) (Carter et al., 2008). Acceptability was good as 93.6% completed all items.

Screening for unmet needs

The application of a screening test for emotional complications is unlikely to be sufficient to facilitate a change in patient outcomes: clinicians usually require additional help to pinpoint the cause of distress. Clinicians can use their own clinical skills to ask about physical, practical, emotional, family or spiritual problems but it is unlikely that all domains will be covered. It may also be advisable to ask patients formally if they wish to receive input from clinical services (and to clarify why, if patients decline) because only the minority of patients with emotional complications want professional help at any point in time (Baker-Glenn et al., 2011); however, the 'help question' (simply, 'Do you want help from a health-care professional?') must itself be used with care (Baker-Glenn et al., 2011; Lombardo et al., 2011). Needs assessment is a strategy that focuses on identifying the unresolved concerns that patients are experiencing and determines if they require further assistance, as well as the level of assistance they require (Sanson-Fischer et al., 2000). A surprising number of tools have been developed to assess the unmet needs of patients with cancer (see the following box). In an up-to-date review, Carlson et al. (2012a) found 38 studies investigating psychometric qualities of 29 needs assessment tools. The majority of tools were developed for use with patients diagnosed with any type of cancer; however, some were proposed as specific to advanced stage of disease, clinical settings or survivors. The number of items in reviewed tools ranged from 13 to 138. Tools such as the PNPC, NA-ACP, CNAT, SCNS and CARES include more than 50 items and are likely to be too burdensome unless computerized and given at home or in the waiting room.

Evidence of validity and reliability vary considerably between tools. Like distress, there is no accepted gold standard, and therefore, construct validity will in effect be convergent validity against a previous method. No attempt at validity, however, was available for some tools (3LNQ, PNAS, SNST and the SPARC) and no reliability data for the PCNA, SNST, SPARC or SPEED. Four reported on inter-rater reliability (3LNQ, NAT: PD-C and PNAT) and nine on test–retest reliability (CaNDI, CARES, CARES-SF, CaSUN, CCM, NA-ACP, NEQ, PCNQ and PNAT). At the current time, unmet needs tools are probably best chosen on the basis of ease of application and interpretation, possibly with consideration of reliability.

Tools for unmet needs in cancer settings

3LNQ

Three-Levels-of-Needs Questionnaire

CaNDI

Cancer Needs Distress Inventory

CARES

Cancer Rehabilitation Evaluation System

CARES-SF

Cancer Rehab Evaluation System Short Form

CaSun

Cancer Survivors Unmet Needs measure

CaTS

Cancer Treatment Survey

CCM

Cancer Care Monitor

CNAT

Comprehensive Needs Assessment Tool in cancer

CNQ-SF

Cancer Needs Questionnaire Short Form

CPILS

Cancer Problems in Living Scale

NA-ACP

Needs Assessment of Advanced Cancer Patients

NA-ALCP

Needs Assessment for Advanced Lung Cancer Patients

NAT: PD-C

Needs Assessment Tool: Progressive Disease-Cancer

NEQ

Needs Evaluation Questionnaire

(Continued)

significantly more frequently in the intervention than in the control condition, but there was little effect on patient management and patient-reported QoL. Subgroup analysis showed there was improvement in HRQoL domains, namely involving better identification in mental health and role functioning over time. In the Velikova et al. (2004) study, 28 oncologists treating 286 cancer patients were randomly assigned to an intervention group who underwent screening along with feedback of results to physicians, a screen-only group who completed questionnaires without feedback and a control group with no screening at all (Velikova et al., 2004; Velikova et al., 2010). The questionnaires used were the EORTC QLQ-C30 and a touch screen version of HADS. A positive effect on emotional wellbeing was seen in the intervention versus control group, but there was little to differentiate intervention and the screening-only no feedback group. Although more frequent discussion of chronic non-specific symptoms was found in the intervention group (without prolonging encounters), there was no detectable effect on patient management.

Several new studies have now revisited screening with the simple DT with or without additional QoL ratings. Carlson et al. (2010) examined the effect of screening on the level of psychological distress in lung and breast cancer patients randomized to minimal screening (no feedback), full screening (with feedback) or screening with optional triage and referral (Braeken et al., 2011; Furukawa et al., 1999). This was one of the largest studies to date with over 1000 patients, 365 in minimal screen, 391 in full screen and 378 in screening with triage. Results differed by cancer type. In patients with lung cancer receiving full triage, continued high distress at follow-up was reduced by 20% compared to other groups. In breast cancer, the full screening and triage groups both had significantly lower distress at follow-up than minimal screening. Recently, Hollingworth et al. (2012) used the DT and problem list to rate distress and discuss its sources as applied by a trained radiographer/nurse, and compared this with treatment-as-usual (Boyes et al., 2006). Psychological distress (POMS-SF) and disease-specific quality of life (EORTC QLQ-C30) were measured at baseline, one and six months. Two hundred and twenty patients were randomized with 107/112 in the DT arm. Both groups improved by six months and there was no evidence that patients randomized to the screening condition had better outcomes. Results pertaining to uptake of resources have not yet been reported.

Summarizing the rather complex results so far, across all 21 studies published to date, only six of the randomized controlled trials actually reported direct benefits on wellbeing or distress (five as a direct result of screening), although an additional eight non-randomized studies showed partial benefits. Benefits appeared to be more significant in those depressed at baseline (Rosenbloom et al., 2007), those followed frequently (Velikova et al., 2004) or given linked input for unmet needs (Boyes et al., 2006), and possibly in lung cancer (Velikova et al., 2004; Braeken et al., 2011). Looking at the design of these implementation studies, six were randomized applications of the screening tool itself, whilst the remainder randomized feedback of the results. Contrary to expectations, both Velikova et al. (2004) and Carlson et al. (2010) found that screening without feedback of results to clinicians appeared to be more beneficial than no screening at all (Carlson et al., 2010; Braeken et al., 2011); however, this is contradicted by Sarna (1998) and McLachlan et al. (2001), who found screening with feedback was more beneficial than screening without feedback, and Mills et al. (2009), who found screening without feedback was potentially harmful (Braeken et al., 2011). It is worth highlighting that some studies compared standard feedback with enhanced (personalized) feedback (Hollingworth, 2012), and many studies varied on what intervention(s) followed screen positive results (Hollingworth, 2012). From the non-randomized studies, most benefits were in the areas of communication, clinician behaviour/referral. Overall, five studies reported that screening helped with patient-clinician communication (Mills et al., 2009; Carlson et al., 2010; Hilarius et al., 2008; Ito, 2011; American Psychiatric Association, 1952). Four studies noted a benefit on referral rates or referral delay (Grassi et al., 2011; Mitchell et al., 2012b; Velikova et al., 2010; World Health Organization (WHO), 1948). However, even with screening, the referral rates did not exceed 25% thereby allaying concerns that screening would lead to an excess of referrals to specialist services.

CLINICAL CASE-FINDING OF PSYCHOSOCIAL WELLBEING

ICD10 and DSM-IV/DSM-V criteria

The criteria for major depression, minor depression, dysthymia, adjustment disorder and anxiety disorders (including PTSD) are listed in ICD10 and DSM-IV/DSM-V. Ideally, clinicians should make reference to the official criteria when making a diagnosis but evidence shows that in reality this rarely happens. A complication is that ICD10 and DSM-IV differ and clinicians should therefore probably choose a preferred method. For example, the DSM-IV criteria for GAD are excessive, including difficult to control anxiety for at least six months and at least three of the following symptoms: restlessness or feeling keyed up or on edge, easily fatigued, difficulty concentrating or mind going blank, irritability, muscle tension and sleep disturbance. ICD10, on the other hand, requires 4 out of 22 possible symptoms. Major Depressive Disorder (MDD) is defined by depressed mood or loss of interest for at least two weeks, accompanied by an additional three (from a total of five) symptoms. The criteria for minor depression are identical but require only two symptoms. Dysthymia requires three symptoms and a chronic course lasting at least two years. In ICD10, the core symptoms of depression include decreased energy or increased fatigue, in addition to low mood and loss of interest. Further, only four symptoms are required for a mild episode and six (five in early versions) symptoms qualify as moderate depressive episode. Thus DSM-IV major depression is broadly analogous to ICD10 moderate or severe depression concept. Both ICD and DSM suggest a minimum number of typical and associated symptoms and a minimum two-week duration of symptoms. In DSM-IV, an important qualifier is that all of these disorders should cause significant distress or impairment in social, occupational or other important areas of functioning. Clinicians should, therefore, ask patients routinely about distress and impaired daily function with a question such as 'how difficult is it to do your work, take care of things at home, or get along with people?'.

Accuracy of clinical judgement habits

Several studies have examined how cancer professionals look for depression or anxiety. Mitchell and colleagues (2008) found that only 5.9% of all staff reported using a formal questionnaire with the majority (62.2%) relying on their own clinical judgement. Regarding the accuracy of unassisted judgement, Sollner et al. (2001) examined the accuracy of eight oncologists who had evaluated 298 cancer patients. Against moderate or severe distress on the HADST (a 12v13 cut-off), oncologists' sensitivity was 80.2% and specificity 32.8%. Fallowfield's group (2001) compared cancer clinicians' ratings using visual analogue scales with an independent GHQ12 score (cut-off 3v4). In this high prevalence sample, detection sensitivity was only 28.9%. Notably, patients who were identified had longer consultations than those who were missed, suggesting that giving patients more time is a key factor that can improve care.

Improving clinical judgement (clinical case-finding)

Many factors are known to influence the accuracy of clinical judgement. These include training, confidence in mental health, willingness to discuss mental health concerns and awareness (index of suspicion) of such concerns. Detection is easier in high prevalence settings where mental health problems are common. Here the challenge may be to allocate sufficient time to deal with regular mental health issues. In a low prevalence settings, it may be useful to watch out for 'red flags', that is, symptoms such as tearfulness, isolation, trouble sleeping, irritability, agitation, which may reveal a more serious disorder. In all patients, it is reasonable to ask generic questions such as 'how are you feeling?' or 'how are you coping at the moment?'. If there is a positive response, or if the patient has persistent concerns or is clearly distressed, move on to ask about symptoms of depression. Even in the absence of a formal scale, a positive answer to either persistent low mood or loss of interest is enough to suspect possible depression and would warrant further questions. At the end of an appointment, it may be useful to ask 'is this out of the ordinary for you' and 'are things generally getting better or worse at the current time'. Lastly, clinicians should not be afraid to see the patient again in order to clarify a diagnosis. This has been quantified in that a second assessment increases unassisted accuracy by about 15% (from 79–93%) (Mitchell et al., 2009).

CASE STUDY

A previously healthy 50-year-old man has been struggling to cope with a new diagnosis of bowel cancer, which has been responding to chemotherapy alone prior to planned surgery. He is distressed and has mouth sores following chemotherapy. A scale or tool can help clarify whether he is depressed, as well as careful clinical assessment. Application of the distress thermometer reveals a score of 8/10, which is a high score, well above the usual threshold of 4 or more. This may be sufficient grounds to address the problem area (mouth sores) and offer support. However, application of either ICD10 criteria or DSM-IV/DSM-V criteria or application of the PHQ-9 would furnish additional valuable information:

Table 19.1   ICD10 and DSM-IV core symptoms of depression

Core symptoms	ICD10	DSM-IV
Persistent sadness or low mood	Yes (core)	Yes (core)
Loss of interests or pleasure	Yes (core)	Yes (core)
Fatigue or low energy	Yes (core)	Yes
Disturbed sleep	Yes	Yes
Poor concentration or indecisiveness	Yes	Yes
Low self-confidence	Yes	No
Poor or increased appetite	Yes	No
Suicidal thoughts or acts	Yes	Yes

Core symptoms	ICD10	DSM-IV
Agitation or slowing of movements	Yes	Yes
Guilt or self-blame	Yes	Yes
Significant change in weight	No	Yes
Distress or daily dysfunction?	Yes	Yes
Duration required?	Yes	Yes

On further assessment, it is clarified that he complains of five symptoms he has been experiencing for the last three weeks – low mood, loss of drive, low energy, poor appetite and insomnia. These, along with distress, are sufficient for a diagnosis of major depression. There is no need to disqualify any symptoms because of cancer; this approach has not proven fruitful in the literature. The severity of the depression can be further quantified using a depression scale, and this also provides a baseline for tracking change. Overall, the depression would warrant further psychological help or referral to a colleague with mental health experience. Supportive counselling and self-help can be considered. Often patients feel alone with their condition or fear specific issues (e.g. having a stoma) and this can be helped by peer support options, such as group therapy (see also Chapter 22). Input from the clinical nurse specialist in this area is highly recommended.

DISCUSSION AND FUTURE DIRECTIONS

A large body of work has attempted to develop and validate tools for psychological wellbeing and emotional distress. This has been largely successful with numerous tools available to improve upon the clinician's unassisted judgement; however, adoption of these tools into clinical practice has been largely unsuccessful in terms of reach (very few centres) or effect (proven added value over and above clinical routine) (Jacobsen and Ransom, 2007; Vodermaier and Linden, 2008). In a national survey of US oncologists, 65% reported screening patients for distress routinely, but only 14.3% used a screening instrument (Pirl et al., 2007). Out of 84 Canadian cancer institutions, only 36.5% routinely screened patients for emotional distress at the time of admission (Moller, 2000). In short, there is no country that has mandated routine screening and this may be because the evidence base for distress screening in cancer is by no means overwhelming and has been limited by methodological considerations. In our analysis, only 6 of 12 (50%) randomized and 8 of 9 non-randomized trials showed a positive effect on psychological wellbeing and numerous questions remain. As an example, the question of whether emotional complications require a different approach in palliative settings is completely unresolved. Screening for emotional complications has often focused on depression and overlooked other emotional domains. Screening for depression, although important, cannot encompass the whole patient experience (Mitchell et al., 2011). Further, most groups have overlooked evaluation of unmet needs and practical concerns, clarification of a desire for help and the acceptability of the treatment offered. These may be essential rate-limiting steps in determining the effectiveness of screening in the real world.

A fundamental issue even for a successful screening method is long-term acceptability. That includes acceptability to both clinicians and patients. Programmes appear to show enhanced acceptability when assisted by dedicated funded researchers, but maintaining this in the clinical environment is extremely difficult. Indeed, it is not certain whether systematic screening can actually be accomplished in busy clinical environments. An alternative to systematic screening is targeted screening of pre-selected high-risk groups, such as those with troubling physical complications or those whose family members ask for help. Targeted screening is theoretically more efficient than systematic screening because the prevalence of the condition under study is higher and hence fewer screens are needed for each identified case. In addition, psychosocial treatment is more successful when the baseline severity is high (Schneider et al., 2010); yet targeted screening is more likely to overlook many individuals occupying low risk status, but with unmet needs nevertheless. For widespread use in clinical practice, tools that take less than two minutes to apply are preferred, especially when trained mental health specialists are not available (Jones and Doebbeling, 2007; Moller, 2000). Currently, the most popular type of short tools for screening for distress are visual–analogue scales, which include the 'distress thermometer', the 'impact thermometer' and the 'emotion thermometer'. Even here, certain patient groups may struggle in completing self-reports, particularly those with visual problems, severe fatigue or cognitive impairment. Language and cultural barriers must also be considered. A brief alternative to visual–analogue methods is simple verbal query, although surprisingly no studies have been conducted to validate it against distress in cancer patients. A comparison of these newer methods with older methods (like the HADS) appears to show that their accuracy is similar, although there has not been comparative research.

Following on from screening, a key question is what happens to patients who screen positive and those who screen negative. Generally, a **distress management plan** is important to ensure that staff act systematically on screening results. It also implies that the healthcare system has resources for handling distress. Thorough clinical assessment and competent management should follow a positive screen (Williams and Dale, 2006) and clinicians should be able to override screening protocols if needed. Depending on the needs identified for specific populations, the actions that follow screening could involve, for example, a stepped approach, ranging from group-based psycho-education for people with mild–moderate distress, to structured individual therapy for those with high distress.

Future studies will clarify the optimal methods that bring added value to clinical practice. They will also clarify the best mode of delivery (e.g. computerized, paper, verbal). Future studies should use representative samples, offer staff training and track staff and patient use of subsequent interventions. New trials addressing some of these methodological issues are currently underway in oncology settings but few, if any, have been conducted in palliative care. Successful distress screening tools could be incorporated into screening programmes that also contain elements for measuring unmet needs, desire for help, clinical responses and longitudinal outcomes. Screening that is accurate, acceptable and has added value will have the more likelihood of being seen as an integral part of essential cancer care.

CHAPTER SUMMARY

Psychological issues are common in cancer and can be expressed in various types of symptoms and disorders, but these are often the least likely component of patient wellbeing to be addressed. A large number of screening tools exist and, in principle, many are accurate enough to rule out those without a clinical depression or anxiety disorder. Most will also help point towards those with a clinical disorder, but here a second step confirmation (case-finding) is usually required to confirm the diagnosis. Given that many people who suffer distress do not have clinical depression, there has been increasing awareness of subtypes of depression, anxiety disorders, adjustment disorders and PTSD. Screening for each condition individually can be cumbersome in the clinic or in hospital without a computer-based algorithm (or perhaps excellent clinical skills). An alternative, therefore, is to screen for broadly defined distress using a unidimensional or multidimensional thermometer (such as the distress thermometer or emotion thermometers). The evidence base for screening is accumulating, but is still subject to debate. Screening may not have a dramatic effect on recognition, but may have secondary benefits on communication and reducing addressable unmet needs.

Key learning points

- Psychological complications of cancer are common and too frequently unaddressed.
- Psychological complications are associated with negative outcomes of cancer, including reduced compliance with medical treatment.
- Patients with psychiatric illness receive lower quality medical care in cancer settings.
- Screening may help to enhance timely recognition and treatment of mental disorders, as well as broadly defined distress.
- Screening can be a burden to staff, but this can be reduced using simple tools, a two-step approach and waiting room screening where possible.

Recommended further reading

- Mitchell, A.J. (2012) *Rapid Screening for Depression and Emotional Distress in Routine Cancer Care: Local Implementation and Meta-Analysis.* MD thesis. University of Leicester, UK.
- Mitchell, A.J. and Coyne, J.C. (2009) *Screening for Depression in Clinical Practice: An Evidence-Based Guide.* Oxford UK: Open University Press.
- Grassi, L. and Riba, M. (2012) *Clinical Psycho-Oncology: An International Perspective.* Hoboken, NJ: Wiley-Blackwell.

20 THE IMPACT OF CANCER ON FAMILY MEMBERS AND FAMILY CAREGIVERS

EILA WATSON AND MARY BOULTON

Chapter outline

- Who are family caregivers
- What does family caregiving involve
- Psychological, physical, social, financial impact of cancer
- Positive effects
- Childhood cancer – the impact of cancer on parents
- Parental cancer – the impact of cancer on children
- Interventions for family members
- Policy and practice implications

INTRODUCTION

A diagnosis of cancer can be devastating. It often happens suddenly and unexpectedly, and family members may feel its effects as much as the patient. Family members play an important role in providing emotional support to patients and, as many cancer treatments occur in outpatient settings, may also be drawn into providing care during and following treatment. They take on these roles whilst having to deal with their own emotions and striving to maintain family life, education, work and other responsibilities.

As diagnosis and treatment services continue to improve, and increasing numbers of people live longer with cancer, more families are having to cope with the impact of the disease, and over a longer period. In the USA, 4.6 million people are reportedly caring for someone with cancer at home (National Alliance for Caregiving, 2009). In the UK, Macmillan Cancer Support report that an estimated 15% of people have given some unpaid, informal support to a person with cancer in the last 12 months, with 1 in 20 (5%) doing so currently (Macmillan Cancer Support, 2011a). Family members who are directly involved in providing care or support to someone with cancer are often termed 'family caregivers' and this is the term that will be used throughout this chapter. Not all 'family caregivers' see themselves in these terms, however, particularly in the early stages of illness when patients often do not require any personal care (Thomas et al., 2002). But cancer can affect family members across the whole trajectory from diagnosis, through treatment and into survivorship, at recurrence and during palliative and end-of-life phases. The effects will vary from family to family and will likely change over the course of the illness.

WHO ARE FAMILY CAREGIVERS?

While the main **family caregiver** for children with cancer is likely to be their mother, for adults with cancer it is most likely to be their spouse or partner, although other family members may also take on this responsibility. All will face a range of challenges associated with their particular circumstances.

The partners of elderly people with cancer may themselves be physically frail, which may make caring more difficult and mean that they require more help from other carers, including those outside the family, if their partner with cancer is to continue to live at home (Bee et al., 2008; Kotkamp-Mothes et al., 2005). Working-age partners of cancer patients are likely to have a range of responsibilities towards others, including their children and their employers, which will have to be managed as they take on new caring responsibilities, as will their relationship with the person with cancer. Parents of a child with cancer are also likely to be of working age and may need to alter their patterns of employment and domestic responsibilities to accommodate the needs of their child (Long and Marsland, 2011).

Adult children of cancer patients may also take on significant caring responsibilities, particularly if the patient has no partner or spouse who can provide care. In the context of increasing mobility and globalization, this may mean 'caring at a distance', which places a unique set of demands on the carer (Carers UK, 2011). Changing family patterns also mean that adolescents and young adults are now more likely to take on significant caring responsibilities for a lone parent with cancer, which may alter their relationship with their parent and siblings, affect their school performance and limit their opportunities for socializing and personal pursuits (Gates and Lackey, 1998; Rose and Cohen, 2010).

What care is given by family caregivers?

Caring for a family member with cancer can encompass a wide range of activities. A distinction often made in relation to caring is between the practical tasks of **caregiving**, often referred to as 'caring for' or '**care work**', and the emotional dimensions, which involve both 'caring about' and '**emotion work**' (Ribbens McCarthy and Edwards, 2011).

'Care work' typically involves assisting with additional domestic tasks arising as a consequence of the patient's condition (e.g. cooking special meals, doing additional laundry), personal care (e.g. washing, toileting, including dealing with bedpan, catheter bag, colostomy bag), administrative/instrumental tasks (e.g. navigating the complexities of the care system, transportation to and from appointments) and clinical care related to the patient's medical condition (e.g. administering treatments, monitoring and managing side effects, changing dressings). Not all family caregivers will engage with all these tasks and the quantity and intensity of tasks is likely to change across the cancer trajectory. Nevertheless, even basic care work can be time-consuming. In a study of caregivers of people recently diagnosed with lung and colorectal cancer, Van Ryn et al. (2011) found that 17% provided care for over 40 hours a week, and a further 20% provided care for 21 to 40 hours a week, with those providing care for 'high-need' cancer patients spending significantly more time caring than other caregivers. This included providing cancer-specific care, with 68% of carers watching for treatment side effects, 47% helping manage pain, nausea or fatigue, 29% deciding whether medicine was needed and 19% changing bandages. However, between a half and a third of caregivers reported that they had not received the training they felt they needed to perform these tasks.

The demands of care work are greatest when the patient is having aggressive treatment, or is very ill or close to death. Additional care tasks may emerge at these times and other tasks may be reallocated to other family members. Thomas et al. (2002), for example, carried out a large mixed-methods study of carers that included partners/spouses, parents, children, siblings and friends. They found that more than half of the main carers called on other informal carers to help with care work at difficult times. This may result in considerable changes in the nature and distribution of care work within households and families, which may in turn disrupt existing relationships and create challenges for those who have not previously been involved in such activities. For example, the husband of a woman who develops breast cancer in her early fifties, in addition to dealing with the impact of the diagnosis and providing support to his wife, may have to take on additional responsibility for childcare, domestic and household responsibilities, and elderly relatives, whilst also holding down a job to maintain financial security for the family.

Thomas et al. (2002) found that specific groups of family caregivers also expressed their own need for help with particular aspects of care work, including carers who themselves had health problems and/or disabilities, those who looked after patients that required extra help with basic activities of daily living, and those who did not have use of a car. Female carers reported higher levels of need than male carers across a number of areas. The reasons for this are not known, and this is an area that warrants further exploration. Spira and Kenemore (2000) also suggest that when children are involved, caregiving, which is undertaken voluntarily, is less likely to result in additional strains on the family than situations when the child feels compelled to provide care.

Thomas et al. (2002) define 'emotion work' as 'managing feelings in order to sustain a sense of control over events, to stave off the nightmares of death, loss and major life change and to promote healing' (2002: 538). Emotion work is carried out in relation to the patient's feeling states, the carer's own feeling states and, through managing information on the patient's well-being, the feeling states of friends and relatives in their wider social network. A key aspect of emotion work in relation to the patient is ensuring that they do not feel alone or abandoned. Thomas et al. (2002) give examples of the efforts made by family caregivers to share symbolically in their illness, to construct the shared reality of their plight and to reassure the patient that they were 'facing cancer together'. In terms of managing their own emotions, carers were guided by a common view that they should put the patient first and hide their own distress. For the carers in Thomas et al.'s study, this meant having to 'be strong' and to avoid 'giving way' to their feelings. Although they often worried about the future, they did not share these thoughts with the patient.

THE IMPACT OF CANCER ON ADULT FAMILY CAREGIVERS

Psychological and emotional impact

Studies have shown that partners and family members experience equivalent or sometimes even higher levels of **psychological distress** than the patient with cancer (see also Chapter 18). Anxiety and depression are two of the most commonly reported problems, although other emotions such as feelings of fear, uncertainty, hopelessness, powerlessness, resentment and mood disturbances have also been reported (Stenberg et al., 2010).

Rates of **anxiety** and **depression** vary according to the phase of the patient's cancer trajectory. In the advanced stages of disease, there is a high prevalence of psychological distress in family caregivers. For example, in a study of spousal caregivers of patients with advanced cancer, almost 40% reported significant symptoms of depression (Braun, 2007). This study found that the caregiver's **subjective assessment of the burden** of care was particularly important and a better predictor of depression than an objective assessment. A study conducted by Fridriksdottir et al. (2011) looked at family members of patients with a range of cancers at different stages who had been admitted as an inpatient for three or more days, or who were scheduled for their third (or more) outpatient clinic appointment. They found that 41% of the sample were possible or probable candidates for a diagnosis of clinical depression and 20% experienced possible or probable symptoms of clinical anxiety (measured using the Hospital Anxiety and Depression Scale (HADS) (Zigmond and Snaith, 1983). Anxiety scores were found to be higher in women, and there was a significant relationship between levels of anxiety and both unmet needs and quality of life. In another study, 13% of caregivers of patients with advanced cancer met the criteria for a psychiatric disorder (Vanderwerker, 2005).

Studies have also begun to focus on the impact of cancer on family members during the survivorship phase. In one Australian study (Hodgkinson et al., 2007), partners of long-term cancer survivors (up to eleven years post-diagnosis) reported significantly higher rates of anxiety than population norms (the rates of depression expected in a random sample of the population). Conversely, however, a study of the partners of long-term survivors (five to fifteen years post-diagnosis) in the UK found levels of anxiety and depression that were consistent with population norms (Turner D. et al., 2011).

In addition to reports of anxiety and depression in caregivers, several studies have looked at broader emotional reactions. Feelings of uncertainty and fear of what the future holds and whether the cancer will recur are commonly reported, as well as feelings of hopelessness, powerlessness and mood disturbances. Further work has also identified socio-demographic variables that are predictive of psychological distress in family members, for example cancer type, younger age, female age, spousal relationship, lower socio-economic status and lack of personal and social support (Kozachik, 2001).

Physical impact

Although the evidence base is relatively sparse, some studies have demonstrated that the physical wellbeing of family members can also be affected as a consequence of their caregiving role. Commonly reported problems include fatigue, sleep disturbance, pain, loss of physical strength, loss of appetite and weight loss (Stenberg et al., 2010). For example, Carter et al. (2000), in a small study of caregivers of people with advanced cancer, found that 95% experienced moderate to severe sleep disturbance, and also reported a correlation between their sleep problems and levels of depression. Caregivers, who are often elderly, also often have health problems of their own, which may be exacerbated because of their caregiving role resulting in additional stress and a lack of time to take appropriate rest, engage in health promotion activities and seek medical advice when necessary.

Relationships

Diagnosis and treatment for cancer can also have a significant impact on relationships. For couples, there may be a change in the nature of sexual relationships (see Chapter 21). For other family members, caring for a loved one with cancer may also require providing assistance with intimate tasks such as dressing, bathing and toileting. While this is likely to cause embarrassment or a perceived loss of dignity, little research has been conducted on this topic.

Social impact

Family members may also experience changes to their education, employment and financial situation. Amongst those of working age, concerns with employment are not uncommon. Those who do not have flexible working conditions and do not have support from their employers may be forced to take sick leave and holidays and suffer loss of income as a result. This can be in addition to loss of income from the patient. A study of patients with cancer aged 18–55 in one area of England and whom the GP considered suitable for return to work, found that 20% were not able to return to their place of work and, of those who did return to work, one-fifth reported deterioration in job satisfaction and career prospects (Amir et al., 2007). A recent report by Macmillan Cancer Support highlighted that almost one in three people living with cancer experienced a loss of income as a result of their diagnosis equivalent to an average monthly loss of £860. Day-to-day living costs also tend to increase (e.g. additional heating, paying for help, travelling to and from hospital appointments): on average this is estimated to be an extra £63 per month for those affected (Macmillan Cancer Support, 2013b).

Some family members also report feelings of social isolation because they are unable to engage in the same activities they did prior to the cancer diagnosis (perhaps, for example, as a result of lack of time, lack of enthusiasm or feelings of guilt that the patient can no longer join in). In one study of caregivers of individuals with a range of cancer types, 60% indicated they did not see friends or have hobbies (Rossi-Ferrario, 2003). In another study of family caregivers of women with ovarian cancer, isolation emerged as a prominent theme, with the importance of support from others in a similar situation emphasized (Ferrell, 2002). Grbich et al. (2001) found that caregivers without other family members or close friends nearby expressed considerable loneliness as they cared for a loved one with terminal cancer. Some report that they have lost contact with friends who appear to have chosen to avoid them following their diagnosis of cancer.

Unmet needs

A few studies have assessed unmet needs in family caregivers. In one UK study, partners and close family members of long-term cancer survivors of breast, colorectal and prostate cancer reported information on familial risk, a coordinated approach to care for their partner, and help managing fears of recurrence as their most commonly unmet needs (Turner D. et al., 2011). Information is important to caregivers and they have a wide range of information requirements. A recent review of information needs of a wide range of family caregivers (Adams et al., 2009) suggested that whilst information regarding diagnosis and treatment is clearly very important to caregivers at the time of diagnosis, further along the trajectory information about supportive care aspects became a greater need than medical information, for example information on coping with cancer and the effects on relationships.

Positive effects

There is also a growing literature on the positive effects of cancer on family members, sometimes termed **benefit finding** or **post-traumatic growth**. Some family members find that the caregiving role is satisfying, increases their self-esteem and provides meaning to life. For example, Grbich et al. (2001) found that family members caring for a patient with terminal cancer expressed strong positive emotions regarding the opportunity that providing care gave them to express their love. Families can also become closer as a result of the diagnosis, and learn to appreciate time spent with one another, as well as developing a greater appreciation for the 'smaller things in life'. In the study by Turner D. et al. (2011), two-thirds of respondents reported a greater appreciation of life, almost half felt they had become a stronger person and a quarter felt the way in which they related to others had improved. The nature of the attachment between patient and carer may play a role in this, with attachment security providing a protective buffer during stressful times, (Nicholls, Hulbert-Williams and Bramwell, 2014). It has been suggested that a focus on benefit finding interventions may be useful, but that this would need to take into account the relationship between the carer and the patient (Cassidy, 2013). Similarly, in a large US study of caregivers, Kim et al. (2013) concluded that carers may benefit from interventions that help them to accept the situation they are in and find meaning in their experience, which in turn may reduce symptoms of depression.

THE IMPACT ON CHILDREN OF A PARENT WITH CANCER

Based on evidence from the US National Health Interview Survey (2000 to 2007), it is estimated that about 2.54 million children of minor age in the USA live with a parent who has or has survived cancer (Weaver et al., 2010). These survivors are likely to be female, married and less than 50-years-old. Having a parent with cancer affects children in a number of ways, which are specific to their **developmental stage**. Whilst research with pre-school children is limited, there is some evidence that they show increased crying, clinging and difficulty sleeping, probably in response to **non-verbal cues** from distressed parents or as a result of separation from their mother (Visser et al., 2004). Considerably more research has focused on school-aged children and adolescents, however, and this suggests that although both groups are affected, the effects are greatest amongst adolescents.

For younger school-aged children, parental cancer poses a threat to their sense of security and of the predictability of their world, and can give rise to a number of distressing fears and anxieties. These include fears that the parent may die, feelings of guilt that they are responsible for their parent's cancer, concern about the vulnerability of the healthy parent and anxiety about parental anger, withdrawal or lack of affection (Visser et al., 2004; Lewis, 2006). Visible symptoms of the illness or of treatment side effects, such as vomiting and hair loss, and unexpected events and emergency admissions to hospital were found to be particularly disturbing. School-aged children were also distressed by disruption to their usual routines and activities and their relationships with their friends, which arise as families attempt to cope with the additional demands of caring for an ill parent. Such disturbances and disruptions may also lead to increased conflicts with parents, siblings and peers, and to anxious behaviours, such as seeking closeness to and withdrawing from the ill parent and paying attention to parents' needs and wanting to support them (Visser et al., 2004). Despite these experiences, however, quantitative studies have not found significant differences in levels of emotional, behavioural and social functioning between school-aged children of parents with cancer and other school-aged children (Visser et al., 2004).

By contrast, there is evidence that adolescent children of parents with cancer have a particularly difficult experience, with higher rates of emotional problems compared to other adolescents (Visser et al., 2004) and a higher proportion reporting anxiety and depression than children at other stages (Welch et al., 1996). For these adolescents, parental cancer creates tensions between their attempts to become more independent from their family (a developmental task of adolescence) and their need to return to it to deal with the threat to important personal relationships. These tensions may be expressed in a range of sometimes contradictory responses and coping behaviours. Participants in a study of African–American adolescents (Davey et al., 2011), for example, described discomfort in managing family relationships, as well as fear and uncertainty about the mortality of their parent and their own unpredictable future without them. Changes in the parent's mood, fatigue and physical frailty increased both conflict within the family and a desire on the adolescent's part to protect the parent by taking on more domestic responsibility. They also **coped** by distracting themselves from their anxieties at home by engaging in sports and other activities outside the home, and by engaging in pro-social behaviours, such as school attendance and homework, so as not to add to the family's problems. This greater engagement with family activities also appeared to be balanced by a sense of personal growth and development of strengths for independence.

Sheehan and Draucker (2011) similarly found that the adolescent children of parents with advanced cancer in their study experienced conflicting feelings about spending more time with their family and wanting to establish independence from it. Having limited remaining time together was a key issue for this group of families, and Sheehan and Draucker found that the adolescents attempted to deal with the conflict it created by 'seeking greater intimacy with their parents and doing tangible tasks for them but also by retreating to their lives with their friends and doing "normal activities" when necessary' (2011: 1114). Kristjanson et al. (2004) also found that adolescents had a need for more information and support both from family members and from persons outside the family.

Gender differences have also been found amongst adolescents, with daughters of women with breast cancer reporting fear of developing breast cancer themselves, fear of losing their mother, anger, and guilt related to their wish to get on with their own lives (Visser et al., 2004).

Adolescent girls were also concerned that caring for their mothers would permanently alter their relationship with their mother, which caused further anxiety (Spira and Kenemore, 2000).

As well as dealing with the psychosocial consequences of parental cancer, children may also be required to take on caregiving responsibilities for their parent. '**Young carers**' have been defined as

> children and young persons under 18 who provide or intend to provide care, assistance or support to another family member [and who] carry out, often on a regular basis, significant or substantial caring tasks and assume a level of responsibility which would usually be associated with an adult. (Becker et al., 2000: 13).

Research on young carers, including those caring for someone with cancer, suggests that they are more likely to provide care to a parent, particularly their mother (Dearden and Becker, 2004), and to provide a wide range of types of care. In an Australian study to develop a scale of care tasks performed by young people in the context of family illness/disability (which included cancer along with other conditions), Ireland and Pakenham (2010) identified four distinct dimensions to care tasks performed by young carers: instrumental care, social/emotional care, personal/intimate care and domestic/household care. Using this scale, they found no significant differences in the care provided by boys and girls but a significant difference according to the age of the carer, with more care tasks performed with increasing age (Ireland and Pakenham, 2010). They also found that (1) more care tasks were performed by children and young people living in single-parent households than in two-parent households, most likely reflecting the lack of alternative help; and (2) that more instrumental, social/emotional and domestic/household care tasks were performed when it was the mother rather than the father who required care, most likely reflecting differential responses of mothers and fathers in taking on additional demands for care within the family. Greater levels of caregiving on the part of young carers were also associated with greater levels of functional impairment of the patient and poorer prognosis. In a qualitative study of young carers of parents exclusively with cancer, Gates and Lackey (1998) reported similar findings, adding that when there was more than one child in the family, caring responsibilities tended to be shared, but that this could lead to bickering amongst siblings.

In relation to the impact of caregiving on young carers, Ireland and Pakenham (2010) found evidence of both positive and negative effects. Overall, they found that higher levels of caregiving across all care task dimensions were related to more adverse effects, including activity restrictions, worry about parents and caregiving compulsion, but also to more positive effects such as perceived maturity and caregiving confidence. In a similar vein, Gates and Lackey (1998) characterize the experience of young carers as 'hard but gratifying'.

Ireland and Pakenham further suggest that these findings 'have clinical implications with respect to the need for interventions that mitigate adverse and cultivate positive caregiving experiences' (Ireland and Pakenham, 2010: 729). They also speculate on the role of parental attachment in shaping adjustment outcomes, suggesting that greater parental attachment may foster both increased caregiving and increased risk of health problems.

IMPACT ON PARENTS AND SIBLINGS OF A CHILD WITH CANCER

While cancer is less common in children than in adults, every year about 10,400 children in the USA (www.cancer.gov/cancertopics/types/childhoodcancers) and about 1600 children in the UK (www.cancerresearchuk.org/cancer-info/cancerstats/childhoodcancer/incidence) are diagnosed with cancer. The demands of treatment, as well as the possibility that the child may not respond to treatment or will face further risks subsequent to treatment, mean that childhood cancer is a highly stressful experience for parents and other members of the family, and may also bring about more fundamental changes to their lives (Long and Marsland, 2011).

In a Swedish study by Norberg and Steneby (2009), parents of children who had completed treatment described their experience of childhood cancer as a profound psychological and **existential** challenge, so that not only had their daily lives changed, but they had also acquired a different view of life. Similarly, Björk et al. (2005), in a Swedish study of parents of children newly diagnosed with cancer, described the consequences as 'a broken life world' (p.269) and as precipitating an immediate 'striving to survive' (p.270) as fear, chaos and loneliness took over their normal lives. In a Canadian study of children with a range of cancers and at a range of stages in the cancer trajectory, Woodgate and Degner (2003) described a similar response as 'the process of keeping the spirit alive' (p. 108) while enduring the 'rough spots' they experienced, which they 'got through' but did not 'get over' (p.112). In a later in-depth, longitudinal study of two families, Woodgate (2006:11) described her core narrative (Bury, 2001) as 'life is never be the same', reflecting the extent to which they felt their experience had altered their life stories.

On a more pragmatic level, childhood cancer alters responsibilities and intensifies demands on parents and other family members. For mothers, this includes the obligation to stay close to their child as much as possible in order to provide comfort and 'keep watch' over them (Young et al., 2002). Amongst the caring tasks that may come to greater prominence are (1) managing their child's cooperation with treatment, (2) rehabilitating children with severe impairments, and (3) supporting less impaired children to catch up with their peers (Young et al., 2002; Norberg and Steneby, 2009). Emotional labour may also be heightened as parents attempt to manage their own and their child's emotions by keeping their child entertained or occupied, and by maintaining a cheerful demeanour themselves and shielding children from their own emotions. As a consequence, their daily routines change, their parenting roles become more demanding and everyday family life becomes more restricted (Young et al., 2002; Norberg and Steneby, 2009; Woodgate and Degner, 2003).

Disruptions to their daily routines and the shifts in roles and responsibilities appear to be more pronounced in the early stages of diagnosis and initial treatment, when parents face the need to incorporate hospital visits and intensive treatment regimens into their daily schedules (Patterson et al., 2004; Svavarsdottir, 2005; Long and Marsland, 2011). A common pattern is for mothers to assume primary responsibility for looking after the child with cancer while fathers are left to assume responsibility for other children and general domestic duties alongside their responsibilities in their paid employment (Svavarsdottir, 2005; Long and Marsland, 2011). This may be followed by a period of family conflict before a new 'normality' is eventually established (Woodgate, 2006; Woodgate and Degner, 2003, 2004; Long and Marsland, 2011).

Parents may also experience difficulties in balancing the needs of the ill child with those of other family members and with work commitments. Norberg and Steneby (2009), for example, found that parents described siblings as feeling envious, jealous or bitter about the amount of time and attention given to the child with cancer, and that they did not find it easy to redress the balance. In an American study of parents of a child with cancer two to five years after the end of treatment, Patterson et al. (2004) reported similar findings, but added that some parents indicated that siblings felt overly responsible for the child with cancer. Svavarsdottir (2005), in a longitudinal questionnaire study of parents of children with cancer in Iceland, reported that parents found providing support to siblings and meeting their demands as amongst the most difficult aspects of their roles. In addition, she reported that fathers found managing work outside the home while also organizing care for other children and providing emotional support for their spouse, to be both difficult and time-consuming.

Studies of siblings themselves report that they experience negative emotional reactions, (including feelings of shock, loss, fear, grief, guilt and helplessness) and disruption to schooling and family and social relationships, particularly in the early period following diagnosis (Björk et al., 2005; Grinyer and Thomas, 2001; Patterson, 2004; Alderfer et al., 2010). There is little evidence, however, of significant differences in levels of clinical anxiety or depression or behavioural problems between siblings of children with cancer and population norms, although significant distress may continue beyond diagnosis for a subgroup of children (Barrera et al., 2005; Houtzager et al., 2004; Alderfer et al., 2010).

Factors that helped parents cope with the demands of caring for a child with cancer included timely information about their child's health status from healthcare professionals, emotional support from family and friends, flexibility and accessibility of clinical services and regular help with domestic tasks and child care (James et al., 2002). Several studies also reported that, when they were able to do so, parents reduced their working hours or gave up employment altogether in order to care for their child with cancer (James et al., 2002; Patterson et al., 2004; Norberg and Steneby, 2009).

Parenting practices have also been shown to shift following the diagnosis of a child with cancer. Overall, parents of a child with or surviving cancer tend to be more overprotective, to set fewer limits on their child and to spoil them (Long and Marsland, 2011). In an Australian study of parenting children two to five years after treatment, Williams and colleagues (2013) found differences in **parenting styles** according to the age of the child, but identified three as common for both adolescents and younger children: increased intimacy, closeness and emotional support; parental protectiveness; and differential parenting. Parental protectiveness included withholding information about their disease, controlling aspects of their health not related to cancer and hyper-vigilance in monitoring their health. Differential parenting included giving additional time and attention to the cancer survivor, which in many cases resulted in competitiveness, jealousy and animosity on the part of siblings. In an American study of parents of children two to five years after the end of treatment, some participants reported that their child with cancer viewed their parenting patterns negatively and as putting a strain on their relationship (Patterson et al., 2004).

Although the emphasis was on the difficulties parents faced, most studies also reported some positive consequences of caring for a child with cancer, including a feeling of greater family closeness and a greater priority given to family life. Norberg and Steneby (2009), for example, reported a closer unity in the family, and especially a closer bond between the parents and the cancer survivor. Woodgate (2006) reported that siblings also felt closer to their families, but only if they had provided active support during the treatment stage.

IMPACT OF CANCER ON THE FAMILY AS A WHOLE

Whilst the most common approach to understanding the impact of cancer on family members has been to describe its effects on individuals, particularly partners, parents or children of people with cancer, this approach has been criticized as providing too narrow a perspective and not capturing the inter-relationships amongst family members or the relationship between the family and other systems such as healthcare services (see also Chapter 18). Within nursing, this has led to renewed interest in examining the impact of cancer on the family as a whole, and understanding how the experience of any one family member, and others in the family, is affected by their relationships with healthcare professionals.

One framework for looking at the impact of cancer on the family as a whole is **Family Systems Theory**. Although there are many versions of Family Systems Theory (Wright and Leahey, 2005; Mehta et al., 2009; Harris et al., 2010), the central tenets include:

- The family is a system, comprising interdependent and inter-related elements, so that a significant change or event in one member affects all other members and the system as a whole.
- The family is composed of subsystems – the husband–wife, parent–child, sibling–sibling dyads – and individuals are members of more than one subsystem.
- The family is part of a large social system, which is also composed of many subsystems.
- Each system has boundaries that may be more or less rigid or permeable to exchange with other systems.
- The family as a whole is greater than the sum of its parts, so that the family system can only be understood 'holistically', and individual members cannot be understood without understanding how all family members relate, communicate and behave.
- As individual family members continue to develop and change, families must be able to adjust and reorganize to regain a balance between change and stability.

Although few recent studies have looked at the family system as a whole, those that have done so report findings consistent with this approach. For example, more open communication between the family members and greater marital satisfaction between the parents has been shown to have a positive effect on the wellbeing and functioning of children (Visser et al., 2004). Similarly, better psychological functioning of the parent with cancer has been found to be associated with better psychological functioning of the child (Nelson and While, 2002) and higher self-esteem (Siegel et al., 2000). Studies that explored the relationship between patient and caregiver distress found interdependency in the responses (Hodges et al., 2005; Hagedoorn et al., 2000), which also supports the view that families respond as an integrated system.

INTERVENTIONS TO IMPROVE OUTCOMES FOR FAMILY MEMBERS/CAREGIVERS

As evidence grows regarding the impact of cancer on family caregivers, there is increasing interest in interventions to promote the health and wellbeing of family caregivers. A number of recent reviews have provided useful syntheses of the available literature on the range of interventions for caregivers, and current evidence on the effectiveness of these interventions in improving caregiver outcomes (e.g. Northouse et al., 2010; Hudson, 2005; Harding and Higginson, 2003; Candy et al., 2011).

Northouse et al. (2010) described three classes of family caregiver interventions that have been tested in studies using a randomized controlled trial design: (1) **psycho-educational**, where the primary focus of the intervention was to provide information on symptom management and physical patient care (e.g. administering medication, changing dressings), as well as to address the emotional and psychosocial needs of patients, caregivers and/or to address marital/family relationships; (2) **skills training**, where the focus of the intervention was primarily on developing coping, communication and problem-solving skills, with some focus on behaviour change; and (3) **therapeutic counselling** interventions (see also Chapter 22). Most of these interventions were delivered to both patients and caregivers, with considerable range in terms of duration and intensity of the intervention and some combined psycho-educational and skills training into one intervention package. The mean number of sessions over which interventions were delivered was 6.7 and most were delivered in a face-to-face setting, although some used telephone delivery and group sessions. Interventions were most commonly delivered by nurses, but social workers and psychologists also delivered them. These studies measured a range of caregiver outcomes, including appraisal of caregiving burden and benefit; information needs; coping strategies; self-efficacy; and physical, psychological and social functioning.

The findings of the meta-analyses conducted by Northouse and colleagues were encouraging. Although the effect sizes found were small to moderate, they suggested that interventions aimed at caregivers significantly reduced their perceived burden, improved their ability to cope, increased their self-efficacy and improved aspects of their quality of life. Many of the existing published studies, however, are small, do not include patients from minority ethnic groups, do not adequately address caregivers' self-care behaviours and physical health outcomes and do not provide long-term follow-up or cost-effectiveness information. There is therefore a definite need for further research in this area to address these shortcomings. It is also important that researchers, policymakers and clinicians come together and establish the best ways of implementing interventions that have been shown to be effective into practice, thereby enhancing the wellbeing of caregivers and, in turn, the people with cancer themselves.

Reflective activity

Reflect on situations from your own practice where the impact of cancer on family members and caregivers (e.g. children or adolescents whose parents have cancer, spouse, partner, sibling) was clearly evident.

How can healthcare professionals ensure that different family members and caregivers are supported throughout the illness trajectory?

CHAPTER SUMMARY

Given the vital role family caregivers play, it is important that healthcare professionals communicate effectively with family members and provide information and support throughout the illness trajectory as and when necessary. At the time of diagnosis, and throughout treatment, survivorship and end-of-life care, healthcare professionals should assess/address the following:

in practice settings because they require privacy, time and skill (White et al., 2013). Without these in place, conversations risk becoming awkward or overly superficial, and may be avoided by both clinicians and patients/partners. This chapter will focus on the impact of cancer on the body and personal relationships, including those of an intimate nature.

CANCER AND ITS IMPACT ON BODY IMAGE AND RELATIONSHIPS

'Cancer leaves people alone with their body.' (Schilling, 1993: 167).

The changes in physical appearance brought about by cancer treatments can alter how a person feels about their body, which in turn may impact negatively on their **identity**. These effects will also impact on those around them, including those with whom they share close relationships. If professionals do not feel confident talking about the impact of cancer on body image and relationships, then holistic supportive care will be compromised.

In times of good health, the body is often taken for granted and its workings may seem invisible to most people; however, the introduction of a serious and potentially life-threatening illness, such as cancer, forces attention directly onto the body. Identity in cancer survivors is imbued with notions of discontinuity of the **embodied self** and memory (Little et al., 2002: 170). Cancer may arise in the most private of body areas, such as the rectum, breast, prostate and cervix, meaning that these areas become the focus of professional, rather than solely personal, attention. Other cancers located in less intimate places also carry with them the potential for significant physical impact. The treatment of laryngeal cancer and bone sarcomas, for example, may result in loss of the voice box or of a limb, thereby leaving lasting and observable physical markers.

Sociologists draw a useful distinction between *the body* as a physical entity that matures, ages and dies over the life course, and *embodiment* as the experience of everyday life that occurs via our bodies. Essentially, embodiment refers to the 'lived body' (Turner, 1991). Cancer care professionals must move between treating the physical, objective body (through the use of scans and other tests to detect changes in tumours) as well as attending to the embodied experience of cancer, with its daily impact on human experience. A balance must therefore be struck in the way professionals work with people's 'bodies' that does not dehumanize or diminish cancer as a uniquely emotional human experience.

There is a dichotomy between objective constructions of a medicalized body and the impact of cancer on body image. Whilst a diagnosis of cancer focuses attention via the 'medical gaze' on the *tumour* (that is, the site of the illness such as the breast or stomach), the impact on *body image* is only revealed via the *embodied impact* of cancer treatment (such as hair loss, scarring or weight loss). Importantly, not all body image changes will be so immediately visible. Despite their lack of visibility, however, they can also result in changes that impact on the patient's embodied experience (such as dealing with incontinence or reduced libido due to hormonal therapy for prostate cancer), and each will need to be explored with sensitivity. Research has demonstrated that some men living with prostate cancer stated that they would rather die than live with body image changes such as incontinence or impotence (Kelly, 2004), while **lymphoedema**, caused by cancer treatments, has been described as worse than breast cancer itself (Ridner et al., 2012).

Consequently, embodiment and the impact of changes to body image are important dimensions of the cancer experience. Some elements of body image care are now mainstream, such as breast reconstruction following mastectomy. Other aspects of body image care, however, remain more taboo For example, dealing with stomas following resection surgery for colorectal cancer has been described as 'dirty work' (Twigg, 2000: 389). The embodied and intimate nature of some aspects of care can be problematic for both patient and professionals:

> Bodywork is ambivalent work. At times it verges on areas of taboo in connection with sexuality or human waste. It is potentially demeaning work, and when undertaken by high status individuals it is typically accompanied by distancing techniques. (Twigg, 2000: 391).

The **distancing techniques** that Twigg (2000) refers to are those most often employed by clinicians, such as the use of technical language and adopting an unemotional, detached demeanour. Each are intended to limit the **embarrassment** that may be present in such situations. Other tactics that may be used include humour and distracting attention away from the procedure by encouraging conversations about other, less embarrassing, topics. By exposing what are normally private body functions to another's gaze, such as faecal waste, the person with cancer may feel at risk of exposure to such an extent that could further damage their already fragile sense of self. It is useful for nurses and other professionals to consider how they manage embarrassment in their own practice and whether this limits the possibility of understanding embodied experience and the impact of cancer on the individual.

Importantly, perceptions about body image changes do not always occur at the same time as alterations to physical status. Although the physical impact of cancer surgery may be immediate, there may be a time lag between the event itself and the psychological adaptation required to cope with the social impact of such changes. Both weight loss (Helms et al., 2008) and weight gain (Demark-Wahnefried et al., 1997) are also established side effects of cancer treatments that can impact on people's perceptions of their body in the short, medium and longer term. Research has further indicated that the impact of cancer on body image for adolescents may not become apparent for several years (Pendley et al., 1997): adolescents in this study reported less than half the social activities, lower levels of self-worth, more social anxiety and a more negative body image than healthy controls at 17 months after cancer treatment.

The timeframe of adaptation to changes in body image is inextricably bound up with appearance and attitudes toward health and wellbeing. A study of older women (aged between 60–69) in the USA demonstrated that participants engaged in a continual process of cognitive adjustments to ongoing body changes, including adaptations in line with physical changes over the life course (Liechty and Yarnal, 2010), therefore, when experiencing periods of ill health, adaptations occurred alongside existing adjustments to anticipated levels of pain, movement or energy. These shifts at an individual level are reflected in cultural norms about ageing bodies that impact further on how people internalize their own sense of dynamic embodiment. Whilst normal ageing may allow such gradual adaptations to occur, cancer treatment may lead to changes that are more immediate and lead to a new body image that must be adapted and presented to others relatively quickly.

Over the past two decades, research studies seeking to measure body image changes in people affected by cancer have revealed several methodological flaws (Hopwood, 1994), resulting in no leading tool that practitioners can use for all patients across the treatment

Despite a widespread stereotype that older people gradually lose interest in sex, research evidence suggests that this group often remains interested in intimacy (Gott and Hinchcliffe, 2003). In their study of people aged 50–92-years-old, these researchers identified that every participant who was in a relationship attributed some importance to sex; indeed many rated sex as very or extremely important. Whilst the age range for their study also included working-age adults, the researchers concluded:

> Only when the barriers to remaining sexually active were seen as so insurmountable as to be completely prohibitive did sex assume no importance, regardless of age. (Gott and Hinchcliffe, 2003: 1626).

Treatments for cancers that are more prevalent in older age can result in specific problems, such as erectile dysfunction, vaginal dryness or hormone changes. Despite such side effects being widely recognized, research evidence demonstrates significant levels of unmet psychosexual support needs for couples affected by prostate cancer (Forbat et al., 2011; Steginga et al., 2001) and breast cancer (Hellwig, 2011).

It is known that open discussion of such topics can be challenging for practitioners, particularly when it is difficult to find a common language for sexual practices. The following quotation comes from a 63-year-old man, who was interviewed about couple adaptation to prostate cancer:

> He [the Consultant] said 'Have I had sex' and I said 'Oh I'd had a shag twice' and he said 'Don't talk like that' or something ... so I said 'Oh well, better call it sexual intercourse. (Kelly et al., 2010: 44)

The challenges in finding a common and comfortable language to explore sexual function and intimacy issues, combined with stereotypical attitudes towards older people as having less interest in sexual activity, may explain the paucity of support services in this area. Indeed, as important as sexual intimacy may be for a positive body image, identity, relationships and emotional wellbeing, one published survey indicates that only 58% of nurses feel comfortable leading discussions about these issues (Cartwright-Alcarese, 1995). Another more recent study in general practice about human papilloma virus (HPV) vaccination found that the term a 'can of worms' captured participants' views that issues related to sexual practices were highly problematic because they were considered sensitive and complex (McSherry et al., 2012).

At the heart of these findings is one explanation for the difficulty in providing effective relational support. Professionals find it challenging to identify with the intimate relational needs of patients – especially with those who represent some degree of difference from the professional's own life experience, such as a different sexual orientation (Horden and Street, 2007). The situation is likely to be just as important, if not more so, in cancer care settings, especially when dealing with diverse populations and significant body image changes as a result of disease or treatment. Indeed, the UK NICE recommends the need for more research into the impact of prostate cancer on masculinity, highlighting the impact of treatments for localized disease on sexual function and intimate relationships in particular (NICE, 2008).

The literature on the experience of human ageing also suggests that the interaction between the mind and the body can be understood as a culturally determined 'performance' (Laz, 2003). Part of the performance of 'body work' (such as sexual expression) is the discrepancy between the outer appearance of advanced years and the inner sense of a younger 'true self' (Featherstone and Hepworth, 1991), described by these social researchers as the 'mask of ageing'. The 'mask of ageing' concept suggests that for some older people, there may be dissonance between what they feel about themselves as sexual beings with the need for relational interactions and their outer physical appearance. This is brought into sharp relief when cancer demonstrates the physical frailty of the human body; that is, there can no longer be a clear distinction between an inner youthfulness and outer older age when feeling fatigued, experiencing cachexia or being in pain.

Reflective activity

Consider a man in his early 70s who has been diagnosed with locally advanced prostate cancer. What physical symptoms might you expect him to experience, first in relation to his age and then in terms of the symptoms of his disease?

As a healthcare professional, how might you support him in adapting to the embodied changes he is experiencing to help him make sense of them and learn ways to cope?

Some of the symptoms considered in this reflective activity may include **polyuria**, fatigue, **erectile dysfunction** and mood changes. Each of these symptoms may be a consequence of the normal ageing process, but they are also frequently seen in men with prostate cancer undergoing the various treatments available.

Normalization of embodied change is one approach to help people adapt to changes in physical functioning, offering reassurance that such changes are not out of the ordinary. Since the aetiology of the changes may not always be clear, there may be more information needed before the experiences can be normalized as a result of the ageing process or cancer. Ascertaining the man's own understanding and belief system about the varied impacts of ageing and cancer is likely to be fruitful.

An opening conversation might therefore include some discussion about how he feels about changes to his body and the extent to which he believes different treatments (and associated side effects), if available, might be most acceptable to him. It may also be useful to discuss whether he has already made adjustments to how he perceives his body at this point in his lifecycle, including his expectations about sexual function. The relational impact of the cancer can then be explored to assess the emotional support mechanisms that he might be able to draw upon (such as partners, friends or psychological support services).

In the next section, the needs of a young patient population are discussed in order to compare their needs in a different relational context.

SUPPORTING ADOLESCENTS AND YOUNGER ADULTS WITH CANCER

Cancer had stifled my life when I was 14–17-years old: it had hijacked what should have been formative years. I could not go back to the life I led before cancer: life had moved on. Neither was I equipped to build a contemporary life as if cancer never

happened. [...] I was a lost boy, lost to cancer. Chemotherapy saved me but, in the life
it granted, I still had to find myself. (Pitcairn, 2008: 166).

This statement is from an adolescent cancer survivor, now in his late 30s, who was treated for
sarcoma of the pelvis at the age of 13. The sentiment suggests an acceptance of what was gained
from cancer treatment (survival) weighed against the costs that he paid (enduring physical
and emotional disability). He reports that many of his enduring problems stem from a sense
of isolation and separation from peer groups and friends due to cancer in his teenage years.
Importantly, these problems can be understood as relational in nature.

Adolescence is characterized by a gradual process of separation from parents and a developing sense of **individuality**; however, the anxiety and distress caused by cancer may disrupt
usual processes of individuation and separation between the young person and their parent(s),
resulting in maladaptive attachment patterns. As well as separation from parents, there is also
a need for a sense of relational belonging with peer groups that may be accompanied with particular social symbols, such as challenging fashion trends, new forms of music and rebellious
behaviour (Kelly and Gibson, 2008).

A diagnosis of cancer is likely to disrupt these processes and evoke both fear and uncertainty for most young people. In this age group, there is the additional impact of cancer on a
body that is already in a state of change. A unique feature of cancer at this time, therefore, is
that it is will be experienced alongside intense physical growth, emotional development and
formation of body image and social role. Jacobs (1990) describes this as:

> A time of awkwardness, of disproportions, of frightening sexual maturation, of pimples,
> and of new and untried feelings ... Everything is in flux and change. (Jacobs, 1990: 109).

One important feature of adolescence and young adulthood is the importance on the
formation of independent, non-familial relationships. For young people undergoing cancer
treatment, however, this may be more difficult due to prolonged periods of hospitalization
and recovery. This disruption can result in intense emotions such as anger and frustration and
the desire for relational support from non-cancer friends hampered as a result of being singled
out as 'different'. Cancer in adolescence, therefore, brings not only the risk of death at a time
when the future is normally anticipated eagerly, but also the threat of being 'different from
the crowd.' For example, baldness, amputation, weight loss and fatigue all lead to restricted
independence and diminished physical, social and sexual capacity. Research is currently
underway to understand better the extent of these problems in young cancer populations.
Once again, relational concerns lie at the heart of this sense of difference and may help to
suggest a way forward.

Treatments that young cancer patients commonly undergo include radiotherapy, surgery
(including radical amputations) and chemotherapy. All can have a profound impact on body
image, confidence and a sense of embodiment as a 'sick adolescent'. As a result of such treatments, young people are marked out as different and may find it easier to relate to others
undergoing the same experience (Kelly et al., 2004).

Relationships, body image and sexuality are concerns that are defining dimensions in the
lives of many young people, and these issues can be expected to assume greater importance
during cancer. Adolescence and young adulthood covers a wide age range, extending from
12-years-old to the mid-20s, and is highly disparate in terms of physical, emotional and social

maturity. For example, the rate at which sexual maturity is reached does not follow a fixed pattern, reinforcing the need for individual patient assessment being at the heart of personalized supportive care programmes (Kelly, 2013).

Addressing concerns about the impact of cancer on sexual intimacy that may arise during treatment will have to be matched appropriately to the age (both chronological and emotional) of the young person involved. Awareness of the importance of age-appropriate relational approach to psychosocial care can help to ensure that other issues, such as maintaining links with education, returning to employment or developing new interests, are considered alongside treatment of the cancer itself.

As with studies in adult cohorts, research has demonstrated that the informal support provided by family members can be linked directly to the illness experience of younger adults (Decker, 2006a; see also Chapter 20). This suggests that successful relational support can help balance the challenge of living with cancer and its treatment with healthy familial relationships, achieving success with careers and other key life events (including success in the formation of intimate relationships).

Reflective activity

Joe is 18-years-old and recently started studying drama at university. He had been feeling unwell for some time with pain in his leg that was worse at night. During the second week of his course, he fell over. When his leg was examined under X-ray, an abnormality was discovered and he was referred to a specialist who diagnosed osteosarcoma of the upper tibia. Joe was admitted for further staging investigations and possible treatment with chemotherapy with the aim of limb-sparing surgery. He was accompanied by his mother and father who live 300 miles away.

- What might be the key concerns for Joe discovering that his pain was due to cancer?
- How might his past experience of working hard to get into university be used to help him think about his treatment journey?
- By using a relational approach, how might you help ensure that Joe receives the necessary age-appropriate information and support?
- What resources could be accessed to help Joe and his family at this time?

This exercise may have suggested how this young man might also go about maintaining existing friendships, as well as intimate relationships, and how and when he might talk with his partner about the impact of cancer on his body. The impact that the situation will have on his relationship with his parents is also worth considering.

Adolescence and young adulthood are times of intense sexual development. A life-threatening disease does not necessarily always halt this process. Instead, sexual function can become a focus of particular and, at times, unspoken concern for young people. For instance, young men may struggle to come to terms with the loss of a testicle from testicular cancer (Kim et al., 2012). Fertility-preserving techniques, such as sperm banking, will also require a thoughtful and delicate conversation. Quinn and Kelly (2000) identified that although this is an everyday procedure for healthcare professionals, it can be highly embarrassing.

Discussing such topics can be very difficult for parents and healthcare professionals; however, when compared with other cancer groups, there is a lack of research evidence to support effective psychosexual interventions for young people in this situation (Kelly, 2013). The final section of this chapter explores some strategies for engaging in conversations or using specific interventions about these issues.

Despite the presence of cancer, adolescents may still develop new physical and emotional attachments and attractions. Such feelings may be directed towards those in closest proximity, including healthcare professionals, which can become problematic when boundaries become blurred. Supervision and debriefing sessions may be helpful for professionals to respond to these occurrences appropriately (Pearce, 2008).

THE NEED FOR EMOTIONAL SUPPORT

The central message in this chapter is the need for awareness of the negative impact that cancer can have on people's identity and their need for emotional support and human connection. Cancer can impact negatively by altering a person's body image that, in turn, may have negative consequences on close relationships (which may or may not include disruption to sexual function with partners).

When considering the impact of cancer on different age groups, it is evident that there are differences, but also remarkable similarities. Both young and old have need for information and support, and both require to be acknowledged as having unique relational needs by professionals in practice contexts.

A diagnosis of cancer magnifies the need for emotional support, but close relationships may actually be put at risk due to psychological withdrawal or isolation by the patient or those closest to them. **Protective buffering** is a core psychological and relational process that may emerge. This is the process whereby individuals choose not to speak of their concerns and worries in order to protect those around them from further worry, and may be particularly apparent in partners with low self-efficacy (Kuijer et al., 2000). This protection, however, leads to others feeling cut-off and excluded from developing a full understanding of emotional needs. Consequently, although some patients may believe that choosing not to verbalize worries is protecting their loved ones, it can actually lead to increased distress and relational distancing.

Practitioners have an important role in facilitating adaptation by both patients and family members. Adopting a relational approach to adaptation and supportive cancer care requires an understanding of the interconnections between cancer, its impact on self, intimate relationships and body image. Addressing the complex psychosocial support needs of every cancer patient within busy workloads, however, is a challenge to practitioners: referral to other members of the team with more time or expertise might be the most valuable skill to develop.

Reflective activity

How might a relational approach to care be promoted in your own setting? Think about how you might use this to enhance awareness of patient's needs when they go home, or how it might help you support patients better during treatment.

- Can you identify how you currently use such information, or how it might be used better?
- Does the depersonalized nature of healthcare clash with the promotion of relational approaches? Is intimacy/relationships valued in your service as a supportive resource during the cancer experience?
- You may wish to consider the needs not just of the patient, but also of their close relatives who are also impacted by the disease.

Thinking about these questions, it is possible for clinicians to promote a greater sense of awareness about an individual's supportive relational resources. A first step might be to ask people about their lives and to map the support available to them from family, friends and within the clinical environment. The range of available supports can then be recognized within an individual's plan of care. Sometimes interventions are requires when the impact of cancer on relationships requires skilled expertise.

INTERVENTIONS TO SUPPORT BODY IMAGE AND SEXUALITY POST-CANCER

Relational interventions

Research evidence demonstrates that psychosocial support services could help address unmet needs (Street et al., 2010). A number of core relational components are drawn upon in interventions for different cancer patient groups. In a recent systematic review, Hubbard, Knighting, et al. (2013) identify three core relational mechanisms that are evident in the breast cancer literature: (1) couple coping, (2) relational functioning and satisfaction, and (3) communication. Taken together, these three features indicate that individuals' and partners' experience of cancer can be seen as part of an interdependent relational system. As highlighted in the introduction, relationships mediate the experience of cancer and, consequently, intervening at a relational level can support both parties in their adjustment and coping.

Relationship-based interventions have been applied to serious illness, including disability, cancer and palliative care. In his work focused on chronic illness, Rolland (1994) outlines his theory for the interaction between illness and relationships. His approach proposes the need to understand the psychosocial demands of illness on the wider family, and how this interacts with the lifecycle of family members. Rolland (1999) commends consideration of key features of the disease that will influence the family's adaptation and identify the resources necessary to cope, for example the onset (chronic or acute), prognosis (curable or palliative), course (steady, decline with plateaus, or episodic) and incapacitation (e.g. fatigue or limb amputation). Different patterns in each of these domains will lead to different relational adaptations. For example, chronic bone pain stemming from curable osteosarcoma may lead to considerable incapacitation through lower limb amputation. Such a situation is likely to herald a period of rapid change in family dynamics at the point of diagnosis and treatment; the family will have little time to adapt to the initial symptoms before having to manage the treatments and resulting impairment. Over the longer term, however, there is the potential for a new equilibrium to emerge as the illness is eradicated and prostheses are integrated into the patient's functioning.

Recommended further reading

- The Teenage Cancer Trust supports and funds specialist units to help young people facing cancer (www.teenagecancertrust.org). They also provide online information and support resources.
- CANO-ACIO (Canadian Association of Nurses in Oncology) provides a useful summary of sexual health interventions and resources for healthcare practitioners in oncology (www.cano-acio.ca/~ASSETS/DOCUMENT/CANO_SM_UNIT%207.pdf).
- Macmillan Cancer Support provides information about different types of cancer and the impact relationships (www.Macmillan.org.uk/Cancerinformation/Livingwithandaftercancer/Relationshipscommunication/Relationshipscommunication.aspx).

22 PSYCHOLOGICAL CARE AND SUPPORT FOR PEOPLE AFFECTED BY CANCER

ALEX KING, NICHOLAS HULBERT-WILLIAMS AND SAMANTHA FLYNN

Chapter outline

- Counselling approaches
- Cognitive-behavioural therapy
- Solution-focused therapy
- Cognitive-analytic therapy
- Mindfulness and acceptance-based approaches
- Systemic family therapy
- Cancer support groups

INTRODUCTION

The previous four chapters have outlined what is known about the psychological impact of cancer, the adjustment process that people go through, and how clinicians might best screen for adjustment difficulties and distress in the clinical setting. Yet there is little point in screening if there are no services to address the needs of distressed patients. This chapter will provide an overview of the theory, practice and evidence for commonly used psychological interventions for people with cancer. It would be impossible to give an overview of every different type of intervention possible in one chapter, and so this chapter focuses on the main therapeutic modalities, their rationale, application and evidence base.

More than one-third of people with cancer will experience significant **distress** as a result of their illness, but far fewer will actively seek out **counselling** or **psychological support** (Nekolaichuk et al., 2011). This may be for many reasons: they may be too preoccupied with treatment and rehabilitation, unaware such services exist, or apprehensive about being perceived as 'not coping' or being a 'mental health' patient. Patients and their healthcare professionals may also be sceptical about whether **psychotherapeutic intervention** can be effective or not. The evidence for effectiveness is equivocal and most review articles tend to sit on the fence, not only because of mixed outcomes, but often because of poor methodological quality (Newell et al., 2002). Review articles that exclude poorly designed studies and only include studies with rigorous methodology, tend to yield better effect sizes (Andrykowski and Manne, 2006). This is not surprising as interventions will only result in significant changes where patients are already considerably psychologically distressed, white in less rigorous designs, where screening with clear clinical criteria is not used, effectiveness can be diluted (van Scheppingen et al., 2014).

A recently published Cochrane meta-analysis even goes so far as to suggest that evidence is now emerging for a moderate one-year survival benefit of psychological intervention for women with metastatic breast cancer (Mustafa et al., 2013). Although this finding is relevant and important, it should be considered within the broader debate and literature on the impact of psychological interventions on survival and, indeed, whether this should even be expected – surely it is good enough for psychological interventions to be effective against their primary intended outcome, that of reducing psychological distress.

NICE (2004b) guidelines recommend the appropriate and tiered use of psychological interventions for distress in people with cancer, and suggest a four-tier model based on the complexity of intervention required. Level 1 refers to universal care and support behaviours, such as active listening, providing information and signposting, which all professionals in cancer care will routinely provide. Level 2 refers to the screening, assessment, first-line interventions (e.g. breathing relaxation for panic, active listening, goal setting, supported self-help etc.) and support of an ongoing relationship with a key worker (most often a clinical nurse specialist), and these require additional training and regular supervision. It is expected that the support needs of the majority of patients will be met by Level 1 and 2 input. Level 3 refers to adjustment-focused interventions, such as counselling or solution-focused brief therapy, whilst Level 4 refers to more intensive interventions based on specific models to deal with mental health problems, such as significant mood disorders, risk, personality

Table 22.1 Four-tier model of psychological interventions for distress in people with cancer

Level	Group	Assessment	Intervention
1	All health and social care professionals	Recognition of psychological needs	Effective information giving, compassionate communication and general psychological support
2	Health and social care professionals with additional expertise	Screening for psychological distress	Psychological techniques such as problem solving
3	Trained and accredited professionals	Assessed for psychological distress and diagnosis of some psychopathology	Counselling and specific psychological interventions such as anxiety management and solution-focused therapy, delivered according to an explicit theoretical framework
4	Mental health specialists	Diagnosis of psychopathology	Specialist psychological psychiatric interventions such as psychotherapy, including cognitive–behavioural therapy

Source: NICE (2004b: 72)

disorder, post-traumatic stress disorder and so forth. These more complex interventions require specifically trained and accredited professionals, such as clinical or counselling psychologists and liaison psychiatrists, with specific expertise in cancer. NICE (2004b) estimate that 15% and 10% of cancer patients will require Levels 3 and 4, respectively, for raised and clinical levels of distress.

This four-tier model is summarized in Table 22.1.

It goes without saying that all health professionals need to work within the limits of their knowledge and training. This chapter provides an overview of a range of approaches, each requiring its own specific training, accreditation, ongoing supervision and continuous professional development. Some require a relevant professional background (e.g. clinical psychology or psychiatry), whilst others can be open to a wider range of professionals. Even those who don't go on to train in or use these approaches may find that simply knowing more about them will help in the day-to-day communication with patients and understanding their experience. This knowledge will make it clearer for health professionals to know when, and to whom, onward referrals need to be made for patients within their care.

COUNSELLING

The term '**counselling**' is broadly used as a reference to the *format* of a confidential, face-to-face interaction where a professional aims to help the patient resolve difficulties in their life. This chapter will focus on counselling as a psychological therapy, although other strands also exist, for example genetic counselling for individuals who are carriers of genetic cancer risk (Butow et al., 2003). What happens *within* a counselling session will vary depending on the theoretical model that the counsellor is adopting and might include **humanistic, person-centred, gestalt, transactional, existential–phenomenological, integrative** or **psychodynamic** approaches. These vary considerably in their assumptions about the causes of distress, the process of change and the role and activity of the therapist (Dryden and Reeves, 2013). There is also broad variation in counselling training, from relatively brief single-model courses to professional doctoral-level qualifications, which develop expertise in multiple models; however, it is possible to outline some key aspects that most counselling models share, including a focus on the therapeutic relationship, clear therapeutic boundaries and a broadly supportive ethos. The counsellor typically espouses values of empathy, acceptance, genuineness and flexibility and *being with* the patient, rather than *doing to*. As a process, counselling seeks to bring change through reflection, exploration and insight (Dryden and Reeves, 2013), rather than a focus on goals, skills or symptoms.

As we have seen in previous chapters, people with cancer face significant and rapidly emerging threats and demands, to which they have to rapidly adjust. The strain and distress inherent in adjusting to cancer at different points through treatment and survivorship is expected and normal, and usually time-limited; however, for a variety of social and psychological reasons, some people find this process particularly difficult, feel 'stuck' and remain more distressed for longer than they can tolerate. Counselling can be useful to give the person with cancer a safe, confidential space where the counsellor's empathic, person-centred and accepting attitude can help them to access and consider their thoughts and feelings without trying to suppress them – at times out of concern for 'burdening' or 'disappointing' others. People often experience considerable emotional relief from this process of talking openly, and then find themselves more able to 'move forward' and take appropriate actions.

Counselling is listed in the NICE (2004b) guidelines as a 'Level 3' level intervention for cancer-related distress, and is supposed to be delivered by counsellors with professional body accreditation and specialist supervision. All members of a healthcare team, however, may benefit from training in basic skills derived from counselling, such as active listening and summarizing, to improving communication (Maguire and Faulkner, 1988a; Moore et al., 2013; see also Chapter 17) and even potentially in the screening and triage process for psychological distress. Indeed, in the UK, clinical staff in cancer multidisciplinary teams are required to undertake courses such as Advanced Communications Skills (Connected) training or SAGE & THYME training (Connolly et al., 2010), which include such core skills.

There are very few published studies that provide empirical evidence for the effectiveness of counselling interventions for people with cancer because most explore the benefits of more structured therapies, such as **Cognitive–Behavioural Therapy** (CBT). However, there is broader evidence across general health populations for the effectiveness of counselling approaches. Gibbard and Hanley (2008), King et al. (2013) and Glover et al. (2010) all show equivalence for counselling with other psychological therapies in primary care settings.

We are aware of just one empirical study – Moorey et al. (1998) – that compared counselling with other types of psychological intervention for patients with cancer meeting criteria for an abnormal adjustment reaction. This study's results suggest counselling to be a less effective method of improving psychological adjustment. This finding, however, may be related to entrance criteria into the study: although structured and complex psychological interventions are probably more suited to patients meeting clinical levels of psychological disorders, counselling may work well for those who are experiencing symptomatic distress and simply need an opportunity to talk about their feelings. The following case study exemplifies this.

CASE STUDY

Ms G

Ms G was a lady in her 60s with an advanced cancer that would likely remain relatively stable for a period. She was referred when, several months after a very intense chemotherapy, she spoke to her nurse specialist about feeling upset about being criticized by friends. In an initial session, she came across as a proud, direct, self-sufficient and determined lady with good overall functioning. She told the counsellor she had grown up abroad, had decided in her 20s not to have children, and had until recently been working in a demanding senior commercial job. She breezily said she had always been good at 'sweeping things under the carpet' and carrying on a full life of work, travel and broad interests. All through her treatments she had jumped back into work, days later, and tried to carry on as normal. It was clearly hard for her to talk about losing her standing and position, and facing the prospect of being on the sidelines of the business and the shock of limited health. She had withdrawn, seeing others as abandoning and critical, and felt she could not bear to address the financial and procedural stresses of taking early retirement through ill health. Over the course of five sessions, and as more trust was established in the counsellor, she showed brief and fleeting moments of emotion when really touching on difficult feelings of anger and vulnerability. She was surprised that she had allowed these through, and reported a lot of relief and feeling that she had 'moved on'. The counsellor adopted a person-centred position of active listening, prompting her to stay with feelings, and reflecting back key emotional themes. In the final session, Ms G said that she was now aware to expect moments of vulnerability, but instead of withdrawing and fearing criticism, she would reach out to trusted friends to receive support.

COGNITIVE–BEHAVIOURAL THERAPY (CBT)

The key concept in CBT is that distress and dysfunction is maintained by persistently **distorted thinking** (cognition), for example **black-or-white thinking** ('Either I can cope perfectly, or I'll be a total mess') or **catastrophizing** ('This pain will never stop and will drive me crazy') (Beck, 2011). These thoughts, beliefs and expectations about the self, others and the world are '**automatic**' and not fully conscious, and can lead to unhelpful behaviour such as withdrawal, avoidance, aggression and so forth. CBT suggests that different difficulties are linked to distinct patterns of distorted thinking. Depression is linked to distorted thoughts about being helpless and worthless, for example 'I can never get anything right', while health anxiety will be linked to thoughts such as 'I must be on constant alert for symptoms to avoid a serious illness'. A CBT **formulation** involves pointing out how automatic thoughts influence feelings, physical sensations and behaviours, which then can confirm or reinforce the thoughts. For example, in panic, an errant physical sensation may be interpreted as 'I'm having a massive heart attack', thus triggering intense fear and a cascade of autonomic arousal responses (sweating, shallow breathing, muscle tension, etc.) which are in turn seen as confirming evidence of a heart attack, and so forth. It is very important to notice that CBT is never about creating 'positive' thinking or stopping 'negative' thinking. When the stress of cancer brings about thinking that is persistently fixed, distorted and unbalanced, this can trigger and maintain depression and anxiety (Greer, 2008). For example, at diagnosis, a person who persistently thinks 'There is nothing anyone can do to help me' is likely to feel low, helpless and withdrawn.

Beyond the broader distress issues discussed in the previous section, cancer and its treatment also bring a range of more severe threats and real losses. Thinking about one's cancer situation with a balanced perspective, especially when physically weakened and fatigued, can be very difficult. CBT therapy in cancer care consists of the therapist and the person working together to identify automatic thoughts and their influence on day-to-day life and coping with cancer. Between sessions, the person may use self-monitoring diaries to track how they think, feel and behave moment-by-moment. In sessions with their therapist they will analyze these patterns to identify unhelpful and distorted thinking, and try to come up with more balanced and helpful thoughts (Horne and Watson, 2011). To help the person shift their thinking, the therapist may use a variety of techniques, such as '**behavioural experiments**' where the person tries to think or behave differently and notices the different feelings this creates (Westbrook et al., 2011). The therapist may also be teaching the person helpful coping techniques such as relaxation, sleep hygiene, problem solving and so forth. When CBT is effective, people usually report that it has helped them to understand their thoughts, take a step back and be more balanced, and challenge themselves to confront things they are avoiding.

CBT is a specialist intervention that requires specific training. This is often undertaken as part of clinical or counselling psychology training; however, healthcare professionals from other backgrounds such as nurses, psychiatrists and allied health professionals can train specifically in this model, and qualify and practice as CBT therapists. CBT is considered a suitable intervention for patients across the full spectrum of severity and NICE (2004b) guidelines list it as an example of a 'Level 4' intervention for clinically significant cancer-related mental health difficulties, such as anxiety, depression or post-traumatic stress.

In an effort to make CBT more accessible and cost-effective, Kathryn Mannix, Steven Moorey and colleagues have recently developed Cognitive Therapy First Aid (CTFA), a short and intensive training package of basic CBT skills for cancer and palliative care nurses. Results from randomized controlled trials are somewhat mixed to date and whilst their findings do not demonstrate significant improvement for depression, patients with advanced cancer receiving nurse-delivered CTFA reported lower anxiety (Moorey et al., 2009; Mannix et al., 2006).

The evidence for the effectiveness of CBT for these kinds of psychological outcomes is encouraging, particularly when compared with other therapeutic modalities. In their comparative meta-analysis of CBT versus **patient education** for adult cancer survivors, Osborn et al. (2006) concluded that CBT treatment results in improved depression and anxiety (in the short-term only) and improved quality of life (both shorter and longer term). They suggest that one-to-one delivered CBT is more effective than group delivery, but that more informally delivered CBT can assist in reducing survivorship-related distress. These effects are also applicable for patients with advanced cancer – Uitterhoeve et al. (2004) reviewed literature on CBT trials for people with advanced cancer and found a positive improvement on multiple different indicators of quality of life. Similarly, Mustafa et al. (2013) in their recently updated Cochrane Review conclude that not only is CBT more effective than **supportive-expressive group therapy** across a variety of outcomes in women with metastatic breast cancer, but also that there is emerging evidence for a survival benefit, in the short-term at least.

More recently, there has been an increased attention to using CBT for coping with and managing specific treatment-related side effects, and the evidence here is also positive. One such focus has been on fatigue, whereby CBT is found to have positive, and long-lasting (up to two years) beneficial effects upon fatigue reduction and functional impairment in cancer survivors (Gielissen et al., 2007). Similar improvements following CBT (above and beyond treatment-as-usual controls) are reported for persistent insomnia (e.g. Espie et al., 2008) and menopausal symptoms in breast cancer survivors (e.g. Hunter et al., 2008).

CASE STUDY

Chris

Chris recently completed radiotherapy for throat cancer and had eight weeks to wait before scan results. He sought help with feeling very anxious, afraid of being alone at home, sleeping poorly and feeling useless and a burden to his family. He described how he had been a confident businessman, with no past experiences of anxiety. He spoke about how his cancer had taken a very long time to diagnose and how, during treatment, he had had to come into hospital with pain and dehydration.

Taking a CBT perspective, the therapist helped Chris identify automatic thoughts such as 'I was always in control - now nothing is in my control' (black-white), 'This fatigue will not get better - I will never get back to work' (catastrophizing), 'If I'm not getting checked frequently, I can deteriorate quickly - but I don't trust doctors because they missed it' (overgeneralizing). Together they tracked how these thoughts, plus the post-radiotherapy fatigue, led Chris to feel helpless and vulnerable. He was demanding of others to stay with him and reassure him all the time - then feeling a burden for doing so. He received medical reassurance but would not trust it. Going to sleep was disrupted because he kept thinking of all the things that would go wrong.

Chris had not realized he was thinking that way, but when this became clearer he started to see how it related to his problems. With the therapist, they looked at finding a more balanced perspective, for example speaking to the doctors he did trust, realizing that he had some control over his recovery, and challenging his fear that he would be vulnerable without others to watch over him. His anxiety gradually settled and he was able to reconnect with his more independent self, whilst he waited for results.

SOLUTION-FOCUSED THERAPY

The key concept in Solution-Focused Therapy (SFT) is that it is much more important to pay the most attention to the way a person is *already addressing* a problem, rather than to delve too far into *the problem* itself (as might be the tendency in CBT) (De Shazer, 1985; Iveson, 2002). By not assuming that people's difficulties require a complex and thorough analysis of their backgrounds and developmental experiences, or a reworking of their ways of coping, SFT is a pragmatic, accessible and typically brief approach. In SFT, there is no sense of an 'expert' therapist that 'analyzes' the disorder and selects the right treatment for the patient. The solution-focused consultation is a 'meeting of experts' where the therapist guides the patient in exploring and mobilizing their own values, hopes, strengths and resources to overcome their difficulties. The actual SFT intervention, therefore, is in the therapist's distinctive, skilful questioning that will draw these out, rather than any new skills or techniques they impart to the patient.

From an SFT perspective, to help people with cancer or advancing disease, it is important to look beyond the problem posed by the cancer to the person's experience with overcoming adversity, and to their hopes and values for life ahead – even if time is limited. SFT can be a particularly good fit for unwell inpatients with little energy or will to engage in complex discussions. In the inpatient context, a solution-focused conversation can be a quick(er) route to pragmatic solutions – what keeps a person going, what makes for a slightly better day, how have they learnt to cope with the ward's quirks, what advice would they give to others about coping on the ward, what are they hoping for when they get home. Additionally, SFT can also be a good fit for people who, before cancer, had never considered seeing a psychologist or counsellor, and would not expect to be talking about their early life and past difficulties; for them, it feels much more appropriate that SFT focuses on the present and future instead. When SFT is effective, people come away with a much clearer sense of how to apply their personal strengths and resources to cancer-related problems, and a renewed confidence in themselves, despite the limitations of the cancer and its treatments.

SFT is listed in the NICE (2004b) guidelines as an example of a 'Level 3' intervention in cancer and palliative care, and Bray and Groves (2007) set out its key benefits and attractions in this context. Although its use as a psychological intervention requires specific training and supervision, key concepts and basic skills drawn from an SFT perspective can be drawn usefully into many aspects of routine clinical practice by any specialty, for example in setting rehabilitation therapy goals.

Although the chapter's authors are not aware of any specific studies that evaluate the effectiveness of solution-focused therapy in a cancer setting, a review of the evidence for SFT practice across many clinical areas (mostly in educational settings) suggested positive effectiveness (Gingerich and Peterson, 2013), however, the variability in study quality was noted to limit the reliability of the results.

Mrs J

Mrs J was a lady of Eastern Asian background who had just been diagnosed with an advanced pancreatic cancer. She was on the inpatient ward when she requested a consultation to discuss how she could prepare her two sons (both in their early 20s) about her dying. She came across as very composed and revealed a background as a successful businesswoman, with a very matter-of-fact attitude. The psychologist felt that a solution-focused approach would best respect this lady's strong work ethos. He asked how she would know that the consultation had been worth her time, and she said that she would know 'the right way' to do it. The psychologist was curious about what she saw as the 'right way' and it emerged that it was about self-sufficiency, struggling through adversity and 'not having it on a plate'. She expressed her concerns that her sons had not shown as much drive as she had hoped, and would 'go soft' if she was not there to prompt and push them. The psychologist asked, 'What would they have learnt from you about how to cope with losing you?'. She talked about how she dealt with separating from her husband when he was gambling and failing to contribute to the family, and took full responsibility for her children. When prompted to summarize the session, she said that it had reminded her that she could not control how her sons led their life, but felt good about having been a good example, which she hoped they would one day emulate.

COGNITIVE–ANALYTIC THERAPY

Cognitive–Analytic Therapy (CAT) is a pragmatic integration of ideas from **psychodynamic theory** and early CBT in a package specifically adapted for use in an NHS context (Ryle, 1991; Ryle and Kerr, 2002; Kerr and Ryle, 2006). CAT focuses on the repetition of patterns of interpersonal interactions as the core element underlying emotional distress. Ryle (1991) suggests that early life interactions with caregivers shape our internal, mental models of relationships (e.g. a child feeling safe in relation to a parent being caring) that later become internalized (e.g. as self-caring). This is the element that derives from psychoanalytic theory. Problems arise in life when early difficulties lead to rigid, limited and harsh ways of relating to oneself and others; the person is then likely to use unhelpful patterns of planning, thinking and behaving as an attempt to compensate and cope – this is the cognitive element. In a typical 16-session CAT therapy, the therapist and patient work together to explore and visualize these patterns in a diagram, with the aim to achieve better insight and perspective, and start to identify and practice alternative patterns. The relationship to the therapist is a core element for the patient to experience and practice more balanced and respectful ways of relating, but an eclectic range of other techniques can be used as well to change patterns.

Within a cancer context, CAT is a very practical tool for understanding how a person's interpersonal past and present can interact with the complexities of cancer care to result in distress or undue conflict with carers and professionals. For example, seeing an authority-figure doctor to discuss toxic chemotherapy can bring up painful early experiences of a cruel or abusive parent and trigger angry or defiant responses, leading to mistrust, rejecting advice and erratic treatment decisions; or the cancer itself can be seen as a repeat of the dominating and overpowering parent, and the person may adopt a passive, helpless position, leading to depression.

Studies of CAT in emotional and personality disorders have been promising (Clarke et al., 2013). No specific research has taken place in a cancer context, although some are reported to be underway (Pitceathly et al., 2011). A recent survey of UK psychologists working in cancer care reported that CAT is perceived by these therapists to be a relevant and helpful approach to intervention for some people with cancer (Charman and Hulbert-Williams, 2013).

MINDFULNESS AND ACCEPTANCE-BASED APPROACHES

The term **mindfulness** refers to focusing the mind's attention in a particular way: with purpose, in the present and non-judgementally (Wilson and DuFrene, 2009). It is about alert perception, and quite distinct to states of **relaxation** or **hypnosis**. This focus can be applied to the internal world of thoughts, feelings and bodily sensations, or the external world of nature, people and so forth. Although simple as a concept to understand *logically*, it is demanding to achieve in practice because our minds are typically used to flitting rapidly and often randomly between thoughts, impressions, judgements, the past and the future, nice and unpleasant feelings, ourselves and others. Another way to describe mindfulness is as a constant process, *a way of paying attention*, rather than a 'state' of perfect unbroken attentiveness, which is not attainable (Kabat-Zinn, 1994).

There are several approaches to cultivating and practicing mindfulness; some are forms of meditation that developed within the prayer practices of religious traditions, particularly Buddhism, and some are adaptations from a modern perspective. Other contemporary therapeutic models have also incorporated mindfulness into their practices, for example **mindfulness-based stress reduction** (MBSR) (Kabat-Zinn, 2003, 2013) and **mindfulness-based cognitive therapy** (MBCT) (Teasdale, 1995).

MBSR is typically delivered as a group programme for people with a range of health conditions, including cancer, who are led by a mindfulness teacher over eight weekly sessions through a series of exercises to develop their mindfulness skills. The group sessions are supported by daily home mindfulness exercise practice and an all-day group session. People who attend MBSR (and similar programmes) report a better developed ability to keep a 'mental balance', notice and stand back from rumination and worry, focus on the present, tolerate unpleasant experiences and live 'a day at a time' (Kabat-Zinn, 2013). These skills can be particularly helpful when dealing with persistent cancer-related symptoms, such as pain or nausea, and related stresses and distressing thoughts. It can be particularly helpful for people who may be averse to typical individual psychotherapeutic approaches, as a gentler way of overcoming unhelpful avoidant coping.

A newer wave of CBT has recently emerged, referred to as **'third-wave'** therapies, many of which integrate mindfulness as both a key construct and therapeutic technique. Of these approaches, **Acceptance and Commitment Therapy** (Hayes et al., 2011) is suggested to be especially relevant to the psychological wellbeing of patients with cancer (Hulbert-Williams et al., 2014).

ACT proposes that improvement in psychological wellbeing is best achieved through learning to let go of ineffective efforts to control, avoid or suppress distress, because often these efforts in themselves cause additional loss and restriction (Hayes et al., 2011), for example not going out with friends to avoid feelings of anxiety. Instead, it focuses on guiding people to *radically* accept pain and suffering (in the broadest sense, including the physical and emotional) as part of living, and to look beyond pain to the pursuit of one's values in life. Therefore, ACT is less concerned with reducing symptoms per se, and much more about addressing the **behavioural impact** of perceived suffering, distressing cognitions and emotions (Greco, Lambert and Baer, 2008).

There is mounting evidence for positive effects from mindfulness-based interventions on general emotional distress (Fjorback et al., 2011) and specifically in cancer (e.g. Schroevers and Brandsma, 2010; Shennan et al., 2011). A recent randomized controlled trial of MBSR in breast cancer using wait-list controls (Hoffman et al., 2012) demonstrated clear benefits in mood and quality of life for women on this programme, with effects maintained for up to three months post-intervention. Of further interest is a growing body of findings demonstrating improvements in biological outcomes following mindfulness-based interventions, including both **hormonal** and **immune function** improvements (e.g. Carlson et al., 2004; Witek-Janusek et al., 2008).

Empirical evidence for the effectiveness of ACT within cancer samples is not so extensive, but is still of significance. Feros et al. (2013) recently published on a non-randomized trial of patients with a range of cancer diagnoses and severity levels. Participants were entered into the trial only if they had previously been screened as highly distressed. The findings demonstrate clear and significant improvement in not only distress, but also in quality of life and mood. A more methodologically powerful randomized controlled trial in patients with late-stage ovarian cancer demonstrated not only significant improvements in mood and quality of life for the ACT group, but also that these improvements were significantly larger than control participants who had received standard CBT (Rost et al., 2012).

Though a formal mindfulness or ACT intervention requires specific training, accreditation and supervision, it's possible to encourage people to use specific components as simple self-help routines. The 'mindful breathing' technique given in the box below is one example of this. There are as many wordings of this as there are practitioners, with the essential elements being the tuning and re-tuning of attention onto the physical act of breathing. This may be somewhat similar to relaxation, but the intention is different: this is about training one's attention, rather than lowering autonomic arousal levels in the moment.

A mindful breathing meditation

- Assume a comfortable posture lying on your back or sitting. If you are sitting, keep the spine straight and let your shoulders drop.
- Close your eyes if it feels comfortable.
- Bring your attention to your abdomen, feeling it rise or expand gently on the in-breath and fall or recede on the out-breath.
- Keep your focus on the breathing, 'being with' each in-breath for its full duration and with each out-breath for its full duration, as if you were riding the waves of your own breathing.

- Every time you notice that your mind has wandered off the breath, notice what it was that took you away and then gently bring your attention back to your stomach and the feeling of the breath coming in and out.
- If your mind wanders away from the breath a thousand times, then your 'job' is simply to bring it back to the breath every time, no matter what it becomes preoccupied with.
- Practice this exercise for fifteen minutes at a convenient time every day, whether you feel like it or not, for one week, and see how it feels to incorporate a disciplined meditation practice into your life. Be aware of how it feels to spend some time each day just being with your breath without having to *do* anything.

Source: www.getselfhelp.co.uk/mindfulness.htm

SYSTEMIC, COUPLES AND FAMILY THERAPY

We know that cancer has considerable effects on the family (see also Chapter 20). Many of the therapeutic models mentioned earlier focus on the individual, and conceptualize distress as internal, *within* the person. From these perspectives, therefore, the impact of cancer on a family would be considered by focusing on one person at a time. In contrast, systemic approaches place distress as *between* people, in the context of multiple relationships that interlink and can become stuck in unhelpful, imbalanced patterns (Dallos and Draper, 2010). This system is often the family (thus the approach is often known as **family systems therapy**), but in a broader sense, any system of relationships, including with health professionals, workplace colleagues, a religious community and others, can be the focus of attention. The impact of cancer from a systemic perspective would therefore be seen in the pattern of interactions and communications, and how these change and adapt.

As with counselling, there are several strands of theory and practice within the broader domain of **systemic approaches**, such as **structural** (Minuchin, 1968), **Milan** (Palazzoli et al., 1978) and **narrative** (White and Epston, 1990; Roberts and Holmes, 1998). These do share common principles, mainly in the position of the therapist, who does not assume an 'expert' role but instead facilitates the exchange between multiple equal perspectives, focusing on the pattern and sequence of interactions in the present rather than looking at past causes, considering culture and difference as primary factors, and looking out for imbalances of power. Systemic therapists often see their role as bringing about change through introducing *difference* – that is, new and different ways of looking at and talking about stuck patterns of interaction, for example by side-stepping blaming and critical language (Carr, 2012).

In a cancer context, systemic thinking in the broadest sense can be particularly relevant on multiple counts. At the level of the family, the roles of the person with cancer will change, as will the roles of the people around them. These changes may create strain for all involved, but often it is the patient who is the focus of attention and may be identified as the one having 'the problem'. Furthermore, considering the sheer number of people involved in cancer treatment, which the patient and family have to navigate, we can see broad scope for strain, conflict and power imbalances with medical and nursing professionals, extended family, workplace hierarchies, culture and social subgroups, welfare systems and so on. Again, the patient may be identified as 'having' the distress, even if it is linked to a complex set of interactions with powerful others.

The Smith family

A teenager with leukaemia was seeing a counsellor while undertaking treatment. Soon, her mother and father separately requested counselling, and one of her two brothers also. The team recognized the potential for the strain the family was going through to be 'broken up' into individual pieces that failed to connect, and instead proposed they all be seen as a family. The sessions brought all the family together with a systemic therapist who ensured a balanced discussion, taking all perspectives on board. The family expressed their frustrations with each other and their ways their coping was causing strain on others, for example father's drinking, mother's over-control, the teenager's helpless stance, the brother's disengagement. A 'reflecting team' of two co-therapists sat in, observing the discussion and towards the end fed back directly to the family about how they clearly wanted to pull together as if to release a car from the mud, but ended up pulling apart as if in a tug-of-war, by sometimes competing for attention and care. This different language, which linked them all together and avoided blame, was a significant point for the family, who gradually came to see each others' positions and efforts more compassionately.

Systemic models are not the only way to address the issues that cancer poses to couples and families. Many of the other models outlined here, including counselling and CBT, can be adapted for use with couples and families. For example, Collins et al. (2011) recently reported a pilot study of the application of **Cognitive Existential Couple Therapy** for men with prostate cancer and their spouses. They concluded from this mixed-methods investigation that couples therapy is not only desirable and acceptable but feasible and effective too, reducing overall distress, especially for the spouses. Zaider and Kissane (2010) offer an extensive review of the range and evidence of couple and family interventions in cancer care that may be of interest to the reader wishing to learn more about these types of intervention.

Debate on diagnosis-based versus formulation-based therapy

By this point, the reader will have picked up that psychological therapies are not always designed to treat specific diagnoses such as 'depression' or 'health anxiety', but seem to aim more broadly. This is a significant distinction, a point of vivid current debate, and well worth knowing about.

You will be familiar with the medical concept of diagnosis (the label that describes a list of symptoms and points to the underlying pathological cause) and so that probably needs no further explanation here. But in mental health, things are not quite as straightforward.

On one side, many feel that a diagnostic approach can be applied in mental health in the same way as it is in medicine. This approach can be seen in systems of psychiatric classification, such as the DSM (Diagnostic and Statistical Manual) of the American Psychiatric Association, now in its fifth revision (DSM-V; American Psychiatric Association, 2013). They argue that we can distinguish and classify the various types of mental health problems and reliably apply labels such as 'bipolar depression type II', 'schizophrenia', 'borderline personality disorder' etc. They argue that this is the best way to ensure that mental health is approached in a standardized, rigorously scientific way because it allows testing specific formulas of step-by-step psychological (or biomedical) interventions in controlled clinical trials, in the same way as in medicine.

On the other side are those who argue that psychological distress is quite fundamentally different. They argue that classifications of human behaviour can never be objective and free of cultural values (a key example was the psychiatric classification of homosexuality as a disorder in DSM-III); categories often have large overlaps, which brings into question their distinctiveness (e.g. high rates of co-morbidity between depression and anxiety); and that in contrast to most of medicine, no mental health diagnosis has, to date, a proven singular cause. They counter with the view that people will vary in their resources and opportunities, and emotional problems are linked to how people use these resources to resolve difficult circumstances. They suggest that we should therefore focus on describing difficulties (rather than classifying symptoms), explore their coping procedures and create individualized interventions tailored for each person in each circumstance (Hallam, 2013).

In other words, should the therapy be tailored to each individual's unique history and context (a formulation-based or person-centred approach) but risk being too subjective, or should every person be offered the set treatment protocol that on average works best for their diagnostic category, and risk being too rigid? There is certainly no firm answer to this – which way do you lean towards?

CANCER SUPPORT GROUPS

Although cancer is a common disease that affects most families, many people feel that cancer isolates them and distances others, and they talk about feeling very 'alone with it' and not understood by others around them. They often say that they find great relief and kinship with others who have cancer – not purely for seeking information from more experienced patients about their condition and treatment, but more fundamentally about living through a shared experience (Flynn et al., 2013).

Irvin Yalom is well known as an eloquent writer on group therapy and existential issues (Yalom, 2011), as well as key professional texts about psychotherapeutic groups (Yalom and Lesczc, 2005). His summary of the twelve themes in which people feel benefit from therapeutic groups includes instilling hope, sharing information, finding common ground, belonging, having the satisfaction of helping others, learning and practicing new social skills, and 'letting out' painful feelings (Yalom and Lesczc, 2005). Cancer support groups draw on the general principles and practices of therapeutic groups to address these needs for people with cancer. There is wide variety in the model underlying cancer support groups, and they may range from supportive–expressive groups and expert patient programmes to cognitive–behavioural groups (e.g. on sleep and stress management) to psychodynamic group therapy. Accordingly, groups may be *open*, where people can join or leave at any point (for example, an open support group for people with myeloma), or *closed*, where the group stays together for a defined period, which can range from a few sessions (for example, a group for young women dealing with hot flushes post-chemotherapy) to many years (for example, a therapeutic group for people with advanced disease). As well as organized and professionally moderated groups, people often report coming together in a variety of situations in the course of cancer treatment, for example as one-off groups (e.g. a pre-surgery preparation and education day) or ad hoc groups (e.g. in an outpatient clinic waiting area or in the community setting). The outcome of such activities are based mostly on improved knowledge and perceived social support (Hulbert-William et al., under review) and whilst these are clearly important and relevant, other aspects of distress (such as anxiety or depression) require group interventions with clearer therapeutic frameworks, such as CBT, existential or meaning-centred group psychotherapy.

Recent years have also seen significant growth in the provision of online or internet-facilitated supported groups and these have the advantage that they may be more accessible when travel is a financial, practical or health barrier (e.g., due to to compromised immunity). There is only a limited literature on the support provided by online groups, but this suggests that these resources may be helpful in cancer rehabilitation (e.g. Winzelberg et al., 2003; Høybye et al., 2005).

Peer support groups, where the main focus is to provide a forum for knowledge exchange are widely available and acceptable to people with cancer in the UK and worldwide. A systematic review of 43 publications on group-support programmes for patients with cancer (Hoey et al., 2008) concluded that participants reported high satisfaction, increased perception of social support, and improved knowledge (Hulbert-Williams et al., under review). These groups act to **empower** patients in their coping and adjustment efforts (van Uden-Kraan et al., 2009) and this is clearly important, however if is important to appreciate that this is not sufficient to address other aspects of distress (such as anxiety or depression) where group interventions with clearer therapeutic frameworks, such as CBT, existential or remaining-centred group psychotheraphy are needed.

CASE STUDY

A prostate cancer men's group at Guy's Hospital, London

The nurse specialists for prostate cancer put together a team to set up and run a support group for men with prostate cancer. Between them, the team attended a specific training programme for cancer support group facilitators, sought input from patients and observed other support groups. The nurse specialist, clinical psychologist, prostate radiographer and a patient volunteer formed the group of moderators. They aimed for an open-access group that would offer reliable information, which the men highlighted as a priority, as well as an opportunity for social contact and support.

The group was set up to meet monthly and alternate between an information topic presented by a specialist and small group discussions. Presenters have included dieticians, oncologists, cancer researchers, continence nurses, psychologists, complementary therapists, surgeons, physiotherapists, pathologists, etc. The men in the audience often ask the speakers about their personal situations and their answers help clarify things because the men come to understand the terminology and variations in the cancer and its treatment. In small group discussions, patients get together with one of the moderators to tell their stories, ask each other questions and generally catch up; and then there was the banter about continence and erections, love of gadgets and a good dose of dark humour – the group dubbed itself the 'Glee Club'.

Over the course of several years, attendance has remained persistently high, with new people attending every time and many attending regularly for a period. There have also been deaths, as well as people saying a natural goodbye after being in extended remission. Several from the group developed their confidence and engaged with charity work, research panels and in advocacy, with the issue of prostate specific antigen (PSA) screening always prompting debates. When asked about their experience, the men said that attending the group was highly valuable because it gave them a sense of belonging, reliable information about prostate cancer, helped them collaborate better with health professionals and gave them a way of being helpful to others in the same boat.

CHAPTER SUMMARY

The diagnosis, treatment and ongoing impact of cancer can lead to major psychological difficulties. Modern healthcare, with an emphasis on holistic and person-centred care, includes specialist psychological input as a core, embedded aspect of clinical cancer services. This chapter reviewed some of the main psychological models and interventions used in this context. It also highlighted their distinctive aspects to offer an insight into how clinicians match the needs of each individual patient with the most relevant model. Whilst specific evidence for effectiveness is mounting, more comparative trials are needed to clarify which approaches are better for which people in which circumstances.

Key learning points

- For most people, the diagnosis and treatment of cancer is distressing, and has significant impacts on quality of life.
- People with persistently increased distress can benefit from referral to cancer psychological care services.
- There is a broad range of psychological approaches to cancer-related distress, drawn from a range of psychological theories with distinct rationales.
- The emerging evidence base is supportive of structured approaches such as CBT and MBSR to address clinically significant distress, and there is also a clear role for a broad range of approaches to address the diverse adjustment challenges for people with cancer.

Recommended further reading

- Watson, M. and Kissane, D. (2011) *Handbook of Psychotherapy in Cancer Care.* Chichester, UK: Wiley-Blackwell.
- Moorey, S. and Greer, S. (2012) *Oxford Guide to CBT for People with Cancer (Oxford Guides to Cognitive Behavioural Therapy).* 2nd edn. Oxford, UK: Oxford University Press.
- Carlson, L. and Speca, M. (2011) *Mindfulness-Based Cancer Recovery: A Step-by-Step MBSR Approach to Help you Cope with Treatment and Reclaim your Life.* Oakland, CA: New Harbinger.
- Hulbert-Williams, N.J., Storey, L. and Wilson, K. (2014) 'Psychological interventions for patients with cancer: psychological flexibility and the potential utility of Acceptance and Commitment Therapy', *European Journal of Cancer Care*, Doi: 10.1111/ecc.12223
- van Scheppingen, C., Schroevers, M.J., Pool, G., Smink, A., Mul, V.E., Cogne, J.C. and Sanderman, R. (2014) 'Is implementing screening for distress an efficient means to recruit patients to a psychological intervention trial?', *Psycho-oncology*, 23: 516–523. doi: 10.1002/pon.3447.

23 SURVIVORSHIP AND SELF-MANAGEMENT IN CANCER CARE

CLAIRE FOSTER

Chapter outline

- Life as a cancer survivor
- The changing context of follow-up care
- Self-management of consequences of cancer and its treatment
- Self-management support

INTRODUCTION

This chapter focuses on supporting patients with cancer to self-manage the impact of cancer and its treatment on their lives once primary treatment is over. Many people report feeling isolated at the end of their treatment and may also feel low in confidence, which can affect their management of problems and access to support. It is increasingly being recognized that consequences of cancer and its treatment can have a significant impact on people's daily lives, and some consequences may persist for years. The quality of people's lives may be enhanced by support to self-manage problems and concerns in the short and longer term following treatment.

By 2040, around 1 in 4 people aged 65 and over will have had a diagnosis of cancer and the number of people living with and beyond cancer is set to double by 2030 (Maddams et al., 2012). Rising survival rates are due to improvements in detection and treatments, with many people faring well after treatment; however, cancer and its treatment can have a considerable and long-term impact on everyday life (Corner et al., 2007; Hewitt et al., 2003; Foster et al., 2009). With an ageing population, around 23% of the UK population will be over 65 by 2035 (UK National Statistics, 2013), and with a stretched healthcare system, there is growing concern about how best to support cancer survivors. The current **aftercare** system does not meet the needs of patients (Armes et al., 2009) and the National Cancer Survivorship Initiative (NCSI) has been established to investigate new models of aftercare (DH, 2010b). As a consequence, aftercare for people with cancer is radically changing.

There is currently no clear definition of what is meant by the term **cancer survivor**. The term is often used broadly to refer to all people who have had a cancer diagnosis at some point in their lives. This, therefore, includes both individuals who are living with cancer and those who have had cancer in the past. The focus of the NCSI has generally been on the care and support given to patients and their families from the end of **primary treatment** onwards (DH, 2010b).

Primary treatment is defined as the **curative intent treatment** individuals receive following their diagnosis of cancer. This may include (although not exclusively) surgery, radiotherapy, chemotherapy or a combination of these. This period of treatment may be short-term or last for many months with regular and frequent hospital visits.

The NCSI is testing new models of aftercare using the framework depicted in Figure 23.1 (DH, 2010b). Patients will be stratified to one of the three layers of follow-up: (1) self-care with support and open access; (2) shared care; or (3) complex case management through multidisciplinary teams (MDT). The amount of professional care a person receives will vary according to the type of follow-up the person is allocated to. This allocation will be determined by a **risk assessment** and patients will be stratified according to level of risk and follow-up care organized accordingly. Those with highest risk of problems, for example due to advanced cancer or complex needs, will receive complex case management through MDT, which will involve a high level of professional intervention. Those with least risk, for example many of those patients who have had treatment with curative intent, will be allocated to **supported self-care** and open access with less professional intervention. This latter form of follow-up is sometimes referred to as **patient triggered follow-up** or **supported self-managed follow-up**. As a consequence, routine follow-up appointments for all will no longer be the norm; instead, follow-up care will be tailored to individual needs. Patients' needs will be assessed and many patients will be allocated to supported self-managed follow-up.

The proportion of patients allocated to different types of follow-up will vary by cancer type. For example, early estimates suggested around 70% of breast, 40% of both colorectal and prostate, and 15% of lung cancer patients would be risk stratified to supported self-managed follow-up (NCSI, 2012) following an assessment by their clinical team that they are able to self-manage. They will be given information about self-management support; signs and symptoms to look out for, and who to contact if they notice any; what scheduled tests they may need (e.g. annual mammograms); and how they can contact professionals if they have any concerns. The type of information and support offered will vary across cancer types within hospitals and across hospitals.

Self-management by cancer survivors has been defined as 'awareness and active participation by the person in their recovery, recuperation, and rehabilitation, to minimize the consequences of treatment, promote survival, health and wellbeing' (DH, 2010b). Self-management, therefore, will involve people with cancer:

- Managing consequences of cancer and its treatment, including physical, psychological, social, practical problems that can arise, for example managing to live with cancer-related fatigue and fear of recurrence;
- Understanding how and when to seek support to access aftercare;
- Recognizing and reporting signs and symptoms of possible disease progression; and
- Making lifestyle changes to promote health, wellbeing and survival (see also Chapter 24).

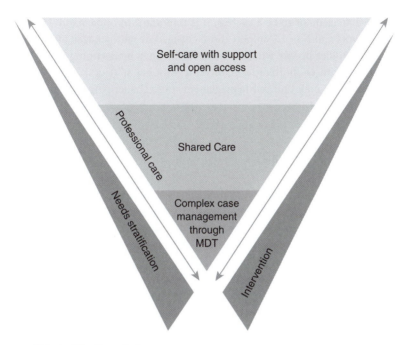

Figure 23.1 Risk stratification of aftercare

Source: DH (2010)

Lorig and Holman (2003) have suggested that in the context of chronic disease the goals of **self-management support** are to enable patients to perform three sets of tasks: (1) medical management of the illness (e.g. taking medication, adhering to a special diet); (2) carrying out normal roles and activities; and (3) managing the emotional impact of their illness. In the case of cancer, these goals may be different to other disease groups because the problems for cancer survivors may be more about managing the long-term effects of disease and treatment and health promotion, rather than management of active disease, although this may be the case for people with metastatic disease.

Cancer survivors in supported self-managed follow-up will be supported in a variety of ways and will receive regular **surveillance tests**, but the onus will be on them to initiate contact with healthcare professionals and others to support their self-management (DH, 2010b). For example, healthcare professionals will need to support cancer survivors to make lifestyle changes and recognize and act on signs and symptoms of possible disease recurrence. Responsibility for aftercare will shift from the clinic to the patient (May et al., 2009). Those in shared care will work together with healthcare professionals to support their aftercare and will also engage in self-management. Figure 23.1 depicts that those in complex case management will not self-manage; however, evidence suggests that even those with advanced cancer who are approaching end of life can find it very important to self-manage aspects of their condition (Hopkinson and Corner, 2006). This means that those in palliative care may gain great value in being supported to self-manage aspects of their cancer and its treatment that are interfering with their daily lives (see Chapter 28 for more about end-of-life care).

There is a risk that **inequalities** in access to healthcare and support may be exacerbated by changes in aftercare (National Cancer Equality Initiative, 2010). For example, for supported self-management to be a success, it is important to understand what is involved for cancer survivors and how to support those engaged in self-managed aftercare. Cancer is more common in older people whose general health may be declining and who are more likely to be living with co-morbidities (Office for National Statistics, 2006). Those who are older and living alone may find self-management more challenging than those living with others (Foster et al., 2014).

CANCER SURVIVORSHIP

Following primary treatment, cancer survivors can face a number of challenges that impact on everyday life (Hewitt et al., 2003) and these may continue for years (Foster et al., 2009). These may include fatigue, concerns about recurrence, dealing with others' expectations that life should be 'back to normal', having to adjust expectations about physical ability and concerns about leaving the hospital system (Jefford et al., 2008), as well as concerns about the impact on family and friends and unmet supportive care needs (Armes et al., 2009).

Cancer is largely regarded and treated as an acute condition and the realization for cancer survivors that cancer and its treatment can be chronic and have long-term consequences may be unexpected and generate new challenges. Expectations within an acute medical framework that people should return to 'normal life' can become the symbol of a valued self (Charmaz, 1983; see also Chapter 18). A person who is unable to 'return to normal' or takes longer than expected (Rasmussen and Elverdam, 2007), can experience suffering in the form of restricted lives, social isolation, being discredited and becoming a burden to others (Charmaz, 1983). Further consequences of chronic illness can include loss of productive function, financial crises and family strain.

For many, the problems of cancer survivorship are broader than the physical consequences and psychological distress of cancer diagnosis and treatment. Similar to people with other chronic illnesses, cancer survivors may need to rebuild and integrate their disrupted identities into new and changed identities (Bury, 1982). The emerging picture is of people living after a diagnosis of cancer, free from active disease, yet having similar health and wellbeing profiles to people living with a long-term condition (Elliott et al., 2011) with high usage of health services (Hewitt et al., 2003; Nord et al., 2005). Until recently, however, the experiences and needs of those who have completed primary cancer treatment are poorly understood and relatively neglected (DH, 2007a). Health professionals may be unaware of who is struggling with problems (Maher and Makin, 2007), and interventions to help relieve or prevent problems following primary treatment are just beginning to be explored.

In the current aftercare system, routine appointments present opportunities to discuss problems and concerns; however, transition from treatment to follow-up can leave patients feeling abandoned, vulnerable or without a 'safety net' (Ward et al., 1992) and many become 'lost' in the transition from patient to survivor (Hewitt et al., 2005). At this time, cancer survivors may take stock and realize that life may never completely return to normal (Allen et al., 2009). Not only may they grieve the loss of their previous life, but they also need to adapt to fundamental changes that have taken place in their lives. They can also experience significant barriers to accessing care and support, which may be exacerbated by vulnerability and low confidence following primary treatment (Foster and Fenlon, 2011).

THE CHANGING CONTEXT OF FOLLOW-UP CARE

For supported self-managed follow-up to work, cancer survivors will need to identify and self-manage problems caused by cancer and/or its treatment, take responsibility for seeking help and support, and articulate their preferences and needs for support in managing such problems, as well as identify and act on early signs and symptoms of possible disease progression. Healthcare professionals will also have to change established ways of working to accommodate this change in follow-up care.

Reflective activity

- How will you know who is feeling vulnerable at the end of treatment?
- What implications might a sense of vulnerability and low confidence have for cancer survivors?
- How will you know who is struggling to manage the consequences of their cancer and treatment when their primary treatment is over?
- How will you respond to requests for help to self-manage problems in daily life that are a consequence of cancer and its treatment?

Whilst many patients will be risk stratified to supported self-managed follow-up, what this self-managed follow-up looks like will vary considerably within and between hospitals. For example, patients with one type of cancer may participate in self-management workshops or programmes, whereas others may receive follow-up phone calls from their specialist nurse. Different models of cancer follow-up are being evaluated as part of the NCSI.

It is important to understand how this change in care will impact on patients, particularly what factors promote or inhibit contact with health/support services and the consequences for individual patients. This may have serious implications for the success of self-managed follow-up, and the work survivors feel able to undertake in order to identify problems and gain timely access to health/support services. There is a risk that with the new approach to cancer follow-up, those most in need of help will not receive it, which will have implications for their health and wellbeing, including early detection of recurrence and reporting of signs and symptoms. Inequalities exist in help-seeking behaviours and the use of health services (National Cancer Equality Initiative, 2010) and it is important that these are not exacerbated by the new approaches to follow-up (see Chapter 8 for more on diversity and equality).

Primary care will have an increasingly important role in cancer follow-up with the introduction of **cancer care reviews** within six months of diagnosis and the implementation of care plans to summarize treatment and identify the potential needs of cancer survivors (DH, 2007a). Watson et al. (2010) have reported general practitioner (GP) views on the content and usefulness of the cancer care review and GP and oncologist views around discharge of patients from secondary care follow-up and generation of survivorship care plans. Half of the GPs in the online survey reported undertaking the cancer care review opportunistically; 40% felt the cancer care review was useful for the doctor; and 60% felt it was useful for the patient. At discharge from follow-up, less than half of the oncologists responding indicated that they provide information on potential late effects or symptoms of recurrence. GPs indicated that information on these areas was important, but that the information they receive is often inadequate.

SELF-MANAGEMENT OF CONSEQUENCES OF CANCER AND ITS TREATMENT

It has long been recognized that there is considerable variation in how people respond to objectively similar stressful life events, such as a diagnosis and treatment for cancer (Bandura, 1977b; Lazarus and Folkman, 1984). Lent's (2007) model of **restorative emotional wellbeing** suggests that two key facets for restoration of emotional wellbeing are (1) the individual's characteristics, and (2) the environmental supports and resources available to them. Drawing on Bandura's (1986) concept of **self-efficacy**, Lent (2007) suggests that the ability of the individual to cope with their perceived problems depends on personality and affective dispositions, and that people's emotional wellbeing will depend on their dispositions, as well as their environmental supports and resources. The model recognizes that through their different dispositions, supports, resources and coping efficacy, people will differ in their level of restoration of emotional wellbeing.

Foster and Fenlon (2011) have developed a conceptual framework of recovery of health and wellbeing following cancer treatment – informed by Lent's model (2007) and their own research – which proposes psychosocial, physical and emotional factors, as well as the availability of supportive resources, have an impact on recovery of health and wellbeing. This framework is directly shaped by the experiences and priorities of patients with cancer and survivors to inform how health professionals and others can support recovery and self-management by recognizing the importance of **confidence** in the management of problems following primary treatment. Many people want more help in a variety of forms to manage the impact of cancer on their lives, but the cancer diagnosis and treatment leaves them vulnerable and lacking in confidence (Foster and Fenlon, 2011). We know from chronic illness research (e.g. Bury, 1982; Charmaz, 1983) that many cancer survivors are likely to need to rebuild their lives and identity, but diminished confidence may leave them ill-equipped to do this. Foster and Fenlon (2011) suggest that rebuilding confidence is an important part of recovery and, if patients can be supported as they rebuild their confidence following primary cancer treatment, they will be in a better position to self-manage problems and access self-management support as required. This in turn will influence recovery of health and wellbeing following cancer treatment and ultimately whether individuals 'live well' after treatment. The fundamental principle informing the conceptual framework is that confidence to manage problems arising from cancer and its treatment is key, and that some people want and need support to help them become more confident to self-manage problems that impact on everyday life (Corner et al., 2007; Foster et al., 2010).

The conceptual framework makes two assumptions. One is that cancer diagnosis and treatment disrupt an individual's subjective sense of health and wellbeing, and the other is that this is restored over a period of time (although not necessarily to the same/similar level as pre-diagnosis). The linear nature of the model reflects the passage of time. For many people, however, restoration of health and wellbeing is likely to be accompanied by a life free from cancer, whereas others may experience long-lasting problems as a consequence of cancer and its treatment or may face cancer recurrence. The phase of **problem resolution** and restoration of health and wellbeing may therefore be protracted or repeated.

Shippee et al. (2012) have developed a model of **cumulative patient complexity** identifying two areas where complexity can disrupt effective care and outcomes: (1) the workload placed upon the patient (e.g. medical and non-medical demands placed on patients in supported self-managed follow-up); and (2) the patient's capacity to do this work (e.g. being able to manage the consequences of cancer/treatment once primary treatment is over, and accessing care and support as required). Managing aftercare following primary cancer treatment is complex and patients will need to be supported to manage this complexity and enhance their capacity to take on the work involved in aftercare. If they are not adequately supported, then evidence suggests that they will be less likely to self-manage and may have inappropriate access to health services (Shippee et al., 2012). Failing to support individuals living with physical, psychosocial and practical problems associated with cancer and its treatment is likely to prevent survivors from returning to fulfilling lives (Corner, 2008).

WHAT DOES SELF-MANAGEMENT SUPPORT LOOK LIKE?

People can be unprepared for the impact that cancer and its treatment can have on their lives, and the resultant vulnerability and lost confidence can act as barriers to seeking help (Jefford et al., 2008; Hewitt et al., 2005; Foster and Fenlon, 2011). People generally manage problems associated with cancer and its treatment as part of their daily lives. Patients have highlighted the need for support in managing the impact of cancer on everyday life (Corner et al., 2007) and many want an active role in tackling them (Brennan, 2004; Hopkinson and Corner, 2006), but little is known about how people affected by cancer manage to live with persistent problems once primary treatment is complete, and how they can be supported to do this. With rising numbers of survivors, the need to understand problems faced following treatment, how they are resolved, and how to support people to manage them are becoming increasingly important for cancer survivors, service planners and health policymakers.

Self-efficacy – a component of Bandura's **Social Cognitive Theory** (Bandura, 1986) – refers to the confidence one has to achieve particular goals in living with or managing problems associated with illness. Low self-efficacy is associated with poorer quality of life and more symptoms experienced, but importantly self-efficacy can be enhanced by intervention (Lorig et al., 2001; Kennedy et al., 2007).

Karnilowicz (2011) argues that chronic illness identity work is mediated through psychological ownership of illness, and that the experience of owning an illness is fixed in the idea of **control**. The greater the level of control, the more likely control is experienced psychologically as part of self, and there is a close and ongoing interaction between an individual's psychological state and his or her social environment (Shaw, 1999). Regan-Smith et al., (2006) suggest that self-care behaviours are integral in re-establishing ownership, and people with high levels of self-efficacy are more likely to engage in self-care behaviours. High self-efficacy is associated with a greater effort and persistence to cope with obstacles (Bandura, 1977b) and enhanced wellbeing (Lev et al., 2001). Where there is a high degree of self-efficacy in people affected by cancer, a number of improvements in healthcare outcomes result, including increased **self-care behaviours** and decreased physical and psychological symptoms (Egbert and Parrott, 2001;

Luszczynska et al., 2007). The terms self-care and self-management are often used interchange-ably. Self-care is generally regarded as a broader term encompassing all actions that individuals take to care for themselves to maintain health and wellbeing, whereas self-management is more focused on the ability to manage day-to-day problems that result from long-term and chronic health conditions (Coulter and Ellins, 2006).

Managing everyday problems brought about by cancer and its treatment is likely to be enhanced by a collaborative partnership between patients and healthcare providers, both of whom are considered to be experts of the condition, albeit from different perspectives (Von Korff et al., 1997). A collaborative approach that delineates how the healthcare system and healthcare professionals can support patients in their self-management has been referred to as self-management support. The Health Foundation (www.health.org.uk/areas-of-work/top-ics/self-management-support/) describes self-management support as those things that can be performed by health services to aid and encourage people living with long-term conditions to improve or maintain their own health and wellbeing. It can be viewed in two ways: (1) as a portfolio of techniques and tools; and (2) as a fundamental transformation of the patient–car-egiver relationship into a collaborative partnership. This has been described as a **whole-sys-tem approach**. It involves far more than providing a one-off expert patient course, although these can be useful. Clinical services, systems, processes and environments must all convey to patients the message: 'You have a part to play. We are partners. We respect your role and will support you to be part of the team' (Grazin, 2007: 28–29). Thus, the principle of supporting self-management through partnership working reverses the focus on telling patients what they 'should do', to one where the patient is supported in addressing their own agenda.

Self-management programmes, such as the Expert Patient Programme, established to provide people with a generic set of skills to self-manage successfully, have been shown to improve self-efficacy and health status (Kennedy et al., 2007). The central tenet of many such programmes is that patients can be educated to self-manage their condition (Lorig, 2002), thus increasing their self-efficacy to manage their own illness, and consequently improve their quality of life and reduce health service utilization. Such programmes have, however, come under some criticism for drawing on sociological research into the everyday realities of living with chronic conditions and 'transforming what patients do into what patients should do' (Bury, 2010).

Kralik et al. (2004) have suggested that although 'self-management' is key to the identity work required by people with long-term conditions, they highlight that 'self-management' is conceptualized quite differently by health professionals and people with long-term health con-ditions. Health professionals identify self-management as structured education, but those with long-term health conditions identify self-management as a process initiated to bring about order in their lives (Kralik et al., 2004). Creating the conditions to enable people to self-manage this transition and restore order in their disrupted lives will be necessary, rather than simply turning patient actions into directives for others to follow. Programmes for self-management may be part of a culture shift towards creating these conditions, but there also needs to be a more fundamental shift in the way that healthcare is delivered.

Self-management support is broader than that provided by health services, and also includes support from other sources such as other cancer survivors, family and social networks, third sector organizations, the workplace, the community, online resources and so on. These may or not be cancer-specific resources, but they can provide great benefit to those building confidence and managing consequences of cancer and its treatment in their everyday lives.

Social support is associated with higher self-efficacy to self-manage problems associated with cancer and its treatment (Foster et al., 2014) and cancer survivors may be more inclined to turn to alternative sources of support, rather than healthcare professionals, once their treatment is over. A major source of support for many is that provided by family caregivers (see also Chapter 20). A longitudinal Australian study of patients and their partners shows that feelings of being on an emotional rollercoaster persist beyond the end of treatment and reactions include shock, uncertainty and distress (Girgis and Lambert, 2009). In some contexts, partners and other caregivers have been reported to experience emotional reactions more intensely than patients (Lambert et al., 2012). High rates of distress in caregivers are of concern because evidence suggests patients and partners can exacerbate each other's distress (Lambert et al., 2012). Moreover, distress will adversely affect the caregivers' ability to support patients, which in turn will impact on patients' recovery (see also Chapter 18). A better understanding of caregivers' cancer experiences is needed to inform the design of effective healthcare services and the development of resources for patients and caregivers.

Reflective activity

Are you aware of organizations or groups that may be of value to cancer survivors in your area?

HOW CAN SELF-MANAGEMENT BE SUPPORTED?

Drawing from evidence in the chronic illness literature, Fenlon and Foster (2009) have made seven recommendations to the NCSI to support self-management. These are currently being tested through the NCSI test communities:

1. *Survivorship care plans:* People who have come to the end of active treatment or are newly diagnosed with recurrent disease should have one-to-one assessment by a healthcare professional and a survivorship care plan drawn up, in conjunction with goals as expressed by the cancer survivor.
2. *Topic-specific programmes of care:* Cancer survivors have many, varied needs and they have expressed the need for programmes of care to be more targeted towards their specific needs. A variety of programmes of care should be made available covering specific topics, such as management of lymphoedema; management of chronic pain; fatigue management; healthy eating programmes; carers' programmes; cognitive–behavioural therapy and skills for communicating with health professionals. There is some evidence that individual topic-specific programmes are effective in cancer survivors.
3. *Programmes for socially disadvantaged groups:* There is evidence that some groups are disadvantaged when delivering care in programmes. Where programmes have been developed to address the specific needs of minority ethnic and socially disadvantaged groups, there is evidence that these have been welcomed and effective use made of them. There is the potential to have greater benefit amongst these groups when programmes are appropriately targeted.

24 LIFESTYLE CHANGE AND HEALTH PROMOTION IN CANCER SURVIVORSHIP

LEE HULBERT-WILLIAMS

Chapter outline

- The evidence for lifestyle risk factors in occurrence and recurrence
- Simple psychological variables associated with behaviour change
- Complex psychological models of behaviour change
- Intervention approaches

INTRODUCTION

Health professionals working in cancer care often wish to encourage clients to change certain **behaviours** in order to mitigate the risk of **recurrence** or to increase the likelihood of good treatment outcomes. What evidence is there that adopting a healthier **diet**, taking more **exercise**, giving up **smoking**, or reducing **alcohol** intake result in better health outcomes for cancer survivors? What is known about the psychological processes associated with these sorts of health behaviours? How might a health professional intervene in a time-limited fashion to encourage healthier lifestyle choices? This chapter will begin to answer these questions and to provide concrete tools for use in clinical practice.

To begin, it is worth noting that health professionals know that adopting a healthier lifestyle reduces the risk for ill health, but doesn't *guarantee* health. Patients too should be given this information in a spirit of informed consent.

RISK FACTORS

A good deal is now known about **health behaviours** that increase and decrease risk for incidence of cancer (see also Chapter 2). Tabloid newspapers make a handsome living out of publishing the findings of studies on these sorts of **risk factors** (though with dubious veracity). At the point of writing, however, rather less is known about the extent to which similar behaviours might affect the risk of **survival** or **recurrence**. Such knowledge is of direct clinical relevance: if a given behaviour doubles the risk of recurrence for a specific cancer type, patients will want to know, and what's more, many will want help in changing that behaviour. There follows a brief summary of the evidence as it currently stands on four major risk factors and their relationship to survival and recurrence.

Smoking

In 1950, Doll and Hill published retrospective **epidemiological** evidence showing an association between carcinoma of the lung and a history of smoking (Doll and Hill, 1950). This led directly to the establishment of the *British Doctor's Study*, a prospective epidemiological survey that, over the course of fifty years, followed a sample of several thousand British doctors, asking about smoking habits, and providing further evidence of a link (Doll, 2004). Over the years, similar (less ambitious) epidemiological studies have shown that smoking is also a risk factor for a number of other diseases, including cancer of the mouth, larynx, pancreas and urinary tract (Sasco et al., 2004). It is now uncontroversial that smoking is a risk factor for cancer at a number of sites. Only recently have methodologically sophisticated attempts been made to examine the effects of smoking on survival and recurrence, however, and the results are much as one might expect. For example, the prospective study of Warren et al. (2012), reporting on 5185 patients, found smoking at the time of diagnosis to be associated with increased mortality in lung, head/neck, prostate and leukaemia in men and breast, ovary, uterus and melanoma in women. Overall, current smokers were 1.38 times more likely to die (this is called a **hazard ratio**) than patients who had never smoked, and that this occurred 1.17 times faster than those who had recently quit. A number of other studies have associated smoking with decreased survival for other sites, including head and neck, kidney, prostate, colorectal, breast, vulvar, leukaemia and malignant melanoma (see Tammemagi et al. (2004) for a very brief review). There is also tentative evidence that continuing to smoke may increase the likelihood of recurrence for some cancers, for example bladder cancer (Chen et al., 2007).

Alcohol

Evidence on the link between alcohol consumption and cancer incidence follows a similar pattern, with a large number of well-designed epidemiological studies producing consistent results (International Agency for Research on Cancer Working Group on the Evaluation of Carcinogenic Risk to Humans, 2009). The idea that one drink a day is healthy is probably a myth, at least so far as cancer incidence is concerned (Tramacere et al., 2010). Alcohol consumption has been shown to increase the risk for cancer of the breast (Seitz et al., 2012), liver (Stickel et al., 2002), and bowel (Fedirko et al., 2011) with a straightforward dose response. A meta-analysis published in 2012, combining the results of 49 studies, found that alcohol consumption and smoking might have a **synergistic effect**, increasing the risk of cancer even further (Turati et al., 2012).

Post-diagnosis, there may be acute clinical reasons for recommending abstinence, for example in patients with reduced liver function, but the evidence for effects on mortality and recurrence is less well developed. For cancer sites other than the breast, there is almost no evidence. A non-systematic review of breast cancer studies published in 2002 (Rock and Demark-Wahnefried) reported a mixed evidence base, with a few studies suggesting alcohol may increase risk of recurrence, but most failing to find such a link. However, since then a small number of further studies have been published that do suggest a link between alcohol consumption and recurrence of breast cancer. For instance, Kwan and colleagues (2010) recruited 1897 patients on average two years after diagnosis, and assessed their alcohol intake. An intake greater than 6 g per day (approximately one-quarter the current UK safe drinking limit for women) was found to be associated with an increased risk for both recurrence (hazard ratio = 1.35) and mortality (hazard ratio = 1.51), although both of these findings were only just statistically significant. At present, there appears to be insufficient evidence to answer the question conclusively.

Diet and exercise

There is a great deal of published evidence on the links that diet, exercise and **body mass** may have with cancer incidence. The question is confused by the nature of the variables. Healthy diets, high in vegetables, have been investigated, but is it the nature of the food or the resultant reduction in body mass that leads to the beneficial effect? **Obesity** is consistently linked with increased risk of cancer. A large recent systematic review (Ma et al., 2013) meta-analyzed 54 prospective epidemiological studies on body mass and cancer incidence, finding that participants classified as obese using body mass index (BMI) carried an increased risk (hazard ratio = 1.33) of colorectal cancer. Similarly, Harvie et al. (2003) published a systematic review showing that central obesity (assessed using waist–hip ratio) may increase the risk for breast cancer in post-menopausal, but not premenopausal women. Similar findings have been reported for thyroid, renal, endometrial, oesophageal, pancreatic and other cancer sites (Renehanet al., 2008). Beside overall body mass, a number of studies have linked dietary composition to cancer risk (Aune et al., 2013; Tantamango-Bartley et al., 2013) and there is some evidence that regular physical exercise may reduce risk for some cancer types, independent of body mass status (e.g. Behrens and Leitzmann, 2013).

The effects of diet and exercise on recurrence and mortality are fairly well established too. Rock and Demark-Wahnefried (2002) published a review of 26 studies on the association between body mass before or at the time of diagnosis and recurrence or survival from breast cancer. Seventeen of the included studies reported that higher BMI or body weight was significantly associated with recurrence, poorer survival or both, seven found no association and two found a significant inverse association. A subsequent, broader review provided evidence of a deleterious impact of higher BMI on survival for breast, prostate and colorectal sites (Parekh et al., 2012). The World Cancer Research Fund and the American Institute for Cancer Research (2007) conclude that whilst there is considerable evidence linking low-fat and other specific diets to better outcomes for survivors, it is currently impossible to say whether the effects are in fact due to the participants having lost weight, rather than to the specific macronutrient make-up of the diets tested. It is also worth noting that exercise improves quality of life for survivors and patients (McNeely et al., 2006).

The quality of the evidence

Before proceeding to ask how healthcare professionals might help patients to change these lifestyle factors to better their own outcomes, a cautionary note is warranted. Nearly all of the evidence in relation to lifestyle factors and recurrence or mortality is epidemiological in nature. Although many of the studies have been excellently designed, one cannot confidently conclude that increasing exercise, changing diet or losing weight at the point of diagnosis will have salutary effects without intervention studies. To date, most intervention trials have reported a diverse set of other outcomes, including self-reported functioning and symptoms, psychological wellbeing and overall health-related quality of life (Knols et al., 2005), but not usually recurrence, which requires longer-term follow-up. There is some evidence that diet and exercise interventions improve biomarkers of recurrence, such as **oxidative stress** (Pekmezi and Demark-Wahnefried, 2011). More work needs to be done. Much of the evidence of post-diagnosis lifestyle risk factors is beset by a number of methodological difficulties, not least the timing of assessments of lifestyle factors relative to diagnosis and treatment. For a fuller discussion, see Land (2012).

PSYCHOLOGICAL PHENOMENA ASSOCIATED WITH HEALTH BEHAVIOURS

Demographic differences and personality

The environments in which people live (and have lived) affect their habits and lifestyles. The effects are legion. For example, socio-economic status affects a range of health behaviours. Across the industrialized world, it is often reported that people with lower socio-economic status tend to drink more (Van Oers et al., 1999), smoke more (Laaksonen et al., 2005) and exercise less (Ford et al., 1991). These differences are likely to account partially for the socio-economic differences in morbidity and mortality often reported (e.g. Mackenbach et al., 1997). To take another example, men may engage in heavy drinking (de Visser and Smith, 2007) and avoid consulting health professionals (Marcell et al., 2007) because these behaviours fit societal preconceptions about masculine identity. In trying to explain and alter such behaviours, psychologists are not content simply to accept a genetic-deterministic model where being male results necessarily in heavy drinking. It would be silly to suggest that the Y chromosome has a 'heavy drinking' gene on it. The effect of sex is surely being brought to bear on drinking behaviour via some intervening and more general behavioural phenomena.

The huge number of influences impinging upon the individual throughout childhood and adulthood from all conceivable sources gives rise to considerable individual differences. To aid research and practice, psychologists group and label naturally co-occurring behaviours and in doing so produce summary constructs, often called **traits**. The most commonly used nomenclature is the **'big five'** (Costa and McCrae, 1988), which attempts to summarize variation between people's personalities according to the following constructs: **neuroticism**, **extraversion**, **openness** to experience, **agreeableness** and **conscientiousness**. The 'big five' has received empirical support over the years, and there is some evidence that these aspects of personality are related to observed differences in health behaviours. Harakeh et al. (2006) conducted a cross-sectional survey of 832 Dutch adolescents and found that the 'big five' personality constructs accounted for 4.3% of the variance in smoking behaviour. Personality may also help to measure motivational differences that result in similar observable behaviour patterns, as illustrated by Cooper and colleagues' (2000) study in which extraverts tended to use alcohol to increase positive moods, whilst those high in neuroticism used alcohol as an anaesthetic for negative moods. Whilst it is interesting to know how personality constructs might be related to specific behaviours like drinking, there has not really been any successful behaviour change techniques developed to take advantage of this knowledge.

Locus of control

The 'big five' is not the only way to conceptualize individual psychological differences. In 1966, Rotter developed the concept of **locus of control** beliefs. His analysis suggested that people tend either to consider themselves responsible for and capable of influencing outcomes, or else believe that external factors – even happenstance – are most influential in determining what happens in their lives. He named these orientations *internal* and *external*. Wallston and colleagues (1978) later developed the Multidimensional Health Locus of Control (MHLC) scale to measure people's beliefs about their control over their own health, and in doing so discovered three types of locus of control orientation, adding a *powerful others* dimension to the two orientations identified in Rotter's work. Those with a *powerful others* orientation believe that the power to affect their health lies with medical professionals, and to some extent one's family.

In cross-sectional studies, locus of control measures, including MHLC, are reliably associated with both health behaviours and health outcomes, but the effect sizes are generally very small. For example, Norman et al. (1997) recruited a sample of 13,000 participants in Wales and found health locus of control dimensions predicted only 0.6% of the variance in exercise behaviours. Some fourteen years after the development of the concept of health locus of control, Wallston (1992) reviewed a number of such studies and found that locus of control measures regularly account for less than 6% of the variance in health behaviours. It is understandable therefore that few sustained attempts have been made to develop interventions that take advantage of the construct of health locus of control.

Self-efficacy

Another psychological construct used to predict health behaviour is that of **self-efficacy**. Introduced by the social psychologist Albert Bandura (1977a), self-efficacy is defined as the sum of one's beliefs about one's own capabilities in managing a specific prospective situation. For instance, someone who thinks, 'I'll never be able to give up smoking because I'm just not strong enough,' would be considered to have low self-efficacy in regard of smoking. Across a number of health behaviours, self-efficacy has been found to be predictive of the degree of effort people put into planning and carrying out health-enhancing behaviours, like losing weight or giving up smoking (see Schwarzer and Fuchs (1996) for a review). Whilst certain interventions, including **Cognitive–Behavioural Therapy**, have been shown to increase self-efficacy, to date there has been no sustained effort to develop a health promotion intervention based on self-efficacy theory.

Risk perception and unrealistic optimism

In 1982, Weinstein coined the term **unrealistic optimism** to describe his finding that most participants considered themselves to be at a much lower risk of experiencing a number of health- and safety-related problems than their peers. Unrealistic optimism tends to occur when the person has no direct experience of the risk, a belief that one's own actions can affect the risk and the belief that if the problem has not developed to date, then it is unlikely to do so in future

(Weinstein, 1987). Whilst unrealistic optimism has not led to the development of any intervention strategies in and of itself, it has become part of **Health Beliefs Model**, discussed in the next section.

Social influences

Our social environments affect our behaviours profoundly, and often without our realizing it. Peer groups, be they friends, family or co-workers, bombard us with cues as to what is **normative** and what is acceptable. The influence of **social norms** on a number of health behaviours has been well documented. To take an example, alcohol consumption in college students has been especially closely studied. College students in the UK, Canada and the USA amongst others, tend to overestimate the quantity and frequency of alcohol consumption amongst their peers, although of course individual students vary in their estimations (e.g. Perkins, 2007). An individual's perceptions of their peers' drinking habits have frequently been shown to be highly predictive of personal drinking habits, even more so than other likely predictors such as religious affiliation (see Borsari and Carey (2001) for a review).

The influences of peer groups are by no means restricted to student populations, or to drinking behaviour. Choi and colleagues (2003) found that a perception that one's peers approved of smoking was predictive of subsequent initiation of regular smoking. In one of the most sophisticated analyses to date, Christakis and Fowler (2007) analyzed data on 12,607 participants recruited into the *Framingham Heart Study*. Since many of the participants are friends, siblings or parents of other participants in the study, the researchers were able to assess patterns of influence and to watch obesity 'spread' through **social networks**. They concluded, for example, that a participant would have a 57% increased risk of becoming obese if he or she had a friend who had become obese in a given time interval.

Interventions based on these findings have been trialled, wherein participants are presented with accurate data on social norms. For instance, presented with data showing that their peer group drink less than the participant, participants tend to reduce their own drinking thereafter (e.g. Haines and Spear, 1996; see Perkins (2007) for a brief review).

PSYCHOLOGICAL THEORIES OF HEALTH BEHAVIOURS

A number of researchers have combined several **cognitive** constructs into **process models** that attempt to predict health-related behaviours, and to inform intervention design. The models generally adopt a boxes-and-arrows approach to describe the putative causal links between phenomena. The theorists who build these models recognize that there are many thousands of factors that might influence whether or not a person performs a certain behaviour or adopts a particular health-related habit. In an attempt to explain behaviours, and to identify places in this interlinked network of causes to focus intervention work, these factors are separated into **distal** ones (e.g. whether or not you were given sweets as a child) and **proximal** ones (e.g. whether you intend to eat sweets in the next hour). The assumption is that distal factors will have their effect *through* proximal ones (i.e. whether you were given sweets as a child is only relevant because it might influence your intentions in the present moment, but it doesn't *directly* affect behaviour). This is called a **mediated model**. This section will briefly review a number of such models, and talk about the key proximal factors they postulate as important to the adoption of healthy lifestyles.

The Health Belief Model

The **Health Belief Model** (HBM) was one of the earliest attempts to explain and predict health-related behaviour change, devised in the 1970s (Rosenstock, 1974) and further developed in the 1980s (Becker and Rosenstock, 1984). The model postulates six proximal factors (or variables) through which things like age, socio-economic status, schooling and gender have their influence. These are summarized in Figure 24.1 with example cognitions.

Harrison et al. (1992) conducted a meta-analysis of 51 empirical studies to test the predictive power of the HBM. The HBM was generally supported, but overall, the effect sizes were small, indicating that the HBM accounted for only a small proportion of the variance in the outcome measures and was thus a mediocre predictor.

Theory of Planned Behaviour

By contrast, the **Theory of Planned Behaviour** (TPB) (Ajzen, 1985) and its predecessor, the **Theory of Reasoned Action** (Fishbein and Ajzen, 1975), are based on social learning theory. They combine a number of psychological constructs to attempt to explain people's engagement and disengagement in health behaviours. The model centres on three constructs, with some subcomponents, as shown in Figure 24.2.

Over a number of reviews, the TPB has been shown to explain between 26–35% of the variance in health behaviours (Sutton, 2004). Given the measurement error involved in such studies, such results are encouraging. No sustained efforts have been made to develop specific intervention types based on the TPB, although one might reasonably hypothesize that the three factors (attitude, subjective norm and perceived behavioural control) could be at the core of useful interventions.

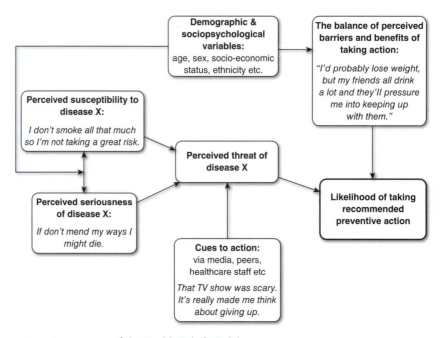

Figure 24.1   An overview of the Health Belief Model

Source: Adapted from Rosenstock (1974) and Becker and Rosenstock (1984)

Transtheoretical Model

Psychology has more than its fair share of stage theories, which claim that a series of linked behavioural phenomena occur in discrete stages, through which one moves in a more or less linear manner. In 1984, Prochaska and di Clemente published such a model for health promotion, describing five main stages, as summarized in Figure 24.3.

The **Transtheoretical Model** (or **Stages of Change Model**) suggests that any health promotion intervention ought to be tailored according to the stage the client is currently in. Many trials have been published , testing the effectiveness of these interventions. Several systematic reviews of these trials have concluded that there is very little evidence that interventions based on the Stages of Change Model are any more effective either than alternative interventions or placebo (e.g. Bridle et al., 2005; Tuah et al., 2012).

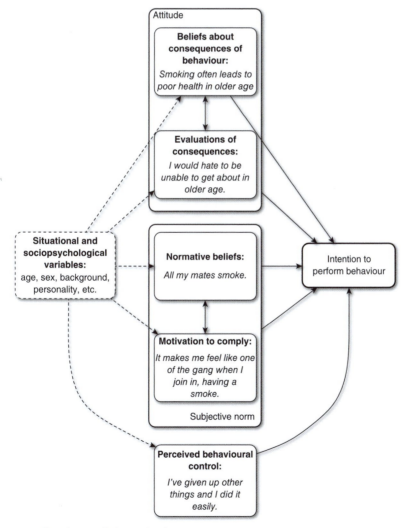

Figure 24.2   The Theory of Planned Behaviour

Source: Adapted from Ajzen (1991)

Health Action Process Approach

The **Health Action Process Approach** (HAPA) combines static and stage elements, and might be seen as a direct descendant of the theory of planned behaviour (Schwarzer, 1992; Schwarzer and Luszczynska, 2008). It separates, for instance, a **motivation** phase wherein a person is considering whether to act, from a **volition** phase, where the person plans when to act and makes

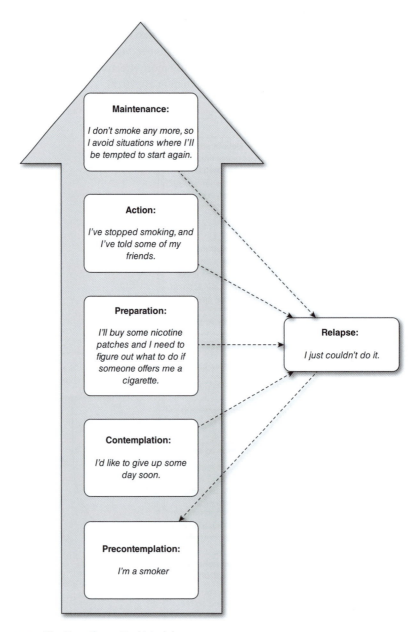

Figure 24.3   The Transtheoretical Model

Source: Adapted from Prochaska and di Clemente (1984)

plans for action. The HAPA suggests that action planning is an important step, without which no changes in health behaviour are likely to succeed. Whilst the HAPA represents a number of improvements over previous models, it is still in its infancy. Renner et al. (2007) reported that the HAPA was poor at predicting the health behaviours of younger people.

Mindfulness and acceptance-based approaches

One of the most talked about problems in relation to all the foregoing models of health behaviour is the so-called **intention-behaviour gap**. This phrase describes an everyday phenomenon – you say you are on a strict diet but you eat more than you say you will. Some theorists have claimed that the poor ability to account for and deal with impulsivity or 'urges' might be the main problem with these health psychology models (see Hofmann et al. (2008) for an extensive review). **Mindfulness-based approaches** first made an impact in medicine with Kabat-Zinn's (1990) Mindfulness-Based Stress Reduction, developed in the 1970s. The programme is loosely based on Eastern philosophical insights about the impermanence of psychological states and how the extent to which a state is pleasant or unpleasant is malleable according to the perceiver. Other programmes have also been developed along these lines, taking traditional mediation practices into the clinic.

Acceptance and Commitment Therapy (ACT) adopts similar techniques, but goes a step further. ACT draws on **Relational Frame Theory** (RFT), which is a theory of how humans learn and use language (Hayes et al., 2001). RFT theorists have identified a number of interesting phenomena with direct clinical relevance. For instance, humans can learn to perform certain complex behaviours more rapidly than other species because of the ability to use language to establish and communicate rules (Hayes, 1989); however, these rules can make us inflexible. Humans develop such rules for themselves. The thought, 'When I feel like this I have to have a cigarette', can function as a rule and lead to **inflexibility**, regardless of how strong or weak the physiological urge for nicotine is in the present moment. ACT deliberately establishes rule-based learning for personal values and other things that might be associated with desirable behaviour, and helps clients to disengage from verbal rules that are keeping them stuck (see Chapter 22 for more information about mindfulness and ACT).

PSYCHOLOGICAL INTERVENTIONS FOR HEALTH BEHAVIOURS

This section will summarize some **psycho-educational** and **psychotherapeutic** approaches that can be incorporated into clinical practice, based on the earlier theoretical perspectives. The more complex interventions that have been developed from the Transtheoretical Model will not be reviewed, given the poor evidence of efficacy (see earlier).

Information giving

The simplest health promotion intervention to incorporate into routine clinical practice is simply giving information about the risks associated with certain lifestyle factors, and the benefits of altering them. For example, given that people are generally inclined to fit in with social norms, they will attempt to smoke or drink less if they believe that they currently engage in those behaviours more than their peers (e.g. Choi et al., 2003). The point here is that personal perception drives behaviour. One may have some success in reducing a person's drinking, for example, by sharing data showing that they drink more than is average for their peer group (Perkins, 2007). It can readily be seen that providing information of this sort might affect risk perceptions and unrealistic optimism.

Motivational Interviewing

Motivational Interviewing (Miller and Rollnick, 2002) is an approach for encouraging a person to contemplate the possibility of change. It is best thought of as a technique to engage a client at the **precontemplation** stage (to borrow terminology from the Transtheoretical Model). In brief, the client is encouraged to consider thoughts and beliefs both for and against the potential behaviour change. Beforehand, presumably, the balance is for the status quo, or else the client would already have made the change. The intention, therefore, is to encourage the client to explore quite fully both sides of the argument. Thoughts and beliefs such as, 'I enjoy a drink with my friends', 'I know I should give up', 'I don't really drink in moderation', and so on, can be elicited and perhaps written down. The idea is to bring the client's existing thoughts and beliefs into sharp relief and so engender **cognitive dissonance**, which is an unpleasant state of being conscious of holding conflicting beliefs (Festinger, 1957). The client should not be coerced, but rather the therapist expresses **empathy** for the client's position. A number of studies have now been conducted, comparing Motivational Interviewing to **treatment as usual** for substance abuse, smoking and other health behaviours (e.g. Carroll et al., 2001; Lai et al., 2010) with generally positive results. Motivational Interviewing is relatively simple to incorporate into routine clinical evaluations run by physicians or nurses (Lai et al., 2010).

Planning

The HAPA describes planning as a crucial step in health behaviour change (Schwarzer, 1992; Schwarzer and Luszczynska, 2008). In that model, the planning phase is usually described as 'post-intentional planning', to highlight the idea that for a person to be ready for planning they must already have established a clear intention to change a given health behaviour. Planning is as simple as setting out a number of discrete steps necessary to achieve a given goal. For example, in adopting a healthier lifestyle, one might make the following action plan: (1) find a number of healthy, tasty recipes; (2) develop a weekly meal plan; (3) write out a shopping list for the ingredients in those recipes; and (4) sign up for online shopping so as to avoid the tempting offers present in physical supermarkets. Coping plans can also be developed, where the person is encouraged to envisage barriers that might arise to prevent the adoption of the healthy behaviour, and to think of things that might be done to overcome that barrier.

Planning is simple and there is some good evidence that without planning, good intentions do not turn into good behaviours (e.g. Scholz et al., 2008). It is a generally accepted principle that the client should take an active role in the planning; however, for some clients, this can be difficult because they focus on previous attempts and on problems that have arisen in trying to achieve a goal. This is dealt with next.

Problem solving

Good intentions often conflict with the circumstances of life. A person with a strong desire to lose weight is unlikely to succeed if he has never learned to cook and is thus reliant on fast food. A smoker who believes she needs cigarettes to help with social anxiety is unlikely to quit unless another coping technique is found. A number of approaches have been developed to help people overcome these sorts of problems.

Egan (2009) has developed a three-stage model for **counselling** and other helping professionals. First, the helper supports and encourages the client to explore and clarify the problem. Second, the helper encourages the client to set his or her own goals. These should be concrete and behaviourally defined ('I will smoke no more than …'). Third, the helper facilitates action by encouraging the client to develop clear plans and strategies through which the goals can be achieved. Egan recognizes that clients will differ in their need for these stages. Some will skip some stages. Some will move through all three in one session. Others will need time to reflect in between. In fairness to Egan, it should also be made clear that he does not propose that these stages are strictly linear, where the client moves from one to the other; rather they are a conceptual framework for the helper.

A similar approach, developed by De Shazer and Berg (1997), is known as **brief solution-focused therapy** (BSFT). Counsellors using BSFT assume that a person's circumstances are complex enough that a great deal of time might be needed in order for a therapist or counsellor to understand enough to generate valid solutions. The model also presupposes that the client is stuck in habits of thinking, and that these habits are preventing the client from coming up with solutions. BSFT recommends the use of a discrete number of well-described techniques to help the client to describe what life would look like after a solution to the problem has been found. Similar techniques are used to help the client identify strengths and resources that he or she might use.

Mrs B

Mrs B expresses a desire to quit smoking. After multiple failed attempts, her self-efficacy is low, and she has very little hope that she can find a solution. During a follow-up consultation, her nurse asks what techniques she's tried in the past. She's had some success with nicotine patches and other pharmaceuticals, and has even resorted to acupuncture, but each of these techniques fails when she tries to venture into a social situation. Mrs B explains that she first started smoking to calm her nerves and that the main thing that makes her nervous is being with a group of people.

Nurse: Are you always nervous in social situations?

Mrs B: No. Usually. Not always. For instance, it's really bad when …

Nurse: [interupts] Sorry, but can you give me an example or two of when it's better?

Mrs B: Uh … well, it's OK if it's people I know. If there's no strangers there. Or if I'm with my sister. I know it sounds ridiculous but she's always pushed me into things all my life and I still feel a bit safer having my big sister around! Though there's only two years between us!

Nurse: Are there any other times when you don't feel such an urge to smoke?

(Continued)

CASE EXAMPLE

(Continued)

Mrs B: I don't think about it as much if no one else is smoking.

Nurse: Anything else?

Mrs B: I don't think so.

Nurse: Do you think you could maybe use any of those things to help you quit? For example, what would your sister say if you asked her to be your quit-smoking buddy for a few weeks until you've got used to it?

Mrs B: I don't know. She'd probably want to help.

Nurse: And what about social situations where no one else is smoking?

Mrs B: Well, I've joined a book club and no one smokes there. It's not allowed in the bookshop where we meet. And I'm really enjoying that. I could go out there more.

Here, the nurse is using 'exception questions' to help the client think outside of her current mental habits. In a brief interview, the client has begun to formulate plans, including how to draw upon her social support network. She may also have gained a little hope and confidence.

Reflection activities

- How could you routinely work exception questions into your work with clients who might benefit from losing weight or quitting a habit?
- What other questions can be posed to help a patient identify their own strengths in relation to a health behaviour?
- How can these sorts of questions be posed without seeming careless or confrontational to the patient?

BFST has been recommended as particularly suitable for busy health professionals, given its lower demands in terms of time and training (Greenberg et al., 2001). For an excellent introductory text, see Macdonald (2008).

Cognitive interventions

Cognitive Therapy and **Cognitive–Behavioural Therapy** (CBT) are currently the dominant models in NHS mental healthcare (Baker et al., 2008; see also Chapter 22). The founding idea of these models, developed by Aaron Beck in the 1960s, is that events themselves do not dictate psychological outcomes; rather it is how one interprets those events that has the power to alters one's mood and outlook on life (Beck, 1979). Whilst one person might interpret the smoking of a cigarette as 'only a little slip', another might consider it hugely significant and become distressed, thinking, 'I'm never going to give up, I haven't the willpower. I'm such a failure.' Beck's contention is that by challenging and changing these ways of thinking, especially by challenging unhelpful cognitions, a professional might bring about positive behavioural change. Modern CBT is a complex and multifaceted edifice, with well-developed manual treatments for a dizzying array of problems and disorders. There is evidence from systematic reviews for the effectiveness of CBT in a range of situations, including with substance use (McHugh et al., 2010) and eating disorders (Murphy et al., 2010).

Intervention manuals are generally complex and most authorities suggest substantial training. For example, the British Association for Behavioural & Cognitive Psychotherapies (BABCP) accredits therapists who have undergone 450 hours of training in cognitive and behavioural therapeutic approach (BABCP, n.d.). And to confuse the novice still more, there is considerable controversy over the method by which CBT works. For example, although the Beckian model maintains a central role for unhelpful cognitions, there is little evidence that challenging thoughts accounts for the salutary effects of CBT models (Longmore and Worrell, 2007).

Third-wave behavioural approaches

As described earlier and in Chapter 22, **contextual behavioural scientists** make different assumptions about the role of thoughts in the causation of other behaviours. This different perspective has given rise to a number of novel empirical findings about how behaviours are caused and maintained. These findings can be applied in clinical settings to support a client in changing behaviours in line with the client's own wishes. Together, these approaches are known as **third-wave behavioural approaches** (Hofmann and Asmundson, 2008). The principal examples are Acceptance and Commitment Therapy (ACT) and Dialectical Behaviour Therapy. Space will not allow a full exposition of the clinical techniques employed in these approaches, but because they differ so dramatically from the other approaches described here, some brief examples are warranted.

A number of central techniques in ACT are intended to change the believability or perceived literality of a thought. For instance, clients sometimes get stuck in a pattern of thinking. A phrase such as 'I'm a failure', or 'I just don't have the will power', can have powerful emotions associated with them, and might come into the client's mind unbidden each time they try to plan how to quit cigarettes. Some traditional CBT models would encourage the therapist to challenge that thought, perhaps by having the client generate examples of personal successes (see Longmore and Worrell, 2007). Another common sense approach might be simply to encourage the client not to think that way – in other words to suppress the thought – although there is now evidence that the attempt to suppress a thought makes related thoughts more likely to occur in future (Wenzlaff and Wegner, 2000). Contrariwise, in ACT, the therapist might encourage the client to use techniques to make the thought less literally believable. For instance, much of the emotional tone of a word can be stripped away simply by repeating the word, very quickly and loudly, in a rather silly way. This is not too dissimilar to 'exposure' techniques used since the 1950s to reduce fear of a stimulus through repeated experience. The client might otherwise be encouraged to give the thought a ridiculous voice, perhaps that of a squeaky cartoon character. These ideas might seem whimsical, but studies have shown that these techniques make thoughts less believable, although they have no short-term effect on the frequency with which the thoughts occur (Blackledge, 2007).

Human beings are able to learn much more quickly than other animals, and we develop and communicate rules as a result of our linguistic abilities, whilst other animals learn more slowly by trial and error. Behaviour governed by verbal rules is relatively inflexible, and humans can maintain old patterns of behaviour due to these rules, even when the physical and social environments have changed so as to support new and different behaviours (e.g. Hayes et al., 1986 ; Hayes and Gifford, 1997). ACT includes a number of techniques to encourage **psychological flexibility** by directing the client's attention toward the physical world in a non-verbal manner. Chief among these is the practice of mindfulness, borrowed from ancient Eastern teachings (and used by a number of other schools of psychotherapy), which involves the client noticing experiences without judgement and without deliberate verbal elaboration (Hayes, 2002).

One concrete example of a mindfulness-based approach to addiction is known as **urge surfing** (Ostafin and Marlatt, 2008). In a sense, this technique has developed in response to the intention–behaviour gap. A number of scholars have explained the gap between intention and actual behaviour by reference to urges or cravings (McKay et al., 2006). Acceptance of experiences (an element of mindfulness) has been shown to reduce the power that urges have over the control of behaviour (Ostafin and Marlatt, 2008). A client who finds the urge overwhelming to smoke cigarettes, imbibe alcohol, or engage in a chocolate binge, can be taught techniques to disengage somewhat from the thoughts associated with the feeling. Rather than **ruminating** and becoming agitated or distressed over thoughts such as 'This won't go away until I have a cigarette', the client can be taught to 'watch' the physical sensations and to remind themselves that such cravings and desires naturally ebb and flow.

CHAPTER SUMMARY

This chapter has briefly reviewed the evidence on the relationships between three specific lifestyle factors and both recurrence and mortality subsequent to an initial cancer diagnosis. There is sound evidence that smoking at time of diagnosis is linked with mortality, and perhaps recurrence. There is evidence also that being overweight or drinking alcohol can increase mortality for some cancer types. Whilst NICE has briefly recommend that healthcare professionals discuss modifiable risk factors with, for example, those at increased familial risk of cancer (NICE, 2013b), there are no similar guidelines to date for cancer survivors.

A frank (and appropriately tentative) discussion of the current state of knowledge would be in the spirit of informed decision-making; however, changing health behaviours is no simple matter. Each of us has had a personal experience of what health psychologists refer to as the 'intention–behaviour gap' when we have declared our intention to forego the extra slice of cake, only later to indulge. The social environment, both now and in the past, plays a powerful role in determining these behaviours. It is impossible to measure the multitudinous influences on health behaviours, and so health psychologists have developed models that attempt to measure and account for the most proximal or immediate causes of health behaviours. To date, these models have received reasonable support in cross-sectional studies, but have fared much less well in randomized intervention trials. Much of the work on behaviour change in healthcare settings borrows not from these theories, but from general psychotherapeutic and psycho-educational models. This chapter has reviewed some of these too. Most require lengthy training to be delivered properly as therapies, but many also provide basic techniques that can safely be applied in routine healthcare practice.

Reflective activity

- It has long been known that some patients with cancer will blame themselves for their illness (e.g. Bard and Dyk, 1956). It is plausible that this might be exacerbated by the giving of information on the strength of the link between health behaviours and cancer risk. How might you best support a patient to move past self-blame and make productive behaviour changes?
- Which of the behaviour change techniques described in this chapter seem to fit best with your current practice? What practical steps might you take to develop clinical competencies relevant to these approaches?

Key learning points

- Psychologists have identified a number of constructs or variables that are associated with behaviour change, some of which are proximal and some of which are distal.
- Complex models are built from a number of proximal variables to predict behaviour change.
- Randomized controlled trial evidence for interventions designed from these models is somewhat mixed.
- Brief Solution-Focused Therapy, CBT, Motivational Interviewing and third-wave techniques have reasonably sound evidence bases, and some techniques from these approaches can safely be used by healthcare professionals without extensive training.

Recommended reading

- Rollnick, S., Miller, W.R., and Butler, C.C. (2012) *Motivational Interviewing in Healthcare*. London: Guilford Press.
- Harris, R. (2009) *ACT Made Simple*. Oakland, CA: New Harbinger Publications.
- Macdonald, A. (2008) *Solution-Focused Therapy*. London: Sage Publications.

25 THE USE OF COMPLEMENTARY AND ALTERNATIVE THERAPIES IN CANCER CARE

LESLEY STOREY

Chapter outline

- Definitions of complementary and alternative medicine (CAM)
- Identification of the main challenges being faced by survivors that CAM may help with
- Examples of the use of CAM in cancer survivorship

- Evidence base for CAM therapies in cancer care
- Consideration of some important debates about methods for and ethics of researching CAM in cancer

---

INTRODUCTION

The aim of this chapter is to attempt to apply the limited research evidence for **complementary and alternative medicine** (CAM) to the needs identified for cancer survivors. The aim is to do this critically and to include a discussion of the controversies around this area of research from both an academic and practical perspective.

The *NHS Cancer Plan* (DH, 2000) highlighted the need to improve supportive and palliative care for people with cancer. Complementary and alternative therapies have been shown to be effective at providing symptom relief, reducing anxiety and improving quality of life (Wilkinson, Barnes and Storey, 2008), and were amongst the package of psychosocial measures for adults with cancer evaluated by the NICE (2004c). Much of the focus in policy guidelines for cancer is on the active treatment and palliative care phases of the cancer journey and, until recently, the survivorship phase had been relatively neglected by researchers and policymakers. Foster et al. (2009) carried out a systematic review of research on survivorship and found that there were relatively few interventions for this population and that methods used tended to be poor. They identified a number of key issues facing survivors and researchers interested in this area, including the variation in the definition of '**survivor**'. The Macmillan Cancer Support leaflet *Life after treatment* (2009) identifies a number of challenges that people may face at the end of their cancer treatment and these are summarized in Table 25.1. Devane (2009) identifies the gaps in research and the possible opportunities for nurses to support cancer survivors.

Much of the research activity in CAM has focused on symptom relief during active treatment, for example the use of acupuncture to alleviate chemotherapy-induced nausea or the use of relaxation techniques to support emotional wellbeing during treatment. This chapter provides a critical discussion of the research evidence for complementary therapies that may be useful in addressing some of the challenges for survivors.

Table 25.1   Issues most affecting cancer survivors

Emotional issues	Physical concerns	Social problems	Other
Anger	Peripheral neuropathy	Isolation	Eating issues
Depression	Pain	Isolation from medical care	Fertility
Uncertainty	Fatigue		Sexual function
Negative feelings	Lymphoedema		
	Late effects from radiotherapy		
	Vaso-motor symptoms (men and women)		

WHAT ARE COMPLEMENTARY AND ALTERNATIVE THERAPIES?

Definitions

In order to discuss and evaluate the contribution that CAM can make to the wellbeing of cancer survivors, it is important to be clear about what we mean when we use the term. Several professional bodies have attempted to define CAM with varying degrees of success. The British Medical Association (BMA) report *Complementary Medicine: New Approaches to Good Practice* (1993) suggests that although the term '**complementary therapies**' is familiar to the public, a more accurate term for research purposes might be '**non-conventional therapies**'. The BMA defines these as: 'those forms of treatment which are not widely used by the conventional healthcare professions, and the skills of which are not taught as part of the undergraduate curriculum of conventional medical and paramedical healthcare courses' (1993: 15). This definition is sufficiently fluid to accommodate the changes in both medical training and CAM practice (for example, the increasing use of acupuncture in general practice) but it defines CAM in oppositional terms; in other words, what it is not, rather than what it is.

A very different approach was taken by the *House of Lords Select Committee on Science and Technology report on Complementary and Alternative Medicine (HL Paper 123 2000)* (House of Lords, 2000). The Committee categorized specific approaches and therapies into three groups:

- **Group 1: Professionally organized alternative therapies** (acupuncture, chiropractic, herbal medicine, homeopathy and osteopathy)
- **Group 2: Complementary therapies** (Alexander technique, aromatherapy, Bach and other flower remedies, body work therapies, including massage, counselling stress therapy, hypnotherapy, meditation, reflexology, shiatsu, healing, Maharishi ayurvedic medicine, nutritional medicine, yoga)
- **Group 3: Alternative disciplines 3a:** Long-established and traditional systems of healthcare (anthroposophical medicine, ayurvedic medicine, Chinese herbal medicine, Eastern medicine, naturopathy, traditional Chinese medicine); **3b:** Other alternative disciplines (crystal therapy, dowsing, iridology, kinesiology, radionics).

The National Center for Complementary and Alternative Medicine (NCCAM, 2002) identify one of the problems with attempting to categorize specific CAM therapies: 'The list of what is considered to be CAM changes continually, as those therapies that are proven to be safe and effective become adopted into conventional healthcare and as new approaches to healthcare emerge' (2002: 1). A patient-centred and needs-based definition, on the other hand, attempts to also look at the aims and ethos of CAM practice, which also specifies how CAM differs from conventional medicine: 'Complementary medicine is diagnosis, treatment and/or prevention which complements mainstream medicine by contributing to a common whole, by satisfying a demand not met by orthodoxy or by diversifying the conceptual frameworks of medicine' (Ernst et al., 1995: 506).

A more encompassing temporal definition of CAM is provided by the Cochrane Collaboration as: 'a broad domain of healing resources that encompasses all health systems, modalities, and practices and their accompanying theories and beliefs, other than those intrinsic to the politically dominant health systems of a particular society or culture in a given historical period' (Zollman, 1999: 695). None of these definitions is specific to CAM in cancer care, but they provide a sense of the fluidity of the concept as well as a basis for the discussion in the rest of this chapter.

Training and accreditation

Another area of controversy is the issue of **training** and **accreditation**. There is no single body that provides accreditation or training for the use of CAM therapies in cancer care. Each therapy has its own professional body, some of which provide training and others do not. For some therapies, there are multiple professional organizations. It is possible for individuals to undertake relatively short courses in some therapies and then set up in practice, and there is no requirement for any consideration of issues specific to cancer survivors in these courses. In the UK, the Complementary and Natural Healthcare Council (CNHC) is a voluntary regulator for complementary therapists. The CNHC was set up with Government support to protect the public by providing an Accredited Voluntary Register by the Professional Standards Authority for Health and Social Care. Therapies registered include Alexander Technique teaching, aromatherapy, Bowen Therapy, craniosacral therapy, healing, hypnotherapy, massage therapy, microsystems acupuncture, naturopathy, nutritional therapy, reflexology, reiki, shiatsu, sports therapy and yoga therapy.

As O'Regan et al. (2010) point out, education about complementary therapies is not part of nurse training. Halcón et al. (2003) further highlighted that most nurses are not knowledgeable about complementary health and healing practices. Sohn and Loveland Cook (2002) also identified that the source of nurses' knowledge about complementary therapies comes from the individual's own personal experience, which may be sporadic and unreliable in nature. More information for nurse practitioners may assist in successful and safe integration of complementary and conventional approaches to supporting those affected by cancer.

CAM PROVISION AND USE IN CANCER CARE

Who uses CAM?

Corner et al. (2009) undertook a large study to explore patterns of CAM use in people with cancer: out of a total of 304 newly diagnosed UK cancer patients, 100 had used CAM before their diagnosis, and of these, 59 continued post-diagnosis. Twenty-nine who had not used CAM previously commenced use following their diagnosis. The most commonly used therapies were reflexology, aromatherapy and herbal medicine. The patients who used CAM following their diagnosis were more likely to be younger, female and with a diagnosis of breast cancer; have a higher level of education; not currently working; used CAM before; and perceived their illness as affecting their everyday lives. Independent factors that predicted continuing CAM use following diagnosis were younger age, female gender and early stage disease. Survivors' motivations for CAM use were categorized as:

- Perceived increase in chance of cure from cancer;
- To deal with the stress of having cancer, which in turn was perceived as enhancing the probability of treatment being successful; and
- To reduce side effects of cancer treatment.

Evans et al. (2007) explored the use of CAM by men with cancer. The men in this study had used a wide range of therapies, including mind–body therapies, such as healing and visualization; homeopathy; nutrition; psychological therapies; physical therapies; herbal remedies and a range of alternative therapies, such as **cyto-luminescent** therapy, which uses whole body irradiation and claims to eliminate tumour cells. Her qualitative study found that for these male survivors, the main motivations for CAM use were:

- Improving quality of life;
- Fighting the disease; and
- Possibly prolonging life.

She also found that these men seemed to be using CAM to meet the gaps perceived to be left by conventional healthcare. These 'gaps' included a lack of empathy and support, poor continuity of care and a lack of lifestyle advice for self-help. She concluded that the CAM practitioners seemed to have been better able to tap into the underlying needs of the men in a way that time and resource constraints meant was not possible for the mainstream healthcare team.

While there is no specific information on CAM utilization following the end of active treatment, it is likely that those whose primary motivation was informed by a perception of increasing their chances of a cure are likely to continue CAM use on the basis of also perceiving this as a way of preventing recurrence.

CAM provision for cancer survivors

CAMs are not routinely available within most branches of the British NHS, and many patients have to make their own arrangements. One of the main arguments for why CAM is not routinely integrated into NHS care is the lack of a strong evidence base. There has, however, been a move to integrate CAM provision into conventional cancer treatment centres, to make it easier for patients to access appropriate supportive and palliative services (Egan et al., 2012). A recent study found that 16% of patients with cancer (broadly defined) visited a CAM unit that was located within a regional conventional cancer treatment centre for information and informal support over a six-month period, and that 9% of visitors accessed at least one of the twenty CAM therapies that were available (Egan et al., 2012). The lack of provision within mainstream healthcare settings means that many individuals access their CAM provision through private practitioners who may not have sufficient cancer-specific knowledge to ensure that the treatments they offer are safe for both cancer survivors and those still undergoing active treatment for cancer; for example, some therapists still believe the myth that massage 'spreads' the cancer. The dominance of private practice also means that accessing CAM is dependent, for most, on the ability to pay for private sessions when it is provided by a therapist.

CHALLENGES OF RESEARCHING COMPLEMENTARY THERAPIES

Josephine Briggs, the Director of NCCAM in the USA, has suggested that CAM research should follow the classic sequence of cancer research, starting with basic research, via translational studies and randomized controlled trials, to studies of effectiveness for each treatment modality in order for CAM to have research-based credibility. In reality, much of CAM research bypasses the early phases and starts with effectiveness studies. One of the reasons for this is that often the mechanisms of action for specific therapies are unknown and this lack of information makes basic and translational research particularly challenging.

The lack of information about these mechanisms or '**active ingredients**' also has an impact on the ability to design an appropriate **placebo-controlled randomized trial** because there is insufficient information to inform the design of an appropriate placebo. If we are not clear on how change is effected, then how can we be sure that a convincing placebo is not also activating the mechanism of change? This is particularly a challenge in touch-based therapies such as massage. For example, when reviewing evidence for a systematic review of reflexology, one of the issues that became apparent was whether the intervention being provided in both the intervention and the control arms of the randomized controlled trials were sufficiently different: 'Reflexology is defined as "a method of using thumb pressure with a walking motion on reflex areas of the feet which correspond to the glands, organs, and systems of the body"' (Wyatt et al., 2010: 3).

As an example, a study by Ross et al. (2002) found that patients requiring palliative care seemed to benefit more from the 'sham' reflexology than from genuine reflexology. The fact that there were no positive differences in favour of reflexology between the sham and authentic modalities was attributed to the non-specific effects of the intervention with both groups; participants seemingly benefited most from the opportunity to discuss their concerns and fears. These findings were not dependent on sample size or methodological quality.

These kinds of studies raise important questions about non-specific effects that may be common to all practitioner-based complementary therapies, primarily about what the active ingredient in reflexology is and, therefore, what the relative cost effectiveness of the use of trained reflexologists might be.

Other challenges of researching CAM identified in a report by the UK-based Kings Fund (Smallwood, 2005) include:

- How to take account of the context in which the intervention is made;
- How to reflect the importance attached to treating the whole person;
- How to accommodate the fact that the relationship between cause and effect may not be straightforward; and
- How to understand 'placebo' or non-specific effects.

There are other systemic issues that also act as barriers to building a solid research base for CAM. Often, CAM practitioners have limited understanding of research practice and are suspicious of both the research agenda and the research community. Many are looking to research to provide the 'proof' that their therapy 'works'. Concepts such as **scientific equipoise** (i.e. that there is genuine uncertainty about whether a treatment is likely to be beneficial), although important to the scientific community, have less resonance amongst CAM practitioners.

One of the key arguments within CAM research is the call by practitioners for research that replicates the 'real life' characteristics of their practice set against the demand by researchers for a standardized and replicable research protocol. In a UK NHS context, this debate becomes more heated: the 'real life' holistic practice of many complementary therapists is rooted in a history of private practice in which consultations last for an hour and take place in a calm, relaxing, fragrant setting. This is a setting that is almost impossible to replicate within the constraints of an NHS cancer unit.

For clarity, acupuncture will be explored as an example. Broadly speaking, acupuncture consists of inserting needles at specific points around the body with a view to manipulating Chi or the energy forces of the body. Particular points are associated with particular complaints, for example the Pericardium 6 (P6), or Neiguan, is the most commonly used **acupuncture point** to control nausea and vomiting (Dundee, 1988). There is a broad spectrum of acupuncture practice within the UK. Most are generally affiliated to one of two broad theoretical bases, which are not mutually exclusive: traditional acupuncture, based on traditional oriental medical principles, and Western acupuncture, a modern interpretation of acupuncture based on anatomical, physiological and pathological principles (Hughes, 2009) These have some differences in training and practice: traditional acupuncturists generally complete longer periods of training and administer lengthier treatments incorporating a greater range and number of needle insertion points than Western acupuncturists (Hughes et al., 2007). Traditional acupuncturists also draw distinction between the 'energy work', which they perceived themselves as doing, and the process of inserting needles. For them, acupuncture treatment encompassed the entire patient experience, with all aspects of that experience being seen as capable of impacting on the patient's condition (Hughes et al., 2007). The relationship and interactive process between practitioner and patient was seen as being of crucial importance to treatment success. In particular, traditional acupuncturists saw their role as facilitators, educating and empowering patients to assume responsibility for their own health and adopt a healthier lifestyle. By contrast, many

reduction by 6 points on a 10-point scale. This patient regained movement and was able to walk and resume work as a bus driver. There were no adverse effects reported. Methodologically, a far stronger study was reported by Alimi et al. (2003) who carried out a randomized, blinded placebo-controlled trial of auricular acupuncture (AA) for neuropathic pain in ninety cancer patients. AA is a form of acupuncture carried out on the ear rather than on any other area of the body. Nogier (1981) has suggested that all internal organs are represented on the ear and that stimulation of specific points has a corresponding effect on that area of the body. One of the advantages of this form of acupuncture is that it does not require the patient to remove any clothing. In this study, Alimi et al. (2003) observed a statistically significant reduction in pain between the AA and placebo groups.

There is clearly a need for more research into acupuncture, especially for peripheral neuropathy, and ideally this research should explore which form of acupuncture is most effective and most acceptable for the cancer survivor population. The research also needs to ensure that it is methodologically appropriate and that findings can stand up to critical examination in order for it to be 'prescribed' by healthcare practitioners or for cancer practitioners to be able to access safe private acupuncture treatment with confidence. It is possible that other therapies may also provide relief and this is an area that needs to be explored further.

Vasomotor symptoms (patients with breast cancer)

When vasomotor symptoms (hot flushes and night sweats) appear as part of menopause in the healthy population, GPs usually prescribe a pharmacological form of oestrogen replacement. This form of treatment is, however, not considered safe for many patients with breast cancer and this means that women with breast cancer often look to alternative forms of treatments. Some alternative treatments, which work in a similar way to boost oestrogen production, are also problematic for those with a history of breast cancer (e.g. the black cohosh herbal supplement). A number of studies (e.g. Filshie et al., 2005; De Valois et al., 2010) suggest that acupuncture might provide a safe and effective source of relief. Filshie et al. (2005) carried out an audit of acupuncture and self-acupuncture via a retrospective audit of electronic records. Their dataset included patients treated for as long as six years, and 79% of patients were found to have gained a 50% or greater reduction in hot flushes. This evidence of long-term use suggests a value in this approach to self-care for the survivor population.

Similarly, De Valois et al. (2010) explored whether traditional acupuncture (TA) is effective in the treatment of vasomotor symptoms experienced by 50 women taking tamoxifen as a maintenance treatment for breast cancer. The study also aimed to improve physical and emotional wellbeing. Participants received eight weekly individualized TA treatment using a core standardized protocol based on the usual acupuncture treatment for natural menopause. The study required participants to keep a diary in which they recorded the frequency and intensity of hot flushes and night sweats over a 14-day period. Other outcome measures included the Women's Health Questionnaire (WHQ), which assessed physical and emotional wellbeing, and the Hot Flushes and Night Sweats Questionnaire (HFNSQ). The mean frequency of hot flushes and night sweats reduced by a statistically significant 50% from baseline to the end of treatment. Long-term trends indicated that these benefits were sustained when assessed up to 18 weeks after the last treatment session. Perceptions of hot flushes and night sweats as a problem reduced by 2.2 points, also a statistically significant reduction. Additional improvements were seen across the seven domains measured by the WHQ, including anxiety/fears, memory/ concentration, menstrual problems, sexual behaviour, sleep problems, somatic symptoms and vasomotor symptoms. It is important to note that this paper reports on a pilot study only, which did not have a control group; however, the use of robust, validated measures seems to show promising benefits for the use of CAM for this distressing physical symptom. The fact that the benefit was sustained for some time following the end of treatment is a particularly important finding for the survivor population because it suggests that acupuncture may provide long-term rather than transient relief.

Vasomotor symptoms (prostate cancer patients)

The vast majority of research into cancer-induced vasomotor symptoms has been carried out in women with breast cancer; however, the same symptoms are a side effect of ongoing **androgen-deprivation therapy** (ADT) treatment for men with prostate cancer, and it is possible that men may find such symptoms more distressing than women. Gommella (2007) suggests that 50–80% of men on ADT experience these symptoms. Women, after all, may expect to encounter some of these symptoms at the time of the menopause, but for men, the experience of these traditionally female symptoms may feel like an additional and ongoing attack on their masculinity, which may make them reluctant to report them to healthcare professionals and seek help.

Harding et al. (2009) report findings from a pilot study of AA for men with vasomotor symptoms in a UK NHS hospital. This study used the National Acupuncture Detoxification Association (NADA) protocol, which involves the insertion of sterile single use needles at five points on the ear bilaterally. These were left in place for 40 minutes with treatments given in a group setting once a week for 10 weeks. They used two main outcome measures, including the Measure Yourself Concern and Wellbeing (MYCAW) scale, which has been specifically developed for use in complementary therapy settings. This allows the patient to specify their primary 'concern' rather than having it pre-determined by the researcher or healthcare professional, and also includes a general wellbeing question. MYCAW has been validated (Paterson et al., 2007) and found to be acceptable and easy to use. MYCAW measurements were taken at baseline and at the end of the study. In addition, patients were asked to keep a diary specifically to measure their hot flushes (both frequency and intensity) at day and night. They were asked to do this at weeks 0, 4 and 10. The results of Harding et al.'s (2009) study bore out the assumption that the experience of vasomotor symptoms was a significant problem for the participants. When asked to identify their primary concern on the MYCAW scale, 62% of the men identified hot flushes and night sweats. Other concerns also likely to be related to their vasomotor symptoms include depression, anxiety, sleep disturbance and fatigue. The reduction in primary concern scores, frequency and intensity of hot flushes and night sweats, and improvement in general wellbeing were all statistically significant.

Lee et al. (2009) conducted a systematic review of acupuncture for the relief of hot flushes in men with prostate cancer and found that the evidence base was poor quality, with very few randomized controlled trials and work that had been undertaken had limited small sample sizes, which are likely to be underpowered. The paper argues for randomized controlled trials including a placebo; however, they also recognize that there are problems with an effective placebo for acupuncture (e.g. either inserting needles into non-acupuncture points or using a form of sham acupuncture, which does not puncture the skin but is not obvious to the participant).

They discuss the possible mechanisms of action for acupuncture, such as the release of **beta-endorphin** and **serotonin** activity, operating to regulate the **autonomic nervous system** but do not come to any definite conclusions.

Despite this hypothesis, the actual mechanism of action for AA for vasomotor symptoms remains unclear. What is clear, however, is that in a healthcare context in which there are very limited conventional healthcare solutions for this type of treatment side effect, anything that improves both physical and psychological symptoms is to be welcomed by patients. Personal experience of informal discussions with the participants (during their treatment) was that they found it a universally positive experience. Indeed, rather than finding the record keeping burdensome, they took great pleasure in reporting their logbooks and enjoyed both the 'enforced' relaxation and the opportunity to receive informal social support from their peers. Harding et al. are currently carrying out a larger scale study as a follow-up to their pilot study.

Lymphoedema

Cancer treatments, specifically surgery and radiotherapy, are the main cause of secondary **lymphoedema** in the developed world (Lymphoedema Framework, 2006). It consists of chronic swelling affecting the limbs, trunk, head, neck, breast or genitalia and arises when reduced capacity of the **lymphatic transport system** causes accumulation of fluid in the tissue spaces (International Society of Lymphology, 2003). Secondary lymphoedema is a common side effect caused by treatments for many cancers, including breast and head and neck cancers (Keeley, 2000; Withey et al., 2000). Studies report occurrence ranging from 3–89% of patients with breast cancer (Williams et al., 2005), with prevalence of arm oedema calculated to be 29% of breast cancer patients (Moffatt et al., 2003). Secondary lymphoedema is also reported in 10–40% of people with head and neck cancer (Bjordal et al., 2000).

There is currently no cure for lymphodoema and standard treatment consists of wearing pressure bandages in the affected area (e.g. a sleeve for an affected arm). Lymphoedema is therefore widely considered to be a distressing condition. Disfigurement and the wearing of specialist bandages may cause social embarrassment, body image problems and possibly low self-esteem (De Valois, 2012). In their exploratory study with survivors of breast and head and neck cancers who had clinically diagnosed lymphoedema, De Valois et al. (2012) attempted to assess whether treatment with a combination of acupuncture and moxibustion improved wellbeing (this is a form of traditional acupuncture enhanced by the application of heat produced by the burning of the moxa herb). The study did not set out to treat the lymphoedema itself, and it was controversial in that most patients with lymphoedema are advised to avoid any activity or treatment (including vaccination) that punctures the skin because this can precipitate lymphoedema in individuals who have had lymph nodes removed.

The inclusion criteria for this study was a diagnosis of mild-to-moderate uncomplicated lymphoedema for more than three months for individuals who were more than three months after active cancer treatment maintenance. Participants received seven individualized treatments and six optional additional treatments. Measure Your Medical Outcome Profile (MYMOP), SF-36 and Positive And Negative Affect Scale (PANAS) were administered at baseline during each series, and at follow-up 4 and 12 weeks after end of treatment. The primary outcome was change in MYMOP scores at the end of each series. MYMOP is a variation on MYCAW, which again allows participants to specify their own area of concern. The mean MYMOP profile change scores for breast cancer participants were a statistically significant 1.28 points improvement on a 7-point scale; head and neck cancer participants showed a greater improvement of 2.29 points and no serious adverse effects were reported in either group.

This small-scale study also included six focus groups, which were carried out with six head and neck cancer survivors and seventeen breast cancer survivors. They discussed a range of physical and emotional benefits, which included reduced pain, improved sleep, increased energy levels, reduced stress levels and reduced medication. In terms of the lymphoedema itself, they also reported a perceived reduction in swelling, as well as increased mobility. Participants reported variation in the duration of beneficial effects, which could be short term or long lasting. Several participants reported increased motivation to manage their long-term health issues, such as attempting to lose weight or making more effort to maintain self-care routines.

The combination of qualitative and quantitative findings in this study suggests that this approach has benefits both for a physical symptom (e.g. lymphoedema), which has long been an intractable burden for survivors, but also for a population (patients with head and neck cancer) who are traditionally under-represented in research and whose socio-demographic profile suggests that they may derive a disproportionate benefit from holistic interventions that address a variety of wellbeing issues as well as physical challenges.

Emotional concerns

Macmillan Cancer Support (n.d.) has identified a range of emotional concerns that may contribute to reduced quality of life for cancer survivors. Many of these will be best addressed by counselling or other psychological therapies (see Chapter 22). In some cases, however, the use of touch therapies may also be useful. An unpublished Grounded Theory study of women diagnosed with breast cancer looked at the early stages of transition from patient to survivor (Downing et al., 2012). The core category identified illustrated the process of 'finding a new identity and normality'. Physical problems, such as fatigue, were conceptualized in terms of the search for a 'new me' and the interaction between physical limitations and the need to incorporate the cancer experience into a new sense of self (which allowed for continuity with the past but still respected the impact of the social, psychological and physical changes wrought by the disease and its treatment). Many of these women found that touch-based therapies, such as massage, were helpful as part of this process. Reflexology and aromatherapy massage have also been used to treat emotional distress in patients undergoing active cancer treatment (Corner et al., 2009). Systematic reviews (Wilkinson, Barnes and Storey, 2008) of the evidence for both reflexology and aromatherapy massage for a range of physical and psychosocial symptoms highlighted some of the challenges involved in researching CAM in cancer, but produced no conclusive results about the benefits. For example, the absence of a suitable control group for these touch therapies and the inability to double-blind the treatment limited the research designs that could be used.

Aromatherapy massage has also been trialled using randomized controlled trial methodology in people with cancer who require palliative care, demonstrating statistically significant reductions in anxiety and improved scores for the psychological and quality of life subscales of the Rotterdam Symptom Checklist (Wilkinson et al., 1999). Again, this was a relatively small study with no follow-up data and, given the nature of the intervention, it was impossible to blind the participants to the intervention; however, the results are promising: if such a therapy is effective in addressing emotional and psychological distress in people at the end of life, it might be effective in survivors who are experiencing some of the negative emotions associated with the transition to the survivorship phase of the cancer journey.

DIETARY CHANGE AND SUPPLEMENTS AS POSSIBLE CAM APPROACHES

Foster et al. (2009) identified fear of a cancer recurrence as one of the key stressors for people during the survivorship phase. It is likely that one of the ways in which people may attempt to manage that fear is by adopting appropriate health protection measures in terms of lifestyle change towards healthier choices; however, such changes need to be supported by appropriate and specific guidance, and it is this information that is very often lacking. For example, Maskarinec et al. (2001) highlight the uncertainty pervading dietary advice in cancer and recognize that much of the guidance for cancer survivors (National Cancer Institute, 1998) has its basis in the healthy eating guidelines aimed at the general population. Cancer-specific nutritional recommendations are limited to the management of treatment side effects, such as chemotherapy-induced nausea and vomiting (National Cancer Institute, 1998, 2000). Maskarinec et al. (2001) report a range of 4.4–57% of reported dietary change in patients with cancer. This was often based on the belief that nutritional changes would increase wellbeing, maintain health and prevent recurrence, but it was also mediated by beliefs about the cause of cancer. This link was also evident in the consumption of supplements (Maskarinec et al., 2001).

The effect of this uncertainty was evident in an unpublished study carried out with post-menopausal survivors of breast cancer. This was a qualitative interview study exploring the eating habits of survivors of breast cancer. There were two key linked findings from this study. First, the women felt that they had no information or guidance from healthcare professionals about diet following the end of active treatment. A number compared this lack of guidance with the level of input received when undergoing chemotherapy. The consequence of this information vacuum was that the women prioritized continuity in their food choices with phrases such as 'that's the way I've always done it' coming up repeatedly in the interviews. This meant that rather than their cancer diagnosis being an important factor in how they lived their lives following treatment, they reverted to behavioural patterns that were familiar and comfortable, including the importance of the nurturing role of wife and mother when making choices about food shopping, meal planning and preparation. In light of a relatively healthy diet, this can be considered to be an effective coping strategy. There is clearly a need for information about what cancer survivors can do to live healthily once they have completed active treatment. This information may also need to explicitly address the lack of strong evidence in this area.

CONCLUSIONS AND RELEVANCE FOR PRACTICE

The worth of CAM depends on the criteria by which it is judged. It has been argued that the non-medical touch and holistic care, which are core characteristics of CAM, meet a need that was traditionally provided by nursing. In survivorship, CAM appears to offer options for chronic cancer-induced problems for which conventional medicine is ill-equipped to cope with. The downside is the lack of a strong evidence base to support these options. This is an issue for all CAM users, but it is particularly a concern for those who have experienced cancer. There are safety issues and contraindications for cancer survivors that may not be obvious to either CAM users or CAM practitioners who have not been specifically trained in the care of cancer survivors. For example, women suffering from vasomotor symptoms following treatment for breast cancer may follow a recommendation from a female friend who had similar symptoms during menopause, but although the menopausal woman is unlikely to be harmed by taking the herb, black cohosh, it is strongly contraindicated for women who have had particular forms of breast cancer. More research on both the efficacy and the safety of CAM throughout the patient journey into survivorship is much needed.

The issue of the lack of knowledge about the specific mechanisms of action in CAM clearly poses significant challenges for carrying out traditional-style research about efficacy and effectiveness. The Medical Research Council framework for the evaluation of complex interventions offers guidance for researchers attempting to do research that both respects the holistic ethos of most CAM interventions as well as producing results that will be meaningful and have credibility with the research and healthcare communities (Craig et al., 2008).

One of the issues that CAM researchers have to address is the degree to which the observed changes following a CAM intervention are a result of the placebo effect or non-specific effects around the treatment. For example, massage involves pleasant non-medical touch, the focused and interested attention of a therapist and often takes place in a non-clinical environment, which is scented and playing ambient music. The argument is, therefore, that any relaxation effect comes from a combination of all of these additional factors, as well as the therapy itself, rather than specifically from a physical effect of the massage or other therapy.

This is an important consideration when policy decisions, which have public funding implications for treatment options, are being made. Although less of an issue for self-funding cancer survivors, it is still important that people have sufficient information about these issues in order to make informed choices about their self-care and wellbeing.

Nurses and other healthcare professionals are likely to encounter cancer survivors in a variety of contexts during follow-up care. These are likely to offer a good opportunity to check how effectively survivors are dealing with post-treatment physical and emotional issues and whether they are using complementary therapies in the survivorship phase for issues relating to their cancer. These meetings might also enable cancer care professionals to remind individuals that they need to bear their cancer diagnosis in mind when making these decisions (e.g. mentioning acupuncture when discussing lymphoedema risk). In terms of continuing professional development, efforts to stay abreast of any ongoing research into the use of complementary therapies for conditions such as peripheral neuropathy, which are not currently well dealt with by conventional medicine, will ensure that cancer care professionals are able to have informed discussions with patients, and to ensure that any advice they offer is both safe and supported by available evidence. It is likely that this, in turn, will lead to patients being more open about their complementary therapy use and provide a better basis for consultations that promote holistic care, which is at the heart of good nursing practice.

CHAPTER SUMMARY

This is a chapter that evades a neat summary. The concept of survivorship is loose, ill defined and historically under-researched. CAM is equally subject to multiple definitions and is also under-researched. There are a number of significant methodological challenges involved in carrying out research into CAM in any disease, but also particularly during the survivorship phase when target populations may prove more elusive.

In terms of therapies, acupuncture is over-represented in CAM research in general, and in cancer research in particular. This is because acupuncture (compared with other therapies) lends itself better to symptom management and is thus easier to research, and it also meets patient-led priorities. As with many areas of cancer, women with breast cancer are over-represented within the research populations.

Despite the limitations of the research evidence in this area, there are promising areas of research where CAM may offer support for life-limiting conditions that are currently not well-served by mainstream treatments, which may improve quality of life and emotional wellbeing. Touch-based therapies in particular may have something to offer those struggling with negative emotions and social isolation. Acupuncture seems to offer relief for those symptoms that act as a daily reminder of the experience of cancer and cancer treatment at a time when patients are hoping to move on to a period of more robust physical and emotional health.

Key learning points

- Cancer survivors have ongoing physical and emotional concerns.
- Some complementary therapies seem to be effective for dealing with the ongoing legacy of treatment.
- Acupuncture is over-represented in research on complementary therapies.
- There needs to be much more research on the use of complementary therapies in the survivorship phase.

Recommended further reading

- Macmillan Cancer Support (www.Macmillan.org.uk/Cancerinformation/Cancertreatment/ Complementarytherapies/Complementarytherapies.aspx).
- National Center for Complementary and Alternative Medicine (NCCAM) (http://nccam. nih.gov/health/cancer/camcancer.htm).
- Ernst, E. (ed.) (2006) *The Desktop Guide to Complementary and Alternative Medicine: An Evidence-Based Approach*. 2nd edn. Maryland Heights, MO: Mosby.

26 ART AND MUSIC THERAPY IN CANCER CARE

FAY MITCHELL AND LESLIE BUNT

Chapter outline

- Introduction and historical context of art and music therapy
- Definitions, areas of practice and theoretical perspectives that are shared between art and music therapy
- In-depth analysis of the application of these two therapies in cancer care

- The art therapy section is written very much from a clinical perspective with examples drawn from individual sessions
- In contrast, the music therapy section is more general in tone and incorporates an adult group example

---

INTRODUCTION TO ART AND MUSIC THERAPY

Historical perspective

The use of the arts to alleviate **pain** and **distress** is not new. It can be found throughout history in most cultures, but it is only from the second half of the last century that the specific professions of art and music therapy became increasingly established. In the UK, the British Association of Art Therapists (BAAT) was set up in 1964 and the Association of Professional Music Therapists (APMT) in 1976 (there had been a general British Society for Music Therapy since 1958). In 1982, these two professions were awarded a Career and Grading Structure within the Whitley Council, by what was then the Department of Health and Social Security. Fifteen years later, in 1997, art and music therapy joined drama therapy by becoming registered within the **Health Professions Council**, a move towards protecting the public and setting up standards and proficiencies of training and practice. The titles are now legally protected (Waller, 1991; Bunt and Hoskyns, 2002; Bunt and Stige, 2014). In 2012, the Council was renamed the **Health and Care Professions Council** (HCPC) and one of the roles of the HCPC is to validate and monitor training programmes. Since 2006, all such training in art and music therapy in the UK has needed to be at the Master's level, with practitioners graduating with either an MSc or MA.

What is art therapy?

Art therapy is a form of **psychotherapy** using art making as a fundamental means of **communication**. It 'offers the opportunity for expression and communication and can be particularly helpful to people who find it hard to express themselves verbally' (BAAT, 2014a: 2). The creation of an image provides, in concrete form, something of the patient's experience with which both the therapist and patient can engage. The image provides a tangible record of change. In making a picture, previously unacknowledged feelings can be given shape, which may lead to those feelings being shared and reflected upon.

Art therapy, along with other arts-based therapies, was for many years embedded within **psychiatric services**. Towards the end of the last century, art therapists began to establish themselves in hospitals and to move into more community-based settings, such as day centres and hospices, local residential settings and the probation and prison service. This growth, tentative at first, has been augmented by an increase in therapists writing for publication and embracing the need for evidence-based research. The Art Therapy Practice Research Network (ATPRN) is a group of art therapists who collaborate on practice-led research and evaluation. Gilroy (2007) looked at the literature related to evidence-based practice in art therapy. She acknowledges that there is a need to research art therapy with various client groups, and also to present rigorous literature and hard data as to its efficacy. In doing so, we should also strive to preserve and present: 'Art therapy's differing forms of evidence and argue that it be judged according to the values and norms of the discipline' (Gilroy, 2007: 150).

What is music therapy?

Music therapy, as a resource, can provide people of all ages with a wide range of creative actions, connections and relationships. It can be defined as, 'the use of sounds and music within an evolving relationship between client/patient and therapist to support and develop physical, mental, social, emotional and spiritual well-being' (Bunt and Hoskyns, 2002: 10–11). Music therapists work in individual or group contexts with three main areas of activity:

- Active music making, both vocally and instrumentally, with the emphasis on **improvisation** (Wigram, 2004);
- Listening or receptive approaches, including incorporating **guided imagery** (Grocke and Wigram, 2007); and
- **Songwriting** (Baker and Wigram, 2005).

Traditionally, music therapists have worked with children and adults with some form of communication problem resulting from learning difficulties, physical disabilities, neurological problems, visual or hearing impairments, mental health or other emotional and social issues. Music therapists have a history of working in hospital settings, specialist units, nurseries and schools for children with learning difficulties. In parallel with the developments in art therapy, music therapists are increasingly working outside of the institutional context, bringing the work to more community-based contexts (Pavlicevic and Ansdell, 2004; Bunt and Stige, 2014).

Some shared theoretical perspectives

The professions of art and music therapy straddle many artistic and scientific disciplines. First, both are creative arts therapies with their own historical and philosophical links to a study of the **humanities**. The amount of importance attached to the actual artistic or musical processes within the therapy is borne out by the ongoing debate as to whether to describe the professions as art or music **therapy** or art or music **psychotherapy**. Therapists need to be well qualified in their perspective artistic traditions, although any previous training in either art or music is not required of patients participating in the therapy.

Second, art and music therapists underpin their practice with reference to a range of other theoretical perspectives and approaches, such as **psychoanalytical**, **physiological/medical**, **neurological**, **cognitive/behavioural**, **humanistic** or **transpersonal** (Silverstone, 1997; Bruscia, 1998; Schaverien, 2000; Bunt and Hoskyns, 2002; Wigram et al., 2002; Edwards, 2004; Bunt and Stige, 2014). Some music and art therapists work in an **integrative** fashion, drawing on different perspectives depending on context, for example in short-term brief therapy (Balloqui, 2005).

Art and music therapy in cancer care

Over recent decades, greater numbers of art and music therapists have been establishing services in physical health and, in particular, cancer care. Camilla Connell introduced art therapy to the Royal Marsden Hospital in 1987 and Professor Michael Baum spoke positively of the contribution of her work: 'As far as I am concerned, art therapy is the most direct line into a patient's experience of illness, and I feel almost ashamed that I do not make use of it in the day-to-day practice of my own clinic' (Baum, 1998: 8–9). A participant in a music therapy group summed up the experience: 'I think music is definitely fundamental in one's search for one's self. As far as cancer patients or any other illnesses [are] concerned, listening to music or communicating through music or making music even plays a very crucial role' (McClean et al., 2012: 404).

Art and music therapists working within cancer care in the UK practise in a variety of settings: hospital oncology units (Heywood, 2003; Bocking, 2005), cancer care centres and hospices (Aldridge, 1998; Thomas, 1998; Duesbury, 2005; Pavlicevic, 2005; Wood, 2005; Daykin et al., 2006; O'Kelly and Koffmann, 2007). The work within these establishments is with inpatients, day-care or outpatients. Patients can be also seen on a domiciliary basis (Bell, 1998).

The evidence for art therapy is documented in a recent NHS London (2012) publication titled *Allied Health Professionals* (AHP) *Cancer Care Toolkit*. In this toolkit, an AHP cancer framework is outlined and the efficacy of art therapy with cancer patients in the management of depression, anxiety disorders and altered body image is acknowledged. Evidence for effective music therapy practice has also been included in two systematic literature reviews published by the Cochrane Collaboration (Bradt and Dileo, 2010; Bradt et al., 2011; see later for further discussion).

ART THERAPY IN CANCER CARE

The following section of the chapter will describe the place that art therapy in particular can occupy within the provision of psychosocial support in cancer care. This is an area where an increasing number of arts therapists are gaining a foothold. There is a slow but progressive recognition of the value in a creative approach to ameliorate the difficulties of living with a life-threatening or life-limiting disease (see Wood et al., 2011; NHS London, 2012; Wood et al., 2013). There will also be an insight into how to use the time and space offered, with an illustration of a typical session. The section concludes with case material, and imagery and words produced by patients engaged in art therapy.

The following words of a patient[1] living with cancer who had spent time in art therapy were documented during an unpublished audit of the art therapy service and articulate the benefit she derived from the process:

> 'I have drawn myself a new horizon, it has helped me focus my thoughts and address my fears. It isn't as frightening in the picture as it is in my head.'

Referrals

There is a place for referral to art therapy at all stages of the patient's cancer experience:

- **Assessment and diagnosis**: the psychological impact of a cancer diagnosis can generate **adjustment disorders, anxiety** and **depression** manifesting in feelings of **anger, guilt** and **fear**. Art therapy has been effective in enabling people with cancer to **express** anxiety after diagnosis, which helps prevent the onset of depression. A pilot complementary creative art therapy intervention, for example, showed enhanced psychological wellbeing in women with breast cancer (Puig et al., 2006).
- **During treatment**: Cancer patients undergoing painful and/or unpleasant treatments and procedures may benefit from art therapy interventions. Nainis et al. (2006), for example, reported reduction in distress and anxiety from participation in art therapy sessions for this group of patients.
- **At the end of life**, when expression of feelings can sometimes be considerably more difficult (see, for example, Jones, 2000).

Cancer treatment centres are stretched to full capacity, and will continue to be so as this patient population grows. Diagnostic tools will become ever more sophisticated and attuned, and physical illness outcomes will improve. As the research progresses and the efficiency of better targeted pharmacology increases, so do patients' chances of survival. This in turn heralds a further development in patients' needs: having to live with the changes and disabilities that

---

[1]Please note that consent has been obtained from patients for the inclusion of direct quotes throughout the chapter. Those that appear in the art therapy section, within quotation marks, come from an unpublished audit; in the music therapy section, they are reproduced from earlier publications.

disease has brought can be challenging. Cancer services, which were developed to treat a disease of the **soma**, are arguably poorly served to safeguard the **psyche**. Art therapy can offer a creative way to address this. Luzzatto and Gabriel (2000), for example, described directive, theme-based groups that facilitated self-expression using art materials. Group members completed post-intervention questionnaires, which documented increases in feelings of freedom, peace and of their self-awareness.

Art therapy may be especially useful for:

- Those needing support, but who find it difficult to articulate **verbally**.
- Those whose **cognitive abilities** have been impaired by disease or treatment and may therefore find it a difficult to put into words how they may be feeling. For example, those who have cancer in the brain, either primary tumour or metastatic disease.
- Those who have cancer of the head or neck whose ability to physically speak has been compromised may also find an alternative way to express themselves helpful.
- Those with a **learning difficulty** as a useful mode of communication.
- Those who may have an age-related organic degeneration of brain functioning (e.g. **dementia**).
- For those individuals whose cognition has been affected by medication.

In many of these patients, it may be the case that discovery of cancer and the resulting tumult can act as a catalyst, catapulting patients back to unresolved issues from their past. Memories long repressed can resurface and old wounds reopen. These can hinder adjustment to diagnosis and compound a patient's already fragile emotional state. An individual may find it a struggle to accept diagnosis and find it exhausting navigating themselves around all that is demanded of them regarding therapy choices. Patients can, in some cases, face not only the disease and its resulting treatments, but also the difficult feelings that it has conjured up from the past. Art and its production can prove a vital alternative for expression of the spoken word.

The structure of the sessions

Art therapy sessions are generally weekly, one hour in duration and delivered one-to-one or in a small group. There is initial introductory assessment in which any difficulties, emotional or psychological, that patients are experiencing are identified. Realistic goals can then be discussed regarding desirable outcomes to therapy. A number of sessions are offered, after which a review is undertaken as to whether the time and space made available has been of benefit. If art therapy is useful to the patient, further sessions can be offered and support continues. The therapy thereafter is reviewed regularly until discharge. For a reasonable proportion of the patients seen for art therapy, between six and twelve sessions are required; however, for some patients who may have more complex needs, it is appropriate for art therapy to be offered for a longer period. Guidelines have been developed for art therapists working in various settings and with different patient populations in the UK. These are outlined in *Code of Ethics and Principals of Professional Practice* (BAAT, 2014b).

A sample art therapy session

An extensive variety of materials should be made available to the patient to make use of, such as:

- Paints: oil, acrylic or watercolour
- Pens
- Inks
- Pencils
- Crayons
- Pastels
- Paper
- Canvas
- Clay
- Glue

When patients commence art therapy, they are invited to use the space and time in the way that feels most comfortable. Some patients like to paint quietly, engaging with the varied art materials primarily; others may find the need to talk more.

An image is produced or worked on during the session that is witnessed by the therapist, whose role is that of a **facilitator** and **listener** – a therapist as opposed to a teacher or tutor. As mentioned earlier, the trained therapist has knowledge of a range of theoretical approaches such as psychoanalytical, humanistic and behavioural/cognitive (Schaverien, 2000; Edwards, 2004). The theory informs the practice in an art therapy session, and the therapist has the benefit of an added tool: the art. The creative process is the focus and this provides the framework for any powerful feelings that may emerge to be acknowledged, contained and worked through. The patient has the total and undivided attention of the therapist who needs to be empathic and sensitive without being obtrusive.

If the patient is apprehensive and finds it difficult to begin, the therapist may suggest that they start by simply choosing a colour that appeals to them and make a mark on the paper (Coote, 1998; Bocking, 2005). It is vital that trust is established and this is reinforced by clearly defined boundaries and codes of confidentiality. Patients may be surprised by what they produce. If long suppressed emotions are triggered by the imagery, the therapist is experienced in containing these securely, enabling the patient to process them constructively. Difficult feelings that may have been damaging to the patient can surface through the artwork, which releases the patient from the pain of holding them.

Patients may not wish or need to relate to the therapist, but instead opt to engage with the materials and the art making entirely. They may not choose to reflect on their imagery, but benefit solely from the process. Mastering the materials to make a picture in and of itself may help to boost morale (Connell, 1998).

At the onset of therapy, the patient's permission is obtained by way of a consent form should the therapist wish to use their imagery for education and research. Anonymity is at all times safeguarded.

Those individuals referred for art therapy bring with them their own unique narrative, which may be important to explore. The image may hold clues to this narrative and this can be reflected upon, along with the memories or feelings evoked. This can be on an individual basis or in a small group (Luzzatto, 2005). For some patients, their challenges lie in the **internal landscape** rather than the **interpersonal**.

Cancer and depression

When patients with a cancer diagnosis appear low in mood, a common response has been to **pathologize** this reaction and to offer medicative treatment. This pharmacological reflex reaction may, for some, provide welcome relief from the symptoms of depression; however, for many this response is far from helpful. NHS London (2012) documents the evidence of the efficacy of art therapy in reducing depression in people with cancer. Patients may find that engaging with the art materials lifts their mood, and being able to reflect over time on the imagery signals movement that counterbalances the inactive feelings of despondency. Bar-Sela et al. (2007), for example, report the results from a study that indicated that art therapy improved depression and fatigue levels for cancer patients undergoing chemotherapy. Using the artwork produced during therapy, particular reasons for depressed mood can be identified and worked with. Over time, these images can be reflected upon and movement forward signposted:

> 'It captured my thoughts at that moment and together showed a progression of my state of mind.'

> 'I know I have cancer but now I'm being told I am depressed' or ' I thought I was coping well but now I'm not, others seem to manage so why can't I?'

Cancer and anxiety

> 'The art graphically illustrated the turmoil and confusion within me. We were able to start untangling so that it seemed more manageable and less frightening.'

Externalizing the chaos of the mind, which can be brought about by serious illness, by depicting it in imagery and framing it within the confines of a picture can help to contain it. This in turn can reduce its disabling impact on the patient's psychological health. It opens up to the light the anxieties that thrive in the dark. The image, a portrayal of the patient's experience, can then be regarded and reflected upon. The use of metaphors within the imagery can be illuminating in terms of imagining the unimaginable. The symbolic content can also be of great significance in enabling the individual to feel less isolated:

> 'For the sake of mental stability and even physiological health, the unconscious and the conscious must be integrally connected and thus move on parallel lines. If they are split apart or "dissociated," psychological disturbance follows. In this respect, dream symbols are the essential message carriers from the instinctive to the rational parts of the human mind, and their interpretation enriches the poverty of consciousness so that it learns to understand again the forgotten language of the instincts' (Jung, 1978: 37).

The process of making external the internal, whereby the patient puts down their concerns, makes them concrete and then attempts to shape something useful from them, can be a daunting task. Accompanied by a trained therapist and contained by the materials, space provided and time constraints, however, it can be made manageable.

The images produced can be used over time as tangible signposts towards recovery and equilibrium. Words disappear into the ether, whereas pictures act as solid reminders of change and growth. In some circumstances, patients can appear stuck and psychological movement can be difficult to identify. Day-to-day living with a serious illness is burdensome and, at times, patients may not feel emotionally or psychologically robust enough to cope. With images to reflect upon, patterns may emerge and triggers identified that may offer reassurance. Individuals can be alarmed by the strength of the emotional response that their illness evokes within them, occasioning the threat of being overwhelmed.

Wood and colleagues (2013) collated available literature concerning art therapy and psychosocial issues. They identified twelve studies with methods that included interviews, questionnaires, therapists' observations and stress markers in saliva. They concluded that art therapy 'is considered useful for people who find verbal expression difficult, particularly where disease, surgery or treatment impedes communication and disrupts self image'(Wood et al., 2013: 42).

In the words of a patient:

'The art reflects very strongly my emotional life. And has helped me make sense of it and the very mixed up and powerful feelings I have been experiencing.'

Cancer and cancer treatments are unpleasant and can cause pain and discomfort. For some, the opportunity to create pictures imagining or evoking a time or place free of suffering is welcome.

CASE STUDY

Mike

A concern that has often been explored by patients during therapy is the occasional feelings of ambivalence towards medical professionals. This is illustrated by the image in Figure 26.1 produced by Mike, a young man with bowel cancer.

In this picture, Mike has drawn himself lying on a bed with doctors and nurses in attendance. He drew a circle that encompassed his head and his heart. He stated,

'They are all down there looking at my backside and I am up here.'

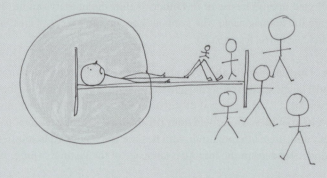

Figure 26.1   Mike's image

In further discussion, it became apparent that he felt as if the process of disease and the resultant treatments had objectified him, and that he was no longer a person with hopes, fears, dreams and desires. In short, he now felt defined by his disease.

Tjasink describes:

> Being poked, prodded and exposed to poisons and radiation is often essential in oncology and can be deeply unpleasant, objectifying and dehumanising. Becoming an object of medical processes can also raise issues of identity. Art psychotherapy can work alongside these medical processes, bringing the humanity and search for and expression of meaning and value back into the equation. (Tjasink, 2010: 75)

Art therapy and the space it provides can be a useful arena to explore patients' feelings around the care and treatment they receive. Patients may wish to be viewed as a 'good' patient, one who doesn't challenge and is compliant with treatments. The art therapist may be perceived as somehow outside of this system and not integral to their physical survival and, therefore, safe to bear witness to any ambivalence towards the medical response.

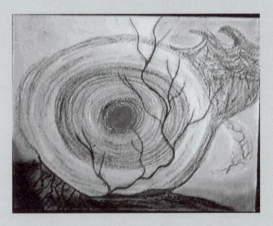

Figure 26.2 Lynne's image

Lynne

Figure 26.2 is a replication of an image produced by Lynne, a woman with bowel cancer.

She said of the painting, 'It's a very bad picture and it causes me pain to look at it but I need to look at it because it's what I'm afraid of. There are lots of tree roots – they are the roots of the cancer spreading out.' Despite the reassurance of the doctors and the positive results of her scan she was very afraid that they hadn't cut it all out and that it would grow again from the roots.

James

The image shown in Figure 26.3 was produced by James, a man with lung cancer.

James found it beneficial to visualize his tumour with the angry pain it caused him. The

(Continued)

(Continued)

grid depicts how he imagined the chemotherapy that he was being treated with was holding his cancer and keeping it in check. He found the effects of the drugs almost intolerable but was determined to continue with the treatment. For him, drawing the medication at work helped reinforce his **coping strategies**.

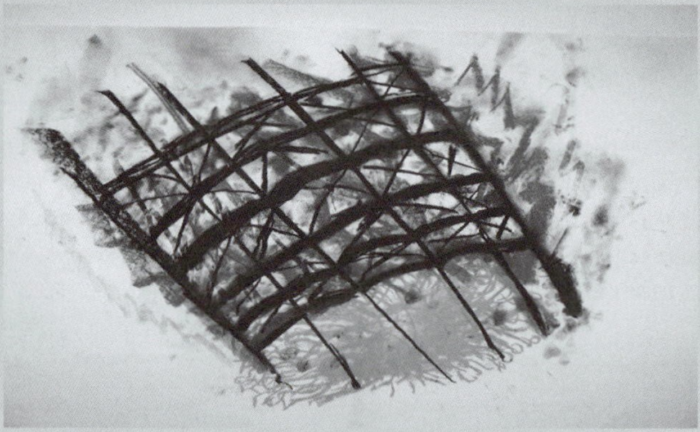

Figure 26.3   James' image

SUMMARY

There is growing evidence for the usefulness of art therapy in the psychosocial support of patients with cancer. Luzzatto and Gabriel (1998) describe the aims of art therapy in cancer care as creativity, communication, catharsis and containment. This section of the chapter ends with the words of patients who speak for themselves.

'Art therapy has been very beneficial to me as it is easier to talk through the pictures and reflect on my depth of mood. It is good to talk but more can be said when talking through the pictures.'

'The pictures stay in my head in a way that's different to words, so I can return to the image and continue to think about it.'

'It feels as if the artwork is a vehicle for talking, it relaxed me and I think over what has been discussed.'

'It started as a decorative flower picture but became a landscape in which I featured. A shadow behind the person captured how I felt about past life experience dragging behind.'

'It gives me something other than the sickness to think about. It calms me down. I feel more in control when I paint.'

MUSIC THERAPY IN CANCER CARE

In today's world, there appears to be an ubiquitous use of music. We are all aware how different kinds of music and musical experiences can energize us physically, aid relaxation, focus attention or shift mood. Music can foster social connections and help build communities; we can actively use music to sing or play out an evolving sense of personal and creative identity in the world (MacDonald et al., 2002). Listening to music or making music can contribute to our ongoing quality of life, sense of health and wellbeing (Ruud, 1998; MacDonald et al., 2012). Above all, music can evoke strong emotional experiences and internal connections within us (Juslin and Sloboda, 2010; Gabrielsson, 2011). At its core, it tells us something about what it is to be human and about our human story. In music therapy, all of these resources and qualities within music are framed within the context of a developing **therapeutic relationship**. As shared with other creative arts therapists, the music therapist has the responsibility to facilitate, attend and witness these wide-ranging potentialities and contributions to health and wellbeing within the client, but although aware of these positive contributions, therapists need to be mindful of the potential risk factors involved in inviting individuals or groups to take part in making or listening to music, given music's capacity to evoke such powerful feelings and emotions (Daykin, 2007).

Music therapy also has its place as part of a broad continuum under the umbrella of 'Music in Health' and as part of a burgeoning 'Arts and Health' agenda (Clift et al., 2009). Within healthcare settings, a range of musical activities is facilitated not only by music therapists, but also by nurses, other allied health professionals, volunteers and visiting musicians, amongst others (Daykin et al., 2006). Bruscia (1987: 9) has differentiated **'music in therapy'**, when music is part of another therapeutic intervention, from **'music as therapy'**, when music is the central agent of therapeutic change. A trained music therapist would, for the most part, be using 'music as therapy'; whereas the use of music by a nurse, for example as a background to aid relaxation during a medical procedure, could be described as 'music in therapy'.

Music therapy and music in cancer care

Music therapy's place in a continuum within the broader role of music in cancer care can be illustrated by a UK-based survey of organizations (the majority from the non-statutory sector) providing music in this context (Daykin et al., 2006). A range of activities was discovered that used music as:

- Calming and relaxing background;
- Enjoyable entertainment;
- A diversionary activity;
- Adjunctive to another therapy; and
- As a specific therapy.

The most frequent activity was 'listening to recorded music', although 60% of the sample also used 'live music' of some sort (Daykin et al., 2006: 407). But there was a lack of clear distinction between the various roles, for example less than half of those organizations in adult cancer care reporting the use of music therapy actually engaged a registered music therapist. Contrastingly, all of the children's hospices that took part in the survey employed registered music therapists. This relates to the work of the charity Jessie's Fund that supports the setting up of music therapy in children's hospices within the UK, although children with conditions other than cancer are also referred (Pavlicevic, 2005; Hodkinson et al., 2014). It is also of interest in relation to the content of this chapter that at the time of the survey a preference was indicated for art therapy, and the offer of music therapy was more likely alongside another intervention rather than being delivered as a unique therapy (Daykin et al., 2006).

Music therapists also use active approaches, and in the UK there is much use of improvisation and live engagement in making music both in individual and group work. The next section of the chapter will relate for the most part to this active use of music facilitated by a professionally trained music therapist. The focus is on work with adults living with wide-ranging cancers at all stages, including those at a **palliative** and **terminal** stage. The range of potential referrals to music therapy is similar to those already outlined for art therapy. But one of the obvious differences between art and music therapy is that whereas an art object can possess a solid form about which different perspectives can be explored with the therapist, the nature of any active musical encounter is its very fluid form, with no two musical experiences, either active or receptive, ever being the same.

Themes emerging from music research on therapy practice

This section incorporates a short description of an adult music therapy group session (see Bunt (2011) for a further example). The description is an amalgamation of the kinds of activities that might take place in a one-off session in a cancer care setting. The emergent themes developed in research on music therapy on cancer care that Leslie Bunt undertook with Norma Daykin and Stuart McClean between 2005 and 2007. The direct quotes from participants, particularly those relating to this section's theme of survivorship, are drawn or abridged from two earlier publications (Daykin et al., 2007a, McClean et al., 2012). The quotes are from 'semi-structured interviews with 23 individuals following their participation in one of six "one-off" group music therapy sessions'. Written consent was obtained for taking part in the research (Daykin et al., 2007a: 353).[2]

Nine adults living with cancer gather together in a well-lit and spacious room for their one-and-a-half hour music therapy session. A range of tuned and untuned percussion instruments from different parts of the world is carefully laid out in the centre of a circle of comfortable chairs. After a brief introduction to set the boundaries of the session, including announcing the length of the session, the music therapist invites each participant to explore an instrument, playing in turn as a kind of introduction and initial expression of individual feelings. These might include any associations with the sounds or evoked memories. It is made clear that people can choose not to play and that taking part does not necessitate musical training or experience: the kinds of instruments available are accessible to all.

Freedom of choice: At the start of session, a sense of curiosity is apparent as each participant explores the various instruments.

'I think what I enjoyed seeing was that there were instruments from many parts of the world ... from many cultures and backgrounds ... he left it to us to choose and pick what

---

[2]The direct quotes from interviewees in this section were originally published in Daykin et al. (2007a) and McClean et al. (2012).

we liked, so everybody went round feeling the instruments ... I liked the wide diversity and I felt very much at home ...'

After the introductions, the music therapist sets up a steady heartbeat pulse on a drum, inviting members of the group to absorb the pulse and join in if and when they wish. As the piece unfolds and people become more comfortable and confident with the instruments, the loudness increases, with some members of the group increasing the tempo.

Group cohesion: At this stage, there are often comments about feelings of group cohesion, with each participant being able to hear their own individual sounds but within the collective group piece. There is often a sense of surprise about how organized and pleasing the improvisation sounds.

'... everybody seemed to realize what the group was doing and not what individuals were doing ... so we were all getting louder and then softer and slowing down, speeding up but not without anybody ... saying that is what we'll do next ... everybody was tuned into each other ...'

But there can be less positive reactions, indicating the potential power of music. This element of risk, and the care involved, must be considered when inviting people to make music.

'... there was a rhythm that was beaten out ... that was picked up ultimately by everybody there, which to a certain extent I found quite alarming ... I thought that this is a good opportunity to demonstrate how easy it is to lead people into war ... because from going from total chaos everybody was following the same tune and marching off ... I just felt that ... everybody lost their individuality and were following the herd ...'

Individual perceptions of music: There is a wide range of what music means to the individuals in the group and the relationship to their own personal history. For some participants, the experience can be releasing, joyful, liberating and empowering; for others, the sounds do not equate with personal perspectives of what constitutes an aesthetically pleasing and enjoyable musical experience. Once again, the music therapist needs to be attentive to this range of individual responses within a group.

After another freer group improvisation with no imposed structure by the therapist, there is a palpable sense of release but also of tiredness in the room. As a change in the level of activity, the participants are invited to play a musical message to another group member, a kind of musical call and response. Spontaneous comments are shared after each short dialogue, ranging from a sense of gratefulness and appreciation at receiving a kind of 'musical present' to a sense of confusion or preferring to not comment and to keep any feelings expressed without words and within the music.

The overall mood changes and the various comments resulting from the dialogues flow into a discussion on the ever-shifting range of feelings that are part of living with cancer. The group members propose to create a longer improvised piece reflecting a polarity of themes arising from the discussion and moving from a place of confusion, darkness and difficulty through to one of more clarity, light and hope. The members of the group choose a range of instruments suited to the different sections of the proposed piece. They settle back into their chairs and after a moment of silent reflection, the first sounds emerge.

On the sense of connection: For some participants, this non-verbal exchange and being played to was 'amazing … like a gift …' and there was a sense of 'communicating beyond superficial, at deeper levels'.

> 'I wanted to give something to one of the people and it was just a peaceful thing … Sometimes you can't express yourself in words, you want to say something special and you can't do that and just playing something to someone can be very special.'

But here again, this activity was not a positive experience for all.

> 'I found that stressful because I didn't really know how to communicate with music like that or to understand what anyone else was saying …'

The themed improvisation lasts for over five minutes and is followed by some space for verbal reflection. Chronological time is running out and the therapist proposes listening to some music as a way of bringing the session to a close. The members of the group are invited to put their chairs into the reclining position, to sit back, use the foot rests and, if they wish, to cover themselves with a blanket. After a short relaxation induction – participants closing their eyes if this feels comfortable – and an invitation for each group member to allow their imaginations to take themselves off to a place where they can feel a sense of quiet rest, a piece of classical music lasting about four minutes is played. At the end, and after some moments of silence, the therapist announces that the music has finished and gently invites each of the nine members of the group to reflect on the listening experience, sharing any images, feelings, memories or reflections that they wish. Comments are also invited on any shifts in energy or feelings from before the session until this point. The members of the group quietly disperse.

On the relaxing, healing and spiritual properties of music: At the end of the session, there are often comments about the relaxing and healing potential of listening to music. There are both highly individual experiences, as well as the emergence of common themes. When taking the time and care to listen to music in this relaxed way, there is also a sense of clarity, focus and concentration, allowing space and freedom for the imagination and spirit to take flight. As in moments of meditative reflection, there are opportunities here to spend some quiet time transcending the intrusion of other thoughts, including the potential of temporary diversion from pain.

> 'I just think it centres the mind and is quite healing …'

This kind of experience and any images, evoked memories or sensations resonating within the psyche, as if part of an ongoing daydream, can also linger after the session.

> '… I think it was one of those uplifting experiences that you carried with you that con-tinued to work after the event …'

> '… music of various types … sort of touches the soul … or it can do … people's moods and people's outlook can be affected by music and obviously tailored by music.'

On the sense of creativity evolving from the session: The end of the session is also a time for comments to be made about the whole experience. Sometimes there is discussion about taking up music again, joining a community music group or learning a new instrument.

'One thing came out of it was that I was going to take up the clarinet once I got the chemotherapy over.'

On the holistic nature of music: A music therapist is privileged to be able to invite participants to explore the totality of a musical experience, one that unites mind, body and spirit.

'Music is symbolic of life and energy and all things.'

Evidence to support the use of music therapy in cancer care

There is an emerging evidence base to support the use of music therapy in cancer care. As mentioned in the introduction, two relevant systematic literature reviews have been published for the Cochrane Collaboration, which summarize a growing research evidence base. Some of the main findings from these two reviews, including reference to a small selection of trials from within these reviews demonstrating work both with children and adults, are summarized next.

The review conducted by Bradt and Dileo (2010) focused specifically on music therapy for end-of-life care. Five studies met the inclusion criteria for this review. Only one of these, a study by Hilliard (2003), had the main focus on music therapy and cancer: the results from this study indicating an increased quality of life for the patients diagnosed with terminal cancer who received music therapy, with further increases as more sessions were taken. The authors concluded tentatively that music therapy may be beneficial for improving quality of life at the end-of-life; however, it should be noted that the review included only a small number of studies and, therefore, carries 'risk of bias'. More research is clearly needed on the role of music therapy for this population of people with cancer.

Bradt and colleagues (2011) published a second review, just one year later, focusing on the effects of a music intervention on psychological and physical outcomes in people with cancer. Thirty studies met the inclusion criteria for this review, including seventeen that employed 'listening to pre-recorded music'; and thirteen that reported interventions encouraging participants towards active engagement. From within this review, there are some particular study examples that are worth a closer analysis. First, in a randomized clinical trial study by Nguyen and colleagues (2010), children with leukaemia who listened to preferred songs were found to demonstrate lower pain scores and improved heart and respiratory rates during and after lumbar puncture procedures. Those children who listened to the music were also less anxious and were less fearful (Nguyen et al., 2010: 146). Similarly, Robb and colleagues (2008) undertook a randomized controlled trial comparing an active music intervention with music/storybook listening in children with cancer. The findings suggest that those in the intervention arm of the trial reported significantly improved coping-related behaviour.

Hanser et al. (2006) undertook a randomized controlled trial in women with metastatic breast cancer, which indicated that after only three sessions of individual music therapy, there were some significant immediate effects in such areas as relaxation, comfort, happiness and heart rate. However, these differences were not maintained over time. Burns et al. (2008) explored the feasibility and potential benefits of using music imagery for patients with acute leukaemia undergoing chemotherapy, reporting that participants in the music imagery programme experienced 'reduced anxiety at discharge'. An earlier study, also by Burns, on the use of guided imagery and music indicated improved quality of life (Burns, 2001). Other beneficial outcomes synthesized in this systematic review included reduced 'mood disturbance' (Cassileth et al., 2003) and greater pain reduction where music therapy was compared to standard care (Clark et al., 2006).

Although Bradt et al. (2011) note a risk of bias once again, they make the cautious conclusion that 'music therapy and music medicine interventions may have a beneficial effect on anxiety, pain, mood, quality of life, heart rate, respiratory rate, and blood pressure in cancer patients' (Bradt et al., 2011: Plain Language Summary). Methodological issues and a small sample made it not possible to compare 'music medicine interventions' with 'music therapy interventions', and effectiveness studies such as these would be good avenues for future research.

SUMMARY

There is growing evidence that both listening to music and active music making can be beneficial for children and adults living with cancer, and that these benefits might include improvements from physiological, psychological and social perspectives. There are positive effects both during medical procedures and whilst coping with the daily patterns of the disease. The holistic nature of music with its potentialities to engage the physical, mental, social, emotional and spiritual within us all can be therapeutically effective in the field of cancer care.

CHAPTER SUMMARY

Both art and music therapy are effective therapies in enabling people with cancer to bypass words in order to access the inner world of the imagination. Participants in art or music therapy can, as it were, scribble with colour or sound in free and very exploratory ways. They can also listen to music, in individual or group therapy, and this can act to initiate or even replace verbal communication about the difficulties they are facing with their cancer.

Key learning points

- Art and music therapy are two categories of arts-based or creative therapies.
- Both are recognized alternative approaches to supporting people with cancer.
- They offer opportunities to explore the inexplicable; to articulate inner feelings in a cathartic way; and allow people with cancer a chance to express the most difficult and powerful of feelings in a safe and contained manner.
- They can provide a chance to come to terms with all the losses associated with cancer and engage people with cancer in an activity that can temporarily transcend current concerns and provide some relief from pain.
- They can allow patients who may feel they have lost control of their health and future regain a sense of autonomy and personal identity by being in control of the materials, artwork or the musical instruments and creative flow and direction.

- For some patients, these therapies simply allow the time and space needed to adapt and make changes to a life, during or post-cancer; for others it may be a place to embrace creativity at a time when other modes of expression may be unavailable.
- For both art and music therapy, although there is a small evidence base of benefits for people with cancer, research to date is limited. It is only by exploring these interventions with more rigorous methodological designs that a more objective empirical rationale will be developed.

Recommended further reading

- Connell, C. (1998) *Something Understood: Art Therapy in Cancer Care*. Wrexham, UK: Wrexham Publications.
- Dileo, C. and Loewy, J.V. (eds) (2005) *Music Therapy at the End of Life*. Cherry Hill, NJ: Jeffrey Books.
- Magill, L. and O'Callaghan, C. (eds) (2011) 'Music therapy and supportive cancer care', *Music and Medicine* (Special issue), 3 (1): 5-63.
- Waller, D. and Sibbett, C. (ed.) (2005) *Art Therapy and Cancer Care*. London: Open University Press.

Useful addresses and websites

The following list summarizes some useful resources for those wishing to know more about the provision of these therapies.

For art therapy

British Association of Art Therapists (BAAT): www.baat.org
Corinne Burton Trust, Parker Cavendish, 28 Church Road, Stanmore HA7 4XR
Creative Response: www.creativeresponse.org.uk

For music therapy

British Association for Music Therapy (an amalgamation of the former AMPT and the British Society for Music Therapy, BSMT): www.bamt.org
Online music therapy journal: www.voices.no
Jessie's Fund: www.jessiesfund.org.uk

27 SPIRITUALITY AND EXISTENTIAL ANGST

MARK COBB

Chapter outline

- Spirituality and the meaning of human existence
- The ways in which spirituality functions in healthcare
- Cancer as an existential challenge and spiritual search
- The role of spirituality in holistic cancer care
- Exploring and assessing spiritual needs
- Supportive interventions of spiritual care

INTRODUCTION

The meaning of life is the apparently simple but evidently problematic issue that will be addressed in the course of this chapter. There are many sources of meaning that nourish and shape our lives, but this chapter will address those that give a point and purpose to life beyond the immediate and ordinary; sources that sustain, inspire and provide an ultimate significance to **human experience**. The problem arises when the meaning by which a person orientates his or her life is questioned, becomes less certain or is entirely lost as a result of a cancer diagnosis and this then impacts on a person's health and **wellbeing**. The resulting uncertainty and disorientation can affect a person's quality of life, capacity to cope, treatment decisions and response to care. This has been recognized by the National Cancer Survivorship Initiative (NCSI), which addresses the full range of issues affecting people living with cancer and aims to ensure these are included in the assessment, care planning and the support and services available. Similarly, the importance of an **holistic** approach to care, which includes the **spiritual** aspects of life, has been articulated in the NICE guidance and more recently supported in the UK National Cancer Programme. What follows in this chapter is an introduction to the place and role of spirituality in healthcare, an explanation of the **existential** and spiritual challenge that cancer may present and an overview of the ways in which cancer services can aim to recognize and respond to the spirituality of patients and their spiritual and existential needs.

SPIRITUALITY IN HEALTHCARE

Spirituality concerns the ways in which people make sense of who they are, their place in the universe and their life's **purpose**. This is an orientation to living within a wider horizon of ultimate significance, purpose and meaning that people embody in a worldview expressed through **beliefs**, **values** and **practices**. Spirituality is, therefore, a way of responding to the intuition that, 'Existence is something tremendous, and day-to-day life, however indispensable, seems an insufficient response to it, a failure of consciousness' (Nagel, 2010: 6). What constitutes a sufficient response is a question that has occupied great philosophers and theologians over many centuries. Some thinkers reject the proposition altogether and more recent responses have followed **secular** and **naturalistic** approaches. **Religions** continue to provide some of the most enduring and widely followed spiritual responses to the question of what it means to exist as a human being. A religion provides a formative framework for an individual's spirituality and orientates the person to a set of claims and commitments about life that are directed to an ultimate reality signified by the divine, the holy or the sacred. Most notably, religions are **social systems** of meaning to which individuals identify and have a sense of belonging that finds expression in established collective acts of observance, ritual and shared narratives. A final category of response to the question of existence is the more defuse forms of spirituality that have been labelled 'new religious movements' or 'alternative spiritualties' with their own associational forms, discourses and practices.

Questions of meaning and purpose are also found in the **humanistic** purposes and responses of healthcare, which itself has a significant religious past that continues to be expressed in some of the discourses, practices and symbols of healthcare. More recently, the language and concepts of spirituality have become folded into healthcare where clinicians and patients face daily challenges to human existence, strive to nourish the human spirit in the face of suffering, participate in collective expressions of the value and purpose of human life and seek a sufficient response to the ways in which people experience illness and injury beyond its immediate physical reality. Spirituality in healthcare is, therefore, often located at the interface of personal, social, moral and existential aspects of healthcare where there is a mutual concern for wellbeing and wholeness. In this particular context, spirituality serves a number of significant functions. First, it provides a way of recognizing a larger human reality that cannot be accommodated by the incomplete and reductionist view of the physical sciences. In other words, it articulates something of the significance and meaning of the person in the midst of a dominant biomedical context where a focus on problematic biology can obscure the humanity in which disease is embodied:

> *Illness* is something beyond mere discomfort, but defined in *my* terms; *disease* is an objective clinical condition, independent of my judgement. So I may feel ill, rotten, 'run down'; but only the doctor can diagnose my disease. Which commonly leads doctors having to focus on bits and pieces – microbes, hormone deficiencies, tumours, lungs, heart, ulcers – while I may experience my illness as the disorder, disruption and apparent disintegration of my life.' (Mayne, 2006: 236).

Second, spirituality functions as an inclusive concept in healthcare premised on a basic and apparently universal human capacity, rather than being a synonym for religion. Spirituality in healthcare is, therefore, a deliberately open term that embraces human diversity and enables clinicians to attend to the particular spiritual histories and needs of patients through appreciative inquiry. Third, spirituality functions as one of the dimensions of personhood in healthcare alongside the psychological, social and physical dimensions, all of which constitute the whole person. Holistic and **person-centred** approaches to healthcare are commonly underpinned by these integrated four dimensions and provide the basis for addressing the needs of the whole person (Sulmasy, 2006). The spiritual dimension, therefore, contributes to overall health and quality of life and represents a distinctive aspect of the person that is not adequately addressed through the psychological and social alone (O'Connell and Skevington, 2010).

A body of knowledge has developed in healthcare about the role of spirituality in the living with and beyond illness, how this can be recognized and what support should be offered by health services. This is substantially clinically derived and applied knowledge informed by disciplines within the broad domain of healthcare and more distally related to academic disciplines concerned with the systematic study of spirituality such as theology and religious studies. Forms of knowledge about healthcare spirituality include practice-based experiential and reflective knowledge; propositional knowledge embedded in policy, guidelines and training; and the research findings of inquiries and empirical studies (Cobb et al., 2012b).

It will be evident that spirituality covers a lot of conceptual ground and this reflects both the diversity of spiritualties that people express, but also the inclusive way that the term is intended to be used in clinical practice. The literature of healthcare spirituality, however, is prone to cluster around two major areas: the patient's experience of spirituality in the face of illness and the ways in which spirituality may function in relation to health outcomes and wellbeing. In particular, the therapeutic role of spirituality in relation to disease prevention, onset, progress, adaptation and coping are significant themes in research literature. For example, in a major review of research about the relationship between religion and health, Koenig et al. (2012) specifically reviewed cancer-related studies, and they concluded that:

> Data are accumulating that indicate R/S [Religion/Spirituality] related to many of the physiological, social, and behavioural factors that influence endocrine and immune function that affect cancer growth. Once cancer develops, R/S beliefs and practices are commonly used to help cope with the disease. Studies show that those who use religion as a coping resource adapt better, experience less anxiety and pain, and are more hopeful … all of which may have endocrine and immune consequences that influence the spread of cancer. (Koenig et al., 2012: 467).

Healthcare research is pulled towards **functionalist** understandings of human phenomena with the aim of controlling them, and intervening to produce a net health benefit. Whatever the merits of this approach, it is important to be aware of the constraints around this form of generalizable knowledge and not confuse its production with the pursuit of other forms of serious and rigorous inquiry that is discerning of contextual knowledge, attentive to particular narratives and inspired by deep understanding and appreciation (Stanworth, 2004). There is also a necessary caveat that we need to enter about spirituality that is typically absent in the healthcare literature when it is either reported as a likely benefit or benignly ineffective. If spirituality involves the essential reference points and absolute realities by which people orientate and find value in their lives (in other words the sacred and the holy), then spirituality will moderate the experience of illness, inform treatment choices and provide resources for adapting and coping. Although these have the potential to be positive and enriching, they can also be disorientating and the location of conflict, distress and suffering. Pargament (2007), writing from the perspective of psychotherapy, describes this problematic form of spirituality at its worst as:

> … dis-integrated, defined by pathways that lack scope and depth, fail to meet the challenges and demands of life events, clash and collide with the surrounding social system, change and shift too easily or not at all, and misdirect the individual in the pursuit of spiritual value. (Pargament, 2007: 136).

A person's spiritual orientation may be latent or unproblematic in the everyday circumstances of life but when faced with a major life challenge, such as cancer, it may be severely tested and found wanting.

THE CHALLENGE TO MEANING

It is easy for human biology to go unnoticed when we are fit and well; however, a simple injury calls our attention to a particular place on our body, for example through pain and bleeding; a strenuous period of exercise or physical work, which makes us aware of our racing pulse and strained breathing; or a bout of flu, which can make our usually fluent and responsive limbs feel heavy and unresponsive. Many of these maladies are short-lived, our health is restored through simple measures and our biology rescinds once more into the background of our lives. Even situations requiring medical assistance focus on the restoration of the human body to its level of normal function by correcting biological faults or traumas through physical and pharmacological interventions. But although who we are and what we experience is dependent on life in a body, we are also much more than our bodies, and illness may be a challenge to these other aspects of who we are as persons:

> … illness is not simply a problem in an isolated physiological body part, but a problem with the whole embodied person and her relationship to her environment. Because the living body is not just the biological body but one's contextual being in the world, a disruption of bodily capacities has a significance that far exceeds that of simple biological dysfunction. (Carel, 2008: 73).

When faced with chronic or life-threatening conditions, such as cancer, physical disruptions can have obvious significance for the ways in which people live out their lives, experience the social and physical world, and face the future. Beyond this, illness can change the ways in which people understand and relate to the world, including the beliefs and meanings that give their lives shape, purpose and fulfilment. At its most significant, we know that cancer is a leading cause of death, and facing our mortality reminds us that our embodied existence is finite. Cancer can, therefore, present an existential challenge to a person because it makes the continuation of life more precarious and can threaten an individual's very existence in the world.

Uncertainty about being in the world and ways of living meaningfully in the face of death has attracted the attention of philosophers, such as Heidegger, Kierkegaard and Sartre (Joseph et al., 2011), and given us the technical term **existential angst** to describe a realization of the banal aspects of life and the possibility (paradoxically) of living an authentic and affirmed life because of our mortality (Malpas and Solomon, 1998). Tillich (1980) explores this human capacity for self-affirmation through the idea of courage in the face of anxiety, and he identifies three types of anxiety related to the threat of non-being: the anxiety of fate and death, the anxiety of emptiness and meaninglessness, and the anxiety of guilt and condemnation. In relation to meaninglessness, this is not just our usual doubt, but what he calls 'total doubt', and he explains that,

> The anxiety of meaningless is anxiety about the loss of ultimate concern, of a meaning which gives meaning to all meanings. This anxiety is aroused by the loss of a spiritual centre, of an answer, however symbolic and indirect, to the question of the meaning of existence. (Tillich, 1980: 47).

This loss of an answer to the meaning of existence, or the failure to find a satisfactory answer to what it means to be a person living with cancer, is the more general sense that shall be considered in this chapter; however, this is more than intellectual exercise because the experience and consequences of living with cancer can profoundly challenge what a person has learnt about the world and the security of their place in it. This sense of dissonance and unfamiliarity with a new reality can leave people experiencing what has been termed 'groundlessness' (Bruce et al., 2011) and be the cause of distress and suffering that can have a significant impact on the way people adapt to living with cancer.

A diagnosis of a serious illness and the experience of invasive treatment can make people acutely aware of their vulnerability and finitude which, in turn, can raise questions about the meaning of their existence, both in the past as well as in the future. Contemplating mortality and an indefinite future is to face uncertainty and question the purpose of living. Lubbock (2012), living with a brain tumour, reflects on this point when he says that,

> What I lose now, most generally, is the indefinite, open-ended prospect of life; not any particular goals but all the unknown imaginable goods, which always fill the edge of your view. Our life is lived on those terms, of ongoingness. They are the assumption. Without them, our life appears alien. (Lubbock, 2012: 47).

Disorientation, disconnection and alienation to life and the world can be the cause of existential **suffering**; equally it can motivate a search for spiritual wellbeing that enriches life with purpose, meaning and hope. The future orientation of ongoing life is commonly expressed in the idea of hope, which in a study of women newly diagnosed with a gynaecological cancer was summarized as '… a belief in the future, an inner willpower to be an integrated human being and an acceptance of being interdependent, being one in relationships with family, friends and God' (Hammer et al., 2009: 278). Similarly, for some people, their lives need re-creating and re-purposing as a result of cancer. McGrath (2003), for example, concludes from her qualitative research that,

> The challenge for [cancer] survivors is to create meaning for a future life in the face of devastating losses. Examples of these losses include infertility, severe educational and employment disadvantage, altered physical self, loss of prior identity, family and relationship pain, fear of relapse, and loss of naivete about life. (McGrath, 2003: 31).

The search for, and the making of, meaning is an existential human concern that is expressed through individual and collective beliefs, behaviours and practices, and shaped through personal experience and social engagement (Cobb et al., 2012a). For some people, the way

Table 27.1 Secular, spiritual and religious meaning-making

Existential meaning-making	Knowing: cognition	Doing: practice	Being: importance
Secular	Secular existential values Secular existential beliefs/concepts Existential knowledge Organization/membership Certainty/orthodoxy/fundamentalism Quest – doubts – seeking Secular views on afterlife Intervention by higher principles	Organized activity/participation/attendance concerning secular values Organization involvement/membership/activity Study/discussion/activity in groups Secular ritual participation Private existential reading Secular television/radio/internet	Salience/self-rated value-commitment Secular existential experience Intrinsic/extrinsic orientation Financial support given/received Existential wellbeing/struggle Coping possibilities/support Personal history of values Development/maturity Attitudes/consequence of attitudes
Spiritual	Spiritual values Spiritual beliefs/concepts Spiritual knowledge Organization/membership Certainty – orthodoxy – fundamentalism Quest – doubts – seeking Spiritual views on afterlife Spiritual intervention	Organized activity/participation/attendance Organization involvement/membership/activity Study/discussion/meditation/prayer in groups Ritual participation Private reading/prayer/meditation/mysticism Spiritual television/radio/internet	Salience/self-rated spirituality Spiritual experience Intrinsic/extrinsic orientation Financial support given/received Spiritual wellbeing/struggle Coping possibilities/support Personal history of spirituality Development/maturity Attitudes/consequence of attitudes
Religious[a]	Religious values Religious beliefs/creedal assent/concepts of God Religious knowledge Non-belief (denial of religion) Certainty – orthodoxy – fundamentalism Quest – doubts – seeking Religious views on afterlife Divine intervention	Organized activity/participation/attendance Organization involvement/membership/activity Study/discussion/prayer in groups Ritual participation Private reading/prayer/devotionalism/non-organized religiosity Religious television/radio/internet	Salience/self-rated religiosity Religious experience Intrinsic/extrinsic orientation Financial support given/received Religious wellbeing/struggle Coping possibilities/support Personal history of religiosity Development/maturity Attitudes/consequence of attitudes

[a] All religiosity dimensions adapted from Hall et al. (2008)

Source: La Cour and Hvidt (2010)

that they understand and represent themselves and their place in the world is related to an ultimate or sacred reality through which they understand what it means to be human. These spiritual identities can be invoked, developed and organized through secular and religious forms and discourses, with the result that people often draw upon multiple sources, practices and authorities. Consequently, we must avoid sharp distinctions between the secular, spiritual and religious, and be careful to understand the terms and contexts by which individuals recognize and present their own existential concerns and spiritual explorations. Readers may find it helpful to refer to the conceptual grid (Table 27.1) developed by La Cour and Hvidt (2010) that aims to provide a level of clarity and coherence to this field by relating the three domains – secular existential, the spiritual and the religious – with the three dimensions of meaning-making – knowing (cognition), doing (practice) and being (importance).

RECOGNIZING SPIRITUAL AND EXISTENTIAL NEED IN CANCER CARE

If cancer services are concerned with the care of patients as persons, the spiritual dimensions of personhood need to be recognized and addressed in the structures, processes and outcomes of care. There is tendency in healthcare for concerns to be pathologized and problem-focused, and spiritual and existential issues can be dealt with in this way, but this ignores the potential for spirituality to also play a positive role in a person's life, which can foster wellbeing and quality of life. It is this balanced approach that allows cancer care to determine the beneficial spiritual resources and capacity that a person already has, whilst recognizing where people may need help and support. In the UK, cancer services are expected to carry out an **Holistic Needs Assessment** (HNA) for people with cancer that provides a consistent means for the multidisciplinary team to identify the physical, social, psychological and spiritual needs of the patient across the care pathway from diagnosis, treatment and into survivorship or end-of-life care pathways (National Cancer Action Team, 2011). Similarly, in the USA, the National Quality Forum includes spiritual, religious, and existential aspects of care in their quality framework for palliative care, and that should be addressed as part of a comprehensive interdisciplinary assessment. (National Quality Forum, 2006). What both of these sets of guidelines point to is the need for a systematic approach to spiritual care at significant phases along the care pathway that should be documented in patient records and included in a patient's care plan. Without this purposeful approach, significant elements of a person's wellbeing and quality of life may be neglected, and spiritual difficulties may be misunderstood and unresolved.

A cancer service needs to give proper consideration to how best to incorporate spiritual assessments into its routines and practices, what its purpose is and how it will respond to and manage the outcomes of an assessment, including care planning and referral. The multidisciplinary team should review their capacity and capability for undertaking spiritual assessments to ensure they can be done safely and competently, and where necessary, they should seek the advice and input of a specialist, usually a healthcare chaplain. This review should identify training and supervision needs of team members, and it should be based upon an holistic model of care that underpins the approach of the service. In addition, the service should review the information it provides to patients, the documentation it uses for patient care and the processes it follows to manage the care pathway to ensure that these support the requirements for effective spiritual care. It is also helpful for services to develop an inventory of available spiritual care resources, including facilities, information and support, and this should pay particular attention to the spiritual and religious characteristics of the patient population.

The assessment of spiritual and existential needs can be approached on a number of levels from the explicit and pragmatic aspects of a person's spirituality, such as the need to meditate or desire to reconnect with a faith community, through to the tacit forms that mediate and disclose spirituality, such as the use of metaphors and symbols (Stanworth, 2004). Objective spiritual needs of patients may be captured by checklists and questionnaires but a fuller understanding will only emerge through relationships of trust, authentic concern and attentiveness. Assessment instruments are, therefore, a starting place and offer healthcare professionals some solid ground on which to begin exploring what can be an extensive territory. The five-item assessment framework for spiritual wellbeing is an example of this approach (National Cancer Action Team, 2007; see Table 27.2). Importantly, clinical assessment instruments developed to support patient care should be distinguished from tools and instruments designed for the purpose of answering research questions and measuring specific items (McSherry and Ross, 2010).

Table 27.2   Assessment framework for spiritual wellbeing

Item	Guidance for assessor and suggested prompts
Faith/belief	An introductory, exploratory question to determine the patient's existing faith/belief, be it 'religious' or non-religious, conventional or unconventional.
Worries and challenges	Identify the person's worries related to spiritual wellbeing, and the challenges they perceive.
	Impact of diagnosis or illness on faith. Coping with impact of diagnosis.
Needs related to spiritual wellbeing	Identify practical, support or other needs related to religion or spiritual matters.
	Religious items (e.g. religious texts or books, prayer mat, religious objects, holy water).
	Someone to speak to: faith leader or minister (e.g. minister, chaplain, vicar, priest, imam, rabbi, spiritual leader, church leader), or other person.
	Help. Things to help you practice. Prayer. Prayer with other people or family. Chapel. Prayer room. Space to pray. Quiet room. Privacy. Private space. Ablution.
Restrictions related to culture or belief system	Practical, support or other restrictions related to person's cultural or ethic background, or belief system.
	Requirements. Restrictions. Diet. Medicines. Treatment products (e.g. blood products). Transplantation.
Life goals	Person's concerns or desires regarding a 'goal' they want to achieve in their life, such as attending a forthcoming wedding.
	Important occasions. Family gatherings. Holidays. Big events.

Source: National Cancer Action Team (2007)

It can be helpful to follow a two-stage approach to spiritual assessment, with the first stage ascertaining the relevance and importance of spiritual and existential issues for the patient, along with information related to their treatment and care. The outcome of this preliminary screening may result in a more comprehensive inquiry about a person's spiritual orientation and its relationship to their experience of living with cancer. One approach to the first stage is modelled on medical history taking, which aims to generate a comprehensive view of a patient's health and wellbeing, concerns and problems. This structured consultation is a purposeful way for initiating discussion about the four domains of person-centred care (physical, psychological, spiritual and social) and exploring issues that the patient wishes to address. **Spiritual history taking**, as it has become known, therefore forms one element of a consultation with the aim of generating salient information for the care team. Services will need to agree on how extensive this first stage should be and may limit it to a simple screening assessment. The following example from an American palliative care context provides a fuller approach to the spiritual history.

Key elements of spirituality in palliative care

- Invite all patients to share spiritual and religious beliefs, and to define what spirituality is for them and their spiritual goals.
- Learn about the patient's beliefs and values.
- Assess for spiritual distress (meaninglessness, hopelessness) as well as for sources of spiritual strength (hope, meaning and purpose).
- Provide an opportunity for compassionate care.
- Empower the patient to find inner resources of healing and acceptance.
- Identify spiritual and religious beliefs that might affect the patient's healthcare decision-making.
- Identify spiritual practices that might be helpful in the treatment or care plan.
- Identify patients who need referral to a board-certified chaplain or other equivalently prepared spiritual care provider.

Source: Puchalski et al. (2009: 893)

Patients should determine the extent to which they wish to explore their spirituality in relation to their healthcare and they should be provided with sufficient information to understand why this is offered as an integral aspect of a cancer service. Following an initial spiritual screening or history taking, patients may wish to follow this with a more in-depth assessment where this is considered helpful. A spiritual assessment, in contrast to a spiritual history, provides a patient with the dedicated space to explore the positive and problematic aspects of their spirituality and to develop with the professional undertaking the assessment an agreed response. Assessment processes of this potential depth and reflexivity need to be contained within clear and consistent boundaries that enable ethical practice within the context of an effective therapeutic relationship. There should be clarity within the care team about the role of the competent professional undertaking this level of assessment, and some form of clinical supervision should be integral to their practice.

There is an emerging picture based on research with patients that is beginning to outline some of the elements of spirituality that may be significant to the lives of patients living with and beyond cancer, but this is currently neither extensive nor critically robust (Stefanek et al., 2005). A recent integrative literature review (Henoch and Danielson, 2009) of qualitative studies that described existential concerns of people with cancer suggests two main themes. The first was the struggle to maintain **self-identity** and included values in life (creating meaning, purpose and hope) and coping in relation to the divine (God). This latter theme was expressed in terms of trust in God, spiritual practice and the making sense of life in relation to the sacred. The second was the threats to self-identity and included loss of life-values (hopelessness), relationships (aloneness) and suffering (guilt, uncertainty and fear of dying) (Henoch and Danielson, 2009). These themes illustrate something of the extensive territory of spiritual and existential issues through which healthcare professionals will be dependent largely on patients to be a guide to their sources of spiritual wellbeing and concerns and struggles.

RESPONDING TO NEED IN CANCER CARE

It has been a major theme of this chapter that cancer can challenge the meaning of our existence and our ability to maintain a sense of who we are, which for some are mediated through existential, spiritual and religious forms. At a practical level, when people face illness they can become dislocated from personal and social sources of meaning due to the demands of treatment and its effects. The experience of being a patient can also diminish people's dignity when healthcare all too easily denies the subjectivity of being a person in all its dimensions. In response to the potential threats to the self and the damage that healthcare services are capable of inflicting, cancer care must place the compassionate understanding of the lived experience of patients central to its purpose. Spirituality for some patients plays an important role in how they understand themselves and live their lives, and cancer services should, therefore, consider how they can offer a positive approach that recognizes, respects and supports spirituality as part of the care they offer.

Against this positive background, and allied with the sensitivity and skills of the care team, a core approach is to foster and promote meaning in – and of – life. The timing and level at which this occurs will be set by the patient and there are a range of practices that can contribute to the spiritual and existential care of patients, from foundational humanistic care to highly specialized therapies and interventions. Relevant therapeutic modalities that have been reported in the literature are largely based upon **psychotherapeutic** interventions. Lethborg and colleagues (2008), for example, have proposed a model of adjustment to cancer in which they construe adjustment as, '… the struggle to achieve meaning in the face of suffering.' (2008: 62). This has led to the development of MaP (meaning and purpose) therapy, a brief individualized narrative-based intervention with the aim of enhancing the cognitive, existential and social components of meaning in the context of the physical impact and treatment of cancer. A small pre-pilot study (Lethborg et al., 2012) that explored the patient experience of MaP reported that:

> Results illustrate how the therapist creates a therapeutic frame that holds up a poignant portrayal of the meaning of life lived and mirrors this to the patient, such that the patient can grasp its rich texture. Participants were buoyed forward as a result with renewed vigor and enthusiasm, despite their illness and any related physical

restrictions. In this sense, they are transcended, spiritually uplifted, and sustained and able to focus on purpose in life alongside the challenges of advanced cancer. (Lethborg et al., 2012: 187).

Another example of a brief individualized intervention to address psychosocial and existential distress in patients with advanced cancer comes from Chochinov and colleagues (2005) and is known as **Dignity Therapy**. A unique aspect of this therapy is that sessions are audio-recorded, transcribed, edited and returned to patients for further editorial corrections and for sharing, if desired, with family members and friends. A multi-site randomized controlled trial (with Dignity Therapy as a study arm) (Chochinov et al., 2011) reported no significant difference across study arms for the primary outcome measures, which included anxiety and depression, spiritual wellbeing and quality of life. The study reported that secondary outcomes, however, measured via a post-study survey showed that patients who received Dignity Therapy,

> … were significantly more likely to report benefits, in terms of finding it helpful, improving their quality of life, their sense of dignity; changing how their family might see or appreciate them, and deeming it helpful to their family, compared to the other study arms. (Chochinov et al., 2011).

A Danish prospective study evaluating Dignity Therapy reported that after immediately completing Dignity Therapy,

> … between 47% and 56% indicated that DT [Dignity Therapy] had heightened their sense of purpose, sense of dignity or will to live, and between 25% and 43% thought DT had made life more meaningful, lessened suffering or expected DT to change the family's appreciation of him or her. (Houmann, Chochinov, Kristjanson et al., 2013).

Interventions that focus more explicitly on spirituality include spiritually integrated counselling (Thorne, 2012) and psychotherapy (Pargament, 2007), pastoral care (Doehring, 2006) and spiritual care (Nolan, 2012), and these draw largely upon well developed clinical or pastoral practices. There is currently a paucity of interventional studies related to these practices, although there are studies that report the significance of spiritualty and religion to the way in which people cope with cancer (for example, Vallurupalli et al., 2012) and the importance of spirituality and spiritual care as a part of end-of-life and palliative care (Edwards et al., 2010). Common to many of these therapeutic approaches is the use of narrative to express, explore and make meaning. Personal narratives are unique **autobiographical** works that help people make sense of their lives, and they are crafted from both internal accounts and external sources. Narrative-based approaches are useful for many aspects of psychological and social issues in cancer care, and in relation to spirituality there are both individual experiences related to people's spiritual beliefs and faith, and collective narratives such as the enduring stories of faith traditions that may provide contexts and resources for meaning:

Not only do language and narrative help sustain and create the fabric of everyday life, they feature prominently in the repair and restoring of meanings when they are threatened. Under conditions of adversity, individuals often feel a pressing need to re-examine and re-fashion their personal narrative in an attempt to maintain a sense of identity. (Bury, 2001: 264).

Spirituality is also expressed and experienced in other forms such as ritual, the significance of place and through belonging to a faith or belief community. An assessment of spirituality may, therefore, identify sources of meaning and support that cannot be addressed through the skills of the care team, or through standard therapeutic interventions, and this may require external referrals with the consent of the patient. This will be made easier for services who have developed some contextual knowledge of the population they serve, including faith communities and their ministers, and who have an extended multidisciplinary team that includes healthcare chaplains and practitioners of psychological therapies.

CHAPTER SUMMARY

Spirituality is a way that people seek meaning and purpose in their lives and respond to the tremendous possibilities of existence. There are many forms of spirituality that help people understand their place in the world and make sense of their experience, and those related to religions are the most prominent. The relationship between health and spirituality is beginning to be explored through empirical research and it may contribute to people's wellbeing and influence their response to disease. However, a person's spirituality may also be challenged or dislocated as a result of a serious or life-limiting disease and this may lead to existential demoralization and suffering. This chapter explored some of the impact that cancer can have on spiritual wellbeing and existential security through the lens of meaning and the challenge of maintaining and creating meaning in the face of human vulnerability and finitude. It looked at a person-centred approach to cancer care that begins with an holistic needs assessment, and explored a two-stage process of spiritual screening and history taking, followed by a more in-depth patient-led assessment. Finally, it considered how cancer services can promote meaning and foster spiritual wellbeing and identified some of the resources and specialist approaches that may be of benefit to patients.

Reflective activity

- What is the extent of your knowledge and understanding of spiritual and existential issues and what are your unmet learning needs in relation to your role?
- How does your practice support the spiritual and existential dimensions of patients?
- In what ways does the organization in which you work positively promote the respect and understanding of spirituality and in what areas are there room for development?

Key learning points

- The beliefs and meanings by which people shape and orientate their lives may be disrupted by a diagnosis of cancer and the illness experience.
- Spirituality can make a positive contribution to wellbeing, and people living with cancer may have well-developed spiritual resources to draw upon.
- Some people living with cancer may be spiritually distressed and benefit from specific support and interventions.
- An holistic approach to cancer care should include spirituality as a dimension of the assessment of needs and planning of care.
- The multidisciplinary team should review their capacity and capability for understanding and addressing spiritual needs.

Recommended further reading

- Gordon, T., Kelly, E. and Mitchell, D.R. (2011) *Spiritual Care for Healthcare Professionals: Reflecting on Clinical Practice*. London: Radcliffe.
- Kliewer, S. and Saultz, J.W. (2006) *Healthcare and Spirituality*. Oxford: Radcliffe.
- Puchalski, C.M. and Ferrell, B. (2010) *Making Healthcare Whole: Integrating Spirituality into Healthcare*. West Conshohocken, PA: Templeton Press.

28 ADJUSTING TO THE PALLIATIVE PHASE AND PREPARING FOR END OF LIFE

ALISON CONNER AND KATHRYN MANNIX

Chapter outline

- Evolution of palliative care
- Key concepts in palliative care
- Palliative phase of disease management

- A model of how patients (and clinician) adjust to end-of-life care
- Working with patients approaching the end of life
- Care in the last few days of life

INTRODUCTION

Palliative care is the clinical science of **holistic symptom management** to improve **quality of life**, and it may be needed at various points over the cancer journey from diagnosis to cure. However, a significant proportion of people with cancer present with cancer too far advanced for cure to be an option. Others are initially treated with curative intent but their disease either relapses or fails to respond to curative treatment. A third group may decline the option of curative treatment because they feel the burdens of treatment outweigh the benefit of extending their lives, or they may have co-morbidities that prevent them tolerating curative treatment, for example advanced respiratory disease may prevent the possibility of major surgery to cure a resectable cancer. These patients with **incurable** disease may be said to be in the Palliative Phase: treatment is now primarily concerned with reducing the symptoms of their illness and maximizing their quality of life.

DEVELOPING THE SPECIALTY OF PALLIATIVE CARE

History and philosophy of palliative care in cancer

In the twenty-first century, oncology and palliative care are closely linked specialities with an obvious symbiotic relationship, but these two specialities have developed this relationship relatively recently. In fact, development of collaborative working between oncologists and palliative care physicians only began in the 1980s; prior to this, there was a tension between these two medical specialties that led to them being seen as mutually exclusive.

The origin of the tension between oncology and palliative care lay in the 'quest for cure' as the model for the development of cancer treatment. This focus of cancer management in the mid-twentieth century was on developing anticancer treatments to prolong life and avoid death, rather than a consideration of cancer prevention or screening. The treatments developed included surgery, radiation and early chemotherapy. Any clinical or philosophical consideration of lightening the **burden of suffering** for the patient was pushed aside in the pursuit of curative therapy, which could possibly eliminate the need for palliation. This approach provided increasingly aggressive treatments and the language of the disease became that of cancer 'victims' who needed to 'fight against' their deadly illness, even to the point that a 'war on cancer' was declared by President Nixon as one of his party's policies in the 1970s (Lewis, 2007). This research-based quest has paid great dividends in the development of new and better anticancer treatments, but sometimes at great cost to those patients whose cancer was not curable, who were often overlooked or even abandoned by their physicians. In the 1950s and 1960s, many patients with cancer reported being told to go home because nothing more could be done.

In response, a few doctors, psychiatrists and social workers began to collect evidence that the drive to cure was failing in many cases, and that it left incurable or dying patients suffering both physically and emotionally. Among these concerned professionals was Cicely Saunders, who went on to found the modern British hospice movement. Initially, she focused on terminal care for those with cancer, building a collection of patients' stories to articulate the relationship between physical and emotional suffering. This led to her concept of 'total pain', which includes physical symptoms, mental distress, social problems and emotional difficulties (Saunders, 1978). This was the beginning of what is now commonly called an holistic approach, an approach that is employed in most aspects of modern nursing care and medicine.

The early palliative care pioneers retained the scientific approach of collecting evidence, developing and refining their treatments based on review, and assessment of their outcomes that had proved so successful in advancing cancer treatment developments. Many clinical and organizational studies provided an evidence base for the development of pharmacological approaches and psychological therapies for symptom management to relieve suffering whilst not hastening death. In this way, a new, symptom-focused approach emerged from the recognition of poor care of the dying and led to the birth of modern hospice and palliative care (Clark, 2007). The thrust of this new speciality of palliative care was to marry scientifically rigorous expertise with a human response to patients' extreme vulnerability.

Both oncology and palliative care shared a regard for evidence-based treatments: cancers often responded initially to newly discovered treatments, then relapsed after a period of remission, leading oncologists to recognize that many oncology treatments are, in fact, palliative in their effect; meanwhile, palliative physicians began to acknowledge that many oncological treatments reduce tumour bulk and thus reduce symptoms. Both specialities recognized that the patient experience is much better when the two specialities work together. To describe this evolving partnership of the specialities in the developed world, Bruera and Yennurajalingam (2012) describe three models of care employed in the last 40 years, beginning with a solo model in the 1970s, when a patient was managed by an oncologist until it seemed no more could be done and then referred to palliative care to manage 'the end'; progressing in the 1980s to a collaborative model with many oncology clinics providing palliative care sessions concurrently; to an integrated model in which oncologists and palliative care physicians run joint clinics where patients can see both specialists at the same time or easily move from one to the other as necessary. The shift from sequential to collaborative care is illustrated in Figure 28.1.

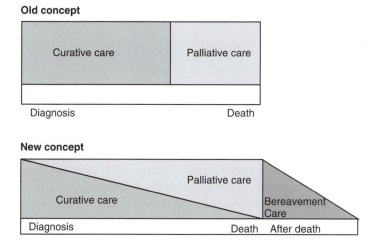

Figure 28.1   Models of palliative care

Source: Adapted from Lynn and Adamson (2003)

Current provision of palliative care

Today, the World Health Organization (WHO), defines palliative care as:

> an approach that improves the quality of life of patients and their families facing the problem associated with life-threatening illness, through the prevention and relief of suffering by means of early identification and impeccable assessment and treatment of pain and other problems, physical, psychosocial and spiritual. Palliative care is applicable early in the course of illness, in conjunction with other therapies that are intended to prolong life, such as chemotherapy or radiation therapy, and includes those investigations needed to better understand and manage distressing clinical complications.' (WHO, 2013a)

This definition shows that palliation is now recognized as being important throughout a patient's illness: oncological treatments and palliative therapies can be administered simultaneously, and both approaches are not only possible together, but can also improve each other. It has been shown that patients who have concurrent oncological and palliative treatments not only experience improved quality of life and mood, but also have **prolonged survival** in some cases (Temel et al., 2010; Bakitas et al., 2009).

The development of a working partnership between oncology and palliative care is clearly beneficial for patients, but it currently represents the experience of a privileged minority. The global picture of cancer is quite different from that of the developed world. In 2002, the WHO estimated that of all cases of cancer worldwide, one-third are preventable, one-third are potentially curable, and the remaining third need relief of suffering and improvements in quality of life through palliative care. They predicted that by 2050 cancer deaths globally will rise to 24 million and that half of all people with cancer will live in developing countries where healthcare systems are under developed or absent (WHO, 2002). Of those countries around the world with healthcare systems, only 34 currently have palliative care integrated into mainstream services. There is still much work to be done to get the right care and treatment to those who need it most.

Palliative care specialist services

Most palliative care services provide holistic care for patients and families via a multidisciplinary team of experts who work together to achieve the best possible quality of living for their patients. This includes doctors and nurses, for whom there is recognized post-graduate specialist training in palliative care in the UK, and also disciplines such as social work, psychology, occupational therapy and physiotherapy. Most teams have access to advisors in the disciplines of pharmacy, chaplaincy, dietetics, speech and language therapy and other specialist advisors as necessary.

In the UK, palliative care originated in hospices and gradually developed to include liaison teams working in the community to advise primary healthcare teams, and hospital teams to advise consultants and ward teams. These teams offer evidence-based advice and support to other clinical teams about the potential for improving patients' quality of life by addressing physical symptoms, attention to emotional needs, offering advice and support about social needs as diverse as preparing children/grandchildren for the patient's death to financial advice to meet bills, access to benefits, etc. Symptom management relies on a careful balance between medical interventions and non-drug measures. Most palliative care nurse specialists have a well-developed knowledge of a range of drug-based interventions, for example selection and careful titration of analgesic drugs including opioids, or selection of anti-emetics depending on the origin of the symptoms of nausea and vomiting.

CASE STUDY

Martin

Martin had bone secondaries from prostate cancer causing a fracture in his pelvis. He was unable to sit up in bed without pain and minimal movement caused excruciating pelvic pain that settled when he was still. His palliative care nurse specialist recognized that drug treatment alone would be unhelpful because his worst pain was short-lived and movement-related. Her recommendations to the ward team caring for Martin included careful positioning in bed and for toileting; referral to a physiotherapist for advice about optimizing mobility including use of aids and appliances; consideration of referral for radiotherapy to his pelvis; a long-acting non-steroidal anti-inflammatory drug monitoring for kidney toxicity;

and the use of a carefully titrated dose of an opioid drug (morphine in this case) by mouth prior to being moved for episodes of personal care or investigations. She was also careful to ensure that Martin understood both the mechanism of his pain and the different treatment approaches to manage it, and that the ward team had the same understanding.

Palliative care specialist teams also have an important **educational role**. By providing advice, support and education to nurses, doctors and others, they can raise the standard of symptom management and holistic care delivered by cancer and primary care staff for patients at all stages of their cancer journey, whilst offering case consultations and direct clinical care for those patients whose physical, emotional, psychological or spiritual needs are more challenging.

The specialty of palliative care is unusual in having developed outside mainstream UK healthcare services, usually supported by charitable donations from the public to establish and maintain hospices. First recognized as a medical speciality in 1985 in the UK, it is now recommended by the UK NHS that access to specialist palliative care support be a mandatory, core element of cancer services (NICE, 2004e).

In North America, palliative care was not recognized as a speciality until 2007. Service development there has followed a different route, with establishment of mostly hospital-based palliative care teams. In 2012, 63% of US hospitals, which have 50 beds or more, had a palliative care team (Center to Advance Palliative Care, 2011). But community outreach, follow-up and development of hospices is generally following more slowly. The North American health insurance system still tends to be based around remuneration for services used and palliative care is aimed at avoidance of service use. Although evidence is emerging to show that combining oncological and palliative approaches both enhances quality of life and reduces overall costs of medical care as people are enabled to relinquish unrealistic 'quests for cure', some US patients may still have to choose between these approaches.

KEY ELEMENTS OF PALLIATIVE CARE

Good palliative care takes an holistic approach including both the patient and their loved ones or carers. It incorporates physical symptom management, function-orientated and psychosocial therapies, as well as spiritual and cultural support. There are many texts that explain the detail of the multiplicity of technologies used by palliative care specialists in the medical, nursing or allied health professions. It is not within the scope of this chapter to cover this area, but recommended reading is given at the end.

Physical symptoms

The experience of physical symptoms like pain, breathlessness, fatigue and nausea can undermine quality of life. Taking a thorough patient history that asks specifically about symptoms in a systematic way is an important part of holistic assessment. There is evidence to suggest that clinicians focus more on symptoms that they are better able to treat (e.g. pain, nausea) than on other symptoms that are harder to manage but cause the patient more concern (e.g. fatigue, anorexia). Nurses can ensure that patients are able to describe all their symptoms by offering time, listening well, offering prompts and using a structured symptom checklist (Conner and Muir, 2007).

Emotional symptoms

Sadness, concern and anger are all normal responses to living with an incurable illness and patients may benefit from telling their story, having their emotions acknowledged and having their experience 'normalized.' Emotional distress is part of the process of adjustment (see later; also Chapter 18), but mood disorders like depression or anxiety should be identified and treated (see Chapter 19). Treatments may include pharmacotherapy, time-limited psycho-therapy such as Cognitive–Behaviour Therapy (CBT), or a combination (see also Chapter 22). Studies have shown that patients with advanced cancer respond to CBT (e.g. Moorey et al., 2009). Applying psychological therapies when patients are weary requires practitioners who are familiar with working in a palliative care context. Training palliative care staff in CBT skills has been shown to be an effective way of providing help and support (Mannix et al., 2006; Moorey et al., 2009).

Social needs

Each patient is an individual belonging to a family, friendship groups and possibly a place of work (see also Chapter 20). Maintaining important social relationships, enabling patients to contribute to loved ones as well as to receive from them, and maintaining their autonomy despite decreasing physical ability are all important considerations in delivering care within a social context. Frailty may reduce a parent's ability to care for their children but does not diminish their desire to help and support; their nurse should seek ways to enable social relationships to be maintained, even if this means adjusting roles or activities.

CASE STUDY

Marion

Marion, 63, was a retired nurse. She was dying of colon cancer, and she so feared incontinence that she required someone (in addition to her husband) with her at home at all times in case she needed to get to the toilet. She adamantly refused to have a commode in her house. She was becoming exhausted.

Her palliative care nurse specialist explored Marion's ideas about the commode and her fear of incontinence. Marion tearfully described her belief that her husband would be disgusted and would cease to love her if he had to empty her commode or wipe up incontinence. This thought made her anxious, which affected her bowels so that she kept feeling the need to go to the toilet. The effort was exhausting her, and she felt too exhausted to enjoy any time with her husband.

Her nurse asked Marion what she would advise a patient in this situation. Marion said she would have advised a patient to come and be nursed by her and her team. The nurse asked her whether she would like to be looked after in this way, and Marion admitted that she was finding staying at home an exhausting struggle. Admission to a hospice was arranged, where Marion was no longer anxious and her constant drive to use the toilet settled down. She was visited daily by her husband and she allowed the hospice nurses to help her at the toilet and to wash her in preparation for her husband's visits. She felt safe in the care of the hospice nurses (several of whom she had trained) and was able to 'feel like a wife again' for the remaining three weeks of her life.

Spiritual needs

The variety of cultural, religious and spiritual beliefs a patient may hold makes each person unique, and their beliefs guide the way in which they find their own 'inner meaning' (see also Chapter 27). This meaning can only be discerned by asking them. Even two patients with the same stated religious affiliation may approach their spiritual practice in very different ways. Some people find spiritual solace in the practice of a faith, others in the cycle of nature and others in music, art or meditation with or without a belief in a deity. Questions like 'What helps you to find strength when times get very difficult?' and 'Do you see yourself as a spiritual person? Can you explain that to me?' can help a nurse to explore a patient's spiritual beliefs. When the nurse and patient are from different cultures, asking patient or family to explain customs and practices that will support or comfort them is very important.

CASE STUDY

Ashoka

Ashoka was a 45-year-old Bangladeshi housewife; she was married to Sanjay and they lived with their two children and Sanjay's mother in an English city. Ashoka and Sanjay spoke good English, as did their British-born children, but Sanjay's mother spoke only Bengali. Ashoka had ovarian cancer. Five years previously, she had had extensive surgery followed by chemotherapy and a good remission that lasted four years. Last year her cancer came back. Despite several different treatments, the cancer continued to progress, causing Ashoka to lose weight and to feel very tired. She appreciated the support of her mother-in-law in looking after her teenage children, but was anxious that the children were being kept away from her. Visiting the family home, her palliative care nurse specialist noticed that although Ashoka's symptoms were well controlled, she kept asking to be admitted to a hospice and asked her to explain why. Ashoka explained that she did not want 'to be a nuisance' to her mother-in-law, who was encouraging her to consider hospice admission even though this was a very unusual request from within the Bangladeshi community.

The nurse arranged another visit, this time with a Bengali interpreter, and she spent some time listening to the mother-in-law's concerns, particularly about the possibility that the children could 'catch' cancer from their mother. This gave the nurse an opportunity to explain that cancer is not a contagious disease, and to ask the mother-in-law what she understood about the patient's illness. With Ashoka's permission, the nurse explained the facts about Ashoka's cancer. In response to the older woman's questions, the nurse confirmed that Ashoka's life expectancy was possibly as short as weeks, and

(Continued)

(Continued)

the nurse asked her what important cultural or spiritual customs should be respected in her Muslim household. Although Ashoka's mother-in-law had been present in previous visits, the necessity of using her son as her interpreter had discouraged her from asking questions or expressing her own distress.

This opportunity for personal communication via a trained health services interpreter enabled a key family member who was not English-speaking, and who had thus become somewhat excluded, to continue her own adjustment and to offer vital support to her family whilst her daughter-in-law died in her own home, as was her wish.

PROVIDING CARE IN PALLIATIVE PHASE

When it becomes clear that a cancer illness is not curable, many patients and families begin to weigh up the costs and benefits of treatments differently in terms of quality of life. Considerations like being at home or spending time with loved ones often become more important. This could be said to be because we all have an idea of what we consider a **'good death'**. This is true for all those involved and is dependent on the value system of the patient, family or professional, as well as their cultural and faith influences (Blank and Merrick, 2005). Finding meaning in their illness, treatment and care influences patients' behaviour, mood, self-esteem and experience of control, and supporting the search for meaning is a key nursing role.

Changing attitudes to dying and death

Attitudes to death in the developed world have changed enormously over the centuries. Aries's (1974) classic examination of the history of attitudes to death explains that in the Middle Ages there was a naïve acceptance of destiny and nature, which was accompanied by practices and rituals for care of the dying and for mourning their death. By the eighteenth to nineteenth centuries, rituals were similar to the Middle Ages but became much more emotional and practices were dramatized. Death was seen as undesirable, yet admirable in its beauty. The twentieth century saw death become re-interpreted as an ordeal, with a public desire to spare the dying person both the strong emotions and the ugliness of dying. The current emphasis is on an 'acceptable death' for the individual, which their survivors can tolerate.

Palliative care practitioners have observed another shift in attitudes in the developed world to a current view that death is undesirable and even preventable, with a belief that healthy lifestyles and scientific developments can protect everyone from death. Dramatic extension of life expectancy coupled with increased likelihood of death occurring in hospitals, rather than at home, has led a whole generation to become unfamiliar with the process of dying, and so familiarity with the rituals and practices both of deathbed and of mourning have been lost. This often means that individuals find being near dying people difficult and uncomfortable, and so they may seek to avoid it both intellectually and physically.

Of course, 'Western' attitudes only represent part of the developed world's approach to illness, dying and death as cultures become more mixed in an age of global migration. In their international survey of end-of-life decision-making, Blank and Merrick (2005) provide a good guide to some important intercultural differences. For example, the cultural expectation of traditional Chinese people, Turkish Muslims, Kenyans and many from India is that children have a duty to care for their dying parents. This will cause some difficulty and distress when members of the extended family live in a distant country, so care of that dying parent needs to be taken on by an institution, such as a hospice or care home. Also, acceptance of death is different for those whose culture is built around beliefs that death is part of a continuum rather than an ending, as in India and Kenya. Culturally, some will be adamant about being fully informed of their illness and prognosis (Jewish and Chinese) and others feel it is right (and even a duty) to protect the dying from these facts (Turkish and some Japanese).

This mixture of views and the multicultural nature of modern society mean that a 'good death' is in the eye of the beholder. Healthcare professionals must discover the individual's values, desires and goals and incorporate these into care if patients are to achieve a meaningful end to their lives.

In addition, there has been a recent upsurge in a desire for personal autonomy in many cultures. There is an increasing popularity of a view of one's self as intertwined mind, body and spirit with an emphasis on the dignity and worth of individuals. This contrasts a view of the body as a machine needing to be fixed using biomedicine alone. Patient choice policies are now on the rise in the UK, parts of Europe and the USA (Blank and Merrick, 2005; DH, 2008c). It is no longer expected that the doctor will decide the treatment and inform the patient; now patients desire information so they can make informed choices for themselves. Such information may be complex, technical and sometimes distressing to hear. It needs to be delivered in language the patient can understand and at a pace that matches their adjustment process. The importance of assessing patients' competence to make such choices is paramount and their autonomy may lead to differences in their wishes from those of their families/carers/healthcare professionals.

Predicting life expectancy

Although the news that cancer cannot be cured is unwelcome, for many patients there may still be considerable life expectancy, particularly if cancer-shrinking therapies can still be employed. This means that for a large minority of patients, chemotherapy or hormone treatments can be used to reduce the size of cancer masses, slow the rate of metastatic spread and reduce the impact of the cancer on the patient's daily life. Some patients may undergo de-bulking surgery; others may have intermittent radiotherapy treatment to reduce their cancer burden or to palliate symptoms such as bone pain.

The availability of anticancer treatment for disease control even when cure is no longer possible makes it difficult to identify for sure when a patient may be entering the last phase of life, and it has been shown that doctors frequently fail to recognize this transition. Christakis and Lamont (2000) showed that cancer doctors routinely overestimate dying patients' life expectancy, and this reduces patients' opportunity to prepare themselves and their families for their decline and death. In the UK, there has been a campaign to identify people who are likely to die in the next year using a simple question for clinicians to ask themselves: 'Would I be surprised if this person dies in the next 12 months?'

Trajectories of decline in many illnesses are difficult to predict, but in cancer there is often a predictable deterioration towards the end of life (see Figure 8.2, from Murray et al., 2005) that can help in advance care planning. This 'trajectory' of decline (see Figure 28.2) may last many

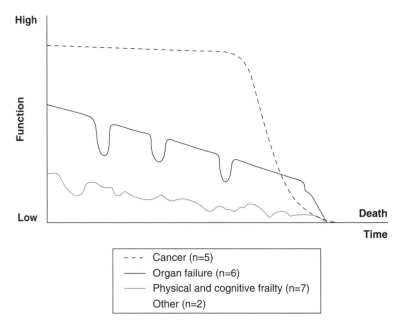

Figure 28.2   Comparison of end of life trajectories in cancer, organ failure conditions (e.g. heart failure; end-stage liver disease) and general frailty with both physical and cognitive decline (e.g. frail elderly)

Source: Murray et al. (2005)

months, or may progress very quickly. Recognizing the pattern of change in energy levels and stamina is often the best guide to estimating the patient's life expectancy. As energy levels are reduced by advancing disease, the patient may notice that they are more tired after completing tasks that previously had no impact; later, they may become unable to perform some tasks or need several attempts with rests in between to complete the task. This gentle decline can be used as a benchmark. If there is noticeable reduction in energy and stamina from one month to the next, then life expectancy is probably measurable in months (possibly enough months to make a year or more); if energy reduction is noticeable week by week, then life expectancy is probably down to weeks into months. Towards the end of life, deterioration in energy levels and alertness can be observed day by day, and this is usually a sign that life expectancy is only measurable in days.

How patients and families adjust to the anticipation of dying

Adjusting to the news that the end of life is approaching is one of the 'emotional tasks' of advanced cancer. Grieving for a lost future with its plans, expectations and time with dear ones becomes bereavement for self that cancer patients work through. Worden's 'Tasks of Grieving' model (2008), initially developed to describe the process of bereavement experienced by widows, is a useful model to describe how patients with cancer deal with this challenge (see also Chapter 29). The following section of this chapter outlines an adaptation of Worden's model for end of life adjustment.

Accept the reality of the loss: For some patients, the news that their disease is incurable and life limiting is a surprise and **shock**. Some are unable to accept the news straight away and need time to reflect, support to review the evidence and opportunities to ask further questions. Other patients are not surprised; they have noticed that they are less well and have often guessed that their symptoms indicate a very serious new diagnosis, or relapse of a previously treated cancer. Some patients, especially those who have been anticipating bad news, feel **relieved** that their uncertainty is over. They prefer to know what they need to deal with; their anxiety about possible scenarios is replaced by a definite answer. Nevertheless, they will encounter the distress of acknowledging the now certain loss of any better news.

Process the pain of the loss: Considering the reality of the poor prognosis involves re-imagining the future. This future will be shorter, involving ill health, the distress of loved ones, the loss of future anticipated pleasures or important roles (particularly poignant when the patient had anticipated being the strong and healthy carer of children, an infirm spouse or relative), the loss of self and the bereavement of loved ones whom they will not be present to console. Health professionals who are breaking bad news would do well to bear in mind that enabling a patient to appreciate the reality of the bad news will allow them to move to the second task (i.e. feeling the pain and distress of their loss). Breaking bad news with sensitivity and skill, at a pace that is suitable for the patient, will open up a new and distressing view of the future that is likely to result in expressions of sadness and anxiety. This does not mean that the news was broken badly.

Re-engage with the remainder of life, from which the lost expectation is missing: Many people with cancer describe the bittersweet sensation of 'the last Christmas' and other occasions traditionally associated with family and happiness. After a diagnosis of incurable cancer, a patient develops a new perspective on the lifetime's collection of objects in the loft, the 'never done' items on their to-do list, the feuds or enmities they have encountered and the apologies they always intended to make. They encounter life with an expectation of foreshortening, and this influences both long-term planning and daily experiences.

Withdraw the emotion invested in the lost expectation, and re-invest it elsewhere: Although emotional distress can be a feature of end-stage cancer, the majority of people do not succumb to major depression or anxiety disorder (Sage et al., 2008). Human **resilience** enables cancer patients to plan for their own death, and for a future for their dear ones without them. This is an example of re-investing their love for dear ones into making their shared end-of-life experience, and the survivors' bereavement experience, as smooth as possible. Professionals who work with patients preparing for death can enable patients to use this resilience, for example, to prepare bereavement support materials for family members like memory boxes for children surviving the death of a parent, or recording **advance care plans**. This is a time when patients may want to prepare statements of their preferences for care at the end of life, including **Advance Decisions to Refuse Treatment** (ADRTs) (enforceable by law in the UK) and **Emergency Health Care Plans**.

Worden's model is useful in enabling professionals to notice how patients and families are adapting to the idea of short life expectancy. Sometimes patients and individual family members may move through the tasks at different paces, and this can lead to misunderstandings.

Bill

Bill was 62-years-old and not terribly surprised when his doctor told him that he had an incurable lung cancer. Bill has smoked for fifty years (from the age of 12), had suffered chest problems every winter for the last ten years and had recently coughed up blood on a few occasions. He was feeling very tired, and was breathless most of the time. He felt he had become a burden to his beloved wife Eileen, who was still 'very young' at 59 years of age. Bill's biggest regret was in leaving Eileen alone, because their children and grandchildren live in Australia. He thought that if he could die sooner, Eileen would be free to travel to Australia so he took an overdose of the morphine tablets he was taking to palliate his breathlessness. Eileen was outraged and angry with him. She did not yet accept that he was too ill to survive more than a few months, and could not comprehend why he would want to leave her when she was just about to retire so that they could fulfil their shared plans to take cruises together in their retirement. When Eileen was helped to explore her understanding of Bill's situation, she understood that he had acted to protect her and also realized for the first time that she would be a widow very soon after her retirement. She decided to retire early; she and Bill took a 'round the world' cruise with their savings and disembarked in Australia, where Bill died a few weeks later with his family around him and his beloved wife safely supported by their children.

What people hope for when cure is no longer an option

Discussion of incurability causes great anxiety for many healthcare professionals and family members, who equate the news of incurability with 'removal of hope'. This can lead them to avoid communicating honestly in an attempt to reduce distress, because patients tell us that hope is an important issue (Conner et al., 2008). Penson et al. (2007) describe hope as a belief in a positive outcome despite the circumstances – an emotional, mood-based, fluid response that overlaps with resilience, adaptation, spirituality and human relationships. It is fundamental to psychological wellbeing and it is, therefore, very important for health professionals to acquire the skills of fostering hope. Advancing disease is usually very obvious to the patient who can become isolated by a well-meaning conspiracy by family and/or professionals to disguise the truth from them. Communicating at the patient's pace, exploring their perceptions and acknowledging uncertainty allows patients to grasp the reality of their situation and adjust to it. The skills of fostering hope include providing realistic, honest information about the disease and emphasizing therapeutic options whilst being emotionally responsive, supportive and facilitating coping (Hagerty et al., 2005). Patients can then move to live with parallel realities: hope for a miracle cure or remission, realization of the terminal nature of the illness, hope of reaching realistic shorter-term goals (e.g. to take a family holiday, to see a special event like the birth of a grandchild, to complete an important task or fulfil an ambition).

Knowledge of incurability enables patients to prioritize their goals in a way that could have felt selfish if they believed they had many years of healthy life ahead. In this way, patients can live in an attitude of 'hoping for the best whilst planning for the worst', calling upon their resilience to work through the tasks of adjustment whilst being able to 'escape' into hopefulness or denial for periods of time.

Carol

Carol is 37, a single mum with two children, works part-time as an administrator for a local factory where she has many friends and is very close to her parents who live nearby.

Carol was diagnosed with ovarian cancer two years ago, which initially responded well to treatment, but a recent CT scan shows multiple abdominal metastases despite a recent course of chemotherapy. She has had recurrent ascites over the last two months, needing paracentesis twice for acute symptoms of abdominal pain, persistent vomiting and constipation. She is waiting for a discussion with her oncologist about the next step in treatment. All treatment so far has been with curative intent.

Dr M began by exploring how Carol had been feeling recently, physically and functionally, as well as 'in her spirits'. He asked how she thought the treatment had been going and what she was expecting from today's consultation. Carol admitted she was worried by the new symptoms and scared that the cancer was spreading. She'd been feeling nervous, shaky, restless and irritable, and having vivid dreams in which she had died and her children were crying and unable to cope without her. In these dreams, the house was a shambles, her son had 'dropped out' and Sarah had stopped going to school. After acknowledging how frightening these dreams must be and that this level of sleep deprivation and worry would lead to irritability, the doctor went on to say,

> Unfortunately you are right – the scan shows that the cancer has spread. But there are ways to manage the symptoms you've been having and there may be more chemotherapy to slow tumour growth without too many side effects. The aim of treatment now is not to cure the disease, it's most important to help you feel as well as possible so you can get on with the things that are important to you.

At this point Carol began to cry and said she had known deep down that this was what he would tell her today. She was so scared about what would happen to her and the children and how soon she would become too ill to look after them.

Dr M sat with her while she cried for a few minutes and then said,

> This is obviously upsetting. It's a lot to take in and it'll take time to think it through. Some of the things you're worried about aren't things that we can address properly in a short outpatient consultation. I recommend that you have some time with the palliative care nurse in the next few days to discuss things in depth and get more information, help or advice.

Over the next few weeks, Carol was very sad about the new situation. She now knew that there was to be no cure, but she was determined to live as long as possible and make the most of her life. Her bad dreams and anxiety symptoms reduced. She decided to cut her working hours so she could have more fun time with her children, yet keep her friends and sense of purpose, which came with her job. With her usual resilience and the support of her parents, friends and palliative care nurse, she was able to focus on her wish to prepare her children for losing her. She found ways to teach her nearly adult son to be domestically

(Continued)

(Continued)

capable (cook a few meals, use the vacuum, pay bills, etc.) and to set up a supportive, caring social network for him because he would probably choose to live independently. She also made legal arrangements for her parents to be guardians for her daughter and told them of her thoughts and desires for her upbringing. In this way, Carol was able to live with parallel realities: planning for how her children would manage after her death but hoping for a long time with her family and friends enjoying life.

As death approaches, hope is adjusted to even smaller and more immediate goals, like place of care and who will be present; relief of symptoms; and hopes based on spiritual or cultural beliefs. Spiritual wellbeing is associated with reduced psychological distress in patients with advanced cancer (McClain et al., 2003).

PROACTIVE PLANNING OF CARE

Facilitating adjustment

If a patient and family understand that cure is no longer possible, then they may need encouragement and support to accomplish the tasks of adjustment. They may all be at different stages in accepting the reality, and may move through adjustment at different paces, which can lead to conflict. Shock and disbelief may slow progress in accepting the reality that death is approaching. Complete denial is unusual but when a patient can maintain complete denial, they can avoid the distress that is a necessary part of the adjustment process (see also Chapter 18). Listening carefully to patients and family members describing how they are currently coping will give the nurse some useful information and insights into how each is progressing in their adjustment tasks. Excellent communication skills begin with the ability to listen: open-ended questions, which invite a patient or loved one to reflect on their situation ('How are things going?', 'How are you managing recently?'), may elicit concerns that a nurse would not guess were important.

Advance care planning

One way to help address concerns is to help the patient express their preferences for future care, thus increasing their sense of control. Planning care in advance is a process that patients and families may engage in fully, partly or not at all. There may be specific health professionals that a particular patient would wish to discuss their preferences with. There may be some days when they find the concept of their ultimate death too troubling to talk about, and other days when they find this discussion easier or even find that such planning gives them a helpful sense of purpose and engagement.

Planning of future care is not a single event or conversation. Patients may use a nurse as a 'sounding board' while exploring many ideas and possibilities. They may change their minds as their disease progresses, so checking their preferences is important. A nurse can support this process by using gentle probe questions, encouraging them to consider pros and cons of each idea, accepting each without judgement and being sensitive to cultural issues. There is no 'right' way to approach the end of life for any individual or family. Summarizing the patient's thoughts at times during the conversation and then at the end also helps them to clarify their ideas, and a written summary for the patient can trigger further discussion with family or significant others.

Listening and eliciting concerns will be part of all interactions between patients, families and health professionals, although some professionals may not feel confident in addressing those concerns and some may find it difficult to deal with the strong emotions experienced or expressed by all involved. It is vital that there are recognized mechanisms to flag any issues that have not been addressed in order that more senior colleagues with the appropriate knowledge, skills and responsibility can offer focused advice, support or counselling and that the patient is not left feeling their concerns have been ignored. In particular, palliative care nurse specialists can offer expertise in symptom management and psychosocial therapies, as well as in end-of-life care. Their specialist expertise and experience of managing patients with progressing disease allows them to anticipate physical and/or psychological events to facilitate holistic proactive planning. They are also familiar with the many ways individuals use their personal resilience to tackle the tasks of adjustment.

Managing the process of advance planning of care in a timely fashion, so that care is given and treatments are accessed appropriately, means the need for skilled communicators in healthcare is more important than ever (see Chapter 17).

Terry

Terry was a 62-year-old man with inoperable stomach cancer and liver metastases. He had a few months relief of symptoms following palliative chemotherapy, but was now becoming frail, weary and anxious. His own mother had died of stomach cancer when he was a young man still living at home, and he remembered that she vomited blood and that he had found this very frightening.

Terry expressed a wish to die at home if this was possible, and to avoid invasive treatments. He was troubled by abdominal pain and occasional vomiting. He had no appetite and was afraid to drink in case he vomited afterwards. His GP and district nurse worked with the community palliative care team to control Terry's pain and nausea, although intermittent retching persisted and occasionally with blood streaks. Terry declined further investigation of his bleeding and said he did not want to be 'dragged off in an ambulance', so his district nurse asked him to participate in making an Emergency Health Care Plan (EHCP).

In his EHCP, the district nurse described the steps that his GP, district nurse and palliative care nurse specialist had agreed with Terry and his wife as follows:

- If Terry vomits blood, family can remind him that we have a plan for this and help him to relax. He may have a cup of tea or other fluids if he wishes. Use dark-coloured towels to catch any blood splashes.
- If vomiting blood continues and/or Terry is very anxious about it, family should phone the district nurse base and ask for a visit. Show the nurse this plan when s/he arrives.

(Continued)

CASE STUDY

(Continued)

District nurse actions:

Terry knows he has end-stage stomach cancer and he wants to die in his own home. If he develops blood-stained vomiting, he wishes to remain at home. There are 'just in case' drugs in a sealed box in his kitchen cupboard. Please refer to the EHCP prescription sheet if these are needed.

- If Terry is nauseated, please give subcutaneous cyclizine 50 mg. This can be repeated up to once in every six hours.
- If Terry has abdominal pain, please give subcutaneous morphine 20 mg. This can be repeated at 30-minute intervals until his pain settles. If several doses are required, please commence a continuous subcutaneous infusion, commencing with morphine 120 mg in 24 hours and STOP his oral slow-release morphine, which is replaced by this infusion. (Learning note: the starting dose of subcutaneous morphine for pain in a patient not already taking opioid pain killers would be very much lower than this.)
- If Terry is restless, anxious or agitated, please offer him subcutaneous midazolam 2.5 mg. This can be repeated at 30-minute intervals until he feels calm or is asleep. If further doses are needed, please commence a continuous subcutaneous infusion, commencing with midazolam 10 mg in 24 hours.
- If bleeding continues, Terry wishes to remain at home for end-of-life care. If appropriate, use End of Life checklist to guide further care.

Terry was very reassured by having a clear plan of action. He also asked for a Do Not Attempt Cardio-Pulmonary Resuscitation order (DNA-CPR) and made an Advance Decision to Refuse Treatment document that declined invasive treatments, even if his life were in danger.

Over the next few weeks, he continued to become weaker. He stopped drinking altogether and became dehydrated, which caused muscular irritability and 'twitching'. His palliative care team arranged subcutaneous rehydration at home, which relieved his symptoms. He died peacefully at home without having a major haematemesis.

Place of care

Much palliative care research in the 1990s focused on the paradox that patients prefer to be cared for or to die at home, but over 50% of deaths occur in hospital despite the development of palliative care services in the community (Hinton, 1994). This preference for home is confirmed by Gomes et al.'s review in 2013 which also found four out of five people do not change their minds about this, even when disease progresses. It has been shown that in the UK, death in hospital is much more likely for patients who are over 75-years-old, male and poor (National End Of Life Care Intelligence Network, 2012). This study also found that 25% of emergency admissions are cancer patients, most people who die in hospital will do so after an emergency admission, and half of these will spend more than 8 days there.

These statistics suggest that there are particular groups of patients who would benefit from practical and/or social support to allow them to remain at home as long as they wish. Forward planning and anticipation of events and circumstances is key to this and should include discussion and documentation in an Advance Care Plan if possible.

PROVIDING CARE IN THE LAST FEW DAYS OF LIFE

Recognizing dying

The last part of life is not always recognized until close to death, and yet the decline towards death is a precious time in the lives of patients and families when it is recognized and managed well. The trajectory of dying is more easily recognizable in cancer than in many other chronic conditions, with a loss of energy and vigour that escalates rapidly over days or a short number of weeks. Reversible causes should be excluded (such as infection, hypercalcaemia, dehydration) before diagnosing dying. Writing an Emergency Health Care Plan enables out of hours medical and nursing services to respond to reversible crises whilst avoiding precipitate and unwanted hospital admissions.

Patients dying from malignant disease will usually be weak and chair- or bed-bound; they have little appetite and will be awake for increasingly shorter periods whilst dozing, sleeping or even slipping in and out of coma for increasingly lengthy periods of time. Although fever, hypoxia or metabolic disturbances can cause **delirium** (disturbance of mind resulting in confusion, poor concentration, inability to form short-term memory), most people dying with cancer who have been cognitively intact during their illness will remain so in their short periods of being awake, remaining able to appreciate the presence or absence of their loved ones.

When they know that they are dying, it can be a great help to patients to have some information in advance about what dying is like. This enables them to have realistic rather than imagined expectations because imagination is usually more frightening. Nurses can use the 'Coma Talk' as a loose script to guide them in a discussion about the end of life (see the following).

An approach to describing what to expect as death approaches

Let me tell you about what we observe as our patients become less well. If you want me to stop at any point, just let me know.

When people are less well, they feel more tired - even having a bad cold does that, doesn't it? If we are really unwell, we may get so tired we can't resist falling asleep. That happens when we have flu, and it can happen if cancer is making us very tired, too.

We can use your energy levels and the tiredness that your illness causes as a kind of guide to how things are going. Early on in the illness, people might not notice much change in their energy levels from one year to the next. This tells us that life expectancy is still measurable in years.

If the illness continues to progress and get more serious, people start to notice their energy levels are dropping, and they can notice the difference between one month and the next. This indicates that now life expectancy is down to months - though this may be enough months to make a year or more.

(Continued)

(Continued)

Later on in the illness, tiredness is more noticeable and energy levels may get worse from one week to the next. This rate of change tells us that life expectancy is down to weeks, and that it is time to make sure that we understand what the person wants their care to be like when time is getting really short.

Towards the end of someone's life, the cancer causes so much tiredness that they find they need to sleep to re-charge their energy batteries, often several times over the day. Gradually, the periods of sleep get longer and the periods of being awake get shorter. While they are awake, they are their normal self – same sense of humour, pleased to see the people they love, irritated by the same things as before – and so they can plan a snooze before doing anything that needs energy and attention, like receiving important visitors or having an important conversation.

Around this time, we start to notice that sometimes the person's sleep is very deep, too deep to wake them up for medications or visitors. This means that for short periods of time the person is not simply asleep, but actually unconscious: in a coma for a short while. When they wake up later, they tell us they have enjoyed their sleep, so we know that being in a coma is not unpleasant and not noticed by the patient.

At the very end of someone's life, they are simply asleep and going in and out of unconsciousness all the time. Then we notice that their breathing starts to change, sometimes going faster and sometimes very slow until, at the very end of their life, they simply and gently stop breathing. There is no sudden rush of pain, no choking or panic, no sign of distress.

This means that if your loved ones are around you when you are dying, they will see something peaceful. We can't stop them from finding it sad, but it will not be frightening for you or for them, and this knowledge can be a wonderful last gift to give them.

Providing comfort-focused care

Once dying is diagnosed, all care is focused on the patient's comfort. Nursing management includes attention to preserving patient autonomy as far as possible, asking permission to deliver care and describing the care as it is given if the patient is not conscious. Attention to mouth care, skin and continence should be regular, and family can be encouraged to join in mouth care and to communicate their presence and care by talking to an apparently unconscious patient, and by touch (e.g. massaging hands and feet). Dying people often express discomfort when they are moved for nursing care; they appreciate being warned by voice and touch prior to being moved, and movement-related stiffness may be relieved by use of regular non-steroidal anti-inflammatory drugs (NSAIDs) administered by mouth, rectum or trans-dermally. The use of a pressure-relieving mattress reduces the need for frequent positional changes to protect skin integrity.

Physical symptoms to consider and address include pain (tumour site, nerve compression, bony metastases, headache, pressure areas, recent onset or longstanding pain unrelated to the cancer); constipation; nausea and breathlessness. If patients are already taking regular medications for symptom control, these must be continued by a non-oral route when the patient becomes unable to swallow easily or when asleep for much of the time. Consider using the subcutaneous route via a small, indwelling cannula for intermittent dosing or continuous infusion; this is easier to maintain than intravenous access and ensures that dosing is not lost if an intravenous cannula becomes displaced.

Emotional distress is not inevitable in the dying. Distress may arise as a consequence of physical symptoms (breathlessness is particularly anxiety-provoking) or may be a consequence of thoughts about loss, separation or even the process of dying. Patients' sense of identity and self-determination is very vulnerable as they become physically less able to do things for themselves; nurses can help by asking patients' permission to give care and asking the patient's priorities (casting the patient as 'manager' even if unable to do a task in person). So if the bed looks untidy but the patient wants it left alone, this is an autonomy issue to be respected.

Spiritual assessment, at this stage, includes asking patient or family about cultural and religious practices, clergy visits and so forth, but also includes reaching a sense of 'acceptable ending' in which a patient can reflect on the meaning of their life, make peace with self or others over regrets, and say goodbye to loved ones with gratitude and peace.

Anticipating care needs

If a dying patient is to remain comfortable, it is vital that they are thoroughly and holistically assessed, their current symptoms are managed and any anticipated symptoms are planned for. Quick and timely access to any medications or equipment that may be required for comfort is very important, such as pressure-relieving aids, infusion devices, analgesics, anti-emetics, drugs for breathlessness, anxiety, agitation, and to reduce respiratory secretions if the ability to cough and clear the throat is lost. The drugs should be prescribed 'as required' if they are not currently needed regularly.

The Department of Health *End of Life Strategy for England and Wales* (2008c) recommends holistic assessment, clear communication with patient and loved ones, and excellent symptom control to support end-of-life care, and to enable best, evidence-based practice and a collaborative multidisciplinary approach. Introduction of an integrated care pathway for the last hours and days of life, translating excellent hospice-based care for use in hospital and community settings, has been subject to controversial criticism and, new ways of ensuring consistency of care are currently in development (NHS England, 2014). Experience suggests that without a tool to guide care, details may be overlooked and care may thus be compromised.

If the patient has been given the opportunity to consider and record their preferences for end-of-life care earlier in their illness, this record should be referred to now. Considerations include whether the patient is in the right place, receiving treatments they do not object to and receiving the spiritual and emotional care they would wish. If competence to make decisions is impaired, autonomy can still be respected by referring to recorded wishes or by asking loved ones' opinion about what the patient would wish (and not what the loved ones wish – a vital distinction that should be explained carefully to them).

Care at home at the end of life is possible but requires planning and availability of staff to support patients' physical and emotional needs, as well as supporting families. The nursing team may become part of an extended family during end-of-life care, and this can be a very rewarding area of clinical practice.

Most patients will reach a stage when they can no longer manage oral medicines; **subcutaneous infusions** of an equi-potent dose of analgesic or other drugs should be prescribed and available in preparation for this phase. Small, battery-driven syringe drivers are ideal and should be checked regularly to ensure the skin site is intact, the infusion is not cloudy and all infusion lines are correctly connected. Spare batteries should be available at all times.

Supporting families and lay carers

Few people in the twenty-first century have seen a death, and this leads to feelings of nervousness or to unrealistic and often frightening predictions about the mode of dying. People may need guidance or prompting in their actions and approach to the dying person even though they are emotionally very close. For example, **reminiscence** is an important component of family communications around a death-bed ('Do you remember when we …?'). In families who are struggling to cope at this time, a nurse can help by asking questions about the patient and family like 'How did you meet?', 'What is the favourite holiday you spent together?', 'What do you love most about him/her?' and so on.

Time spent asking family members about their expectations of dying will allow professionals to explore and correct any misperceptions and allay fearful predictions. It can be very helpful for family members to be with the patient during the 'coma talk' (see 'An approach to describing what to expect as death approaches') so there is mutual understanding of expectations. It may be necessary to repeat some or all of this information for a patient or family fully to absorb it and place their own situation in it.

Support for those who love and are loved by the dying person is an essential part of holistic care. By enabling the loved ones to support the dying person, the nurse provides the patient with the loving support that is most dear whilst providing the carers with opportunities to express their love, make their peace, say farewell and enter bereavement with fewer regrets.

CHAPTER SUMMARY

Palliative care is an approach to patient care that integrates physical, emotional, social and spiritual dimensions and is an essential component of nursing practice at any stage in the cancer journey. Although all cancer clinicians should be familiar with the principles of palliative care and become familiar with managing those symptoms that are common in their field of practice, the help and support of palliative care specialists is a vital part of cancer services that should be available when needed from diagnosis to cure, or to progression and end-of-life care.

The palliative phase of cancer care begins when cure is no longer a possibility. Even then, oncological treatments may be appropriate to achieve best possible disease control and relief of symptoms. An holistic assessment should include physical, emotional, social and spiritual domains and should take into account the patient's culture and personal beliefs. Excellent communication is the key to offering successful palliative care by cancer staff and by palliative care specialists – listening, offering focused probes and summarizing what has been discussed are important components of a good communication skill set.

End-of-life care begins when death is imminent. It is an opportunity for nurses to use compassion, care and knowledge to ensure that a patient's priorities are respected, their loved ones are supported and that symptoms are managed with skill and foresight. A family that is supported in witnessing a 'good death' will move more easily through their bereavement and will have an experience that may help them later in discussing and planning their own priorities for end-of-life care.

Reflective activity

- How could the palliative care needs of a young man undergoing chemotherapy for an advanced but curable testicular cancer be similar to or different from a young woman having palliative chemotherapy for an incurable ovarian cancer?
- Read the box 'An approach to describing what to expect as death approaches'. Can you imagine how you could use the ideas included here in your own words to explain the process of dying to a patient? A patient's relative? A family friend?
- Practice this conversation with a colleague, and give each other feedback about how it feels to be telling and listening.
- If you had only weeks to live, what would be your priorities? How much of that planning could be done months ahead? Years ahead? Now?
- Are you confident that you can complete an holistic assessment of the needs of a patient with advanced cancer? What support might you need before and after the assessment?

Key learning points

- Palliative care is applicable at all points in the cancer journey to address physical, emotional, spiritual or social difficulties. This is not the same as the palliative phase of illness.
- All healthcare practitioners should understand how to deliver simple palliative care support, and know where to access palliative care specialist support for their patients or for themselves.
- Patients and families may make their emotional adjustment to a diagnosis of incurable cancer at different rates; all may need different support.
- Skilled communication is required to enable patients to understand changes in prognosis and life expectancy, and to support them in expressing their preferences about their future place and type of care.
- Even when death is inevitable, human resilience finds new ways to preserve hope.
- Emotional distress may punctuate adjustment, but anxiety and depression should be identified and treated if they arise.
- Planning in advance can help patients regain a sense of control, and helps to reduce the likelihood of unwanted emergency admission to hospital at the end of life.

Recommended further reading

- Dying Matters (www.dyingmatters.org). This is a UK-based public health and education website run by a coalition of palliative care organizations. Dedicated to increasing public engagement and awareness about dying, death and bereavement, it offers practical information and advice, links to Government policies and organizations offering advice and support to patients, relatives and the bereaved.
- Department of Health *End of Life Strategy* (2008) (www.gov.uk/government/publications/end-of-life-care-strategy-promoting-high-quality-care-for-adults-at-the-end-of-their-life). Publications to guide clinicians on anticipating patients' needs as their illness progresses and how to plan care at the end of life.

29 BEREAVEMENT SUPPORT IN CANCER CARE

MARGARET FOULKES

Chapter outline

- Bereavement, grief and mourning
- Theories of grief and loss
- The emergence of policy and practice guidelines for bereavement support
- Bereavement risk assessment
- Interventions to facilitate the expression of grief
- People with special needs
- Practical application
- Care of staff and resources

INTRODUCTION

The care of **bereaved people** has often been overlooked within the health service, or has been seen as desirable but not essential. Different forms of support have been provided by a limited number of statutory organizations, but mostly by the voluntary sector. This has led to patchy, uncoordinated, unmonitored local groups struggling to survive with little financial support, an inequitable distribution of resources and a varying quality of services. The need for support following bereavement is universal and has been recognized throughout all populations. This has taken many forms in different religions and cultures, where rituals have been developed to deal with this. In the UK, many rituals have now been discarded and people are expected to continue with their lives or return to work within a few days or weeks.

Reflective activity

What rituals did/do people observe that may have helped them to cope with their grief?

Hospice and specialist palliative care services have traditionally advocated and provided bereavement support for relatives and carers of patients referred to them for palliative care. It was not until 2004, however, with the publication of the National Institute for Clinical Excellence (NICE, 2004b) *Guidance on Cancer Services: Improving Supportive and Palliative Care for Adults with Cancer* that the importance of assessing the needs of families and carers as well as the patient was emphasized:

> Families and carers have particular needs around the time of death that may only be fully realised after the patient's death ... Bereavement can give rise to a wide range of needs – practical, financial, social, emotional and spiritual. There might be needs for information about loss and grief, needs to pursue particular cultural practices, needs for additional support to deal with the emotional and psychological impact of loss by death or, in a small number of circumstances, specific needs for mental health service intervention to cope with a mental health problem related to loss by death. (NICE, 2004b: 156).

This guidance has been further developed in the *End of Life Care Strategy* (DH, 2008c), which promotes high quality care for all adults at the end of life, and acknowledges that it is essential to provide support for carers, both during a person's illness and after their death:

> Information on how to access comprehensive and culturally appropriate bereavement and support services should be available from all health, social care and other emergency organisations providing care at the end of life and into bereavement. Information on bereavement and support services should be available through a range of formats and channels, including 24/7 helplines and the NHS Choices website. (DH, 2008c: 114).

The Gold Standards Framework, which is part of the End of Life Care Strategy, also identifies the importance of supporting carers with emotional, practical and financial needs and of extending this care into the bereavement phase.

Within England specifically, there are around a half million deaths per year; 99% of these are in adults over the age of 18, and most in people over 65 years of age (DH, 2008c: 24). Of the 16,000 complaints made to the Healthcare Commission between July 2004 and July 2006, approximately half of these related to care given in acute hospitals, and of these, 54% related in some way to end-of-life care.

What happens during end-of-life care, how a person dies and events surrounding and immediately following a death have all been closely linked to bereavement recovery, as well as to other factors, which will be discussed later.

CASE STUDY

Celia's husband, Bill, was attending the local hospice and regional cancer centre for palliative treatment as an outpatient. Celia contacted her GP when Bill became acutely ill at home, but because no one was able to visit immediately, she dialled 999 and Bill was taken to the nearest Accident and Emergency department where he died. Celia was unable to be with Bill during his last few hours and had wanted him to go to the hospice or remain at home. Although Celia and Bill were devout Roman Catholics, no priest had been called.

Celia remained very angry and disillusioned with the GP and ambulance service, and with the care provided in the Accident and Emergency department. She wrote several letters of complaint and during the following five years, refused to go to her GP surgery. At the age of 85, she only agreed to register at another GP surgery following an accident.

- What factors may have impacted on Celia's bereavement recovery?
- Consider other factors which might lead to a perceived 'bad' death, or which could cause a prolonged grief reaction. What might the consequences of these be?

BEREAVEMENT, GRIEF AND MOURNING

John Bowlby (1971: 7) stated that 'the loss of a loved person is one of the most intensely painful experiences any human being can suffer. Not only is it painful to experience but it is also painful to witness, if only because we are so impotent to help'. The only solution a person wants is to be re-united with their loved one and we are unable to achieve this. To fully understand the devastating effect that bereavement can have on an individual, it is important to consider some of the theoretical concepts that have been developed over the years. These explain the process of forming close personal attachments, which bring stability in life, and the major re-adjustments that are needed to ensure personal survival after a significant loss.

The terminology used needs initial clarification:

Bereavement is usually considered to be loss, through death, of a person. This is a condition, not a feeling. It is the state of having lost someone significant. It is sometimes used to include 'something' significant as well (e.g. pet, home, health).

Grief usually means the emotions brought about by bereavement and accompanies any significant loss. It involves a series of powerful emotions, feelings, thoughts, behaviours and, often, physical symptoms.

Mourning is related to the activities associated with bereavement and is a period of recovery from grief. It is often a time when people are expected to fulfil certain duties and rituals. These social expectations vary between different cultures.

Theories of grief and loss

The psychiatrist Lazare (1979) estimated that 10–15% of people who came into the mental health clinics at Massachusetts General Hospital had, underneath their specific psychological condition, an unresolved grief reaction. Other studies examined mortality following bereavement, and found an increase in deaths during the first year of a bereavement (Parkes and Prigerson, 2010). These studies suggest that the needs of bereaved people should be recognized and addressed in a more systematic way in order to prevent serious mental or physical problems.

Grief is universal: it is found in all cultures and all societies. Rosenblatt et al. (1976) observed that grieving people generally experience strong emotions and demonstrate radical changes in their patterns of behaviour. They may feel sadness, anger, fear, anxiety, guilt, loneliness, numbness and tension. Their behaviour may change and they could lose their appetite, lose weight, lose interest in everything and have problems with sleep. However, the authors also argue that different cultures deal with grief in different ways, something that will be covered later in this chapter.

The first formal investigation and attempt to understand grief can be seen in Freud's (1917) work, *Mourning and Melancholia*, where Freud stated that both **mourning** and **melancholia** are caused by the death of someone close. As Freud's work was largely speculative and based on his working experience as a psychoanalyst, it does not, perhaps, represent useful evidence-based knowledge. Lindemann (1944), however, in an early classic and systematic study in the field of loss and grief, demonstrated that the bereaved survivors of a nightclub fire in Boston in 1942, where nearly 500 people died, had similar grief experiences; he had, therefore, identified a **'grief syndrome'**. This was a distinct condition with both psychological and physical symptoms, such as pre-occupation with the image of the deceased person, guilt, hostility to others and loss of established activity patterns. Lindemann's work indicated that all bereaved people share a common experience irrespective of age, gender or cultural background. Having identified grief as a syndrome with specific features, he was able to demonstrate that other people, including health professionals, could then make sense of how bereaved people were feeling and be able to help them to cope with their grief.

Many other psychoanalysts, such as Karl Abraham, Helene Deutsch and Melanie Klein, continued to develop these theories but it was not until the 1960s and 1970s that the work of John Bowlby and Colin Murray Parkes began to promote the importance of working with people in loss and grief situations. Bowlby's (1971) basic theoretical assumption is that all human beings need to form **attachments** to significant people, beginning with parents, which ensures security and safety. When we lose someone through death or separation, a variety of responses occur involving deep distress or **'separation anxiety'**. If the attachment bond is restored, these reactions cease, but when the attachment is completely severed, as in bereavement, the reactions may continue for some time. This is the price we pay for being attached to a person or even a special object.

Reflective activity

Consider the following situations and how these can be related to the theoretical concept of loss and attachment described earlier:

- Young children starting school/nursery
- Loss of a precious, sentimental piece of jewellery
- Loss of a relationship
- Death of a loved person

Most bereaved people will experience similar initial feelings associated with all major losses, but how this continues and is dealt with, depends on a wide variety of other factors.

Colin Murray Parkes (1975) is a British psychiatrist interested in the individual psychological effects of bereavement. In his work, he also considered more of the social dimensions in his theory of **psychosocial transitions**. Most of his early work focused on widows, and he suggested various stages through which a bereaved person progresses until they begin to establish a modified **identity** and **purpose**. These identified stages are still relevant in understanding universal reactions to grief:

1. Shock, numbness, disbelief;
2. Yearning, pining, searching;
3. Anger, guilt, protest, resentment;
4. Disorganization, despair, apathy, depression; and
5. Reorganization, recovery, redefining roles.

These normal responses to grief have been developed over the years into less-structured models, recognizing that bereaved people may experience different grief reactions at different times, and in no particular order or timescale. Similarly, not every stage of the grief reaction may be experienced by each individual. Not everyone will experience anger, for example, or there may be others who will experience anger in the early stages of grief and again, much later on. They can move backwards and forwards between each grief reaction. This understanding of grief has largely replaced staged theories of adjustment.

This pioneering work into the process of grief allowed researchers and healthcare workers to identify what happens when someone is bereaved and to find supportive approaches in response. They provide a framework for understanding some of the overwhelming feelings and reactions that many people experience and that are part of the normal process of grief.

Emotional responses and the resolution of grief

The final phase in each of these models is seen as **recovery, reorganization or acceptance**. Silverman et al., (1992) propose that the term '**accommodation**' is more appropriate because it reflects that the person has found a manageable way of being in the world whilst living with the loss. Many bereaved people say that they have not recovered from their loss, but have learnt to live with it.

Reflective activity

Think about someone who has been bereaved, and consider the reactions and emotions you have witnessed.

Many studies have concentrated on the common feelings associated with grief, such as sadness or distress, but it is also worth considering the reaction of **relief**. Relief is something that many relatives feel after they have watched a loved one suffer during a long illness, and may represent not only relief that the person who has died is now out of pain, distress or suffering, but also relief that that they can now move on with their own lives, free from caring duties and the anxieties/uncertainties surrounding the illness. These feelings of relief, however, are often followed by **guilt** at having felt the relief in the first place. Grief is by no means a simple and straightforward emotional response.

Grief is a time when there is a mixture of feelings, physical sensations, changed behaviour patterns and confused thought patterns:

- Physical sensations may include lack of energy, fatigue, chest pains, digestive upsets, dry mouth, breathlessness and symptoms similar to the illness of the deceased;
- Behaviour changes may manifest as sleeplessness, appetite disturbance, restlessness, crying, searching and sighing; and
- Confused thought patterns may include rumination and preoccupation (going over and over what has happened), hallucinations, dreams, or a perceived sense of presence (feeling the person is still around) and even feelings of going 'mad' (Parkes, 1970). Many people also lose their concentration and confidence.

Parkes (1975) linked these psychological reactions and feelings to the social context in which people live: he discusses the changes that people have to make in their lives when a major loss event occurs. Bereaved people have to change their assumptions of the world and re-integrate into a world that is different because their role and circumstances have changed. Marris (1974) examined the sociological explanation of loss using three key concepts:

The conservative impulse: We are constantly surrounded by change, but we generally prefer predictability and resist change. We need confidence in the predictability of our surroundings and it takes time to change and re-align our world.

Structures of meaning: We relate to the world through familiar patterns, attaching meaning to objects and people throughout our lives. Even though, as humans, we are very adaptable and able to survive in many environments, we need to assimilate new experiences and place them in familiar contexts.

Grieving: Marris equates grieving to our adjustment to loss. We not only lose the person, but also part of our understanding of the world, for example the wife who becomes a widow, or single person again, and all of the changes that this entails.

Bereavement is a complex loss because it is a multiple loss of: (1) a physical presence; (2) a significant relationship; (3) a sense of order or normality; and (4) of ourselves.

Reflective activity

Bereavement has been called the 'shattered dream' or, for children, 'the event that shatters childhood'. Imagine a young married woman with two children who loses her husband when they are both in their late thirties. How would the multiple losses described earlier affect her and what changes would it entail in her life?

Rosenblatt (1983) continued to focus on the importance of the social context of grief, with his **symbolic interaction theory**, which expanded on the concept of loss of one's self (who you are and how you see yourself), and loss of one's world as you knew it and a search for new meaning that then takes place (to dream a new dream). People may turn to religion, or away from it, read books/poems on the subject or seek out people who have had a similar experience in order to understand what is happening and what is normal. Objects and possessions may become important because they hold a special meaning and link to the past. For this reason, wills and distribution of possessions can cause immense distress because the objects are an important source of subjective meaning for each individual involved.

Reflective activity

What examples can you think of where people hold on to things from the past? Some may be quite appropriate (jewellery) but others may stop people from moving on with their lives.

Klass et al. (1996) suggested that there is not always a 'recovery' from grief, but there can be a continuing relationship with the deceased in a different form, through memories, family history, shared interests/professions and mementoes. This is a particularly useful concept when looking at children's grief following a parental death at a young age. Young people will often re-visit their grief at a later stage when it may mean something different to them as they grow older and understand more fully the meaning of that loss.

Two further models that have particular use in explaining grief are the **Dual Process Model** (Stroebe and Schut, 1999) and the work by Robert Neimeyer (2001) on the **reconstruction of meaning**. The Dual Process Model is based on the concept that grief involves two orientations: (1) a loss orientation, and (2) a restoration orientation. In the loss orientation, a person looks back at their grief, holds on to bonds and ties, and avoids changes or moving on. In the restoration orientation, a person looks forward, does new things and takes on new roles and relationships. Bereaved people often oscillate between grieving and clinging to the past, and trying to move on and adjust to new challenges. Such oscillation can be psychologically healthy, but things go wrong when people become stuck in the loss orientation phase or move too quickly into restoration orientation without assimilating their loss and dealing with all that it has meant.

Neimeyer's work is particularly interesting because he uses narrative and identity to reconstruct meaning. He brings together elements of other theories by demonstrating that a person needs to grieve for not only the death of a loved one, but also the changed life of the survivor. The loss event disrupts our sense of autobiographical continuity and coherence (see also Chapter 18 for a discussion of autobiographical adjustment to illness diagnosis). Individuals may become dislodged from a sense of 'who they are' and lose their identity through grief. Maintaining continuity in self-narratives means sustaining connections to those who were part of our life. We sometimes take on the mannerisms, activities, interests, personality and values of the person who has died in order to maintain the connection (Klass et al., 1996). In supporting the bereaved, Neimeyer (2001) suggests several questions to use when constructing a coherent story for the past, present and future:

- What was life like before the event?
- What was the worst thing that happened?
- What is your life like now?
- What do you hope for the future?

For many people, the loss of a close relative or friend can bring enormous unwanted and unplanned changes to their lives that affect aspects such as family life, finances, work, education, home and social structure.

Reflective activity

Consider the effect on families when a parent, partner or child dies. How does life change for the remaining members of the family and how difficult is it to cope with work, school, limited income and society's reactions?

Theories of grief serve as a guide to making sense of the powerful feelings and reactions that bereaved people experience. One of the most important ways in which to comfort a bereaved person is to convey that their emotions and reactions are not unusual.

BEREAVEMENT RISK ASSESSMENT

Theories of bereavement, as outlined in the first section of this chapter, have been useful in distinguishing between normal and abnormal grief reactions, and thus prioritizing who might require support. Many hospices and specialist palliative care units have used some form of risk assessment to identify relatives who may need ongoing support, but there are various issues that arise.

Why should we assess need?

There is a duty of care to minimize the risk to health associated with bereavement by offering support proactively. There is certainly no evidence to suggest that all bereaved people will need help, and support should, therefore, be channelled towards those who are more vulnerable. Parkes and Prigerson (2010) discuss some of the studies in detail that look at family and social support, as well as personal coping strategies and resilience. In short, services need to make the best use of limited resources.

Most bereavement risk assessments have been derived from Parkes' **Bereavement Risk Index** (BRI) (Parkes and Weiss, 1983) and suggest that the following influential factors should be considered in combination:

- Events and circumstances leading up to the death, and the type of death itself (e.g. sudden/ expected, preventability, length of illness and what happened around the time of death).
- Psychological factors (e.g. the personality of the bereaved person, coping mechanisms, past experiences, other concurrent losses and the quality of the relationship with the person who has died).
- Social factors (e.g. support systems, cultural/religious/social background and financial issues).
- Physiological factors (e.g. drug or alcohol dependency, physical health and general wellbeing).

Relf et al. (2008) developed an alternative assessment, suggesting that earlier approaches had limited reliability in predicting bereavement outcome. Instead, they focused on coping styles and argued that 'ways of coping influence individual health outcomes, rather than the presence of risk factors alone. Therefore, an integrative approach to assessment is needed that examines coping as well as risk factors' (Relf et al., 2008: 5). This approach requires detailed knowledge of each person being assessed, however, which is not always possible in the limited time that staff may have with relatives. It is, nevertheless a useful tool for a counsellor beginning bereavement work with a bereaved individual.

There is no conclusive evidence that bereavement risk assessment is totally predictive, but it does ensure that an assessment is made and that the multidisciplinary team identifies those who may be at risk. It is only through this process of initial identification that appropriate support and signposting can be offered to those in need. Agnew et al. (2010) found that most people do not require follow-up after bereavement, but that offering information on resources available did increase resilience and promoted autonomy. Parkes and Prigerson (2010) compared several studies in the USA and the UK, which made similar conclusions.

Abnormal grief

A small number of people with problems resulting from their loss will be referred for psychiatric help. Holland et al. (2009) researched differences between normal and **complicated grief** in a group of widows, concluding that the evidence points to a **grief continuum** where the intensity and duration of grief distinguishes the two categories. There are also more specific subgroups of grief response, including Prolonged Grief Disorder (PGD), which occurs where grief reactions are more extreme and occur over a prolonged period. Evidence shows that there is an increased risk of suicide and major depressive disorder in this group (Parkes and Prigerson, 2010).

Some bereaved people may suffer from symptoms such as anxiety, panic attacks, phobias, guilt or self-blame and **hypochondriasis** (often related to the symptoms experienced by the person who died). Depression commonly occurs following bereavement, often associated with feelings of helplessness and hopelessness. Some of these may be linked to pre-bereavement co-morbidities and personality traits, as well as differences in socio-demographic variables, including age, gender, timeliness or untimeliness of the death, loneliness, isolation and available social support.

Worden (1991) also identified that when grief reactions become abnormal and turn into 'complicated grief', they leave the bereaved individual so overwhelmed by their grief that they can make no progression through it. He identified several forms of abnormal grief:

> **Chronic grief:** This is where grief continues for an excessive period of time and does not come to a satisfactory conclusion.
>
> **Delayed grief:** This may be when grief occurs after a period of time and not immediately. It may be following another loss or even a media event, such as coverage of a celebrity funeral.
>
> **Exaggerated grief:** This may be seen when someone is completely overwhelmed by the grief that they develop co-morbid psychiatric disorder.
>
> **Masked grief:** This is indicated when the bereaved person exhibits physical symptoms or other behaviours that do not appear to be linked to the loss.

There may be times when grief is absent because it is so painful that it must be **denied**. It is also perfectly reasonable that for some people, there may not be any reason to grieve because the loss may not be of personal significance to them, for example siblings in a family may not all grieve the loss of a parent in the same way or degree of intensity because their own personal relationships and contact with the deceased parent may be different. Some people may have been through anticipatory grief (e.g. following a long illness): this long period of pre-death grief often offsets the time taken to grieve for the loss after actual death. Although this process may help families to be able to discuss and prepare for the future, it is by no means inevitable: there are many families for whom a long, expected death still comes as a shock when it finally occurs.

Duty of care

The UK NICE *Guidance on Cancer Services: Improving Supportive and Palliative Care for Adults with Cancer* (2004b) recommends that a three-component model of bereavement support should be developed and implemented within each cancer network. All organizations providing cancer care in the UK should be able to offer the first level seen in component 1 and strategies should be in place to access components 2 and 3.

> **Component 1: Information.** Grief is normal after bereavement and most people manage without professional intervention. Many people, however, lack understanding about the grief experience following bereavement and may benefit from information about this and how to access other forms of support. Family and friends will provide much of this support, with information being supplied by health and social care professionals providing day-to-day care to families.

> **Component 2: Informal bereavement support.** Some people may require an opportunity to review and reflect on their loss experience, but this does not necessarily have to involve professionals. Volunteer bereavement support workers/befrienders, self-help groups, faith groups and community groups will provide much support at this level. Those offering informal bereavement support must establish a process to ensure that when cases involving more complex needs emerge, referral is made to appropriate health and social care professionals with the ability to deliver component 3 interventions.

> **Component 3: Formal supportive care interventions.** A minority of people will require specialist interventions from mental health services or other services that provide psychological support, specialist counselling/psychotherapy, specialist palliative care and general bereavement support or that meet the specialist needs of bereaved children and young people.

Reflective activity

- What services are available for bereaved relatives in your organization?
- Does your organization meet the requirements of Component 1?

INTERVENTIONS TO FACILITATE THE EXPRESSION OF GRIEF

Neimeyer (2006) suggested that '[bereaved people] need to re-establish a life worthy of passionate re-investment'. This may be difficult for many bereaved people and may take a long time. Professional and informal interventions may facilitate the bereavement process and be of benefit to those struggling with this life transition.

There is a wide range of individual and group bereavement interventions, delivered in various forms, which provide support for people who have lost a loved person. These may be via telephone contact, home visiting services, peer support groups or the Internet, and may be provided by volunteers or a range of trained professionals, such as psychologists, social workers, counsellors, nurses or pastoral staff. Schut and Stroebe (2010) examined the challenges of evaluating adult bereavement services and commented that research has shown that intervention is not effective for the bereaved in general, but is effective for those at high risk or for those who are already experiencing complications in their grief. Screening is, therefore, an essential component of bereavement care and may act as an intervention in itself. Most bereaved people find that grief naturally improves with time, but interventions that are aimed at high-risk groups will usually facilitate a speedier recovery to psychological wellbeing (Parkes and Prigerson, 2010).

There may, however, also be a need for practical support to be available for people in the early bereavement period, even when their grief experience is normal. This may include individuals living on their own, or those who do not know what to do about funerals, benefits, wills and financial issues.

Some useful bereavement support organizations

- CRUSE
- Samaritans
- Citizens Advice Bureau
- Age UK
- Compassionate Friends
- Change
- Macmillan Cancer Support
- RD4U
- Winston's Wish
- WAY (Widowed and Young)

For those who need more formal bereavement interventions, many therapists have used the theories of grief as a basis for intervention. One of the most commonly used is Worden's four-task model (1991) discussed in Chapter 28. Littlewood (1992) gives a clear, concise explanation of several other models that could be applied, including:

- Illness and disease models
- Biological models
- Attachment Theory
- Psychodynamic models
- Personal Construct Theory and cognitive models
- Grief as a crisis of coping
- Phenomenological and existential models

These models link in different ways and often overlap in their ideas. They each explore the relationship between the bereaved and the person who has died; the reactions to the loss; the different ways in which people deal with this (often depending on previous experiences and concurrent stressors); support systems available; and how the bereaved person is attempting to and able to re-integrate into a new situation. Some models deal with one or two of these factors in greater or lesser depth and develop their ideas and helping strategies around this. It is, therefore, useful to utilize different models in different situations when trying to help individuals cope with their grief.

Suitably trained counsellors and therapists may use a wide range of interventions and techniques such as client-centred work, **Gestalt therapy**, **behaviour therapy** and **transpersonal techniques**, but, in general, an eclectic approach to grief counselling is advocated.

Counselling and one-to-one therapy are not the only methods of helping bereaved people, and some alternatives are outlined next.

Support groups

Support groups may be professionally or informally run. In either case, they provide beneficial support for those who prefer this form of intervention by:

- Reducing feelings of isolation;
- Providing access to support from others who have also experienced a recent loss;
- Exploring different aspects of grief, and ways of expressing it;
- Developing an individual's natural ability to oscillate between engaging with, and detaching from, their loss;
- Understanding the normality of their experiences of grief; and
- Developing personal resources to cope with their experience of loss. (McGuinness and Finucane, 2011: 38)

Many bereaved people in counselling will express their isolation and feelings that no one else understands or could possibly have experienced the intense emotions they are going through; therefore, a support group can allow people to acknowledge and share their experiences in a safe and understanding environment. Different types of groups may need to be established, so that those experiencing a similar type of loss can share their experiences (e.g. different groups for people losing a spouse or partner, older bereaved people, younger bereaved partners who have children, young adults who have lost a parent, those who have lost a sibling, children who have lost a parent and parents who have lost a child).

Narrative (as an act of healing)

Writing has been used in many therapies and can be a particularly useful tool in bereavement work. One of the early bereavement classics is C.S. Lewis's *A Grief Observed* (1961), which was written immediately following the death of his wife and gives an emotional account of Lewis's feelings at that time. For many bereaved people, this has been a book in which they could identify and find a connection with their own grief. This relates back to Neimeyer's (2001) work on narrative and identity, where the bereaved person needs to make sense of their life story and to process what has happened within their total history and its links to the person who has died.

MacKellar (2010: 31), who is a historian and scholar, turned to writing as a form of release:

> For me, it is the act of writing that unlocks the frame. I pin my tragedy on to paper and with the precision of an anatomist take a scalpel to separate memory from bone. Perhaps if I can peel the layers of skin from its torso, it will stop having the power of a dark shape in the night. By writing, I risk sacrificing my deepest intimacies, but by writing, I control the shape they become.

Regaining a sense of control is one of the most important goals of bereavement therapy. Something has happened over which the bereaved person has no control and life seems to spiral away. By regaining control, the bereaved person becomes secure again. It may mean moving furniture around, decorating the house or making personal choices that suit the bereaved individual and not the person who has died. For some people, this can take a long time, but is an important step in becoming a separate person again. This process clearly relates to Bowlby's (1971) attachment theory (as described earlier in this chapter) and the resultant need to regain security and safety in our world following loss.

Other possible approaches

Other interventions that may be helpful in bereavement support include art therapy, music therapy, drama and other creative activities through which people can express their feelings and find a new purpose in life (see also Chapter 26).

CONSIDERATION OF DIVERSITY AND VULNERABILITY IN LOSS

The *Draft Spiritual Support and Bereavement Care Quality Markers and Measures for End of Life Care* (National Health Service, 2011) identifies children and those with learning difficulties as vulnerable groups for bereavement care. It also stresses the need to offer support at the time of death which is culturally and spiritually appropriate.

Culture and religion

In some of their early work, Rosenblatt and colleagues (1976) explored cultural differences in grief. Although people grieve and express similar emotions, there is a noticeable difference in the way that death is defined and what is an appropriate expression of death. Many cultures have very specific belief systems, which require certain ceremonies, rituals and expressions of grief. Some people retreat and grieve in private; others openly express their feelings in public and weep with others in the streets. Some cultures set a strict time period for mourning and the bereaved person may be pushed into getting on with their life, and considered to be abnormal if they do not conform. People may grieve for varying periods of time and for different losses, and grief may recur throughout a person's lifetime. Walter (2010) highlights the diversity of needs, reactions and rituals associated with grief in different cultures and stresses that in supporting the bereaved, we need to clear our minds of assumptions and really listen to what each individual has to say about how their loss fits into their personal values and belief system. It is also important to recognize that what an individual needs may not be what their culture expects.

Cultures may also change over time, for example Goss and Klass (2005) describe changes in China where respect for senior family ancestors (not children) was shown in the pre-communist era but suppressed during the Maoist regime when funerals were only recognized and acknowledged for important party, rather than family members. More recently, people are reverting back to family values, which include respect and services for both adults and children who have died.

Children and young people

When a parent dies, children are often the 'forgotten mourners'. They are protected from what is going on and thus isolated in their grief. During recent years, the needs of bereaved children have become increasingly recognized and resources are beginning to be put in place to support them. Hospices often take the lead in providing specialist services because, as with adults, bereaved children are more vulnerable to psychiatric disorders than the general population. Winston's Wish was set up by two adult psychologists who came across many adult patients who had suffered a parental loss as a child. They provide a service and resources for families and professionals when a child has been bereaved.

Worden (1996) found that in general, the loss of a mother is worse for most children than the loss of a father and 'is associated with more emotional/behavioural problems including higher levels of anxiety, more acting-out behaviour, lower self-esteem, and less belief in self-efficacy' (Worden, 1996: 95). However, the functioning level of the surviving parent is also an important predictor in a child's adjustment to loss. A more recent study by Tracey (2011) on perpetual loss and pervasive grief examined the impact on daughters of a mother's death and found the following emerging themes: silence in families; the need to 'dig' for information (because no one talked about it); the importance of milestones in their lives (desperately wanting their mothers when they were pregnant); learning to cover your heart (for fear of losing it again); and the incalculable loss (the event that shattered childhood). Tracey noted a common theme from the literature, which was 'the need for children and young people to be listened to, to be supported and to be offered explanations that are age-appropriate' (Tracey, 2011: 17). She quotes Koehler (2010) who states that, 'Honesty from adults is essential. It helps children come to terms with the death and feel honoured as grieving members of the family' (Tracey, 2011: 19).

The need for children and young people to be informed, involved, reassured and allowed to express their feelings is crucial at all stages of end-of-life care and bereavement. Honesty and involvement are essential components of this. During a terminal illness of a family member, children should be given simple, age-appropriate information so that they can share in the family's caregiving and prepare to say their goodbyes. They need some explanations and information in order to make sense of what is happening. Families should be encouraged to include children when visiting parents in care settings. Staff can utilize these opportunities to help families to talk to children about their parent's illness, treatments and equipment or to talk to children themselves.

It is important to recognize the specific needs of children and young adults in bereavement because, unlike adults, they are not able to access or recognize the resources available. They may need to access support individually or in groups, through children's services, school or the Internet. Children also show grief in different ways to adults – usually in short bursts of upset and difficult behaviour or by retreating to their room. They may try to protect adults from grief and adults certainly protect their children. Stability, involvement and inclusion are important at this time and families may need help to recognize these needs and seek support.

> ### Reflective activity
>
> - What can you do in your organization to meet the needs of children and young people at this time?
> - Do you have any leaflets or booklets to give to families?

People with intellectual disabilities

Staff often underestimate the capacity of people with an intellectual disability to understand the concept of death and their need to grieve. This can be particularly difficult if the person who has died was the one who could help them most with communication. The person with an intellectual disability has the right to know what is happening and should be involved in the process, such as talking about the loved person's death and the funeral. It is important to be honest about what is happening and to give them time to express their feelings. They may need to have many conversations about this, with simple, clear explanations in short steps. They will experience the same emotions as those identified earlier, but will also need to be reassured about the future, such as who will care for them if care is required.

The 'unrecognized' bereaved

For some people, there may be '**disenfranchised grief**' where the griever is not recognized and, therefore, is not able to grieve the loss. An example may be in a homosexual relationship that has not been acknowledged or accepted, or may be a mistress in a secret relationship. Sometimes staff working for a long time with a patient may feel a great loss, but may not be able to attend the funeral or have that relationship acknowledged and have to move quickly on to other patients. Doka (1989) wrote extensively about grief and the losses which cannot be acknowledged openly or mourned publicly by the bereaved person.

BEREAVEMENT CARE FOR ALL

This chapter has primarily focused on bereavement support and care for the families, carers and friends of patients who have already died, but it is also essential to recognize that, within a cancer care setting, bereavement affects other individuals too.

Grieving patients: Sometimes, it may be patients who have been recently bereaved and they may refuse treatment because they have no motivation to carry on with life. There may be patients who are about to be discharged and become distressed because there is no one at home to look after them. It can be particularly lonely to face illness and treatment without the support of the person you have shared your life with or depended upon. The patient may need to speak to a counsellor or social worker to support them through this time.

30 SUPPORTING HEALTHCARE PROFESSIONALS IN CANCER SETTINGS

JAN WOODHOUSE

Chapter overview

- Concepts such as stress and burn-out in the occupational healthcare setting
- Emotional labour, a unique aspect of cancer care that may place the greatest demand upon healthcare professionals

- Manifestation and consequences of stress at the personal and interpersonal level
- Strategies and interventions to recognize and prevent stress and burnout

---

INTRODUCTION

In this chapter, it is the wellbeing and care of the healthcare professional involved with patients who have cancer that is the focus of attention. If we have to look after patients then we must also look after ourselves: the two must be in tandem. Often, however, the needs of staff are overlooked and staff may end up feeling expendable to the service, seeking to move on and taking with them the valuable bank of skills and experience. Thus, supporting professional carers has a double objective – maintaining the health of the workforce and maintaining the capacity of the workforce. The Government recognizes that stress, which is linked to mental health problems such as anxiety and depression, needs to be tackled at an organizational level (DH, 2012b).

MODELS OF STRESS

> ## Reflective activity
>
> Draw up a list of things that stress you in your life, especially in relation to your working environment.

Stress is often defined as 'a state of mental or emotional strain or tension resulting from adverse or demanding circumstances' (Oxford Dictionaries, 2014). There are, however, multiple different frameworks and conceptual models of stress (Hanson, 1994).

Stress as a response

The **General Adaptation Syndrome** (GAS) model was first proposed by Hans Selye (Selye, 1953). In response to a potential **stressor**, this model suggests a process of three consecutive phases that the individual will go through. The first is **alarm** (or reaction), which is a state of alertness making us ready for action – essentially the fight or flight response. Our body often enters very quickly into the next phase, which is **adaptation** (or response) and is when the body tries to adapt, adjust and cope with the ongoing presence of the stressor. Normally this occurs without any consequences for the body. The third phase of the model is that of **exhaustion**, and this only occurs when the stressor has continued for prolonged periods of time, and is the recognition that the body's coping reserves have been used up. Exhaustion may be caused by the ongoing presence of one substantial stressor or the multiple, additive effects of many smaller stressors in one period of time. For the cancer care professional, this may be a period of working long hours, not eating regularly, worrying about the things they have done or not done. It may be affected by external factors too, such as catching a cold, which reduces the natural ability to withstand stressors but can be severely debilitating, requiring significant time off work, or worse still even resulting in **diseases of adaptation** or death (Selye, 1953). Healthcare professionals therefore need to recognize the importance, and take notice, of the smaller signs of exhaustion, and prevent their escalation further.

Stress as a stimulus

Stimulus models of stress, such as Holmes and Rahe's Life Events Model (Holmes and Rahe, 1967) recognize that events happening in our lives, such as bereavement or separation, may affect us in ways that make it possible for illness to ensue. It is worth noting that events do not have to be negative or unwanted to be stressful – even positive events, such as a holiday or celebration of Christmas, often cause a similar stress response. A stressor is merely something that requires our psychological and social world to need to be adapted: something referred to as **social readjustment**. If too many events occur in a short space of time, then our personal resources may become depleted and we are then at risk of psychological or physiological ill health. This is sometimes referred to as a **loss spiral** (Örtqvist and Wincent, 2010) and theorists, such as Hobfoll, note that individuals lacking stress coping resources are more likely to lose more from these situations (Hobfoll, 1989). Individuals in such situations, according to Hobfoll's **Conservation of Resources Model**, may strive to 'obtain, retain and protect personal resources' (Örtqvist and Wincent, 2010: 1360) in order to deal with current or future stressors. Many stressors are generally encountered in daily life, but in the context of healthcare stress, attention has been paid to job roles and the nature of employment, which may bring unique stressors.

Stress as a psychological transaction

One of the perhaps best known, and most commonly used models of stress, is Lazarus and Folkman's **Transactional Model of Stress and Coping** (see Folkman et al., 1986; see also Chapter 18). This model introduced the concepts of primary and secondary **appraisal** in an attempt to explain why individuals do not react to stressors in the same way. In this model, the first process in the stress experience is an individual and **subjective** perception of threat, loss or challenge, which may result from the event or situation we find ourselves in (primary appraisal). For some healthcare professionals, working with patients with cancer may seem threatening, whilst others may welcome working in this field. This important distinction helps to predict who may be most at risk of later stress responses. The next part of the model represents the cognitive process whereby the individual considers their personal ability to cope with the potential stressor (secondary appraisal). Once more, the individual will go through a process of cognitive evaluation of their personal resources that can be employed to improve the primary appraisal. In the case of occupational stress, this may include not only personal coping resources, but also how the working environment may be used as a supportive resource (e.g. the level of team work). Although most individuals are not really aware of their appraisals, they will often verbalize explicitly whether they are coping or not, and so this is something quite important to look out for. Maunder (2006: 32) also notes that stress can occur 'when issues perceived to be important to an individual are not addressed or met', thereby, further demonstrating the individuality of stress. Lazarus later expanded on earlier versions of the Transactional Model, noting that emotions, personality and the situation may also affect our appraisal of a potential stressor (Lazarus, 2006; see also Chapter 18).

OCCUPATIONAL STRESS-SPECIFIC MODELS

These models are important to help understand why stress reactions emerge, and what can be done to reduce the stress. Developed for general populations, however, they can sometimes feel a little removed from the occupational setting. For this, models that focus only on the variables and predictors of workplace stress, such as the **Demand-Control Model** (Karasek, 1979; see also Rubino et al., 2012), should be considered. In this model, stress occurs when the demands of the job interact with the degree of **control** perceived by the individual, to an extent that the former outweighs the latter. Issues such as workload, lack of information and time pressures, for example, may bring about various types of strain, such as 'dissatisfaction, psychological strain, burnout, and somatic problems' (Rubino et al., 2012: 457). Such manifestations of underlying psychological stress may alert others to recognize our strain even if we fail to notice it in ourselves.

Reflective activity

How does stress affect you? List all the physical, psychological and social aspects.

MANIFESTATIONS OF STRESS

The manifestations of stress are varied. The typical physical response as outlined in the GAS Model is the 'fight or flight' *response*, which results in an increased heart and pulse rate, raised blood pressure, 'butterflies' in the stomach, nausea, vomiting, diarrhoea, loss of appetite and a hyper-alert state (Rudinger, 1982). Further physical aspects may include tiredness, a lowered immunity, sleep disturbance and aches and pains. Psychological responses may include irritability, an inability to concentrate, indecision, worrying and generally feeling tense, or even co-morbidities such as anxiety or depression. Individuals may attempt to self-medicate in the form of increasing their drinking or smoking (Kovács et al., 2010), and this represents just one form of **coping response** (see Chapter 18). Lambert and Lambert (2008) go beyond the physi-

Table 30.1 Symptoms of stress

Cognitive	Physical	Emotional	Behavioural
Memory impairment	Headaches	Moodiness	Eating more or less
Indecisiveness	Backache	Agitation	Sleeping more or less
Inability to concentrate	Muscle tension	Restlessness	Isolating oneself from others
Poor judgement	Gastric disturbances	Short temper	Procrastinating
Difficulty to think clearly	Nausea	Irritability	Neglecting responsibilities
Thinking negatively	Dizziness	Impatience	Using substances (alcohol, drugs or cigarettes) to relax
Anxiety	Sleep disturbances	Unable to relax	Nail biting
Worrying	Chest pain	Feeling tense	Pacing
Loss of objectivity	Raised pulse rate	Feeling overwhelmed	Teeth grinding
Fearfulness	Weight change	Feeling lonely or isolated	Jaw clenching
	Skin problems	Depression	Overdoing activities
	Reduced libido		Overreacting to unexpected problems
	Frequent colds or infections		Picking fights with others

cal and psychological dimensions distinguishing stress responses according to four categories: cognitive, physical, emotional and behavioural (see Table 30.1).

When this list of symptoms is presented to groups of healthcare professionals, they quickly recognize the range of symptoms that they have experienced and yet have previously considered to be 'normal'. That is probably because they have not experienced the level of distress that can come from repeated exposure to stressors. Distress has been described as: 'An unpleasant emotional experience of a psychological (cognitive, behavioural, emotional), social and/or spiritual nature that may interfere with the ability to cope effectively …' (Waldrop, 2007: 197–8). Originally, this definition was in relation to cancer adjustment in patients, but those working in the field of oncology may also recognize distress in the healthcare professionals. Such distress can lead to higher levels of mortality and suicide, anxiety and depression, unhealthy behaviours and general ill health (Kovács, et al., 2010; Lim et al., 2010). Occupational stress is noted to be related to increasing health costs, reduced productivity, increased sick leave and impacts upon home and family life (McCloskey and Taggart, 2010; Potter et al., 2010). In addition, the resultant absenteeism may cause high staff turnover rates and negatively impact on patient care, administration costs and the efficient functioning of the organization (Lim et al., 2010).

On a broader scale, occupational stress within the healthcare setting is noted to be increasing due to the industrialization of the working environment, increasing working hours and more challenging working conditions. In a worst-case scenario (which happens all too often), this can result in **burnout** and **compassion fatigue**. The notion of burnout, described by Potter et al. (2010), [citing Maslach's original 1982 study] is the 'cumulative stress from the demands of daily life, a state of physical, emotional, and mental exhaustion caused by a depletion of the ability to cope with one's environment, particularly the work environment' (2010: 57), and is suggested to have a risk prevalence of around 33–44% in oncology staff. This compares to a risk prevalence of around 35–37% for compassion fatigue, which is defined as 'a state of tension and preoccupation with the individual or cumulative traumas of clients' (Potter et al., 2010: 57). Both burnout and compassion fatigue can be identified by three indicators: emotional exhaustion, depersonalization and reduced personal accomplishment (Kovács et al., 2010; Potter et al., 2010). The first of these factors, Kovács et al. (2010) suggest, is when you feel 'used up' at the end of the day; the second can be recognized by becoming increasingly cynical, negative and callous; and the third is when self-esteem dips, accompanied by a sense of non-achievement. Kovács et al.'s (2010) study showed that the longer individuals work in the field of oncology, then the less likely they are to experience emotional exhaustion. This seems to suggest that individuals who do not cope may need to move on from working within this challenging setting. However, other work, such as that of Potter et al. (2010) failed to find any significant association between burnout or compassion fatigue and the length of time that individuals have worked in an oncology unit, but they did note that the environment (inpatient versus outpatients) made some difference to scores on a stress measurement tool.

WORK-RELATED STRESS IN THE HEALTHCARE SETTING

Work-related stress can be derived from several sources and you may have identified some of these if you completed the earlier reflective activity. McCloskey and Taggart, (2010) cite six general aspects found in organizations that may contribute to stress levels, and these clearly build on the models outlined earlier: 'demands (workload, work patterns and environment); control (how much say a person has over their work); relationships; role (including role conflict and role ambiguity); change (including how organizational change is managed in the organization); [and] support (how the organization demonstrates managerial commitment)' (McCloskey and Taggart, 2010: 234). It is easily envisaged how several aspects of stress can be found within the fast-paced health service, where change is often a daily occurrence; however, these aspects could equally be found in any workplace, so it is worth considering what it is about the caring professions working in the field of oncology and palliative care that brings the added stress. The study of McCloskey and Taggart (2010) helps to clarify this, and although it was carried out in a children's hospice, its findings resonate with the field of oncology too. The research explored various stressors and found emotional load, ethical conflicts, constraints to the delivery of good care, limited resources, administration and, for those who are community workers, the notion of living and working in the same community, to be especially problematic. Gupta and Woodman (2010) report similar findings, suggesting that stress commonly results from:

> Being short staffed, increased expectations and demands; increased complexity and numbers of referrals; increased numbers of deaths; too many meetings and not having enough time for administrative tasks; job sharing (for part-time working), extra roles and being on call; being reactive, not proactive, crisis driven, short deadlines and the lack of a waiting list; no time to build relationships with families and no time to follow up issues; staff communication problems including not being heard and feeling unsupported. (Gupta and Woodman, 2010: 16).

Part-time workers have reported that it is more difficult to access support, and many individuals speak of taking their work home (Bruneau and Ellison, 2004). It is in instances such as these that individuals may turn to family and friends rather than seek colleague support. As such, the status of an individual within a team may impact upon levels of perceived stress. In their study of oncology and palliative healthcare professionals, Hulbert and Morrison (2006) found that NHS employees were more stressed than those in similar positions at a hospice, citing job demand and perceptions of responsibility as a potentially important predictive factor. One group of personnel that may often be overlooked, yet are found working in oncology and palliative care, are the volunteers (Claxton-Oldfield and Claxton-Oldfield, 2008). They, too, have particular stressors unique to their job role and position within the organization, which have been found to include the attitudes of the trained staff towards volunteers, being underutilized and, over time, their own loss of interest in the position. Role and status ambiguity also played a part in their stress, with the volunteers wondering what their place was in the team, coupled with not knowing what to do or say to patients and relatives. The education and support of volunteers by healthcare professions is vital and may reduce stress and turnover within this beneficial resource.

Comprehending that the workplace can be a source of stress may cause individuals to consider changing jobs or, if old enough, to retire. Yet the resultant loss of a career and potentially the necessity of re-training in another role may be additionally stressful for the individual; furthermore, the consequences of high staff turnover and a loss of valuable expertise within care teams is problematic to a care delivery service, often contributing to risk of increased stress in the remaining workforce.

The unique working environment

A series of quotes presented by previous researchers, may help to exemplify the special nature of the caring professions' relationships and the untoward stress experienced: 'Cancer care providers tend to empathize with patients' losses, resulting in a personal sense of futility or failure in their care' (Potter et al., 2010: 57) and 'You absorb a lot of families' distress and it just wears you down' (McCloskey and Taggart, 2010: 236).

Maunder, on the other hand, comments that '... when nurses put on their uniform, they often put on a performance of behaviour expected of them in their role and do not display emotions in the same way as they would outside work' (Maunder, 2006: 27). This last statement applies to all healthcare professionals, not just nurses, and is supported by the work of Blomberg and Sahlberg-Blom (2007) who consider the conflict between wanting to give a good standard of care and the ability to actually deliver it: 'The most prominent was the tension between the ideal and the reality, i.e. between what the care staff wanted to give and the care that was actually given' (2007: 245).

Kovács et al. (2010) also explored issues commonly found in cancer and palliative care environments, concluding that stress often 'derives from the emotional instability of patients, their anger management, refusal of treatment, talking about bad prognosis and communication with the relatives' (2010: 844). Chaplin and Mitchell (2005), further point out the significance of working internal existential questioning within the oncology setting, which in healthcare professionals may 'challenge us to consider our own spirituality and in particular our beliefs and values and our own mortality' (2005: 194). As Twycross (1995) points out, facing one's mortality is challenging, and healthcare professionals working in this environment may ruminate on serious illness and death, and how prepared they are themselves to face life-threatening illness. In answering such existential questions, they may arrive at making plans for their own future, such as sorting out a will, having a belief system and considering what happens to a person when, and after, they die.

It is easy to see, therefore, that working in healthcare, and in the field of oncology especially, can give rise to particular challenges not experienced in other walks of life. Oncology and palliative care environments bring unique stressors that may act above and beyond the 'usual' predictors of stress outlined in generic stress models and seen in other occupational groups. It makes professionals question themselves and the standard of care being delivered, and it guarantees that no two days will be the same, thus increasing the emotional demands perceived.

Emotional labour

These statements help to illustrate what is known as **'emotional labour'** or 'emotional work', which are terms that are often used interchangeably (Huynh et al., 2008). Emotional labour is defined as 'the psychological processes necessary to regulate organizationally desired emotions as part of one's job during interpersonal transactions' (Kovács et al., 2010: 855). The term was first coined by Hochschild in 1983 when investigating the work of air stewardesses and debt collectors (Staden, 1998). Maunder (2006) explains that emotional work is the suppression of feelings and emotion, pointing out that occupational culture can impact on the level of suppression. When working in an environment such as oncology or palliative care, healthcare professionals are constantly engaged with the processes of 'surface acting' and 'deep acting' or emotional regulation (Martínez-Iñigo et al., 2007; Maunder, 2006). The former, Maunder (2006) suggests, is when professionals perform emotionally as expected by the public, whilst Martínez-Iñigo et al. (2007) state that surface acting is displaying emotions that are not experienced when there is a mismatch between the felt emotion and what is displayed. For example, we may smile whilst at the same time gritting our teeth.

Deep acting, according to Maunder (2006), is our private emotional system that stays hidden from view; Martínez-Iñigo et al. (2007) suggest that this represents a changed inner feeling state in order to display expected emotions. We may say to ourselves, 'I'm not going to cry, I'm not Going to cry' and we succeed in holding back tears. Martínez-Iñigo et al. (2007) comment that there is a third aspect of emotional labour, that of '**automatic regulation**' (previously known as passive deep acting), which is 'the automatic display of an organizationally desired emotion deriving from an emotion that is spontaneously felt' (2007: 32) Hence, a healthcare professional may feel uncomfortable at breaking bad news and may articulate the same to the patient. This may have a positive consequence because emotional work, such as automatic regulation is, as Maunder (2006) and Martínez-Iñigo et al. (2007) contest, a valuable contributor to building trust with patients and families because they pick up on authentic and inauthentic emotional responses. Martínez-Iñigo et al. (2007) note that suppressing emotions, as in surface acting, can be very demanding and lead to emotional exhaustion. This is echoed in the earlier work of Staden (1998).

In a role where there are repeated losses of relationships (e.g. with patients, their families, etc.), involvement in emotional conflicts and absorption of other's anger, it is all too easy to see how the stress being placed on the healthcare professionals' shoulders can intensify through this emotional work (Twycross, 1995). Given that the service relies on teamwork, emotional labour will be experienced by all the team, who may be expected to support each other. Some aspects of teamwork, however, can add to the burden.

McNeilly and Gilmore (2009) remind us that in the fields of oncology and palliative care, there are often a large number of professionals and agencies involved in the care of the patient and their family. The stages of team formation are well known – forming, storming, norming and performing – but McNeilly and Gilmore (2009) point out that there is also 'reforming' that occurs in working environments where there are constantly changing teams, which can be additionally challenging for some people. There are various aspects of teams that McNeilly and Gilmore highlight as potential sources of stress: the size of the team (the bigger the team, the more problems may occur with effective communication); the leadership aspects (a struggle for power may be happening or the style of leadership can affect the team); conflict in the team (personality clashes, differing values, a lack of voice, levels of communication); role ambiguity (lack of clarity of differing roles) and blurring of boundaries within the team (people unsure of their own particular role).

Brunelli (2005) points out that those who work in settings where the patients have a poor prognosis and where there are repeated losses can be subjected to a physical, psychological and spiritual burden being placed upon them. As a result, healthcare professionals may have to work through a process somewhat similar to a grieving process in order to maintain physical, psychological and spiritual health. If this does not happen, Brunelli cautions, then burnout, emotional distancing, anger and depression may occur, resulting in standards of care dropping. It might be useful, therefore, to consider more about coping within the context of stress (see next section).

COPING WITH, AND INTERVENTIONS FOR, STRESS

Coping at the individual level

As far back as 1954, Abraham Maslow (1970) recognized that coping mechanisms were different to free emotional expression. He asserted that coping has several aspects, including:

- Being purposive and motivated;
- Being effortful (the exceptions to this is that of 'artistic expression' where one learns to be spontaneous and expressive, and where one can try to relax);
- Being determined by external environmental and cultural variables;
- Being based on learning history;
- Being controllable (repressed, suppressed, inhibited or accultured);
- Being designed to cause changes in the environment;
- Characteristically a 'means-behaviour', with the end being a need gratification of threat reduction; and,
- Usually being a conscious activity.

Maunder (2006: 30) would concur with this, noting that 'emotional responses can be learnt and used in certain situations' and cautions that emotions can still be unpredictable, taking us off-guard. Free expression, on the other hand, according to Maslow (1970), is often unmotivated and is effortless. Whether an individual expresses themselves freely, rather than using coping, may depend on how they feel on a particular given day for, as Maslow (1970) put it, expression is determined by the state of the organism. Free expression is usually unlearned over time (just watch or listen to an infant, for example) or it is released or disinhibited. It is more often uncontrolled and sometimes even uncontrollable – as anyone who has burst into tears or lost their temper will attest – and is not designed to do anything: if it causes environmental changes, it does so unwittingly. Free expression is often an end to itself and, more often, an unconscious behaviour.

Lazarus and Folkman proposed that, when faced with a potential stressor, individuals engage with coping characterized by eight different approaches (Lambert and Lambert, 2008): confrontative coping; distancing; self-controlling; seeking social support; accepting responsibility; escape-avoidance; planful problem solving and positive reappraisal. These are sometimes grouped together under the terms problem- or emotion-focused coping strategies (see also Chapter 18). Blomberg and Sahlberg-Blom (2007) report that staff working with patients diagnosed with advanced cancer often engage with distancing and closeness as a means of coping: these tactics may be subconscious (spontaneous) or consciously applied. Stayt (2009) found similar tactics for healthcare staff working in the intensive therapy unit setting, where nurses used distancing as a means of self-preservation. Maunder (2006) suggests that distancing may reduce the opportunity to access resources and possibilities for coping that emanate from the patients and their families.

Healthcare professionals actively incorporate **self-control** into their professionalization through education, role modelling and experience. Team members are an important source of support in this endeavour; however, a potential downside to such strategies is that they may appear to be 'hard' to the lay observer, patient or family member.

Accepting responsibility as a means of coping is something that healthcare professionals may perceive as a causative factor of stress, given that concepts of responsibility and accountability are enshrined within the job. **Escape-avoidance** links very closely with distancing and, once again, may not be in the awareness of the individual. However, if it is re-labelled as taking 'time out', then it perhaps becomes a coping strategy that is more likely to be utilized. The idea of working in our 'comfort zone' could also be applied to escape-avoidance coping: individuals usually prefer to work in familiar settings with people they know – this gives a sense of comfort. Being asked to do the unfamiliar, and with strangers as the team, may instil the need to escape ('fight or flight' responses) or avoid the situation altogether.

Lambert and Lambert (2008) reported that **planful problem solving** is a universally popular coping strategy among health professionals. Sometimes it may take external advice (such as a stress management course) to point out the obvious and give stressed individuals the permission that they require to take up stress-reducing activities, such as walking in nature or listening to music, but these can be effective strategies. Whilst many of these coping strategies operate at an individual level, it may be that there has to be a team approach to managing stress as well.

The final aspect, **positive reappraisal**, is one that can be carried out as an exercise. It requires the individual to take time and think about the various issues that cause stress and to review it using cognitive reappraisal skills (see the following).

Cognitive appraisal

As noted earlier, one way to help reduce stress is through the process of cognitive reappraisal; this is something that you may be familiar with as a core component of psychological interventions such as cognitive or cognitive-behavioural therapy.

Using a sheet of paper, reproduce this table.

First take some time to think about the stressors that affect you (as identified in the first reflective activity) in your daily working life, and then, write them in the respective boxes.

Undertaking this exercise helps us to understand that not all the stressors in our daily

Stressors/control	IMPORTANT stressors	UNIMPORTANT stressors
IN your control		
OUT of your control		

life are equally important, and that there are many things within our control, but many more that are not. Cognitive reappraisal helps us to 'let go' of the unimportant and items beyond our control.

Intervening with teams

Being together with team members, either in the workplace or outside it, such as during social events, serves an important function: that of **social support**. It may be as small as sharing a chat and a cup of tea with a colleague to having a full multidisciplinary team debriefing session. As described earlier, however, some aspects of teamwork may also be a source of stress. Addressing issues within a team, therefore, can be especially beneficial; they do not only reduce stressors that may apply to multiple team members, but also provide an alternative means of coping with other stressors.

In their own research, Gupta and Woodman (2010) applied a Solution-Focused Therapy (SFT) model to stress management. This framework '… is a "here-and-now" approach that emphasises the present and future rather than the past' and aims to 'build solutions rather than solve problems and to focus on strengths and resources.' (2010: 16). This strategy was useful in addressing shared stressors between team members and coming up with jointly acceptable solutions. Actions that were taken included re-configuring the frequency of meetings, reorganization of workloads and on-call service, using a 'buddy-system', having a system to take time back where appropriate, having specific working parties, and spending time outside of work with colleagues doing fun and social activities.

McNeilly and Gilmore (2009) propose the following suggestions for resolving issues within a team, structured according to the primary features of teams that most often cause problems in the first place:

- **Team size:** Ensure that the whole team meets regularly, and that the lines of communication are clearly defined and communicated. Use the induction period to familiarize new staff with various meetings, letting them take an observer role.
- **Leadership:** In each team, have a clear leader and someone to deputize in their absence. Lines of responsibility and accountability can help to establish particular roles. Note that if there are dominant characters within a group this may affect intra-team relationships.
- **Team conflict:** Accept that some conflict is normal and can be healthy for a team; however, if personality clashes occur, then resolution should be sought through supervision or mediation. Aim for the allowance of differing values and ensure that all team members are given an opportunity to air their opinions.
- **Role ambiguity:** Carry out an exercise where individual roles are clarified for the team. Repeat the exercise whenever there are changes in the team or a change in working practices.
- **Boundary blurring:** Rather like role ambiguity, individuals may not know where roles stop and start: clarification may help to establish boundaries, knowing what might be a shared task (for example, if the patient is in pain, all healthcare professionals have an obligation to attend to pain relief) and what might be role-specific.

Maunder (2006) notes that care from the work community can provide a supportive structure to the individual and the team. Hulbert and Morrison (2006) support this, noting that groups, such as nurses, '… are observed to have better health and job satisfaction where support groups are provided.' (p. 247). If an individual is feeling stressed, it may be worthwhile to look at how stress is affecting, and affected by, the whole team. Cancer care professionals rarely work in isolation and so an appreciation at this broader level is helpful and effective in stress management. For managers and others in leadership roles, taking a step back from the day-to-day work and thinking about the team structure and functioning, and how to best support it, may provide a platform for shared advice.

The importance of resilience and reflection

Kovács et al. (2010) suggest **resilience** can be especially helpful in resolving and coping with stressful situations in the workplace. Resilience is defined as 'the capacity for recovery and maintained adaptive behaviour that may follow initial threat or incapacity upon initiating a stressful event' (Garmezy, cited by Koen et al., 2011: 2). Training and education may help to clarify roles and responsibilities and other aspects of care in order to prevent burnout (Claxton-Oldfield and Claxton-Oldfield, 2008); equally, they may contribute to the building of resilience at an individual level.

Bruneau and Ellison (2004), for example, utilized a specific stress management course in order to allow time for individuals to identify and reflect on issues of stress. Maunder (2006) suggests that this type of reflection may helps as 'a prop' to emotionally stressful events. Through it, individuals can hone the ability to 'switch on and off' to maintain personal boundaries and prevent burnout.

Twycross (1995) writes that in coping with stress, individuals need a mind that is ready to take on challenges but at the same time is able to accept that mistakes may be made. It is therefore important to have the ability to correct any mistakes: this can be seen as another form of resilience. He suggests that there are opportunities for personal growth, that the focus should move from one of doing things to patients to one of just being there for them (Twycross, 1995). This latter aspect, whilst challenging, can also be the most rewarding and highly valued by the patients and their carers.

Findings indicating that those who have worked in the field of oncology for a long time are less stressed than newer colleagues could reflect the accumulation of resilience at an individual level over time (Potter et al., 2010; Jones et al., 2011). As such, these individuals could be used as role models or mentors for less resilient and more stressed team members, who may be at different stages of their career.

Reflective activity

- Draw out a map of the team members.
- Note the lines of communication between the differing groups – draw unbroken lines between good communicators and use a broken line for those less effective.
- Which way does the communication flow – one-way or two-way?
- Can you state what the role of each team member is?

Rumination and mindfulness

We are accustomed to what Galfin et al. (2011) call **'rumination'** – a recurrent dwelling on abstract concerns. Rumination brings to mind causes, meaning and implications of situations, often without arriving at a solution, which may, in turn, add to perceived stress levels. Altering thought processes and turning rumination on abstract concerns into controlled thought about something more concrete can be helpful – this can be considered to be employing more positive thoughts.

An alternative strategy to resolving unhelpful rumination might be found in mindfulness-based stress reduction (MBSR) (Kabat-Zinn, 2003; Smith et al., 2005). MBSR has already been used extensively to support patients coping with cancer (see Chapter 22), but it can easily be adapted for other groups. Mindfulness is a form of mediation that focuses on moment-to-moment regulation of attention and thought processes, and is found across many settings to be useful in the alleviation of stress. Mindfulness is described as 'being fully present to one's experience without judgement or resistance' (Potter et al., 2010: 57). It requires internal reflection and noticing of the thoughts and emotions that occur. So, for example, if the cause of the stress is an interpersonal relationship, then the thoughts may be about instances of contact with the other person and then noticing the accompanying emotion (irritation, anger, defensiveness, etc.). As such, the use of mindfulness may help enrich the emotional intelligence of an individual. As McQueen (2004) suggests, this 'requires that emotions are recognized and surfaced. The concept provides understanding of how the emotions experienced by individuals affect the work of the team' (p. 106). Mindfulness meditations may not always arrive at a solution for stress and conflict (although they often do), but increasing awareness of thoughts and their concomitant emotions may help in the monitoring and reduction of negative responses to potentially stressful situations.

Other practical steps for stress reduction

Lambert and Lambert (2008) suggest a raft of steps that may help to reduce stress, which they group under five categories (see Table 30.2).

Table 30.2   Five steps that may reduce stress

Steps	Examples
Avoid unnecessary stress	Say 'no' to additional responsibilities
	Make a 'to do' list and distinguish between 'should do' and 'must do' items
Alter the situation	Express or voice feelings
	Compromise
	Be more assertive
	Manage time well
	Know when to let go of control
	Don't over-commit to activities
Accept the things you cannot change	Distinguish between what can and what cannot be controlled. Some stressors, such as illness or death, cannot be controlled or changed.
	Remind yourself that you can only deal with things within your control
Adapt to the stressor	Focus on the positive, such as abilities and talents
	Reframe the problem
	Look at the big picture
	Do the best you can with the available time, resources and expertise
Take care of personal needs	Identify relaxation time
	Connect with others
	Do something enjoyable every day, even if only for a short time
	Use humour and laughter
	Exercise regularly and eat healthily

Source: Lambert and Lambert (2008)

The more we are aware of stress and its potential management, the more resilient to stress we may become.

Stress management courses were mentioned as an example of a learning opportunity earlier in this chapter. For most people, these can be helpful and effective; however, it is possible that some may perceive a recommendation from a supervisor or colleague to attend such a course as a criticism their coping skills and a barrier to seeking solutions. This is partly because they focus almost exclusively on personal coping approaches, rather than the broader context of environmental and organizational factors. Gupta and Woodman (2010) note that solutions are often needed in 'individual, team and service categories, and often required combined commitments' (p. 16).

The solutions and advice that work best are often those that emanate from the team rather than those imposed by management. Having a social gathering, for example, may not suit all. What is important is that team members have an opportunity to contribute to a discussion on stress and how to resolve (if at all possible) or at least reduce the impact of it.

CHAPTER SUMMARY

This chapter has considered what stress is, how it may manifest itself and what strategies may be helpful within the cancer care setting to reduce workforce stress. Oncology (and palliative care) environments bring a recognized number of stressors that are not often seen in other organization settings. These unique stressors within the caring professions require emotional labour and put workers at high risk of compassion fatigue and burnout. In order to promote a healthy workforce, attention has to be paid to how individuals can be supported within that workforce to cope with and mediate against stress. Increasingly, more awareness of the effects of stress has led to the development of a range of stress-reduction strategies, both for the individual and the team, and many of these are supported by commissioning and policymaking bodies.

It is important that healthcare professionals share the responsibility of monitoring not only the patient and their families, but also their work colleagues for signs of stress. Stress does not often happen in isolation: it has a clear interpersonal dimension. Therefore, the team, as well as the individual, can play a crucial role in reducing or alleviating workplace stressors.

Working within a cancer care setting exposes professionals to stressors that are often out of personal control, and accepting that may be a useful starting point to coping with the demands of the job. Equally, though, there are some stressors that can be more easily controlled and the identification of these provides a valuable starting point. Ultimately, if the cancer care workforce is a healthy one that can effectively manage stressors, it will be better placed to help those patients with the support that it is there to provide.

Key learning points

- Cancer care professionals are at high risk of developing stress and stress-related conditions, such as burnout. This can compromise good patient care.
- Stress causes a range of physical and cognitive symptoms, and in chronic and serious cases can lead to psychological co-morbidity and serious physical illness.

(Continued)

A review of literature shows that people affected by cancer have been involved in a myriad of activities, including involvement and engagement in research, policy and planning and practice (Hubbard, Kidd, et al., 2007). The authors note that the biggest gap in understanding the agenda of involvement and engagement is about the impact that it has on care delivery, although one study has attempted to examine impact (Daykin et al., 2007b).

The purpose of this chapter is to highlight the different ways in which patients and the public are, or can be, involved and outline some of the most pertinent issues for readers who wish to take the agenda of public and patient involvement forward in their own practice, whether that is in the policymaking, research or caregiving arena.

Reflective activity

Think about your most recent use of NHS services, as a patient or as a relative of someone using the NHS.

1. Jot down a brief note of what the appointment was for (e.g. *immunization with children? Blood test? Surgery?*).
2. To what extent do you think the practitioner was interested in your experience of that healthcare interaction? (Score from 0-10).
3. How does your experience as a patient differ to their understanding as a professional?

Almost everyone will have experience of using healthcare. These episodes of care can be useful to reflect upon to ensure that the care provided, or the research conducted, upholds the standards that healthcare professionals would expect for themselves. Although it is hard to continually maintain a dual awareness of ourselves as practitioner/researcher AND patient/carer, pausing to consider this can be fruitful in calibrating expectations.

PATIENT EXPERIENCES

Listening to **patient experiences** can be seen as one of the most straightforward ways of involving service users. Patient experience constitutes the person's feelings, their evaluation of their healthcare encounter and their expectations. Patient experience, therefore, takes an explicit focus on what it is like to receive healthcare, adopting a position of interest in patient, not professional, viewpoint. The importance of distinguishing between personal and professional knowledge has been written about for a long time:

> '… "truth learned from personal experience with a phenomenon" rather than "truth acquired through discursive reasoning, observation, or reflection on information provided by others"' (Borkman, 1976: 446).

The definition proposed by Borkman, which has since been taken up by multiple authors, indicates a need to separate out and view differently professional from patient knowledges.

Patient experiences have begun to be collated as a way of measuring the non-clinical elements of care. Although some experiences are likely to be unique, others may be shared by particular groups of people affected by cancer due to their cancer type, age, ethnicity, social class and whether or not they reside in rural or urban locations.

Rather than focusing on satisfaction surveys, questionnaires have been developed to identify overall patient feedback, which have been validated and adopted internationally (Jenkinson et al., 2002). In Scotland, for example, the collection and collation of patient experiences was integrated into the 2008 policy *Better Health, Better Care* (Scottish Government, 2008a). As part of this, *Better Together*, Scotland's Patient Experience Programme, was established and prompted a considerable amount of work in identifying patient experiences. In England, Patient Reported Outcome Measures (PROMs) (Black, 2013) assess the quality of care delivered to NHS patients from the patient perspective. PROMs have been collected by all providers of NHS-funded care since April 2009.

A wide range of other patient-experience resources has also emerged, documenting people's encounters with the health service. Health Talk Online (www.healthtalk.org/) is one exemplar of this and is the work of a health experience research group, which has created a unique database of personal and patient experiences through in-depth qualitative research into over 50 different illnesses and health conditions.

Further websites, such as E-learning for Practitioners (www.e-lfh.org.uk/), provide other avenues for accessing patient experience. E-learning for Practitioners is a free and engaging resource to help clinicians develop understanding of their role in contributing to the management and leadership of healthcare services.

Reflective activity

Consider the evidence in your service or research of the following:

- Staff enquiring about patient experiences.
- What would the response be if you were to introduce ideas of asking for patient feedback?
- How would you go about starting to get feedback on patients' experiences?
- What gets in the way of finding out about the experiences of patients/service users and carers/family members?

Asking patients about their experience does not necessarily require a great deal of skill or expertise, for example Level 1 practitioners should be able to elicit and deal with straightforward pieces of feedback. What is necessary is a genuine interest in the person's experiences.

Practitioners and researchers often worry that they do not have the right resources to engage in these kind of conversations, for example not having a private space to ask for feedback, or indeed having the time or staff to free up to do this. Others worry that it is important to find representative patients. While these are issues to consider, one core principle remains: asking patients to reflect on their care, informally, during the course of routine practice can be a powerful, quick and important way of gaining patient reflections on their experiences.

STRUCTURES TO SUPPORT PATIENT AND PUBLIC INVOLVEMENT

Patient and public involvement has been formalized and supported by a number of organizations. At the time of writing, a number of bodies have been created to champion patient and public involvement:

- The Scottish Health Council
- Board of Community Health Councils in Wales
- HealthWatch in England.

These UK bodies have a very broad remit, which is to promote patient and public involvement in healthcare and monitor whether local NHS services are working well to involve and engage the public.

The Scottish Health Council (n.d.) was established by the Scottish Executive in April 2005 to promote patient focus and public involvement in the NHS in Scotland. This has three core functions:

- **Community Engagement and Improvement Support** – providing proactive and tailored support for NHS Boards.
- **Participation Review** – reviewing and evaluating NHS Boards' approaches to participation.
- **Participation Network** – a centre for the exchange of knowledge, support, development and ideas.

Similarly in Wales, Community Health Councils are designed to:

- Provide help and advice if you have problems with or complaints about NHS services;
- Ensure that your views and needs influence the policies and plans put in place by health providers in your area;
- Monitor the quality of NHS services from your point of view; and
- Give you information about access to the NHS.

Community Health Councils in England were abolished in 2003 and replaced by Patient and Public Involvement Forums, which, in 2008, were replaced by Local Involvement Networks (LINks). LINks were incorporated into HealthWatch, which was established in 2012. HealthWatch is the independent consumer champion for health and social care in England. Working with a network of 152 local authorities, HealthWatch ensures that the voices of consumers and those who use services reach the ears of the decision makers.

Finally, it is worth pointing out that the UK charity 'INVOLVE' carries out research and delivers training to inspire citizens, communities and institutions to take part in high-quality public participation processes, consultations and community engagement. Readers may wish to contact these organizations to find out how members of the public have been involved in local healthcare planning. In doing so, readers will appreciate that involvement and engagement of patients and the public takes many different forms, investing people with power and control about local healthcare to a lesser or greater degree.

POWER AND CONTROL

Traditionally, public involvement has been defined and distinguished by the level of power and control that people have over policy and services. Arnstein's (1969) 'eight-rung ladder of power' was initially designed to understand citizen involvement and the redistribution of political power in decision-making about service planning in the USA. It remains a forceful way of representing involvement and engagement in policymaking but also in any form of involvement and engagement activity. Indeed, Charles and DeMaio (1993) adapted it in their model of lay participation in decision-making about personal care, identifying three degrees of control that patients have ranging from **consultation**, which is the lowest form of control, to **partnership** and **dominant control**.

Hanley (2005) distinguishes between consultation, collaboration and user-controlled involvement in a hierarchy of involvement:

> **Consultation:** people are asked for their views that are used to inform decision-making. These views will not necessarily be adopted, although they may have an influence on decision-making.
>
> **Collaboration:** involves active, ongoing partnership with members of the public/people who use services.
>
> **User-controlled:** power, initiative and subsequent decision-making lies with service users rather than with professionals.

This hierarchy of involvement can be applied to different types of involvement and engagement. Take involvement in treatment decision-making, for example. A doctor may *consult* a patient on the type of treatment that they would prefer but not necessarily act upon it, or a doctor and patient may *collaborate* over the course of an illness and decide collectively upon the treatment and finally a patient may divest doctors of any control over the type of treatment that they have and make the decision alone. In the following section, involvement in treatment decision-making is used as an exemplar of involvement and engagement in care practice.

Reflective activity

Cynthia is a member of a group tasked with developing clinical pathway guidelines for lung cancer. She is the only patient advisor on the group, which includes three surgeons, two general practitioners, a clinical nurse specialist and two service managers. The group meets three times a year. Documents are sent prior to the meeting. Some of these documents are 200 pages long and cover detailed clinical information about the disease.

- What support would you expect Cynthia to need, in order to be able to fully participate in the meeting?
- What would you want the professionals in the room to be mindful of during the course of the meeting itself?

(Continued)

(Continued)

You may have thought that there would be a power imbalance with senior clinicians and managers at this meeting. It is considered best practice to invite at least two service users onto groups, so that they have their own peer group and someone else who can be called upon to give a service user perspective. With so many senior practitioners and managers, this is likely to help ensure that the patients feel like they have a voice within the meetings. This is particularly the case if any of the clinicians were involved in patients' care. Further, the Chair of the meeting might want to meet with the service users before the meeting to ensure they understand the documents and have had a chance to add items to the agenda. This should ensure that power is shared more equally among participants.

You may also have considered whether summary documents would be useful for the patients, alongside briefing notes on some of the more complex clinical information, to augment their knowledge about their own condition.

Of course, Cynthia may well be a powerful individual herself and be used to appraising long, complex documents in her professional life as a Barrister or CEO. The Chair of the group should have determined what she felt she'd need to be able to contribute to the meeting.

There is a move towards greater patient and public involvement and engagement in healthcare. There has been an increased emphasis on patient involvement in decision-making and engaging in self-care. Involvement in one's own care is considered essential and replaces the traditional top–down 'doctor knows best' model of care (Coulter, 1997). Self-care and self-management are examples of patients being involved in actually *doing* care either to prevent illness in the first place or to manage their health when they are ill (see also Chapter 23).

INVOLVEMENT AND ENGAGEMENT IN DECISION-MAKING

There is a vast body of literature on self-care and self-care management in cancer (see McCorkle et al., 2011; Fenlon and Foster, 2009). This chapter focuses on involvement and engagement in treatment decision-making because making a decision about treatment has implications for patients' quality of life, ongoing physiological and psychosocial problems, and survival. It is, therefore, a potentially momentous decision to make.

Patients can be involved in decisions about their care to a greater or lesser degree and the level of involvement and engagement will depend on the power of the patient relative to that of the healthcare professional. This **power equation** will be mediated by the healthcare professional's willingness to adapt (Thompson, 2007). The extent of involvement and engagement will also depend on patient preferences for how much they wish to be involved in making a decision about their treatment. A review of patient preferences for involvement in cancer treatment decision-making suggests that the preferences of patients with cancer vary considerably (Hubbard et al., 2010). While most patients prefer a collaborative role whereby they make the decision jointly with healthcare professionals, a significant minority prefer to remain passive and let the medical profession decide, whereas others prefer to play an active role and make the decision themselves (Hubbard et al., 2010). In 2007, guidance on involving patients in treatment decision-making for medical practitioners was published (General

Medical Council, 2007). Indeed, in recent years there has been a substantial increase in patient involvement in decisions about their care (Tariman et al., 2010). Analysis of 41,441 patients in the National Cancer Patient Experience Survey found that younger patients and ethnic minorities reported substantially less positive experiences of involvement in decision-making and that experience varied considerably between patients with different cancers, with ovarian, myeloma, bladder and rectal cancer patients reporting substantially worse experiences compared with other patients with gynaecological, haematological, urological and colorectal cancers, respectively (El Turabi et al., 2013).

Reflective activity

A 62-year-old man has been diagnosed with prostate cancer. The tumour is confined to his prostate, and the clinical markers of the tumour indicate that surgery is not immediately necessary. The man has the choice between either active surveillance through regular blood tests or laparoscopic surgery. The urologist advises careful consideration of the physical consequences of surgery, including the risk of impotence and incontinence. She also suggests that the patient should consider the psychological consequences of surveillance, for example the risk of increased anxiety and the man's fear of disease spreading.

Consider the position of the patient in this scenario.

- What factors would you want the man to consider when he makes his decision?
- Who else would you expect him to talk his decision over with?
- What other questions would you expect the man to ask the urologist?

One key area to consider might be whether the patient has discussed the treatment choices with a partner. With significant impact on sexual functioning, many men with prostate cancer welcome the opportunity to talk to clinicians and their partner about how surgery might impact their intimate relationships (Forbat et al., 2011). You might also be interested in whether the patient feels well enough informed about either option before they make a choice, and whether they want this responsibility or would rather defer to the doctor.

Research shows that family members can be conduits of information given by health professionals when they are told about their cancer diagnosis or when they discuss treatments and can also help patients make decisions about their care (Hubbard et al., 2010; Illingworth et al., 2010). Other research (Fraenkel and McGraw, 2007; Chewning et al., 2012) has noted that most patients and family caregivers valued and expected family involvement in treatment decision-making. However, there is little explicit agreement in regard to which party in the dyad should take decisional leadership and who should play a supporting role (Shin et al., 2013).

To summarize, involvement in treatment decision-making is a complex process that requires an appreciation of the biopsychosocial consequences of the different options available. Importantly though, involvement also needs to be cognizant of the role of family members in helping in information recall, prompting full disclosure of information from practitioners and assisting in considering the repercussions of the treatment choices made. Relatives have an important part to play in supporting and facilitating the patient to make decisions about their treatment.

INVOLVEMENT AND ENGAGEMENT IN RESEARCH

A review of literature (Hubbard, Kidd, et al., 2007) identified five roles that people affected by cancer have played in research:

1. Advocates
2. Strategists
3. Reviewers
4. Advisors
5. Participatory researchers

Advocacy is when people affected by cancer lobby for research funding or for particular research being carried out. The review found that breast cancer and prostate cancer have strong advocacy movements that have been particularly successful in the USA. Involvement at **strategic** level is evidenced by membership of bodies that make decisions about what research projects are funded or receive ethics approval. Similarly, people affected by cancer may act as **reviewers**, deciding which research proposals are funded or not. People affected by cancer have acted in an **advisory** capacity for individual research projects by, for example, being a member of a project steering group. Finally, people affected by cancer have also been involved as **participatory researchers**, where they have engaged in project planning, study design and conducting studies.

CASES STUDIES DEMONSTRATING PATIENT INVOLVEMENT

This section details two case studies of patient involvement in the work at the Cancer Care Research Centre, University of Stirling. Both examples illustrate participatory involvement.

CASE STUDY

Peter

When people are first told they have cancer, the realization is shock or delayed shock. With me, knowing that I was going to die, because cancer and death were to me synonymous, the shock hit me about two weeks after my diagnosis of prostate cancer.

At first I was a bit blasé about the diagnosis but at a family gathering I suddenly had an overwhelming feeling to cry ... but men cannot be seen to cry, can they? So I left the house and wandered the streets alone, blaspheming and, yes, crying. I don't remember how long it was before I had composed myself and was able to return to my family and friends. It was probably much sooner than I imagine. If any of them had noticed my absence they were kind enough not to mention it.

I knew very little about my prostate. I had an idea where it was and that it had something to do with urinating, but no idea of what its real function was. The Internet helped a bit and I even cheered up when I was told that I was to receive radiotherapy - maybe I was not going to die immediately if 'they' were going to give me treatment. I'd had, up to this time, a healthy life and had little experience of doctors and no experience of health consultants. But events changed a bit when my consultant gave me a letter saying an organization intended to form a support group in the Glasgow area.

I joined the group at its inaugural meeting, met other prostate cancer patients and learned that with a bit of luck I could live quite a long time with the disease, following treatment. I decided that I would make a point of telling as many men as I could that a diagnosis of prostate cancer was not necessarily a death sentence. I was also determined to find out as much as possible about the disease. I ran a prostate cancer support group for a few years, joined the Prostate Cancer Charity (TPCC) as a volunteer helper and was asked to become a patient advisor with the Cancer Care Research Centre (CCRC) at the University of Stirling. I enjoy being involved and truly believe that I have helped many prostate cancer patients overcome their initial fears when told they have prostate cancer just by talking to them.

An example of involvement

The opportunity came to contribute to a research project, headed by Dr Liz Forbat at CCRC, which examined the reasons for the timing of men's diagnosis with prostate cancer. The study (Forbat et al., 2013) investigated the profile of men diagnosed in Greater Glasgow over a two-year period (2008–2009). The team explored the experiences of men before they were diagnosed, including finding out what triggered them to or prevented them from going to their doctor. The study was based on clinical information (pathology records), a postal survey and interviews.

As one of five patient advisors on the team, I had the privilege of sitting in on and contributing my ideas to the whole research process. This included:

- Developing the research method (including suggesting the involvement of male interviewers to put patients at ease).
- Reviewing/assessing the study paperwork (such as survey and interview questions).
- Commenting on the results and conclusions.
- I was also able to be involved in interviewing some of the men who agreed to take part in the study.

In this academic community, the role of the patient advisor is to bring the experience of patients to bear on prioritizing research questions, ensuring the patient-friendliness of any communication or survey, and ensuring the validity of the results and conclusions from a patient's perspective. If well exercised, the role of the patient advisor should enhance the quality and relevance of the investigation, enable the patient advisor to engage effectively in discussions and give the researcher the confidence of knowing that the subject matter has been test-driven. I think that this form of public involvement is very important in reassuring all those involved, especially the research community, that it is an important and valid piece of work.

Was my contribution relevant?

The team believed that more men answered the survey because of the involvement of those affected by prostate cancer (there was a 70% response rate). The involvement of men helped to ensure the survey asked the right questions and was readable/accessible.

Recognition for our involvement

In April 2011, the project won the prestigious Award for User Involvement at the COMPASS Annual Scientific Meeting in Edinburgh for the research team from CCRC. A follow-up article appeared in the Autumn 2011 issue of INVOLVE about involvement.

(Continued)

(Continued)

Peter McAlear was diagnosed with prostate cancer in 1999. His initial treatment was radiotherapy but his cancer returned in 2004. He now has locally advanced prostate cancer and is undergoing hormone therapy. He is a patient representative with CCRC, a volunteer helper with the Prostate Cancer UK and a Prostate Cancer Support Group member.

CASE STUDY

Bill

In the spring of 2000, aged 57, I was diagnosed as having serious, inoperable lung cancer. Following chemo and radiotherapy treatment at the Beatson Oncology Centre in Glasgow, I was able to return to work in December.

After my recovery I was asked to become involved with a lung cancer support group and an advisory board. I think that many people who have been through a serious, life-threatening illness, such as cancer, and survive to tell the tale, have a built-in desire to try and pay something back into the system which saved them. That was the case with me, and I was happy to become involved with these two organizations.

In August 2003, I was asked to be interviewed by a researcher from the Cancer Care Research Centre (CCRC) in connection with my illness and subsequent recovery. I then got involved in their Patient and Carer Advisory Group at the University of Stirling.

This comprised attending focus group meetings hosted by a researcher, designed to encourage those present to engage in meaningful discussion. From the start, it was obvious that the views and points raised by the patients/carers and family members were important to CCRC, rather than just a box-ticking exercise.

Apart from giving me a platform from which to air my views, attendance at the groups made me more aware of the different types of cancer and the difficulties faced by those involved. It also gave me the opportunity to speak with policymakers, the Scotland Health Minister and the media. This allowed people like me to put forward topics that our group were concerned with (like improving patient care) to the people who can make changes happen.

I continued my involvement with CCRC and, when I retired at the end of 2009, I was given the position of Research Assistant/Patient Experience Advisor with the Centre. Becoming an 'official' member of the team allowed me to become involved in more depth, and to learn more about the Centre's work and aims. My attendance at monthly team meetings ensures that there is a patient's viewpoint borne in mind during discussions.

In this capacity, I attended the International Observatory on End of Life Care's International Research Summer School at Lancaster University in summer 2010. This gave me a much broader insight into the work carried out by researchers. I have also attended Research Ethics Committee meetings at the University of Stirling as an observer.

Lately, I have had the privilege of interviewing other cancer patients and family members (along with a senior researcher) in connection with ongoing projects. I feel this has been beneficial to all concerned – the patient, the researcher, CCRC and myself.

The 'been there' theory helps me to build up a feeling of trust between the interviewer and interviewee.

One of the most important things I have learned during my time as a service user involved with CCRC is that the professional researchers really do value the input of patients/carers and family members because they know that we have a wealth of information just waiting to be tapped.

I feel very fortunate to be in this position, and long may it continue.

Bill Culbard, Research Assistant/Patient Experience Advisor

These case studies highlight the profundity of cancer diagnosis, which may be a catalyst for involvement in support groups and patient and carer advisory groups. Involvement is evidently not a one-off event but a process that has small beginnings that mushroom to more intensive and sophisticated forms of involvement. These case studies illustrate that patients can be involved in different activities to facilitate the research process including advocacy and lobbying, advising how to design a study and then conduct the research, and conducting interviews. The involvement of patients improves the quality of the work that is carried out at CCRC and is highly valued. If Bill and Peter had not been involved in the research at CCRC, then the Centre's activities would not be as relevant to patients and the quality of the research would be impoverished.

INVOLVEMENT AND ENGAGEMENT IN TEACHING HEALTHCARE PROFESSIONALS

One of the ways in which patients and the public can influence healthcare is by influencing the current and future workforce by involvement in **education** and **training** programmes for healthcare professionals. Clinical skills training of medical students has a long tradition of using actors to play the part of patients so that students can improve their communication skills. Innovations have been made to these approaches by involving members of the public with healthcare experiences as 'standardized patients' so that trainee medics can hone their skills prior to engaging with patients on the wards.

Patients can have a positive impact on the future healthcare workforce. A randomized controlled study (Klein et al., 1999) was carried out with third-year undergraduate medical students on an interview methods course; one group of students was taught with patients with cancer and the control group was taught with patients with other diagnoses participating. Klein et al. (1999) found that the involvement of patients with cancer enhanced students' ability to elicit psychosocial information and to relate more effectively to patients with cancer. Two years after the course, they found that those students taught by patients with cancer compared to those taught by patients with other diagnoses had a better rating in terms of:

… responding empathically, showing regard and concern for the patient, and assessing the impact of the symptoms on the patient's life. (Klein et al., 1999: 1455)

MODELS AND MUDDLES OF INVOLVEMENT AND ENGAGEMENT

The previous sections have presented case studies of involvement and engagement in research and teaching and illustrated the ways in which patients and family caregivers are involved in treatment decision-making. They illustrate that patients and the public are involved in different activities, but also how involvement and engagement is conceptualized in different ways. This diversity is strength, but it can also cause confusion and there is a lack of clarity about the scope and purpose of involvement and engagement. Should patient and public involvement be about patient care or about making research more relevant? This section describes four different models of involvement and engagement and their ideological drivers. Table 31.1 presents four models of involvement, identifying who is involved, what activity of involvement they participate in and the underpinning ideological driver (Forbat et al., 2009a).

Table 31.1 Four models of involvement

Who	What	Ideological drivers
Consumer	Purchase or choice of service	Free-market economics
Citizen	Policy and service planning	Social democratic
Partner	Care practice	Experiential knowledge
Researcher	Co-research	Emancipation and empowerment

Model 1: consumer

The term '**consumer**' is used interchangeably with the term patient or public in involvement and engagement literature. As a consumer or customer of healthcare services, patients can be aptly described as consumers, and the marketization and privatization of healthcare clearly positions patients as consumers. In private healthcare markets, consumers *buy* healthcare products or services for personal use. Nevertheless, patients can also be positioned as consumer within a welfare state model, particularly if they are conceptualized as choosing different services.

Patient choice is increasingly a key concept within the British welfare state model. The free-market economic doctrine (Needham, 2003) asserts that health services will be developed as a consequence of consumer choice and preference. The underpinning ideology is that consumers form preferences for health services without reference to other people, and make choices in a purely self-regarding and self-interested way. The aggregation of individual consumer actions ultimately decides what health services are available because those that consumers choose thrive, whilst those that are not chosen cease to be offered. Accountability of services is thereby secured by competition and complaint, with the consumer playing the pivotal role. The extent to which consumers are 'free' to exert their influence via purchase and control is a marker for the consumer model.

Reflective activity

Emily has been diagnosed with localized breast cancer. Her preference is to have a lumpectomy, rather than a mastectomy. She asked her local hospital to provide her with information about the number and type of breast operations that each of the surgeons have conducted in the past year so she could make a decision about who would be best placed to do her surgery.

- What is Emily's role as a consumer in her healthcare? How might she make a decision based on the information the hospital gives her?

Having access to information about clinician performance seems intuitively a good thing. Nevertheless, because there are so many influences on performance, comparing different clinician performance is not a straightforward process. For example, one surgeon may take the more complex cases compared to other surgeons, or their patient profile may be much older and with co-morbidity. However, by asking for details of surgical procedures patients can make more informed decisions and take responsibility for choosing procedures, rather than the previous model of accepting what is offered.

Model 2: citizen

Social democratic societies position people as **citizens** and the public as an inter-connected collective of citizens. As a citizen of a society composed of other citizens, individuals form preferences for health services with reference and respect to others and in the interest of the common good. In this model, individuals are accountable to each other. It is not just about what is good for the individual's health and wellbeing, but what is mutually beneficial and good for society as a whole. Choices about services are made collectively and in the context of wider interests than that of the purely personal. Citizens can devolve decision-making about service organization to professionals and politicians who are entrusted to use their expertise and judgement to plan and deliver services. Accountability of services is secured through democratic structures in which citizens participate. Ideological drivers for patients as citizens originate in a form of Government known as social democracy.

Reflective activity

A public meeting is called in a local Health Board where senior members of the management team ask for patient feedback on the closing of services. The press and public unite in vociferous campaigns to keep the services open, citing how closing services will lead to inequities in care.

(Continued)

Model 3: partner

Arguably, people have always been involved in their own care and those of their family and friends. Parents look after their children and children look after their parents in old age. Nevertheless, the policy drive to self-care and self-management has positioned people firmly as **partners** alongside the healthcare professional in being responsible for their own care and decision-making about their care. The ideology underpinning this model is experiential knowledge, which is a conception that patients have a unique perspective on and knowledge about their illness because they are the ones most affected by it. It is a conceptualization that shifts power in the form of knowledge from the medical profession to the individual who has personal and direct experience of the illness or vicarious experience of the illness through looking after someone. It also shifts the nature of the relationship between a patient and a clinician, from passivity and paternalism to shared responsibility and mutual respect for what each person brings to the medical encounter.

Reflective activity

Increasingly, people living with the consequences of cancer may attend rehabilitation courses, aimed to encourage the uptake of healthy lifestyle behaviours such as increasing exercise, smoking cessation and adopting good dietary habits.

● How is responsibility managed in these scenarios, where the practitioner holds expert knowledge about what exercise is safe and what diet is appropriate for someone who has had a cancer diagnosis?
● If this is 'involvement as partnership', who exactly is the patient a 'partner' with?

Although practitioners have undergone extensive periods of training, there is evidence that encouraging people to take an active role in their health and wellbeing has positive impacts for them. Further, those who have personal experience of the disease may be best placed to guide their own recovery, with limited support from practitioners.

Self-care extends beyond the period of treatment and into survivorship. Given the premise that self-care is engaged with in the home/community, changes may well impact on more than just the patient, and shifts in lifestyle behaviours may benefit other family members too. The patient is therefore a partner with the healthcare professionals and their relatives.

Model 4: researcher

The fourth model shows involvement in **research** as a distinct conceptualization. Involvement in research (Hanley, 2005) has been driven by agendas underpinned by ideologies of **emancipation** stemming originally from both disability and feminist lobbies in the 1960s and 1970s. Emancipatory or **participatory research** (Baum et al., 2006) implies, for example, that research about women should be done by or with women as opposed to being done on them. It conceptualizes people as co-researchers rather than just objects or subjects of research, and suggests that research should herald something that is good for the community.

Alongside notions of emancipation is the notion that there are competing truths and that all understandings of history and people's experiences are subjective and can be contested. In this model, a healthcare event can be interpreted and understood in a number of different ways. Traditionally, illness research has prioritized clinicians' concerns, thereby disadvantaging patient perspectives and reinforcing hegemonic knowledge. By attending to patient views and experiences by involving them in driving and contributing collaboratively to the research agenda, the power imbalance is challenged and historical hierarchies of erudition can begin to be dislodged.

Reflective activity

Research agendas are often set by Governments, wishing to increase standards of care, or practitioners who are curious about the impact of different treatments on patients.

- What are the likely impacts on the topics of research if patients are facilitated to help make decisions about what is funded or prioritized?

You may have considered the example from Peter McAlear, in the first case study, and thought that the involvement of patients would help ensure the relevance of research and public funding to patients. You may also have thought about the kind of training and mechanisms that need to be in place so that patients can fully understand the consequences of different kinds of research – to ensure that power is indeed shared and that patients have adequate space in decision-making meetings to voice their views and influence the agenda.

CHAPTER SUMMARY

The agenda of patient and public involvement in health is firmly established and is unlikely to be dismantled. People are involved in a myriad of activities, including healthcare policy, planning and research, as well as in their own and their family's and friends' care. Structures have been established to champion and support involvement. The power and control that people have over their health and services can be conceived along a continuum. Involvement and engagement can include singular activity or occur in a continuous process of engagement. Nevertheless, there is confusion about this agenda because of the different ways in which involvement is conceptualized. Depending on the model of involvement adopted, people are positioned as consumers/customers, citizens, partners in care or as co-researchers.

Reflective activity

Readers should consider the following:

- Is there a tradition of patient and public involvement and engagement in your area?
- What organizations exist to champion involvement in your area and are they effective?
- What attitudes do patients and healthcare professionals in your area have about involvement and engagement?
- What kind of training is available to patients and healthcare professionals to engage fully in user involvement and engagement?
- Where does power and control over healthcare decision-making really lie?
- Who possesses the most knowledge about illness?
- Are different models of involvement mutually exclusive? Can you be a consumer and citizen at the same time?

Key learning points

- There are different structures in the UK to support the involvement and engagement of patients and the public in health.
- There are a myriad of activities that patients and the public can be involved in.
- Power and control over personal healthcare, policy, planning and research varies.
- Involvement and engagement are about relationships between individuals who possess different knowledge, power and control.

Recommended further reading

- Barnes, M. and Cotterell, P. (eds) (2012) *Critical Perspectives on User Involvement*, Bristol, UK: Policy Press.

The following websites may be helpful:

- Involve (www.involve.org.uk/about/)
- HealthTalk (www.healthtalkonline.org) and (www.youthhealthtalk.org)
- Not strictly reading, but the following video describes patient involvement in Harvard Medical School: www.youtube.com/watch?v=jkHOoD_Mc64

32 CLINICAL DRUG TRIALS IN CANCER CARE

PAT GILLIS AND EMMA WHITBY

Chapter outline

- Context of clinical trials and research in cancer care
- Phases (I, II, III, IV) and types of clinical trials
- The role of the research practitioner, especially regarding recruitment into trials
- Patient perspectives and considerations
- Management of clinical trials
- Quality of life assessment

INTRODUCTION

The burden of cancer is predicted to increase by 33% by the year 2020 (Coupland et al., 2010), although more people are now living longer with, and surviving, the disease. Survivors of cancer will need to expect to live with various physical and psychological effects of their illness as the NHS strives to identify improved ways of diagnosing and treating the condition, as well as supporting patients with what is now viewed as a chronic disease associated with long-term management challenges (DH, 2011a).

The delivery of world-class care to patients with cancer is of the highest priority for all professionals working in this field, as set out in the *NHS Cancer Plan* (DH, 2000) and the *NHS Constitution* (DH, 2013). To enable this, the NHS must be in a position to deliver the highest quality cancer research. To continue to improve survival rates and quality of life for those affected by cancer, it is of primary importance to ensure that any developments made though research are expedited and translated efficiently into standard practice (National Institute for Health Research (NIHR), 2013). Research takes many forms, although this chapter will particularly focus on the value of **randomized controlled clinical trials**. In comparison to other research methods, clinical trials are widely recognized as the gold standard approach for researching new treatments and procedures (Bench et al., 2013).

THE UK CONTEXT

In 2000, the UK Department of Health published the *NHS Cancer Plan* (DH, 2000). This document was the result of a strategic review of cancer care delivery within the NHS in England, and subsequently shaped the way cancer services evolved over time. One of the key messages was that, despite having world-class clinical researchers, scientists and equipment, survival rates for cancer in England lagged significantly behind those in other countries. The reason for this was identified as a lack of a sufficiently robust **infrastructure** at frontline clinical level to support the delivery of clinical research. The conduct of research in England was much slower than in Europe or America. This played a vital role in the lack of timely progress for cancer care in this country.

As a result, the Government recognized that coordinated and timely delivery of research is of vital importance to improve outcomes for patients with cancer. The Department of Health re-affirmed its commitment to enhancing the contribution of research to health and social care, whilst minimizing the risks associated with it.

In 2001, the Government commissioned and established the National Cancer Research Network (NCRN), providing investment in infrastructure at the clinical level to support delivery of high quality research programmes. Research practitioners and data managers were employed across the country to provide active support to researchers, enabling them to deliver research results quicker, whilst still ensuring high quality data and information to inform new treatments for the future.

The NCRN became a key component of a number of managed systems and processes that brought together research funders and key professionals to design clinical trials that pose relevant clinical inquiry thereby influencing an improvement in care and treatment. The outcome of these studies will shape the next generation of treatment and will eliminate duplication of effort in multiple smaller trials. The NCRN infrastructure supports recruitment of patients from all over England and has been hugely successful. Prior to the NCRN, only 3.75% of patients with cancer were eligible or recruited into clinical trials, but by 2011/12, this had increased to 23% placing the NCRN as a world leader in clinical trials (Merseyside and Cheshire Cancer Research Network Annual Report, 2012/13)

The success of the NCRN was quickly recognized and provided the model for delivering research in other disease areas, such as diabetes, stroke and mental health; a further five topic networks have been formed since its original inception. The structure of these networks, with a common remit of effective research delivery, is supported by the Comprehensive Local Research Networks (CLRN) and managed at strategic national level by the National Institute for Health Research Clinical Research Network (NIHR CRN). These networks collectively made up the NIHR family of networks.

A national restructure of the NIHR family of networks in 2013/14 has led to a single integrated network operating in fifteen local branches, each mapped onto a specific geographic region of England. Each local research network has six divisions (of which cancer is designated 'Division 1') that incorporate all previous topic networks and clinical speciality groups. This streamlined model of research delivery ensures that there is (1) consistency of geographical coverage across the country; (2) equity of access for patients to trials and other well-designed studies; (3) robust governance arrangements; and, above all, (4) enhanced, timely delivery of research.

The cancer division of the NIHR CRN works synergistically with the National Cancer Research Institute Clinical Studies Groups (NCRI CSGs), Cancer Trials Units (CTUs), grant funders and registered charities. Through this mechanism, it develops and maintains a national portfolio of studies, and secures sufficient resource to ensure effective delivery of research in the NHS in England.

The overall remit of the NIHR CRN is to ensure:

- The integration of research into the core business of NHS organizations via the *NHS Constitution* (DH, 2013);
- That research is embedded within care by working alongside the service network; and
- That all patients, where possible, are aware of the potential trials that might benefit them.

It drives engagement within NHS organizations and key clinical groups to make sure that research is a priority for all NHS Trusts. Within this, it takes responsibility for ensuring that a range of trials are available on the local portfolio, with equity of access for patients, and that patients are not disadvantaged because of where they live.

WHY ARE CLINICAL TRIALS IMPORTANT?

As the gold standard for researching new **pharmacological treatments** and **healthcare technologies**, clinical trials have a key place in cancer care. They have a number of important features:

- They advance treatment in cancer care – today's treatments are a direct result of yesterday's research;
- They are an important way of finding out about new information that will influence better management and treatment for cancer;
- They provide a framework for new drugs, devices and treatments to be tested for safety and efficacy before they are made broadly available for access in the NHS;
- They help to eliminate treatments and devices that would pose a significant health hazard or lack benefit to the population; and
- They provide a framework for drug companies to conduct trials in the healthcare setting to determine the economic viability of their development, and, therefore, to avoid wasting funds on treatments and devices that lack efficacy for patients or are not tolerable due to side effects.

WHAT ARE CLINICAL TRIALS AND HOW DO THEY WORK?

A clinical trial is a research study or experiment that aims to answer a specific question, with identified and measurable **endpoints** that will determine the success or failure of that treatment or intervention. The endpoint might be the effect of the intervention on survival; remission rates after treatment; side effect profiles, quality of life; or cost effectiveness of the proposed intervention. The selected outcome for any given trial will vary depending on the **phase** of the study (Le Blanc and Tangen, 2012).

Well-designed trials generally take many months or even years to develop and need to be scientifically **peer-reviewed** to ensure that valid questions are being asked without duplication of previous work. Ethics review is paramount in order to protect the safety and wellbeing of any potential trial participants. In addition, each NHS Trust is asked to make an assessment of the study to ensure it fits with the proposed patient population and that the NHS service support infrastructure can support the delivery of the research. The *Research Governance Framework for Health and Social Care* (DH, 2005b) and the *Clinical Trials EU Directive* (2004/27/EC) are in place to ensure that all research conducted in the NHS is conducted to the highest safety and ethical standards in order to uphold the safety, wellbeing and rights of the trial participants.

As such, clinical trials tend to be very expensive to design and deliver. They can be funded from multiple sources, including charitable funds, commercial sponsorship or via the NIHR.

Phases of clinical trials

Pre-clinical research: Trials that take place in the healthcare environment are usually managed through four phases of development (see Table 32.1); however, it is important to understand that new drugs and molecules are extensively tested in the laboratory and on animals *prior* to being received by any healthy volunteer or patient.

Sometimes, patients are asked to take part in these Phase 0, or pre-clinical studies. These typically aim to determine if a drug behaves the way that is expected to, following their laboratory exploration. Because the dose of drug that is received is so small, patients are not expected to see any direct benefit, nor are they expected to experience significant acute side effects. The main aim is to speed up the development of potential new drugs because testing on humans yields more information than animal testing alone.

Phase I trials: These studies are sometimes also termed **first in human** (FIH) studies. Outside of cancer, most Phase I trials are conducted on healthy volunteers; however, in cancer, the population of participants is usually made up of people with **advanced cancer** for whom all other conventional treatments have failed, or are no longer a viable option. The patient cohort is not usually within a specific disease group but includes multiple groups, and is usually very small (less than ten). Testing at Phase I proceeds very carefully based upon plans for dose escalation in sequential cohorts of participants.

The dose given to participants will not usually be escalated until the data from the first dosing has been reviewed by a **safety committee** to ensure that side effects are not dose-limiting and that patients remain safe. Patients who participate in Phase I studies often have multiple visits to hospitals to monitor the delivery of drug and their body's reaction to it. Multiple blood tests will be taken and analyzed to look at the **pharmacodynamics** and **pharmacokinetics** of the drug action on the human body. Sometimes these studies are conducted in a purpose-designed **Clinical Research Facility** (CRF), which is equipped to manage high-risk clinical scenarios where there is thought to be a higher risk of **anaphylaxis** and **co-morbidity** associated with the drug. The anticipated level of risk is assessed by scientists and clinical professionals at the study design stage.

Participation in Phase I trials is a big commitment for patients at a time when they may be feeling vulnerable and unwell. It is important that they understand the implications of any proposed trial for themselves and for their families. Whilst patient safety would be a priority for the study team, participants in the trial may experience a whole range of emotions related to their participation as they link it to disease progress, end of life issues and altruism for future generations. There is no predictable personal benefit usually expected for patients in Phase I trials.

Table 32.1 Phases of clinical trial development

Phase of study and key question	Number of participants	Endpoints
Phase I Is it safe?	Small numbers – usually less than 10 participants	Sometimes the first trial in human participants. Usually focuses on safety, tolerability, mode of action, toxicity profiling, dose finding, identifying any action of the drug on the cancer. May be used in many different cancers but not expected to directly benefit the patient.
Phase II Does it work?	Usually less than 50 participants	Primarily dose finding and used in certain types of cancer, or with a focus on ideal **administration route** – the best way of delivering the drug. May also include further toxicity profiling.
Phase III Is it better than the standard treatment?	Large numbers, often including hundreds or thousands of patients. This is the first phase at which full randomization would be expected.	Comparison of the new drug or technology against best-known standard of care. Outcomes of interest usually include disease efficacy, and therefore, patients are expected to benefit from the new treatment.
Phase IV Can we make it safer and work better?	Once again, large numbers similar to those rates recruited in Phase III trials.	Often focuses on longer-term side effects and drug safety; post-marketing evaluation of cost effectiveness; and ongoing further development of the product to improve the efficacy.

Phase II trials: About 70% of drugs tested at Phase I proceed to Phase II testing. Phase II studies include slightly larger numbers of patients (up to 50) and are usually conducted in a tumour-specific cancer group (Centrewatch, 2014). Researchers will continue to monitor dose levels and **toxicity profiling** whilst also observing for some anticancer benefit to that tumour group. They will also want to determine if the efficacy results warrant the drug proceeding into Phase III testing, where there might be an expectation of better outcomes for patients when tested against the standard of care treatment. Valuable information continues to be collected about dose limits and side effects that might need to be managed in a different way.

Phase III trials: Phase III trials are the most commonly encountered in general cancer practice, and all healthcare professionals working within cancer care will encounter patients who are participating (or have done so previously) in Phase III studies.

These trials are mainly **randomized controlled trials** (RCTs), the '**control arm**' being the best-known standard of care, which is compared with the new treatment, technology or intervention. They are often multicentre, multinational trials that recruit thousands of patients in order to determine a discernible **statistically significant improvement** in treatment outcome.

The measurable 'end points' for Phase III studies would typically include:

- Overall survival
- Progression free survival
- Side effect profile

- Time to progression (rate of cancer growth)
- Quality of life
- Economic benefits of the new study treatment versus the best standard of care

Phase III trials are very important to pharmaceutical companies to demonstrate that their product is efficacious, cost-effective and tolerable before they are granted a **medicines license** to market the drug. The process from pre-clinical testing to Phase III trial outcome can often take up to ten years.

Phase IV trials: These trials occur post-licensing and post-marketing of the new drug or technology. Studies in this phase are especially important for the pharmaceutical industry, so that they can measure and report long-term side effects that may not be detected during the previous phases of exploration. They may also look at how the drug can be further improved and used more widely.

Reflective activity

Consider the things that patients would need to think about before deciding whether to participate in any clinical trial. Make a list of these pros and cons that may be associated with clinical trials. Think about:

- What questions the patients might need to ask in order to help them decide?
- How would the interaction between patients and health professionals influence their decision-making about clinical trial participation?

Types of trials

Randomized trials: These include at least two different cohorts of patients. In one, the standard treatment (control arm) is tested against the new treatment or technology (experimental or trial arm). Sometimes there can be additional arms to the study whereby the drug is tested in a variety of combinations or sequences. The patient's treatment is allocated by a random process to avoid introducing **bias** into the allocation of treatment.

Placebo-controlled trials: A **placebo** (e.g. dummy tablet, inactive substance) can be used in a trial where there is no usual standard of care to measure against the new drug or technology. Usually, these studies would be **blinded** (i.e. the patient does not know whether they are receiving the placebo or the treatment in development) or **double-blinded** (where neither the clinician nor the patient know which arm of the trial they have been allocated to). Researchers generally prefer placebo-controlled studies because there is less room for clinician or patient bias in the reporting of data. Patients may be put off, however, by the fact that they may not receive the active substance and the uptake for these studies can be variable, depending on: (1) whether there is any standard treatment available; (2) the way the trial is presented to patients and (3) personal preferences and prior experiences.

Epidemiology trials: These trials are aimed at a particular group of patients and identifies **genetic** or **lifestyle** factors that contribute to cancer. These do not usually involve active treatment and so randomization and blinding procedures are mute.

Screening and prevention trials: These trials aim to either identify those at **high risk** of developing cancer in order to bring them into a **screening** programme (e.g. breast and colorectal screening) or to prevent the onset of cancers in the future by targeting treatments or interventions. Screening trials may improve early detection of cancer and, therefore, have a positive effect on outcomes as patients receive early treatment with better chance of cure than if their disease were to be detected at a later stage.

THE ROLE OF THE RESEARCH PRACTITIONER IN CLINICAL TRIALS

The role of the **research practitioner** will vary considerably depending on the job description of the post holder, location of work and the phase of trial that the individual will be working on. It is important to remember that there are many staff working in clinical trials, including senior medics, research nurses, radiographers, postgraduates with a science background and data coordinators/managers with an IT background. These will be appointed to the trial as relevant to meet the needs of a service or individual protocol. In reality, however, a number of key personnel will make up the core research team to ensure the smooth implementation of the research protocol. All staff involved in clinical research must have been trained in *Good Clinical Practice Guidelines* (ICH GCP, n.d.) and have an understanding of the part or all of the protocol that they will be involved with. It remains the responsibility of the lead clinician, usually referred to as the Principle Investigator (PI), to assess the relevant experience and delegate appropriate duties to members of the research team. This information will be recorded and kept as a legal record.

The research practitioner is an important part of the recruitment process, establishing contact and rapport with the patient and agreeing an acceptable means of communication, such as arranging a separate visit, phone call or clinic appointment to discuss the trial.

Recruiting patients into clinical trials

The *UK National Cancer Patient Experience Survey 2011/12* (NCIN, 2012a), included a question about research for the first time. The results highlighted that most (95%) of the 33% patients who said that some form of research study had been discussed with them, were pleased to have been asked and that of the patients not asked about research, 53% said they would have liked to have been. This suggests that people with cancer want to receive more information than they are currently given.

Each individual trial will clearly outline in the study protocol a list of patient inclusion and exclusion criteria that determine who can be considered for trial entry. This is often presented as a list of clinical questions against which each patient should be assessed. This standardized approach ensures that all patients to whom the trial is relevant have the opportunity to participate. It also limits the trial population effectively in order to:

1. Ensure patients are entered with similar disease profiles to allow effective analysis of data (sample **homogeneity**).
2. Allow safety monitoring of patients. This will have timelines attached and will be only relevant for drug trials.

Research protocols are version-controlled to keep track of any changes made to the document that may or may not affect the delivery of the study; therefore, it is important that the research team are aware of both the inclusion and exclusion criteria from the most up-to-date ethically approved protocol.

Deciding when to approach a patient about entering a clinical trial can be difficult because many patients will be dealing with the devastating, life-changing news that they have cancer. The treating consultant will make the decision regarding a patient's eligibility for the study, and also their physical and emotional fitness to undergo a trial. Ultimately, however, the decision of whether to participate or not belongs to the patient. To support patients through this process, healthcare professionals should pay close attention to the patient's own agenda by taking account of their concerns and issues, and by tailoring information so that it is both understood and remembered (Poon, 2012). All patients are different and therefore require different levels of information to inform their choices (Brown et al., 2011).

Taking informed consent

All ethically approved studies have accompanying written **Patient Information Sheets** (PIS) to assist the patient in making an informed decision about trial participation. These are specific to each individual trial and explain, in lay terms, the required involvement for the patient. When used by the research practitioner to supplement the **informed consent process**, the PIS will detail the currently known risks, benefits and additional visits and tests required. Informed consent should be given freely by the patient without **coercion** from healthcare professionals or other external people. This process is pivotal to the recruitment process and is a legal requirement under the *EU Clinical Trials Directive* (2004/27/EC). Special consideration must be given to obtaining consent for patients who lack **mental capacity** or from children and parents (Kuthning and Hundt, 2013). The *EU Clinical Trials Directive* (2004/27/EC), through *Good Clinical Practice Guidelines* (NCIN, 2012a) advises researchers to allow the patient adequate time to decide, which although not stipulated in law, is generally accepted as a minimum of 24 hours once the patient is in receipt of the information sheet. Exceptions will apply only if the situation is an emergency, thus requiring immediate treatment of a condition. Patients, where possible, should be encouraged to discuss trial entry with others who are independent of the research team, including non-invested healthcare professionals, such as their local GP or a specialist nurse and close family members and friends. Together, these discussions will help the patient reach a decision that they feel comfortable with.

Following a fully informative discussion with the research team, each participant will be required to sign a trial specific **consent form**. Special consideration should be given for processing consent for children and vulnerable adults, but this is outside the scope of this chapter. Each participant will be asked to read through each statement on the consent form, initial each section and then sign and date the consent form in the presence of the PI or nominated co-investigator (usually another healthcare professional) who is delegated the responsibility to take consent. This will vary depending on the trial design and individual hospital trust. Many NHS trusts will only allow medical staff to take consent for a patient taking part in a **Clinical Trial of an Investigational Medicinal Product** (CTIMP: a trial of an unlicensed drug or novel agent), but will allow some nurses to take consent for non-interventional studies or **translational research** providing they have undertaken additional consent training. The advice – if there is any doubt – is to check with the local research and development department and trial sponsor.

Reflective activity

Visit this NIHR link to review the difference between a CTIMP and non-CTIMP (www.crn. nihr.ac.uk/learning-development/).

- Find out your Trust's policy on taking consent. Who can do it and is additional training needed?
- Consider the implications of taking consent from patients for you as a health professional?

Screening for study eligibility: a special case of informed consent

Any assessments or investigations required solely for the purpose of trial entry are referred to as screening investigations. In accordance with *ICH Good Clinical Practice Guidelines* (ICH GCP, n.d.), it is essential that written informed consent is obtained prior to the patient undertaking any trial-related screening procedures.

Patients need to be aware that trial entry can only occur if they meet all the eligibility of the protocol. This can be very disappointing for patients who are keen to participate in a trial and are then not eligible. It is important that the research practitioner notifies the patient that this is a possibility prior to any screening tests, that any information is passed on sensitively to the patient and that the patient is made aware of the alternative treatment options. In certain circumstances, it may be possible to re-screen the patient at a later time. An example could be when a patient has a low haemoglobin level of 8.7 g/dl but the protocol requires haemoglobin of at least 10 g/dl to meet the eligibility criteria. In this instance, with the patient's consent, it may be possible to arrange a blood transfusion to increase the haemoglobin to the required level, thus enabling the patient to enter the study.

Screening investigations can consist of a whole host of simple or complex tests, such as blood tests, 12-lead electrocardiogram (ECG), echocardiogram, eye examination, computerized tomography (CT) and bone scans. If additional imaging such as CT or bone scans are involved, it is important that patients are made aware of the risks of receiving additional radiation. In the UK, an ARSAC (**A**dministration of **R**adioactive **S**ubstances **A**dvisory **C**ommittee) licence will be obtained by the Trust on a trial prior to a patient receiving additional radioactivity. An ARSAC licence is issued to an investigator to permit the use of specified additional radioactivity, only within the specific trial protocol.

Arranging screening procedures may introduce a delay to the start of treatment and patients need to be made aware of this information and kept updated.

The participants' right to withdraw from a clinical trial

Patients must be made clearly aware that clinical trial entry is **voluntary**, and that they can decline entry into a study without fear or concern that any future standard of care will be compromised. Another essential piece of information that must be communicated to the participant is in relation to **withdrawal of consent** at any time-point during the lifetime of a trial. Withdrawal of consent by the patient can occur at any time-point once the written consent form is signed. It can be useful for the healthcare professional to know why a patient has decided not to enter or withdraw from a trial, but a patient is under no obligation to discuss their reasoning if they do not wish to. It is very important that the documentation of explicit refusal to enter or withdraw from a trial is made within the patients' medical record contemporaneously and clearly, and that the decision is communicated to the sponsor so that no further requests are made for patient visits or data.

Reflective activity

Observe a clinical consultation that involves discussion of a clinical trial, paying close attention to:

- Whether the clinician explained the trial logically and simply without jargon?
- How they checked the patient's understanding?
- What, and who, influenced the patient's decision on participation?
- Whether the decision was made freely and with sufficient information?
- How communication could have been improved?

Patient perceptions of trials

Reflective activity

Patients' attitudes to trials will be influenced by a number of factors, such as previous experience of healthcare organizations or cancer, upbringing and personal values and personal circumstances. Consider patients with cancer that you have been involved with in your career.

- Have you been involved in helping them make a decision about participating in a trial?
- What was their reason for accepting or declining participation?
- What was their attitude to being approached?
- How did their previous experiences and attitudes influence their decision-making?

Whilst the clinical research networks have made a significant difference to the recruitment of patients into clinical trials, access to studies and improved patient outcomes, there is still much that needs to be done to ensure that research is available to the majority of patients. Trials are critical to the development of cancer care but typically, recruitment does not tend to exceed 10% of any particular population of patients (Cameron et al., 2013). It is suggested that as many as 81% of patients report that no one has discussed trials with them; this does not compare favourably with the 84% of clinicians who feel that they consistently introduce trials to their patients (Fenton et al., 2009). The reasons for this inconsistency are many and varied, and obstacles to recruitment contribute to the complexity of decision-making about research as a treatment option. These include, but are not limited to, lack of an available study, stringent eligibility criteria, clinicians' personal views on the research question, patient perceptions and practical barriers, such as economic, resource and time factors.

In their qualitative study, Quinn et al. (2012) describe patient-reported influences on their decision-making around trial participation. The authors asked participants to describe images and thoughts that came to mind when they heard the words 'clinical trial'. All of the respondents had heard of clinical trials and research, and all had both positive and negative connotations associated with the concept. For some patients, the overwhelming fear of, and reaction to, the cancer diagnosis prevented them from being able to make a well-informed rational decision. Common descriptions of negative feelings included words such as fear, animal testing, fear of the unknown, scary, like a lottery and anxiety that the trial might not work. Positive associations with trial participation included hope, better outcomes, new cures for cancer and potentially improved healthcare because of close monitoring. Decisions were often driven by an emotional response.

A further study by Kohara and Inoue (2010) was specifically concerned with the decision-making of patients with regard to participation in Phase I studies. They suggest that the key driver in decision-making in this setting is one that facilitates a way for patients to 'live to the end'. Moreover, their decision-making is influenced by having limited other options available to them, and a sense that doing something is better than doing nothing, where the alternative may be waiting to die. They also acknowledge the part played by relatives in the patient decision-making process.

The way in which a trial is presented to patients is crucial to aid decision-making. Patients feel that it is important to understand the purpose of the trial, and the likely benefits and risks, so that they can balance this information against the information on standard care treatments available. Most will be influenced by the level of trust and faith that they have in members of their healthcare team, and the recommendations that these individuals may offer (Ellis et al., 2001; Wright et al., 2004; Cameron et al., 2013). Skilled communication between patients and healthcare professionals is paramount for successful recruitment to clinical trials because low patient awareness and lack of understanding is a significant barrier to participation (Fenton et al., 2009; see also Chapter 17).

Reflective activity

Think about the specific clinical and communication skills that would be required to support a patient on a Phase I trial. Do you think the same skill set will be required to support a Phase IV trial?

Consider, for example, that many Phase I studies will require the researcher to be able to administer any new novel compounds to the patient directly, in a safe and secure environment. The knowledge of any new drugs in Phase I is very limited in humans, and so it is essential that staff are trained in advanced life support and have access to emergency facilities to be prepared in case of a severe adverse reaction to drug.

Phase IV trails, in comparison, include much longer-term follow-up of patients, often observing and managing compliance over a number of years (sometimes fifteen to twenty), and usually once the patient is well and has returned to the routine of normal everyday life.

Key points to consider when discussing clinical trials

The following list offers some useful guidance for those healthcare professionals who may be discussing clinical trials with people being treated for cancer.

- Establish what the patient already knows about their diagnosis/prognosis/disease/condition.
- Describe carefully what the standard of care treatment may be in their particular case.
- Describe carefully what the new treatment will be: what is involved, how long it takes to deliver, what the side effects might be (if known), whether they can expect to see any personal benefit.
- Explain all of the risks and benefits of participating in the trial.
- Explain that participation is entirely voluntary and that care will not be affected if they choose not to participate.
- Explain the practicalities of participating, visits to hospital, arrangements for travel, what is expected of them in terms of compliance with the protocol.
- Use lay language, not medical jargon or abbreviations.
- Give verbal explanations and written information so that the patients may refer back to it when deciding what is best for them and when discussing it with their families.

Reflective activity

You have a randomized controlled Phase II study that has two treatment arms. Arm A involves the currently available gold standard treatment and Arm B involves the addition of a new novel agent. The patient immediately tells you that they want to enter the trial, but only if they are allocated to Arm B. They state that they don't want to attend clinic for the extra follow-ups.

- Based on the information provided, what advice would you give the patient?
- What are the implications for this and for whom?

The insistence of the patient that they wish to be allocated to Arm B implies that they think it is superior to Arm A. It is important that the patient is made aware that it is not known at the time of trial entry which treatment option is superior. You must remember, however, that the patient has the right not to enter the study or to withdraw consent at a later date if not allocated to the preferred arm. It is important that this is also communicated to the patients so that they fully understand the process of randomization should they wish to proceed into the trial.

If patients routinely withdraw consent, it will obviously take longer to collect the required data to answer the research question. High volumes of participant withdrawal may indicate a potential issue with the study design or protocol requirement, and this will need attention by the study research team. Most research **sponsors** will monitor screening and withdrawal rates throughout the trial.

SPECIAL CONSIDERATIONS REGARDING THE RUNNING OF CLINICAL TRIALS

Ensuring protocol compliance

Policies and protocols in standard clinical practice provide healthcare professionals with a clear evidence-based, educational tool to facilitate standardization of practice, reduce variations in care, minimize and reduce risk and improve the quality of patient care.

A research protocol is written to ensure that any results obtained can be scientifically peer-reviewed as resulting from reliable and valid data generated from effective trial delivery. The protocol provides a prescriptive, explicit guide for research staff on how to manage and support participants receiving care as part of the trial. If a participant is receiving treatment, such as chemotherapy or radiotherapy within a clinical trial, the trial protocol will always override the standard of care protocol. It is important for researchers and support staff to understand that trial protocols may sometimes differ significantly from standard of care protocols. The availability of trial information in treatment areas and clear communication of procedures is therefore vital to maintaining safety and for the effective delivery of the trial.

> ### Reflective activity
>
> Imagine that a patient is receiving Oxaliplatin and Capecitabine as part of a clinical trial for the adjuvant treatment of colorectal cancer. The research aims to compare the effects of four versus eight cycles of chemotherapy. On the chemotherapy ward, these drugs would be given to the same patient population as that of the trial. The trial protocol states that the chemotherapy drugs can be given if the platelet count is $>75 \times 10^9$/L. This differs to the chemotherapy unit protocol, which prohibits patients receiving treatment unless they have a platelet count $>100 \times 10^9$/L.
>
> - What are the implications for practice?
>
> There is an increased risk that the patient's treatment may be delayed or omitted due to the low platelet count, if the chemotherapy staff are not made aware of the trial protocol guidelines. In order to minimize errors, it is important for staff to have access to and knowledge of the protocol. In drug trials, it is especially important that any prescription and medication is clearly labelled or identified as for clinical trial use.

Dose reductions in CTIMP

Anticancer treatment can produce significant side effects in patients, which, if not managed correctly, could compromise patient safety. A clinical protocol will always outline the indications for dose reductions, omissions or cessation of therapy.

Deviation: This occurs, quite simply, when the participant's treatment has deviated from the protocol. Reasons for deviation may be that the participant chooses not to comply with study requirements or because the protocol is unclear or misinterpreted by researchers or clinical staff. The sponsor takes any deviation from the trial protocol very seriously and may halt or suspend recruitment at a site pending further investigation if the protocol deviation compromises patient safety.

It is impossible to eliminate the risk of deviations occurring, but sites can reduce the risk considerably by ensuring that:

- Patients are carefully assessed against the inclusion and exclusion criteria prior to study entry;
- The study team ensure that they are fully trained in the protocol and they detail and query any inconsistencies directly with the trial sponsor; and
- Any deviations are reported immediately to the trial sponsor with appropriate corrective and preventive action plans in place to eliminate the risk of the same deviation occurring again.

Trial management and data monitoring

The **Case Report Form** (CRF) is a document (in either electronic or paper format) that is produced by the sponsor for completion by the local trials team. This document allows the research team to send key data on the progress of trial patients to the coordinating trial centre for data analysis. All source data will be documented in the participant's local hospital notes. External monitors, commissioned by the sponsor, will attend sites to monitor data that they receive against the source data written in the notes. Any discrepancies raised by the monitor will be rectified by the research team.

Quality of life assessment

Quality of life assessment is now recommended to be an important component of clinical trials. The assessments are a means by which the participant's symptoms and the subsequent effect on their quality of life on a day-to-day basis can be comprehensively assessed. Quality of life is often a primary or secondary endpoint of the trial design. Assessments will take place at set time-points as specified by the protocol. There are a number of widely used cancer-specific questionnaires available, such as the European Organization for Research and Treatment of Cancer Quality of Life Questionnaire-C30 (EORTC QLQ-C30) and the Functional Assessment of Cancer Therapy-General (FACT-G). Patients may be asked to complete more than one type of questionnaire, depending on their situation and the specifics of the trial.

EORTC QLQ-C30: The EORTC QLQ-C30 is a copyrighted document available in 81 languages and currently used in approximately 3000 studies worldwide (EORTC, 2014). The assessment is in the form of a questionnaire that asks thirty questions, which together assess the quality of life of patients with cancer. Patients are asked to use the scale provided to score their own health and wellbeing over the past 7 days. It assesses quality of life in relation to cancer symptoms, physical fitness, perception of own ability to function in their role, level of emotional wellbeing, alteration to cognitive function and social factors associated with the illness. The patient is advised to complete this independently of others to ensure a true reflection of their subjective perception of their own quality of life.

FACT-G: The FACT-G is another self–assessment patient questionnaire comprising twenty-seven questions. It takes around 5–10 minutes to complete. Similarly to the EORTC QLQ-C30, the measure is split into small categories of specific wellbeing. The four domains assessed by this particular quality of life measure explore physical, social, emotional and functional wellbeing. Participants rate each item within these domains using a five-point scale to report their own health and wellbeing at any particular given point in time.

CHAPTER SUMMARY

Health services, both in the UK and globally, are charged with delivering high quality care and improved patient outcomes through the delivery of well-designed research delivered in a cost-effective and timely manner. This can only be achieved if health professionals work closely with the patient's agenda, responding appropriately to their physical and psychological needs and concerns.

This chapter has provided an overview of the importance of clinical trials as a part of cancer care. As research evolves over time, additional challenges will arise around ensuring that patients are aware of research opportunities and understand the implications of participation in more complex studies. Science delivers improvements in treatment technology, enabling clinicians to tailor treatment to the needs of the individual, but the process of getting to this point necessitates the voluntary participation of people with cancer, at what is already a very difficult time for them.

Key learning points

- Clinical trials are important in the development of effective treatments in cancer care.
- Clinical trials are tightly regulated and monitored.
- Trials may be Phase I, II, III or IV.
- Sensitive approaches to recruiting patients into clinical trials are required.
- Consent to treatment must be informed and patients may withdraw at any time.
- Patients participating in clinical trials are closely monitored according to specific criteria.
- The psychosocial impact of trial participation on the patient and their family should be explored, from initial recruitment through to trial completion (or withdrawal).

Recommended further reading

- Girling, D.J., Stewart, L.A., Parrmar, M.K.B. and Stenning, S.P. (2003) *Clinical Trials in Cancer: Principle and Practice.* Oxford, UK: Oxford University Press.
- The following website may be useful:
- European Organization for Research and Treatment of Cancer (EORTC) website contains many useful information resources about clinical trials within cancer care. (www.eortc.org/)
- National Institute for Health Research Clinical Research Network (NIHR CRN) website (www.nihr.org.uk) contains its structure and function. You will also find further information and guidance on the development and conduct of clinical trials from your local research and development department.

33 PSYCHOSOCIAL RESEARCH IN CANCER CARE

FIONA KENNEDY AND NICHOLAS HULBERT-WILLIAMS

Chapter outline

- An introduction to why continued empirical investigation of the psychosocial impact of cancer is necessary
- An overview of common methods and designs used in psychosocial oncology research, including qualitative and quantitative approaches

- A discussion of commonly reported statistical terminology and how the findings from quantitative research can be understood and interpreted
- A critical exploration of some of the challenges and barriers to conducting research in this area of cancer care

---

INTRODUCTION

As many of the authors in this textbook have emphasized, it is of vital importance that the healthcare community understand the psychosocial impact of cancer and the survivorship issues faced by people with cancer and their families. This chapter is not intended as a fully descriptive training in research methods, but rather to highlight the primary designs that psychosocial oncology researchers use, why these are suited to different research questions, how the findings from such studies might be interpreted and the challenges of undertaking research in this area. For each method, an example of a good piece of published research from psychosocial oncology is provided so that the reader can understand the methodologies in an applied sense.

Why is psychosocial research in this area so important?

The last few decades have witnessed significant advances and developments in the treatment of cancer – more patients are surviving and living longer following their diagnosis and treatment. Alongside this medical progress, it has become increasingly recognized that the personal impact and consequences of a cancer diagnosis and treatment are important to acknowledge and explore.

Psychosocial research in cancer care aims to holistically explore the whole patient, not only how they are affected physically by the diagnosis and treatment, but also how the experience impacts on them psychologically, socially and spiritually (Dolbeault et al., 1999). Furthermore, with continuing advances in medical techniques and treatments, new research areas in psychosocial oncology are continually emerging (Dolbeault et al., 1999; Patenaude and Kupst, 2005), for example palliative care, paediatric oncology and work exploring the needs of healthy individuals at high risk of developing cancer (e.g. women with the genetic predisposition). Of course, it isn't just about the patient either – psychosocial research explores the impact on the patient's families, their friends, their formal and informal caregivers, and even the reciprocal effects that this has on the patients themselves. Research is required to inform each and every aspect of cancer care, and taking an holistic and biopsychosocial stance to this investigative enquiry is of paramount importance.

The next section of this chapter outlines the primary methodological approaches used in both qualitative and quantitative research. These are presented separately because they come from very different philosophical perspectives. Two important concepts that are worth trying to understand at this stage are:

Ontology: a term used to describe *what* there is to be known, what a 'reality' is and, therefore, what can be potentially gained from research

Epistemology: the underlying philosophical beliefs and frameworks that outline *how* new knowledge can be obtained.

QUALITATIVE RESEARCH METHODS

Qualitative research seeks to identify meaning and understanding about how people make sense of their experiences (this is the ontological position), and specifically focuses on exploring narratives, personal stories and language (Holloway and Wheeler, 2010; Kristjanson and Coyle, 2010). Epistemologically, this approach maintains that to eliminate subjectivity from the research process is impossible (Yardley and Marks, 2004), and the methods used should therefore embrace and build upon this, thus tending towards less objective research designs. As a **post-modern** approach to research, qualitative methods tend towards a **constructivist** position (the epistemology), whereby knowledge is inevitably limited by and composed of private and social thoughts, experiences and processes (Yardley and Marks, 2004). The techniques used in qualitative research, therefore, often involve interviews, focus groups, documentary analysis and observation (Kristjanson and Coyle, 2010). There are a wide variety of specific methods that sit within the domain of qualitative research, many of which are applicable to psychosocial oncology research, including (but not limited to) phenomenology, ethnography, grounded theory and framework approaches.

Phenomenology

Phenomenology has its roots in philosophy and aims to discover meaning in individuals' 'lived' or everyday experiences (Polit and Beck, 2004; Todres and Holloway, 2010). There are two schools of phenomenology: descriptive (Husserlian) phenomenology and interpretive/ **hermeneutic** (Heidegger) phenomenology, the latter going further by its emphasis on interpreting and understanding experiences, rather than merely describing them (Polit and Beck, 2004; Lopez and Willis, 2004).

Taking a phenomenological approach, a study would aim to identify 'essences' or '...insights that apply more generally beyond the cases that were studied in order to emphasise what we may have in common as human beings' (Todres and Holloway, 2010: 178). Another key phenomenological concept is **bracketing** whereby the researcher aims to suspend any preconceptions, beliefs or opinions about the phenomenon under study such that the findings from these studies are grounded entirely in what the participants themselves tell the researcher (Polit and Beck, 2004; Todres and Holloway, 2010).

An example of a psychosocial oncology descriptive phenomenological study is that of Worster and Holmes (2009) who explored the post-operative experiences of patients undergoing surgery for colorectal cancer. Bracketing techniques were used and an analytic method was rigorously followed. The findings provide in-depth insight into the personal experience of colorectal surgery and the authors suggest that the work can inform the planning and delivery of care for future patients.

Interpretative Phenomenological Analysis (IPA) is a phenomenological approach that has emerged in the discipline of psychology (Smith et al., 2009). However, whereas traditional descriptive phenomenology emphasizes bracketing any a priori beliefs or values, IPA recognizes the 'central role for the analyst' in making sense of the experiences of the research participants (Smith, 2004). Specifically, researchers will always be influenced by their own experiences and values (Smith et al., 2009). This is referred to as a 'double hermeneutic' as '... the participant is trying to make sense of their personal and social world; the researcher is trying to make sense of the participant trying to make sense of their personal and social world' (2009: 40). Therefore, the understanding gained through IPA is both context specific and influenced by the individual and researcher. IPA is also crucially **idiographic**, meaning that the emphasis is on making sense of the experiences of those individuals, rather than generalizing to wider groups or populations (Smith et al., 2009). An example of a well-conducted IPA study in cancer is a study by Reynolds and Lim (2007), which explored participants' views about the contribution that engaging with art has on their subjective wellbeing in terms of living with cancer. Twelve women participated in semi-structured interviews and the results highlight the powerful positive impact of art in boosting esteem, enhancing social identity and providing a distraction (Smith, 2011).

Ethnography

Ethnography stems from the **anthropology** research discipline (Kristjanson and Coyle, 2010; Holloway and Wheeler, 2010) and specifically focuses on exploring cultural or social groups (Holloway and Todres, 2010a). This focus makes ethnography unique as a qualitative method. In particular, ethnography involves the researcher gaining first-hand experience of participants in their natural setting (Holloway and Todres, 2010a). Direct participant observation is, therefore, one of the main methods used. In health research, ethnography often aims to produce knowledge to inform and improve care and clinical practice (Holloway and Wheeler, 2010). Ethnographic approaches have been a popular method in researching end-of-life care (Payne and Seymour, 2004). For example, Anne-Mei The (2002) studied the experiences of patients with advanced small-cell lung cancer from within a cancer centre. Anne-Mei followed thirty patients from their diagnosis through to their death, spending time observing their clinical experiences. This ethnographic work demonstrates the rich and complex interactions that occur between patients, families and their healthcare professionals in the context of advanced cancer, and how all parties engaged in minimization of the significance of the disease in order to refrain from attending to the long-term outcome of inevitable death.

Grounded theory

Grounded theory originates from the seminal sociological work of Glaser and Strauss (1965) that explored health professionals' interactions with dying patients (Holloway and Wheeler, 2010). A grounded theory approach is interested in social processes and structures (Polit and Beck, 2004) and has its roots in **symbolic interactionism**, which focuses on the process of interaction between people and how it influences their behaviour (Holloway and Wheeler, 2010; Holloway and Todres, 2010b). Furthermore, in contrast to other qualitative methodologies, grounded theory specifically aims to generate concepts and theory from the data collected (Holloway and Todres, 2010b). One of the key principles of a grounded theory approach is the use of a constant comparative method for analysis. Horne et al., (2012) conducted a grounded theory study exploring the views of people affected by advanced lung cancer about their preference for end-of-life care. This method was chosen in order to provide a theoretical model to inform the development of a future complex intervention to support patients and their families. They used a constant comparative analytic method that involved a continuous and iterative analysis throughout the data collection, whereby later interviews were used to theoretically sample and test out the emerging analysis categories. The study presents a theory of 'maintaining integrity in the face of death', focusing on how patients aim to live in the present whilst facing and preparing for the social aspects of death.

Framework approach

The framework approach to qualitative research has been growing in popularity in applied policy health research, and was developed by Ritchie and Spencer (1994). In contrast to other qualitative methodologies, the objectives of the research will often have been established in advance; therefore, although it still acts as an **inductive** methodology (looking for emergent concepts and is grounded in the accounts of the people studied), it can also start **deductively** with pre-set aims and objectives (Pope et al., 2000). The rationale for using this approach in applied or policy research is that often there are tight timescales, there might be a priori issues that funders or other stakeholders want addressing, and there may be a need to link the findings with quantitative results (Pope et al., 2000). A framework analysis involves five stages: (1) familiarization with the data, (2) identify thematic framework for coding data from the interview schedule and initial scrutiny of transcripts/field notes, (3) systematic coding to apply the framework (indexing), (4) organizing coded data into major themes (charting), and (5) mapping and interpreting relationships between themes by exploring the data set as a whole. Iredale et al. (2006) conducted a multi-phase study to explore the experiences of men with breast cancer in the UK. This used a framework approach to analyze the interviews. The theoretical framework they used drew upon the literature and a previous pilot study, although it further evolved through each phase of the research project.

Doing qualitative research and interpreting the data

Whatever methodology is used, qualitative research first involves obtaining a detailed account of participant(s) experiences. Often this is achieved by an interview, whereby open-ended questions are asked by a researcher and the participant is encouraged to give honest responses. Interviews can be conducted on a one-to-one basis or with groups of participants (a focus group). Focus groups can be with participant groups of varied sizes from two upwards, essentially, but normally between five and ten members (Flick, 2002), and they can often be a useful strategy when it is helpful for participants to share and comment on each other's experiences, or to gain a sense of shared opinion from a participant group (for example, in producing a supportive information leaflet). Group-based data collection, however, requires effective moderation, ideally by more than one researcher because the dynamics of group-based discussions can be complex and some participants may lack confidence or efficacy to speak up (Flick, 2002; Brédart et al. 2014). Some consider that one-to-one methods may be favourable for more sensitive research questions to allow participants to privately (one-to-one) express their feelings (Mathieson, 1999), although Kitzinger (2006) considers that group discussions may help to facilitate the discussion of difficult topics. Other qualitative data collection methods may include participant diaries, consultation recordings or research observations notes (Pope and Mays, 2006) – essentially any source that can easily be transcribed or turned into a written, textual account.

The data analysis and interpretation stage involves working with those textual accounts to gain meaning and structure from them (Pope and Mays, 2006). Each method described earlier has specific guidelines for how this should be done, but typically this will involve a lengthy, systematic and iterative process of detailed and repeated readings of the source material, then managing, labelling and grouping the data to build up an account to describe how interpretations emerged from the source material to form overall categories or themes (Pope et al., 2000, 2006; Ritchie et al., 2003). These are then written up as a narrative summary where themes are described and exemplar quotes from the source materials are included as evidence. Typically, the analysis, interpretation and narrative write-up stages are done collaboratively within a research team to ensure that all possible interpretations are considered, and to minimize (as much as is possible) any bias in the analytic process (Barbour, 2001). This is just one marker of good quality qualitative research, and various guidelines have been provided for others that should be considered (Cohen and Crabtree, 2008). Qualitative research is often a very lengthy process and should never be undertaken lightly. To do a good job of a qualitative study is time-consuming and can involve far more person-hours and expense than many alternative research designs (Pope et al., 2000).

QUANTITATIVE RESEARCH METHODS

Quantitative research is a type of investigative inquiry that is used to develop and test '…mental models of the generalizable causal laws that govern reality, using objective methods of analysis such as statistics to ensure that these analyses are not influenced by subjective expectations or values' (Yardley and Marks, 2004: 2–3). This is often referred to as the **hypothetico-deductive** or **scientific** method. Epistemologically, therefore, it feels – and indeed is – very different to the qualitative approaches outlined in the previous section. Quantitative research is hypothesis driven and involves analysis of numerical data to answer research questions. **Research hypotheses** are statements made about the expected outcomes from a research study and are used to guide the types of analysis conducted. Distinction is often made between a **null** and **experimental** hypothesis (where the first is a prediction of a negative finding from the research). Technically speaking, modern statistical techniques have been developed on the basis of testing (and attempting to disprove) the null hypothesis; this is the principle of **falsificationism** and has its roots in the philosophy of Karl Popper.

In order to define a hypothesis, we need a clear definition of what it is that we intend to measure in a study: for this we use the term **variable**. Research variables are perhaps most simply defined as '… things that can change (vary); they might vary between people (e.g. IQ, behaviour) or locations (e.g. unemployment) or even time (e.g. mood, profit, number of cancerous cells)' (Field, 2013: 7). In some designs, we may distinguish between an **independent** variable and a **dependent** variable, whereby the independent variable is something that is manipulated, changed, or deliberately measured to be different between participant groups, expecting it to cause a resultant change in the measured dependent variable.

Quantitative research aims for **replicability** and objectivity, thus research designs are carefully planned to remove (or at least control for) sources of **bias** or **subjectivity**. A statistical or research bias is the existence of some kind of unmeasured influence (e.g. demographic or clinical sample characteristics) that might lead to incorrect conclusions or interpretations being drawn from the data. Bias can be minimized by controlling for possible **confounding variables** or **extraneous factors** in research designs. Unlike qualitative research, subjectivity is considered problematic within the quantitative research tradition, and is controlled for by the epistemological position of the research in and of itself. Rather than collecting a small number of personalized pieces of research data or analyzing findings based on researcher interpretation, sample sizes are calculated precisely to **power** objective statistical tests. In this context, power refers to the fact that the study is designed such that sufficient steps have been taken that if a 'true' effect does exist, the study has a good likelihood of identifying this. There are many types of quantitative research design and it would be impossible to cover them all in this chapter. Instead, we will focus on outlining three predominant designs used in psychosocial oncology research.

There are many types of quantitative research design and it would be impossible to cover them all in this chapter; however, three commonly used designs are outlined next.

Using questionnaires: cross-sectional and cohort studies

One of the more commonly used research methodologies in psychosocial oncology is the questionnaire study. This is sometimes called an **observational design**, but that is a little misleading because it doesn't have to include direct participant observation; **non-experimental** is perhaps a better description. Here, researchers typically recruit large groups of participants (in excess of 100 is not unusual, but some studies recruit thousands) and collect data from them using self-report questionnaires (or **psychometric scales**), in addition to demographic and clinical data. Psychometric scales are measures that have been developed using specific techniques (see later) to assess particular **constructs** (such as a personality trait, coping behaviour or outcome measure) and typically take the form of a number of statements (or **items**) to which participants rate their agreement using **Likert** scales (numerical response categories). Total scores can then be calculated that represent the variables under analysis. If data are collected on just one occasion, the study would be described as a **cross-sectional study**; whereas multiple sets of measures completed by the same participants over a longer period of time would be described as **longitudinal** or a **cohort study.** The following types of statistical analysis are used in this type of research:

- To compare scores on particular variables between subgroups of participants (e.g. between patients with breast and prostate cancer), comparative tests such as *t*-tests, Wilcoxon sign-rank test, ANOVA or Kruskal–Wallis test are used.
- To explore the strength of relationship between two variables within just one group of participants (e.g. to investigate the relationship between psychological flexibility and quality of life), a correlation test (such as Pearson's or Spearman's correlation) or a Kendall's tau would commonly be used.
- When there are more than two variables under analysis, or when the aim of a study is to explore whether scores on one measure are predicted by another, a regression analysis (linear, log-linear or logistic) is most suitable.

A protocol for a particularly impressive cohort study (CREW Study) exploring the long-term recovery of health and wellbeing following colorectal cancer has been published by Fenlon et al. (2012b). This study, which has now closed to recruitment and will be shortly reporting findings, is a longitudinal cohort study of 1000 colorectal cancer survivors. Participants will complete questionnaires prior to surgery and at 3, 9, 15 and 24-month follow-up to identify which variables predict better adjustment in this group.

Developing psychometric tools

In order to undertake a cross-sectional or cohort study, researchers must first identify suitable questionnaire measures to use. If suitable measures don't exist, they might first decide to create a new measure and evaluate it using **psychometric analysis**. The type of design used for data collection in this type of study is essentially a questionnaire study (usually conducted longitudinally), whereby a new questionnaire is developed from observing responses to questions in a large **item pool**, which is compared against other similar measures or relevant clinical data. Psychometric development studies typically analyze the data in the following ways:

- To explore how well new items group together into one (or more) scale(s), **factor analytic** techniques are used. These statistics inform how to score the questionnaire in future uses and what variables it can be claimed to assess.
- Cronbach's alpha tests provide an objective measure of **internal consistency**. This is an indication of how well each of the items appears to be measuring the same underlying construct.

- Correlation tests can be used to explore both test–retest **reliability** (i.e. how consistently the measure performs if administered on different occasions) or the many various forms of **validity** (i.e. how well the new measure is assessing what it was designed to measure).
- In later uses of new psychometric scales, more complex analyses such as **structural equation modelling** can be used to conduct a confirmatory psychometric analysis.

There are many good examples of the development of psychometric scales in psycho-oncology, and indeed the re-analysis and refinement of measures over time. Taking an interesting perspective on how different datasets can be used to improve the Mini-MAC, (a measure of psychological adjustment to and coping with cancer; see Watson et al., 1994), Hulbert-Williams et al. (2012b) used data from 160 mixed cancer survivors to conduct a methodologically rigorous psychometric re-analysis. In addition to suggesting that some items are redundant, their analysis suggested an alternative and arguably more valid and reliable way to score this commonly used psychometric tool, providing subscale scores for cognitive distress, emotional distress, cognitive avoidance and fighting spirit.

Experimental and interventional studies

These studies are essentially a slightly more complicated longitudinal design, with the difference being that between data collection points, participants take part in an experimental manipulation or intervention, allowing a researcher to attempt to **influence** a measured outcome, rather than simply observing and measuring it naturally. This indicates whether an intervention causes a desired outcome. This type of psychosocial oncology study most easily maps onto the clinical drug trial in the previous chapter and, just as the **randomized controlled design** is considered the gold standard for drug trials, so too is it for non-drug-based interventions. Due to the number of variables and time-points of data collection involved in interventional studies, multivariate statistics, such as ANOVA, regression, path analysis or structural equation modelling, are considered ideal analysis methods. The randomized controlled trial of the effectiveness of mindfulness-based stress reduction (MBSR) in mood and quality of life in breast cancer patients, carried out by Caroline Hoffman and her team (2012), is a good example of a psychosocial intervention study. Their findings indicated that the MBSR intervention improved a range of psychosocial outcome measures, and that these intervention effects remained until three-month follow-up.

Interpreting quantitative research findings

There are three important pieces of 'output' information that are common across the findings of most quantitative research: p-value, effect size and estimates of clinical significance.

A **p-value** is essentially a measure of probability and represents **statistical significance**. In quantitative research, investigators want to know whether the finding from a statistical test has arisen purely because the hypothesis is correct and the right thing was measured, or whether the results may have simply arisen by chance. By convention, quantitative research adopts a cut-off p-value of 0.95 (this is called the **alpha** level), which, if met, essentially means to expect statistical tests to give a wrong answer on less that 5% of occasions. Obviously, the smaller the p-value, the more confidence there is in the research findings.

Although researchers still commonly report the statistical significance of their findings, there has been a longstanding debate in research methods literature about whether this is an appropriate value on which to judge the importance of a finding (for those interested, read Meehl, 1967; Lykken, 1968; Meehl, 1978; Nix and Barnette, 1998). Rather than abandoning the *p*-value altogether, research convention is now to also include other metrics that emphasize different aspects of the data.

An **effect size** is an indication of the extent to which the variables being measured have changed as a result of what the researcher has done, or are naturally related to each other. So, for example, to find out how optimism is correlated with depression in cancer survivors in a questionnaire study, running a correlation test will provide an *r* statistic, which is an effect size. The bigger that number, the more 'effect' there is, and therefore, the more important that relationship might be. Similarly, after delivering a support group intervention to reduce fear of recurrence, running a *t*-test between the intervention and non-intervention group will show what difference the support group made: the *t*-value can be transformed into an effect size (for example, **Cohen's *d***), which again provides a **standardized** measure of that effect. In other research designs, there are also standardized **odds ratios**, which suggest that something is more likely in one group than another.

Another type of significance that is especially important in health research is **clinical significance**. There are many different ways that clinical significance can be operationalized (see Jacobsen and Truax, 1991), but simplistically put, it is a term used to indicate whether the effect size reported has any applied relevance, or whether a research study has **clinical efficacy**. For example, in a psychological intervention study, it may be useful to explore whether a change in scores of pre- and post-intervention anxiety are statistically significantly different and if that change represented a substantially big standardized effect size, but what may be *really* useful to know is whether that change has clinical importance, for example has it reduced anxiety in these participants from clinically diagnosable levels to scores that fall within a population normative range? In other words, has the intervention been worthwhile? Clinical significance is not really a 'new' term, but it is one that is only just starting to gain popularity in psychosocial oncology. This could, however, represent an important shift in how findings are reported that will allow for even more objective judgement about whether application and implementation of research findings (e.g. service change) represents good value for money, and would make a big enough difference to patients to justify the costs involved.

CHALLENGES AND BARRIERS IN PSYCHOSOCIAL ONCOLOGY RESEARCH

Gaining necessary approvals to conduct research studies

The dignity, rights, safety and wellbeing of participants must be the primary consideration in any research study. (DH, 2005b: 7).

Professional codes of ethical practice are set out by all major national health and social care organizations, such as the British Psychological Society (2005, 2009), the Health Professionals Council (2008) and the Nursing and Midwifery Council (2010), and these should be referred to where relevant to the researcher's professional role.

In the UK, the *Research Governance Framework for Health and Social Care* (DH, 2005b) is the overarching framework of good practice that should be followed when conducting health and social care research. This framework covers all aspects of research, including whether ethical approval has been granted, financial aspects, health and safety, and the responsibilities of all stakeholders (Thompson and Chambers, 2011).

Most researchers who are based in an academic setting will have access to an ethics committee who can provide guidance, advice and approval for conducting research. In addition, and as part of the research governance framework, formal research ethics approval from an appropriate NHS Research Ethics Committee (REC) is required for all research studies recruiting patients being treated by the NHS (note: this is not always essential for research studies where healthcare professionals, or patients' families, are the desired participants). Ethical approval is not usually required for audit or service evaluation projects (see NHS Health Research Authority (2013) for guidance on the difference between these). Gaining approval, therefore, will usually involve submitting an application to an REC (Gelling, 2010) through the integrated research application system (IRAS). This can be a lengthy process (up to 60 days), but introduction of the proportionate review service means that research presenting minimal risk or burden for participants should be reviewed within 14 days (NHS Health Research Authority, 2014).

All RECs aim to protect research participants and others (e.g. researchers) from harm and try to balance any risk against possible benefits (Gelling, 1999; Gelling 2010). The process also aims to result in high quality, rigorous, ethical research that provides valuable evidence to inform clinical practice (Gelling, 2010). The review process scrutinizes issues such as informed consent and the appropriate use and protection of patient data (DH, 2005b). A useful paper by McIlfatrick et al. (2006) provides a discussion of various ethical issues to consider when conducting interviews with cancer patients (see suggested reading list at end of chapter).

Applying to an REC involves submitting the application form, research protocol and any additional documents such as the participant information sheet (PIS) and consent form (Gelling, 2010). The REC might seek clarification on any of these documents and, if this happens, researchers will often need to resubmit revised versions before a favourable ethical opinion is given. This can obviously cause delays to the process, so careful attention should be taken in the initial preparation and examination of these documents. Templates for the PIS are available on the NHS Health Research Authority (HRA) website, and the input of Patient and Public Involvement (PPI) representatives during the design of any patient resources is recommended. Researchers should also make every effort to attend the REC meeting to discuss the application with the committee, which can often resolve any minor queries (Gelling, 2010).

Researchers should engage with research ethics on an ongoing, reflexive basis (Thompson and Chambers, 2011; Broom, 2006), not just see it as a tick-box exercise at the start of the research process. For example, if undertaking longitudinal research, the participants' rights and what their continued participation entails should be reiterated, and consent reconfirmed regularly at each stage in the research process (Kendall et al., 2007). This is especially important in the context of psychosocial oncology research because a patient's condition and ability or willingness to participate may change over time. Furthermore, certain patient groups may require specific consideration, such as elderly cancer patients (Chouliara et al., 2004b).

The research governance framework also requires that health and social care organizations are informed when a study is planned and that the lead investigator gains permission locally before the study begins (DH, 2005b). If conducting research in an NHS Trust, this involves applying for NHS permission from the Research and Development (R&D), Research and Innovation (R&I) or Research Governance department (DH, 2008d). The process of seeking R&D approval has been streamlined with the introduction of the IRAS form, which now combines the application for ethical and R&D approval (Gelling, 2010). A short site-specific form is also submitted to each relevant Trust R&D office, which details any local details or requirements.

The R&D office will also coordinate the issue of a Research Passport or honorary contract if researchers are not employed by that particular NHS trust (Gelling, 2010; National Institute for Health Research (NIHR), 2010). As part of this process the researcher is likely to need a clear Disclosure and Barring Service (DBS) check, and be screened by the Trust's occupational health department (NIHR, 2010). Some Trusts may also require researchers to have completed an NIHR Good Clinical Practice (GCP) workshop prior to approval being granted. Each of these processes may differ in individual Trusts, but it is important to be aware that they can take additional time, and so should be factored into the timescale of the proposed research.

Accessing patients: issues with gatekeepers

Gaining access to eligible patients and the subsequent recruitment of participants is a crucial part of the research process. Initially, this will require the researcher liaising with appropriate organizations and/or professionals – in cancer care this may include clinical leads or managers in the hospital oncology departments. Other individuals that might need to be consulted include clinical nurse specialists or ward sisters, who might be required to help champion the project or make initial approaches to eligible patients. Successfully gaining access to potential participants requires the researchers to build up good working relationships with these relevant 'gatekeepers' (Kendall et al., 2007). At times, gatekeepers may be concerned about issues relating to the research, for example the burden placed on patients who are going through a difficult experience (e.g. Chiang et al., 2001). These concerns will need to be discussed and negotiated, which may lead to changes to the research protocol. This is why it is advisable that these discussions happen early in the research planning stage (Gelling, 2010).

Furthermore, in sensitive research such as cancer care, recruitment strategies need to recognize and be responsive to the needs of participants (Kendall et al., 2007), for example considering the most appropriate time to initially approach patients about the research. These decisions can be usefully informed by input from stakeholders and PPI representatives who may also suggest different strategies (Thompson and Chambers, 2011).

Retaining participants to follow-up

Longitudinal research will require the consideration of participant retention in order to gain future follow-up data. In most studies, some participant attrition is expected, which is why studies often factor rates of attrition into their initial recruitment targets, for example, in their end-of-life care study, Kendall et al. (2007) suggest factoring in a rate of 30–50%. Significant rates of attrition can be a source of bias, which may compromise the confidence readers may have in the findings and conclusions. Reasons for attrition include death of the study participants, demands of illness and treatments, requirements or duration of study, lack of time, loss of interest, not being randomized to the desired group and loss of contact (Northouse et al., 2006). To some extent, successful retention will involve the researcher building a positive relationship with participants in the initial data collection phase. Various retention strategies have been suggested in the literature (see the following section).

Participant retention strategies

- Reminders (e.g. postcards, phonecalls)
- Advisory panels, including PPI representatives
- Create study identity for participants (e.g. similar colours/fonts in study materials)
- Clear information describing the study, including details of the follow-up process and timetable
- Keep in touch with study participants with newsletters, preliminary findings, etc.
- Offer flexible appointments/methods for obtaining follow-up data
- Financial incentives, reimbursement of expenses or non-financial incentives
- Aim to follow-up drop-outs to identify reasons for withdrawal

Source: Informed by Pruitt and Privette (2001); Robinson et al. (2007).

It is imperative, however, that study participants are not coerced or pressured into participating or continuing at any point during the study or follow-up (Pruitt and Privette, 2001), and they should always have the right to withdraw from a study at any time and for whatever reason.

Multiple roles as a researcher

Another issue to consider is when a researcher has multiple roles, for example both a researcher and nurse, or a researcher and service user (Thompson and Chambers, 2011), perhaps even having previous personal experience on the topic under study (e.g. Johnson, 2009; Hubbard et al., 2001). This has been widely discussed in the literature as a source of methodological and ethical dilemma because the individual might be diverted from their researcher role and into their 'other' role (Allmark et al., 2009). For example, a nurse may feel duty bound to offer advice or guidance to a patient who is struggling with a particular clinical issue, or a service user researcher may become over-involved, offering extensive support or divulging details of their own experience during an interview.

These situations can be intuitively understood, but their handling can impact on the research process. In a qualitative study with researchers engaged in 'sensitive' research, Johnson and Clarke (2003) identified that researchers found this role conflict challenging and, in some cases, it could influence the emotional impact of conducting the research (see next section). Even if a dual role does not exist, researchers may find that they instinctively build up a strong rapport with some participants (Johnson and Clarke, 2003), which could be argued to compromise their professional researcher role.

It is important that researchers are open and honest about how these different roles might influence the research (Thompson and Chambers, 2011). Furthermore, how the researcher's multiple roles are communicated with participants is also valuable to consider

(Thompson and Russo, 2012). Engaging with appropriate supervision and training (including role play) may help to anticipate how a researcher might facilitate these situations (Thompson and Chambers, 2011).

Stress and the emotional impact of undertaking psychosocial research

> If the qualitative researcher is to be the research instrument, then he or she must be fully aware of the nature of that instrument. What is at issue, then, is the impact of immersion in an emotionally charged environment, and the elicitation of painful and inspirational stories, and the telling of these stories. (Gilbert, 2001: 11).

Reflective activity

- What might be the potential impact on the researcher of undertaking psychosocial research in cancer settings?
- What strategies may help to manage the potential emotional impact on the researcher?

As discussed in Chapter 30, working with cancer patients can be both rewarding and stressful: burnout can occur and has been reportedly high amongst oncology health professionals (Grunfeld et al., 2005; Ramirez et al., 1996). This also includes oncology researchers. Emotional work demands have been the focus of recent research (Zapf, 2002; Le Blanc et al., 2001), and concepts such as **emotional labour**, the act of displaying appropriate emotion and managing emotions in order to meet environment expectations (Hochschild, 1983), and **compassion fatigue**, a consequence of interacting with individuals who are experiencing considerable stress (White, 2006), have been proposed as influencing the experience of work-related stress. Hubbard et al. (2001) provide some examples of the emotions (upset, anger, over-empathizing) that can occur during qualitative data collection in a wide range of research topics.

The importance of considering the management of emotions amongst both participants and research staff conducting applied research has been highlighted (Kidd and Finlayson, 2006; Kendall et al., 2007; Lalor et al., 2006); however, generally the focus is on protecting participants, and researchers do not often consider in advance how the research might affect them (Gilbert, 2001, Dickson-Swift et al., 2007). This is very important to do because various personal accounts published by cancer researchers (Rager, 2005; Cannon, 1989; Johnson, 2009) have highlighted the personal impact that undertaking research in this area can have. Research studies by Dickson-Swift et al. (2007, 2009) with Australian public health researchers (some in cancer) also illustrated the potential for researchers to be affected both physically and psychologically. Similar findings were recently found by Kennedy et al. (2013) in a study with UK cancer researchers.

As a researcher working in psychosocial oncology, it is possible to be exposed to highly personal, sensitive information during the interactions with participants. Much of the research and accounts from researchers exploring this area have been from those engaged in qualitative methodology (e.g. Dickson-Swift et al., 2007; 2009; Johnson, 2009); however Kennedy et al. (2013)

emphasize that quantitative sensitive researchers working in psychosocial oncology can also be affected – they can still be involved with patients on a regular basis and the information collected can be potentially distressing.

The issues of stress and the emotional impact on research staff should be considered at the start of any research project, and appropriate strategies and procedures for coping with these experiences established. As Harris and Huntington (2001: 131) state:

> ... if we take emotions and emotional labour seriously into account, then we open a space within which we can explore practical strategies to work with our emotional responses.

The following list is a variety of strategies that might be considered for managing this challenging aspect of being a psychosocial oncology researcher.

Strategies and mechanisms for coping with the emotional impact of research

- Be aware that emotional distress can occur, carry out a risk assessment and plan coping strategies- including guidelines for ending research relationships and how to cope if participants die during the research
- Adequate research training, including discussion of the emotional impact, communication skills, basic counselling skills and education about stress and coping
- Pace the timing of data collection in order to not overburden researchers and provide necessary time after each interview to process information and experiences
- Ensure regular holidays are taken
- Consider the impact on those who transcribe any research interviews
- Keep a journal to record and reflect on the process of undertaking the research
- Regular meetings and open-door policy with supervisors/line managers to offload and gain support. Ingleton and Davies (2004) suggest this might require a change in approach/culture in the supervisory relationship whereby time and space is provided to discuss non-intellectual and non-mechanistic aspects of the research.
- Experienced 'buddy' mentoring system or peer groups
- Consider whether external professional supervision, counselling or psychotherapy is required
- Individualized stress management activities – e.g. relaxation, exercise, pilates/yoga, social events, hobbies.

Source: Informed by Pickett et al. (1994); Ingleton and Davies (2004); Dickson-Swift et al. (2007, 2008, 2009); Johnson (2009); Vachon (2010); Kennedy et al. (2013)

Finding support and funding for research

Conducting psychosocial oncology research is undoubtedly challenging, both in terms of the methodologies used and the emotional impact on the researcher. This isn't made any easier by a comparative lack of research infrastructure for this type of work. Clearly, and understandably, research into treatment and cure of cancer needs to take precedence; however, it is surprising how little is spent on psychosocial aspects of care. The charity, Dimbleby Cancer Care, for example, report that less than 5% of cancer research funds are spent on questions exploring the care needs of patients and their families (Dimbleby Cancer Care, 2014). Similarly, a recent National Cancer Research Institute (NCRI) report suggested that less than 2% of the total budget of UK-based NCRI Partner funding was spent on cancer control, survivorship and outcomes research (NCRI, 2013). This has created a highly competitive funding environment for psychosocial oncology. Funding is essential for most research projects, for example to cover the costs of equipment, travel, personnel, research staff costs or for dissemination and publication costs. In a competitive research-funding environment, psychosocial oncology researchers need to equip themselves with the skills of writing successful grant proposals. There are a variety of potential funders for psychosocial oncology research (see later); however, getting funding for this work continues to be challenging (Travis, 2009; Molassiotis and Jacobs, 2012). Molassiotis and Jacobs (2012) reviewed the current state of cancer research relating to palliative and supportive care in the UK (see suggested reading list at the end of the chapter) and concluded that although an increase in research outputs reflects the promising growth, future research funding was highlighted as a major challenge.

Potential funding sources in the UK

- Government and state-funded health and social care research agencies, such as the NHS and Department of Health programmes, e.g. National Institute for Health Research (NIHR), Research for Patient Benefit (RfPB)
- Research councils, such as Economic and Social Research Council (ESCR) and Medical Research Council (MRC)
- Healthcare and disease-specific charities, such as Dimbleby Cancer Care, Marie Curie Cancer Care, Macmillan Cancer Support, Breast Cancer Campaign, Teenage Cancer Trust, Prostate Cancer Charity, Target Ovarian Cancer, Roy Castle Lung Cancer Foundation, Cicely Saunders Foundation, Big Lottery Fund
- Professional organizations, such as Royal College of Nursing, Burdett Trust for Nursing
- Institutional funding, such as university and hospital sources

---

Obtaining research funding is a time-consuming and skilled activity. Collaboration with more experienced researchers is recommended. The following resources are available to help researchers identify suitable funding sources and develop high quality research grant applications:

- RDInfo (www.rdinfo.org.uk)
- Research Professional (www.researchprofessional.com)
- Research Design Service (RDS) (www.rds.nihr.ac.uk).

Recent work led by the NCRI has attempted to make research in cancer survivorship a little more transparent and effective, for example between 2006 and 2012 they funded two research collaboratives (CECo and Compass), network partnerships between specific UK universities to encourage research collaboration and capacity building; and they have more recently launched a website with advice and guidance for those planning to undertake projects in this area of cancer care (NCRI Grantsmanship Gateway http://grantsmanship.ncri.org.uk).

In addition to funding these one-off projects, the NCRI have recognized the importance of psychosocial oncology research in its structure of Clinical Studies Groups (CSGs). CSGs are appointed committees of national experts who maintain a national Trials Portfolio and oversee recruitment into cancer research, and to encourage and collaborate on new research projects. In addition to a number of site-specific CSGs for individual tumour groups, the Psychosocial Oncology and Survivorship (POS) CSG is one of three cross-cutting groups (the others are Primary Care, and Palliative and Supportive Care) that advance the agenda for psychosocial research in various ways. Between 2004 and 2012, 24,934 UK patients had been recruited into studies on the POS CSG Trials Portfolio, representing the vastly increased opportunities for people with cancer to take part in psychosocial oncology research (Hulbert-Williams et al., 2012c).

The POS CSG currently has three working groups focusing on the following topic areas:

- Patient experience and patient-reported outcome measures (PROMS);
- Developing and testing lifestyle and behaviour change interventions; and
- Interventions to improve psychosocial and survivorship outcomes in those affected by cancer.

Membership of each of these groups is limited, but those interested in getting involved are encouraged to contact the Chair of the relevant subgroups, or indeed, the Main CSG chair. Adverts for new members of the CSG are released frequently because membership duration is limited.

Researchers working in this area might also benefit from networking with other colleagues working in similar research areas, and this is especially helpful for early-career researchers. Academic societies are a great way to do this and they often host regular conferences and seminars where you can meet potential collaborators, learn new research skills and present research findings. The key societies and conferences to consider in psychosocial oncology include:

- The British Psychosocial Oncology Society (BPOS)
- The British Psychological Society (BPS) Faculty for Oncology and Palliative Care (SIGOPAC)
- The International Psycho-Oncology Society (IPOS).

CHAPTER SUMMARY

Conducting psychosocial oncology research is an important part of developing and evaluating holistic and evidence-based cancer care. Compared to some other types of cancer research, a wide variety of research methodologies and designs are used, including both qualitative and quantitative approaches. Understanding the psychosocial impact of cancer, and meeting the needs of this group better, relies upon the use of both types of research, often within the same study (often referred to as **mixed-methods** research; see Beaver and Luker (2005) for a good example of how this can be done). Conducting such research, however, is certainly not easy – on a practical level or an emotional level – and an ongoing reflection on the challenges and personal impact of researching psychosocial issues in cancer care is of vital importance.

Key learning points

- There is a range of different philosophical perspectives that influence the approaches used in various research designs. Those undertaking research in cancer care should be familiar with and have a basic comprehension of how these influence methodology.
- Understanding how various types of research methodologies differ in terms of their design, conduct and how their data are interpreted is important; without this knowledge, interpretations and application of the research data may be inaccurate or inappropriate. This is particularly important when considering differences in the application of qualitative versus quantitative research.
- Conducting psychosocial oncology research is very challenging, from both a practical and an emotional perspective. Overcoming these challenges and continuing to support research into psychosocial aspects of cancer care is important in order to ensure best practice care.

Recommended further reading

- Ritchie, J. and Lewis, J. (2003). *Qualitative Research Practice*. London: Sage Publications.
- Field, A. (2013). *Discovering Statistics Using IBM SPSS Statistics*. 4th edn. London: Sage Publications.
- McIlfatrick, S., Sullivan, K. and McKenna, H. (2006) 'Exploring the ethical issues of the research interview in the cancer context', *European Journal of Oncology Nursing*, 10: 39–47.
- Molassiotis, A. and Jacobs, C. (2012) 'An evaluation of the current state of cancer-related palliative and supportive care research in the UK', *Palliative Care & Medicine*, 2(4): 112–19.

REFERENCES

Aapro, M.S., Tjan-Heijnen, V.C., Walewski, J., Weber, D.C., Zielinski, C. and European Organisation for Research and Treatment of Cancer (EORTC) (2006) 'Granulocyte Colony-Stimulating Factor (G-CSF) Guidelines Working Party', *European Journal of Cancer,* 42(15): 2433–53.

Aaronson, N.K., Ahmedzai, S., Bergman, B., Bullinger, M., Cull, A., Duez, N.J., Filiberti, A., Flechtner, H., Fleishman, S.B., de Haes, J.C. and The European Organization for Research and Treatment of Cancer (1993) 'QLQ-C30: a quality-of-life instrument for use in international clinical trials in oncology', *Journal of the National Cancer Institute,* 85: 365–76.

Abdel-Rahman, M., Stockton, D., Rachet, B., Hakulinen, T. and Coleman, M.P. (2009) 'What if cancer survival rates in Britain were the same as in Europe: how many deaths are avoidable?', *British Journal of Cancer,* 101: 115–125. Available from: www.bjcancer.com.

Acheson, D. (1998) *Independent Inquiry into Inequalities in Health Report.* London: Department of Health.

Adams, E., Boulton, M. and Watson, E. (2009) 'The information needs of partners and family members of cancer patients: a systematic literature review', *Patient Education and Counseling,* 77: 179–86.

Agnew,A., Manktelow,R.,Haynes, T. and Jones, L. (2010) 'Bereavement assessment practice in hospice settings: challenges for palliative care social workers', *British Journal of Social Work,* May 24, 1–20.

Ahmed, H., Naik, G., Willoughby, H., et al. (2012) 'Communicating risk', *British Medical Journal,* 18: 344. e3996. doi:10.1136/bmj.e3996.

Ajzen, I. (1985) 'From intentions to actions: a theory of planned behavior', in J. Kuhl and J. Beckmann (eds), *Action-Control: From Cognition to Behaviour.* Heidelberg: Springer. pp. 11–39.

Ajzen, I. (1991) 'The theory of planned behavior', *Organizational Behavior and Human Decision Processes,* 50(2): 179–211.

Alcântara-Silva, T., Freitas, R., Freitas, N. and Machado, G. (2013) 'Fatigue related to radiotherapy for breast and/or gynaecological cancer: a systematic review', *Journal of Clinical Nursing,* 22(19–20): 2679–86.

Alderfer, M., Log, K., Lown, A., Marsland, A., Ostrowski, N., Hock, J. and Ewing, L. (2010) 'Psychosocial adjustment of siblings of children with cancer: a systematic review', *Psycho-oncology,* 19: 789–805.

Aldridge, D. (eds) (1998) *Music Therapy in Palliative Care: New Voices.* London: Jessica Kingsley.

Alimi, D., Rubino, C., Pichard-Léandri, E., Fermand-Brulé, S., Dubreuil-Lemaire, M.-L. and Hill, C. (2003) 'Analgesic effect of auricular acupuncture for cancer pain: a randomized, blinded, controlled trial', *Journal of Clinical Oncology,* 21(22): 4120–6. doi:10.1200/JCO.2003.09.011.

Allen, J.D., Savadatti, S. and Levy, A.G. (2009) 'The transition from breast cancer "patient" to "survivor"', *Psycho-oncology,* 18(1): 71–8.

Allenby, A., Matthews, J., Beresford, J. and McLachlan, S.A. (2002) 'The application of computer touch-screen technology in screening for psychosocial distress in an ambulatory oncology setting', *European Journal of Cancer Care,* 11(4): 245–53.

Allmark, P., Boote, J., Chambers, E., Clarke, A., McDonnell, A., Thompson, A. and Todd, A.M. (2009) 'Ethical issues in the use of in-depth interviews: literature review and discussion', *Research Ethics Review,* 5(2): 48–54.

All Party Parliamentary Group on Cancer (APPGC) (2009) *Report of the APPGC's Inquiry into Inequalities in Cancer.* London: Macmillan.

Almeida, C.A. and Barry, S.A. (2010) *Cancer: Basic Science and Clinical Aspects*. Oxford: Wiley-Blackwell.

American Cancer Society (2013) *Cancer Facts & Figures*. Atlanta, GA: American Cancer Society.

American Cancer Society (2014a) *Learning about Cancer Surgery.* Available from: www.cancer.org/treatment/treatmentsandsideeffects/treatmenttypes/surgery/surgery-learning-about-cancer-surgery [accessed 18 November 2014].

American Cancer Society (2014b) *The History of Cancer.* Available from: www.cancer.org/acs/groups/cid/documents/webcontent/002048-pdf.pdf [accessed 18 November 2014].

American Psychiatric Association (1952) *Diagnostic and Statistical Manual of Mental Disorders (DSM).* Washington, DC: American Psychiatric Association.

American Psychiatric Association (1994) *Diagnostic and Statistical Manual of Mental Disorders, 4th edition (DSM-IV).* Washington, DC: American Psychiatric Association.

American Psychiatric Association (2013) *Diagnostic and Statistical Manual of Mental Disorders, 5th edition (DSM-V).* Arlington, VA: American Psychiatric Association.

American Society of Clinical Oncologists (ASCO), Griggs, J.J., Mangu, P.B., Anderson, H., Balaban, E.P. Dignam, J.J., Hryniuk, W.M. Morrison, V.A., Pini, T.M., Runowicz, C.D., Rosner, G.L., Shayne, M., Sparreboom, A., Sucheston, L.E. and Lyman, G.H. (2012) 'Appropriate chemotherapy dosing for obese adult patients with cancer: ASCO practice guideline', *Journal of Clinical Oncology*, 30(13): 1553–61. Available from: www.jco.org [accessed 31 May 2012].

Amir, Z., Moran, T., Walsh, L. et al. (2007) 'Return to paid work after cancer: a British experience', *Journal of Cancer Survivorship,* 1(2): 129–36.

Amir, Z., Wynn, P., Chan, F., Strauser, D., Whitaker, S. and Luker, K. (2010) 'Return to work after cancer in the UK: attitudes and experiences of line managers', *Journal of Occupational Rehabilitation,* 20: 435–42.

Andermann, A., Blancquaert, I., Beauchamp, S. and Déry, V. (2008) 'Revisiting Wilson and Jungner in the genomic age: a review of screening criteria over the past 40 years', *Bulletin of the World Health Organization,* 86(4): 317–9.

Andersen, B.L., Kiecolt-Glaser, J.K. and Glaser, R. (1994) 'A biobehavioral model of cancer stress and disease course', *American Psychologist*, 49(5): 389–404.

Anderson, H., Ward C., Eardley A., Gomm, S.A., Connelly, M., Coppinger, T., Corgie, D., Williams, J.L. and Makin, W.P. (2001) 'The concerns of patients undergoing palliative care at a heart failure clinic are not being met', *Palliative Medicine,* 15: 279–286.

Anderson, O.A. and Wearne, I.M.J. (2007) 'Informed consent for elective surgery: what is best practice?', *Journal of the Royal Society of Medicine*, 100: 97–100.

Anderson-Reitz, L. (2011) 'Complications of hematopoietic stem cell transplantation', in C.H. Yarbro, D. Wujcik and B.H. Holmes (eds), *Cancer Nursing: Principles and Practice*. 7th edn. Sudbury, MA: Jones and Bartlett. pp. 513–529.

Andreyev, H.J.N. (2010) 'A physiological approach to modernize the management of cancer chemotherapy-induced gastrointestinal toxicity', *Current Opinion in Supportive and Palliative Care*, 4: 19–25.

Andriole, G.L., Crawford, E.D., Grubb III, R.L. et al. (2009) 'Mortality results from a randomized prostate-cancer screening trial', *The New England Journal of Medicine,* 360(13): 1310–9.

Andrykowski, M.A. and Mann, S.L. (2006) 'Are psychological interventions effective and accepted by cancer patients? Standards and levels of evidence', *Annals of Behavioural Medicine*, 32(2): 93–97.

Annon, J. (1976) 'The PLISSIT model: a proposed conceptual scheme for the behavioural treatment of sexual problems', *Journal of Sex Education and Therapy*, 2(1): 1–15.

Antman, K. and Chang, Y. (2000) 'Kaposi's Sarcoma', *New England Journal of Medicine,* 342(14): 1027–1038.

Anxiety UK (2010) *Injection Phobia and Needle Phobia*. Manchester: Anxiety UK.

Appelbaum, F.R. (2007) 'Hematopoietic-Cell Transplantation at 50', *New England Journal of Medicine*, 357: 1472–75.

Argyriou, A., Koltzenburg, M., Polychronopoulos, P., Papapetropoulos, K. and Kalofonus, H. (2008) 'Peripheral nerve damage associated with administration of taxanes in patients with cancer', *Critical Review Oncology Haematology,* 66(3): 218–28.

Aries, P. (1974) *Western Attitudes Towards Death From the Middle Ages to the Present*. Baltimore, MD: John Hopkins University Press.

Armes, J., Crowe, M., Colbourne, L., Morgan, H., Murrells, T., Oakley, C., Palmer, N., Ream, E., Young, A. and Richardson, A. (2009) 'Patients' supportive care needs beyond the end of cancer treatment: a prospective longitudinal survey', *Journal of Clinical Oncology*, 27(36): 6172–9.

Armes, J., Wagland, R., Finnegan-John, J., Richardson, A., Corner, J. and Griffiths, P. (2013) 'Development and testing of the patient-reported chemotherapy indicators of symptoms and experience: patient-reported outcome and process indicators sensitive to the quality of nursing care in ambulatory chemotherapy settings', *Cancer Nursing*, 37(3): E52–E60. NCC.0b013e3182980420.

Arnstein, S.R. (1969) 'A ladder of citizen participation', *Journal of the American Institute of Planners*, 35(4): 216–224.

Arora, R.S., Alston, R.D., Eden, T., Estlin, E.J., Moran, A., Birch, J.M. (2009) 'Age–incidence patterns of primary CNS tumors in children, adolescents, and adults in England', *Neurological Oncology*, 11(4): 403–13.

Association of Coloproctology of Great Britain and Ireland (2013) *National Bowel Cancer Audit Annual Report 2013*. London: Association of Coloproctology of Great Britain and Ireland.

Association of European Cancer Leagues (2010–2014) *European Code Against Cancer*. Available from: www.europeancancerleagues.org/ewac/european-code-against-cancer.html [accessed 18 April 2014].

Atkin, W.S., Edwards, R., Kralj-Hans, I., et al., UK Flexible Sigmoidoscopy Trial Investigators (2010) 'Once-only flexiblesigmoidoscopy screening in prevention of colorectal cancer: a multicentre randomised controlled trial', *Lancet*, 375(9726): 1624–33.

Aune, D., Chan, D.S.M., Vieira, A.R., Navarro Rosenblatt, D.A., Vieira, R., Greenwood, D.C., et al. (2013) 'Red and processed meat intake and risk of colorectal adenomas: a systematic review and meta-analysis of epidemiological studies', *Cancer Causes & Control*, 24(4): 611–27.

Baade, P.A., Youlden, D.R., Valery, P.C. and Hassall, T. (2010) 'Trends in incidence of childhood cancer in Australia (1983–2006)', *British Journal of Cancer*, 102: 620–626.

Baan, R., Grosse, Y., Straif, K., et al. (2009) 'WHO International Agency for Research on Cancer Monograph Working Group. A review of human carcinogens--Part F: chemical agents and related occupations', *Lancet Oncology*, 10(12): 1143–4.

Baker, C. (2012a) 'Atoms, nuclei and radioactivity', in P. Symonds, C. Deehan, J.A. Mills and C. Meredith (eds), *Walter and Miller's Textbook of Radiotherapy*, 7th edn. London: Elsevier Churchill Livingstone. pp. 3–14.

Baker, C. (2012b) 'Radiation interactions with matter', in P. Symonds, C. Deehan, J.A. Mills and C. Meredith (eds), *Walter and Miller's Textbook of Radiotherapy*, 7th edn. London: Elsevier Churchill Livingstone. pp. 15–32.

Baker, F. and Wigram, T. (eds) (2005) *Songwriting: Methods, Techniques and Clinical Applications for Music Therapy Clinicians, Educators and Students*. London: Jessica Kingsley.

Baker, T.B., McFall, R.M. and Shoham, V. (2008) 'Current status and future prospects of clinical psychology toward a scientifically principled approach to mental and behavioral health care', *Psychological Science in the Public Interest*, 9(2): 67–103.

Baker-Glenn, E.A., Park, B., Granger, L., Symonds, P. and Mitchell, A.J. (2011) 'Desire for psychological support in cancer patients with depression or distress: validation of a simple help question', *Psycho-oncology*, 20(5): 525–31.

Bakitas, M., Doyle Lyons, K., Hegel, M.T., Balan, S., Brokaw, F.C., Seville, J., Hull, J.G., Li, Z. Tosteson, T.D., Byock, I.R. and Ahles, T.A. (2009) 'Effects of a palliative care intervention on clinical outcomes in patients with advanced cancer', *Journal of the American Medical Association*, 302(7): 741–9.

Baldomero, H., Gratwohl, M., Gratwohl, A. et al, for the European Group for Blood and Marrow Transplantation (2011) 'The EBMT activity survey 2009: trends over the past 5 years', *Bone Marrow Transplantation*, 46: 485–501.

Balducci, L. and Ershler, W.B. (2005) 'Cancer and ageing: a nexus at several levels', *National Review Cancer*, 5: 655–62.

Balloqui, J. (2005) 'The efficacy of a single session', in D. Waller and C. Sibbert (eds), *Art Therapy and Cancer Care*. Maidenhead, UK: Open University Press. pp. 128–37.

Bandura, A. (1977a) 'Self-efficacy: toward a unifying theory of behavioral change', *Psychological Review*, 84(2): 191–215.

Bandura, A. (1977b) *Social Learning Theory*. New York, NY: General Learning Press.

Bandura, A. (1986) *Social Foundations of Thought and Action: A Social Cognitive Theory*. Englewood Cliffs, NJ: Prentice Hall.

Bao, T., Zhang, R., Badros, A. and Lao, L. (2011) 'Accupuncture treatment for bortezomib-induced peripheral neuropathy: a case report', *Pain Research and Treatment* doi: 10.1155/2011/920807.

BAPEN (2011) *Nutrition Screening Survey in the UK and Republic of Ireland in 2011*. Available from: www.bapen.org.uk/pdfs/nsw/nsw-2011-report.pdf [accessed 9 December 2013].

Bar-Sela, G., Atid, L., Danos, S., Gabay, N. and Epelbaum, R. (2007) 'Art therapy improved depression and influenced fatigue levels in cancer patients on chemotherapy', *Psycho-oncology*, 16: 980–4.

Barbour, R.S. (2001) 'Checklists for improving rigour in qualitative research: a case of the tail wagging the dog', *British Medical Journal*, 322: 1115–17.

BarChana, M., Levav, I., Lipshitz, I., Pugachova, I., Kohn, R., Weizman, A. and Grinshpoon, A. (2008) 'Enhanced cancer risk among patients with bipolar disorder', *Journal of Affective Disorders*, 108(1–2): 43–8.

Bard, M. and Dyk, R.B. (1956) The psychodynamic significance of beliefs regarding the cause of serious illness', *The Psychoanalytic Review*, 43: 146–62.

Barker, P. and Buchanan-Barker, P. (2012) 'First do no harm: confronting the myths of psychiatric drugs', *Nursing Ethics*, 19(4): 451–63.

Barquinero, J., Eixarch, H. and Pérez-Melgosa, M. (2004) 'Retroviral vectors: new applications for an old tool', *Gene Therapy*, 11: S3–S9.

Barr, R.D., Silva, M.P., Greenberg, M.L. (2007) 'Difficult beginnings – cancer care in infancy', *Journal of Pediatric Blood Cancers*, 49: 1059.

Barrera, M., Chung, J. and Fleming, C.A. (2005) 'Group intervention for siblings of pediatric cancer patients', *Journal of Psychosocial Oncology*, 22(2): 21–39.

Baughan, P., O'Neill, B. and Fletcher, E. (2009) 'Auditing the diagnosis of cancer in primary care: the experience in Scotland', *British Journal of Cancer*, 101(S2): S87–91.

Baum, F., MacDougall, C. and Smith, D. (2006) 'Participatory action research', *Journal of Epidemiology and Community Health*, 60(10): 854–57.

Baum, M. (1998) 'Preface', in C. Connell (ed.), *Something Understood – Art Therapy in Cancer Care*. Wrexham, UK: Wrexham Publications. p. 9.

Baxter, H.L.K., Houston, H., Jones, G., Felce, D. and Kerr, M. (2006) 'Previously unidentified morbidity in patients with intellectual disability', *British Journal of General Practice*, 56(523): 93–98.

Beaumont, J. (2007) 'Breast cancer: what are the issues for young women?', *Cancer Nursing Practice*, 6(9): 36–39.

Beaver, K. and Luker, K.A. (2005) 'Follow-up in breast cancer clinics: reassuring for patients rather than detecting recurrence', *Psycho-oncology*, 14: 94–101.

Beck, A.T. (1979) *Cognitive Therapy of Depression*. New York, NY: Guilford Press.

Beck, A.T., Guth, D., Steer, R.A. et al. (1997) 'Screening for major depression disorders in medical inpatients with the Beck Depression Inventory for Primary Care', *Behaviour Research and Therapy*, 35: 785–91.

Beck, A.T., Steer, R.A. and Brown, G.K. (1996) *Beck Depression Inventory*, 2nd edn. San Antonio, TX: The Psychological Corporation.

Beck, J.S. (2011) *Cognitive Behavior Therapy: Basics and Beyond*, 2nd edn. New York, NY: Guilford Press.

Becker, M.H. and Rosenstock, I.M. (1984) 'Compliance with medical advice', in A. Steptoe and A. Mathews (eds), *Health Care and Human Behaviour*. London: Academic Press.

Becker, S., Dearden, C. and Aldridge, J. (2000) 'Young carers in the UK: research, policy and practice', *Research, Policy and Planning*, 8(2): 13–22.

Beckham, J.C., Burker, E.J., Feldman, M.E. and Costakis, M.J. (1997) 'Self-efficacy and adjustment in cancer patients: a preliminary report', *Behavioral Medicine*, 23(3): 138–42.

Beckingsale, T.B. and Gerrand, C.H. (2010) 'Osteosarcoma', *Orthopaedics and Trauma*, 24(5): 321–31.

Beckman, H.B., Frankel, R.M. and Darnley, J. (1985) 'Soliciting the patient's complete agenda: relationship to the distribution of concerns', *Clinical Research*, 33: 714A.

Bee, P.E., Barnes, P. and Luker, K.A. (2008) 'A systematic review of informal caregivers' needs in providing home-based end-of-life care to people with cancer', *Journal of Clinical Nursing*, 18: 1379–93.

Beeken, R.J., Simon, A.E., von Wagner, C., Whitaker, K.L. and Wardle, L (2011) 'Cancer fatalism: deterring early presentation and increasing social inequalities?', *Cancer Epidemiology, Biomarkers and Prevention*, 20(10): 2127–31.

Befort, C.A., Nazir, N. Engelman, K. and Choi, W. (2013) 'Fatalistic cancer beliefs and information sources among rural and urban adults in the USA', *Journal of Cancer Education*, 28(3): 521–6.

Behrens, G. and Leitzmann, M.F. (2013) 'The association between physical activity and renal cancer: systematic review and meta-analysis', *British Journal of Cancer*, 108(4): 798–811.

Bell, S. (1998)'Will the kitchen table do? Art therapy in the community?', in M. Pratt and J.M. Wood (eds), *Art therapy in Palliative Care – The Creative Response*. London: Routledge. pp. 88–101.

Bellizzi, K.M. and Blank, T.O. (2007) 'Cancer-related identity and positive affect in survivors of prostate cancer', *Journal of Cancer Survivorship*, 1(1): 44–8.

Bench, S., Day, T. and Metcalfe, A. (2013) 'Randomised controlled trials: an introduction for nurse researchers', *Nurse Researcher*, 20(5): 38–44.

Benson, V.S., Patnick, J., Davies, A.K., Nadel, M.R., Smith, R.A., Atkin, W.S. and International Colorectal Cancer Screening Network (2008) 'Colorectal cancer screening: a comparison of 35 initiatives in 17 countries', *International Journal of Cancer*, 122(6): 1357–67.

Bergenmar, M., Johansson, H. and Sharp, L. (2014) 'Patients' perception of information after completion of adjuvant radiotherapy for breast cancer', *European Journal of Oncology Nursing*, 18(3): 305–9.

Berman, R., Campbell, M., Makin, W. and Todd, C. (2007) 'Occupational stress in palliative medicine, medical oncology and clinical oncology specialist registrars', *Clincal Medicine*, 7(3): 235–42.

Berrino, F., De Angelis, R., Sant, M., Rosso, S., Lasota, M.B., Coebergh, J.W. and Santaquilani, M. (2007) 'Survival for eight major cancers and all cancers combined for European adults diagnosed in 1995–99: results of the EUROCARE-4 study', *Lancet Oncology*, 8: 773–83. Available from: www.ncbi.nlm.nih.gov/pubmed/17714991.

Bezjak, A., Ng, P., Skeel, R., et al. (2001) 'Oncologists' use of quality of life information: results of a survey of Eastern Cooperative Oncology Group physicians', *Quality of Life Research*, 10: 1–13.

Bezjak, A., Ng, P., Taylor, K., et al. (1997) 'A preliminary survey of oncologists' perceptions of quality of life information', *Psycho-oncology*, 6: 107–13.

Bhopal, R. (2008) *Concepts of Epidemiology: Integrating the Ideas, Theories, Principles and Methods of Epidemiology*. 2nd edn. Oxford: Oxford University Press.

Bianchi, S. and Vezzosi, V. (2008) 'Microinvasive carcinoma of the breast', *Pathology and Oncology Research*, 14(2): 105–11.

Birchwood, M., Spencer, E. and McGovern, D. (2000) 'Schizophrenia: early warning signs', *Advances in Psychiatric Treatment*, 6(93): 101.

Bjordal, K., de Graeff, A., Fayers, P.M., et al. (2000) 'A 12-country field study of the EORTC QLQ-C30 and the head and neck-specific module', *European Journal of Cancer*, 36: 1796–1807.

Björk, M., Wiebe, T. and Hallström, I. (2005) 'Striving to survive: families' lived experiences when a child is diagnosed with cancer', *Journal of Pediatric Oncology Nursing*, 22: 265–75.

Black D. 1980 *Report of the Working Group on Inequalities in Health* (Chair: Sir Douglas Black) London: Department of Health & Social Security.

Black, N. (2013) 'Patient reported outcome measures could help transform healthcare', *BMJ (Clinical research ed.)*, 346. f167. ISSN 0959-8138 DOI: 10.1136/bmj.f167.

Blackledge, J.T. (2007) 'Disrupting verbal processes: cognitive defusion in acceptance and commitment therapy and other mindfulness-based psychotherapies', *The Psychological Record*, 57(4): 555–576.

Blank, R. and Merrick. J. (2005) *End of Life Decision Making: a Cross National Study*. London: MIT Press.

Bleeker, M.C.G., Heideman, D., Snijders, P., Horenblas, S., Dillner, J. and Meijer, C. (2009) 'Penile cancer: epidemiology, pathogenesis and prevention', *World Journal of Urology*, 27: 141–150.

Bleyer, A., Barr, R., Hayes-Lattin, H., Thomas, D., Ellis, C. and Anderson, B. (2008) 'The distinctive biology of cancer in adolescents and young adults', *Nature*, 8: 288–298.

Blomberg, K., Sahlberg-Blom, E. (2007) 'Closeness and distance: a way of handling difficult situations in daily care', *Journal of Clinical Nursing*, 16: 244–254.

Blumer, H. (1969) *Symbolic Interactionism: Perspective and Method*. Englewood Cliffs, NJ: Prentice-Hall.

Bocking, M. (2005) 'A "don't know" story: art therapy in an NHS medical oncology department', in D. Waller and C. Sibbett (eds), *Art Therapy and Cancer Care*. Maidenhead, UK: Open University Press. pp. 210–223.

Bodenmann, G. (1997) 'Dyadic coping – a systemic-transactional view of stress and coping among couples: theory and empirical findings', *European Review of Applied Psychology*, 47(2): 137–40.

Boffetta, P., Matisane, L., Mundt, K.A., et al. (2003) 'Meta-analysis of studies of occupational exposure to vinyl chloride in relation to cancer mortality', *Scandinavian Journal of Work, Environment and Health*, 29(3): 220–9.

Bohlius, J., Schmidlin, K., Brillant, C., et al. (2009) 'Recombinant human erythropoiesis-stimulating agents and mortality in patients with cancer: a meta-analysis of randomised trials', *Lancet*, 373(9674): 1532–1542.

Bonadonna, G.,Valagussa, P., Moliterni, A., Zambetti, M. and Brambilla, C. (1995) 'Adjuvant Cyclophosphamide, Methotrexate, and Fluorouracil in node-positive breast cancer: the results of 20 years of follow-up', *New England Journal of Medicine*, 332 (14): 901–06.

Bond, M., Pavey, T., Welch, K., et al. (2013) 'Systematic review of the psychological consequences of false-positive screening mammograms', *Health Technology Assessment*, 17(13): 1–170, v–vi. doi:10.3310/hta17130.

Bonner, J.A., Harari, P.M., Giralt, J. et al. (2010) 'Radiotherapy plus cetuximab for locoregionally advanced head and neck cancer: 5-year survival data from a phase 3 randomised trial, and relation between cetuximab-induced rash and survival', *Lancet Oncology*, 11(1): 21–28.

Booth, K., Maguire, P.M., Butterworth, T. and Hillier, V.F. (1996) 'Perceived professional support and the use of blocking behaviours by hospice nurses', *Journal of Advanced Nursing*, 24(3): 522–7.

Borkman, T. (1976) 'Experiential knowledge: a new concept for the analysis of self help groups', *Social Service Review*, 50: 445–56.

Borsari, B. and Carey, K.B. (2001) 'Peer influences on college drinking: a review of the research', *Journal of Substance Abuse*, 13(4): 391–424.

Bosch, F., Ribes, J., Diaz, M. and Cleries, R. (2004) 'Primary liver cancer: worldwide incidence and trends', *Gastroenterology*, 127: S5–S16.

Bowlby, J. (1971) *Attachment and Loss, Vol 1: Attachment*. Middlesex, England: Penguin.

Bowlby, J. (1980) *Attachment and Loss, Vol 3: Loss, Sadness and Depression*. London: Hogarth Press.

Box, V. and Anderson, Y. (1997) 'Cancer beliefs, attitudes and preventive behaviours of nurses working in the community', *European Journal of Cancer Care*, 6: 192–208.

Boyes, A., Newell, S., Girgis, A., McElduff, P., Sanson-Fisher, R. (2006) 'Does routine assessment and real-time feedback improve cancer patients' psychosocial well-being?', *European Journal of Cancer Care*, 15: 163–71.

Boyle, P., Autier, P., Bartelink, H., et al. (2003) 'European Code Against Cancer and scientific justification: third version', *Annals of Oncology*, 14(7): 973–1005.

Bradshaw, T. and Pedley, R. (2012) 'Evolving role of mental health nurses in the physical care of people with serious mental health illness', *International Journal of Mental Health Nursing*, 21: 266–73.

Bradt, J. and Dileo, C. (2010) 'Music therapy for end-of-life care', *Cochrane Database of Systematic Reviews*, Issue 1. Art. No.: CD007169. doi:10.1002/14651858.CD007169.pub2.

Bradt, J., Dileo, C., Grocke, D. and Magill, L. (2011) 'Music interventions for improving psychological and physical outcomes in cancer patients', *Cochrane Database of Systematic Reviews*, Issue 8. Art. No.: CD006911. doi:10.1002/14651858.CD006911.pub2.

Braeken, A.P.B.M., Kempen Gertrudis, I.J.M., Eekers, D. et al. (2011) 'The usefulness and feasibility of a screening instrument to identify psychosocial problems in patients receiving curative radiotherapy: a process evaluation', *BMC Cancer*, 11: 479.

Bramsen, I., van der Linden, M.H., Eskens, F.J., Bijvank, E.M., van Groeningen, C.J., Kaufman, H.J. and Aaronson, N.K. (2008) 'Evaluation of a face-to-face psychosocial screening intervention for cancer patients: acceptance and effects on quality of life', *Patient Education and Counseling*, 70(1): 61–8.

Branney, P., Witty, K. and Eardley, I. (2011) 'Patients' experiences of penile cancer', *European Urology*, 59: 959–61.

BRAP (2010) *Walking into the Unknown*. London: Macmillan Cancer Support www.macmillan. org.uk/Documents/./Walkingintotheunknown.pdf.

Braun, M., Mikulincer, M., Rydall, A., Walsh, A. and Rodin, G. (2007) 'Hidden morbidity in cancer: spouse caregivers', *Journal of Clinical Oncology*, 25(30): 4829–34.

Bray, D. and Groves, K. (2007) 'A tailor-made psychological approach to palliative care', *European Journal of Palliative Care*, 14(4): 141–3.

Breast Cancer Care (2013) *Understanding your pathology report (BCC161)*. Available from: www. breastcancercare.org.uk [accessed 4 January 2014].

Breckons, M., Calman, L. and Foster, C.L. (2012) *An Online Survey to Examine Cancer Survivors' Confidence to Self-manage Problems Arising in the First 12 Months Following Primary Cancer Treatment*. Macmillan Survivorship Research Group Report.

Brédart, A., Marrel, A., Abetz-Webb, L., Lasch, K. and Acquadro, C. (2014) 'Interviewing to develop Patient-Reported Outcome (PRO) measures for clinical research: eliciting patients' experience', *Health and Quality of Life Outcomes*, 12: 15.

Brennan, J. (2001) 'Adjustment to cancer: coping or personal transition?', *Psycho-oncology*, 10 (1): 1–18.

Brennan, J. (2004) *Cancer in Context: A Practical Guide to Supportive Care*. Oxford: Oxford University Press.

Brennan, J. and Moynihan, C. (2004) *Cancer in Context: A Practical Guide to Supportive Care*. Oxford: Oxford University Press.

Brenner, D.J., Curtis, R.E., Hall, E.J., and Ron, E. (2000) 'Second malignancies in prostate carcinoma patients after radiotherapy compared with surgery', *Cancer*, 88: 398–406.

Brenner, M.K., Gottschalk, S., Leen, A.M. and Vera, J.F. (2013) 'Is cancer gene therapy an empty suit?', *Lancet Oncology*, 14(11): e447–56.

Bridle, C., Riemsma, R.P., Pattenden, J., Sowden, A.J., Mather, L., Watt, I.S. and Walker, A. (2005) 'Systematic review of the effectiveness of health behavior interventions based on the transtheoretical model', *Psychology & Health*, 20(3): 283–301.

British Association for Behavioural & Cognitive Psychotherapies (BABCP) (n.d.) *Introduction to training*. Available from: www.babcp.com/Training/Training.aspx [accessed May 2013].

British Association of Art Therapists (BAAT) (2014a) What is Art Therapy? Art Therapy Information London: The British Association of Art Therapists. Available from: www.baat.org.

British Association of Art Therapists (BAAT) (2014b) *The Code of Ethics and Principles of Professional Practice*. London: The British Association of Art Therapists. Available from: www.baat.org.

British Heart Foundation (2012) *Coronary Heart Disease Statistics: A Compendium of Health Statistics*. British Heart Foundation.

British Medical Association (1993) *Complementary Medicine: New Approaches to Good Practice*. Oxford: Oxford University Press.

British Medical Association (2013) *Mental Capacity Toolkit*. Available from: http://bma.org.uk/ practical-support-at-work/ethics/mental-capacity-tool-kit [accessed 9 December 2013].

British National Formulary (BNF) (2012) *BNF 65 September*. Available from: www.bnf.org [accessed 14 June 2012].

British Psychological Society (2005) *Good Practice Guidelines for the Conduct of Psychological Research within the NHS*. Leicester: British Psychological Society.

British Psychological Society (2009) *Code of Ethics and Conduct*. Leicester: British Psychological Society. Available from www.bps.org.uk/sites/default/files/documents/code_of_ethics_and_conduct.pdf [accessed 18 November 2014].

Broom, A. (2006) 'Ethical issues in social research', *Complementary Therapies in Medicine*, 14: 151–6.

Brown, J.E., Brown, R.F., Miller, R.M., Dunn, S.M., King, M.T., Coates, A.S., Butow, P.N. (2000) 'Coping with metastatic melanoma: the last year of life', *Psycho-oncology*, 9: 283–92.

Brown, L.F., Kroenke, K., Theobald, D.E., et al (2010) 'The association of depression and anxiety with health-related quality of life in cancer patients with depression and/or pain', *Psycho-oncology*, 19: 734–41.

Brown, M. (2010) 'Nursing care of patients undergoing allogeneic stem cell transplantation', *Nursing Standard*, 25(11): 47–56.

Brown, M. (2012) 'Understanding haemopoiesis', in M. Brown and T.J. Cutler (eds), *Haematology Nursing*. Oxford: Blackwell Publishing. pp. 3–21.

Brown, R.F., Shuk, E., Butow, P., Edgerson, S., Tattersall, M.H.N., Ostroff, J.S. (2011) 'Identifying patient information needs about cancer clinical trials using a question prompt list', *Patient Education and Counseling*, 84(1): 69–77.

Bruce, A., Schreiber, R., Petrovskaya, O. and Boston, P. (2011) 'Longing for ground in a ground(less) world: a qualitative inquiry of existential suffering', *BMC Nursing*, 10: 2.

Bruera, E. and Yennurajalingam, S. (2012) 'Palliative care in advanced cancer patients: how and when?' *The Oncologist*, 17(2): 267–73.

Bruneau, B.M.S. and Ellison, G.T.H. (2004) 'Palliative care stress in a UK community hospital', *International Journal of Palliative Nursing*, 10(6): 296–304.

Brunelli, T. (2005) 'A concept analysis: the grieving process for nurses', *Nursing Forum*, 40(4): 123–8.

Bruscia, K.E. (1987) *Improvisational Models of Music Therapy*. Springfield, IL: Charles C. Thomas.

Bruscia, K.E. (1998) *Defining Music Therapy*, 2nd edn. Gilsum, NH: Barcelona Publishers.

Brysbaert, M. and Rastle, K. (2009) *Historical and Conceptual Issues in Psychology*. Harlow: Pearson Education Ltd.

Bui, Q.U.T., Ostir, G.V., Kuo, Y.F., Freeman, J. and Goodwin, J.S. (2005) 'Relationship of depression to patient satisfaction: findings from the barriers to breast cancer study', *Breast Cancer Research and Treatment*, 89(1): 23–8.

Bunt, L. (2011) 'Music therapy: a resource for creativity, health and well-being across the lifespan', in O. Edena (ed.), *Music Creativity: Insights from Music Education Research*. Farnham, UK: Ashgate. pp. 165–81.

Bunt, L. and Hoskyns, S. (eds) (2002) *The Handbook of Music Therapy*. Hove, UK: Brunner-Routledge.

Bunt, L. and Stige, B. (2014) *Music Therapy: An Art Beyond Words*, 2nd edn. London: Routledge.

Burkman, R., Schlesselman, J.J. and Zieman, M. (2004) 'Safety concerns and health benefits associated with oral contraception', *American Journal of Obstetrics and Gynecology*, 190(4): S5–22.

Burnet, N. G., Thomas, S. J., Burton, K. E and Jefferies, S. J. (2004) 'Defining the tumour and target volumes for radiotherapy', *Cancer Imaging*, 4(2): 153–161.

Burns, D.S. (2001) 'The effect of the Bonny Method of Guided Imagery and Music on the mood and life quality of cancer patients', *Journal of Music Therapy*, 38(1): 51–65.

Burns, D.S., Azzouz, F., Sledge, R., Rutledge, C., Hicher, K., Monahan, P.O. and Cripe, L.D. (2008) 'Music imagery for adults with acute leukaemia in protective environments: a feasibility study', *Supportive Care in Cancer*, 16(5): 507–13.

Burton, J.L. (2003) 'The autopsy in modern undergraduate medical education: a qualitative study of uses and curriculum considerations', *Medical Education*, 37(12): 1073–81.

Burton, J.L. and Underwood, J. (2007) 'Clinical, educational and epidemiological value of autopsy', *Lancet*, 369: 1471–80.

Bury, M. (1982) 'Chronic illness as biographical disruption', *Sociology of Health and Illness*, 4(2): 167–82.

Bury, M. (1991) 'The sociology of chronic illness: a review of research and prospects', *Sociology of Health and Illness,* 13(4): 451–68.

Bury, M. (2001) 'Illness narratives: fact or fiction?', *Sociology of Health and Illness,* 23(3): 263–85.

Bury, M. (2010) 'Chronic illness, self-management and the rhetoric of empowerment', in G. Scambler and S. Scambler (eds), *New Directions in The Sociology of Chronic and Disabling Conditions: Assaults on the Lifeworld.* Basingstoke: Palgrave Macmillan. Chapter 8.

Bush, N. (2009) 'Post-traumatic stress disorder related to the cancer experience', *Oncology Nursing Forum,* 36(4): 395–399.

Butler, R.W. and Haser, J.K. (2006) 'Neurocognitive effects of treatment for childhood cancer', *Mental Retardation and Developmental Disabilities Research Reviews,* 12: 184–91.

Butow, P., Lobb, E.A., Barratt, A., Meiser, B. and Tucker, K.M. (2003) 'Psychological outcomes and risk perception after genetic testing and counselling in breast cancer: a systematic review', *The Medical Journal of Australia,* 178(2): 77–81.

Butow, P.N. Brown, R.F. et al. (2002) 'Oncologists reactions to cancer patients verbal Please provide all author names cues', *Psycho-oncology,* 11: 47–58.

Byrne, A., Ellershaw, J., Holcombe, C. and Salmon, P. (2002) 'Patients' experience of cancer: evidence of the role of "fighting" in collusive clinical communication', *Patient Education and Counseling,* 48(1): 15–21.

Callaghan, M. and Cooper, A. (2013) 'Alopecia' in C.H. Yarbro, D. Wujcik and B.H. Gobel (eds), *Cancer Symptom Management,* 4th edn. Burlington, VT: Jones and Bartlett Learning. pp. 495–505.

Cameron, P., Pond, G.R., Xu, R.Y., Goffin, J.R. (2013) 'A comparison of patient knowledge of clinical trials and trialist priorities', *Current Oncology,* 20: 193–205.

Cancer Research UK (2011) *People Fear Cancer More Than Other Serious Illness: Survey Commissioned by YouGov.* Available from: www.cancerresearchuk.org/about-us/cancer-news/press-release/people-fear-cancer-more-than-other-serious-illness [accessed 18 November 2014].

Cancer Research UK (2012a) *Cancer Incidence by Age.* Available from: www.cancerresearchuk.org/cancer-info/cancerstats/incidence/age (accessed 9 September 2012).

Cancer Research UK (2012b) *About Cancer.* Available from: www.cancerresearchuk.org/about-cancer/cancers-in-general/what-is-cancer/cells/how-cells-and-tissues-grow (accessed December 2012).

Cancer Research UK (2013a) *Cancer Incidence By Age – UK Statistics.* Available from: http://info.cancerresearchuk.org/cancerstats/incidence/age/ [accessed 9 December 2013].

Cancer Research UK (2013b) *Cancer Mortality by Age – UK Statistics.* Available from: www.cancer-researchuk.org/cancer-info/cancerstats/mortality/age/ [accessed 9 December 2013].

Cancer Research UK (2014a) *Cancer Incidence and Mortality in the UK in 2011: Cancer Statistics Report.* Available from: http://publications.cancerresearchuk.org/downloads/Product/CS_REPORT_TOP10INCMORT.pdf [accessed 27 July 2014].

Cancer Research UK (2014b) *Cancer Incidence in the UK in 2011.* Available from: http://publications.cancerresearchuk.org/downloads/product/CS_REPORT_INCIDENCE.pdf [accessed 27 July 2014].

Cancer Research UK (2014c) *All Cancers Combined, Cancer Statistics Key Facts, September 2014.* Available from: http://publications.cancerresearchuk.org/downloads/product/CS_KF_ALLCANCERS.pdf [accessed 27 July 2014].

Cancer Research UK (2014d) *Cancer Statistics Key Facts Skin Cancer, June 2014.* Available from: http://publications.cancerresearchuk.org/downloads/Product/CS_KF_SKIN.pdf [accessed 27 July 2014].

Cancer Research UK (2014e) *Melanoma Statistics and Outlook.* Available from: www.cancerresearchuk.org/cancer-help/type/melanoma/treatment/melanoma-statistics-and-outlook [accessed 27 July 2014].

Cancer Research UK (2014f) *Statistics and Outlook for Penile Cancer.* Available from: www.cancer-researchuk.org/cancer-help/type/penile-cancer/treatment/statistics-and-outlook-for-penile-cancer [accessed 27 July 2014].

Cancer Research UK (2014g) *Cervical Cancer Risk and Causes*. Available from: www.cancer researchuk.org/cancer-help/type/cervical-cancer/about/cervical-cancer-risks-and-causes [accessed 27 July 2014].

Cancer Research UK (2014h) *Cancer Incidence for Common Cancers*. Available from: www.can cerresearchuk.org/cancer-info/cancerstats/incidence/commoncancers/#Twenty [accessed 27 July 2014].

Cancer Research UK (2014i) *Thyroid Cancer Incidence Statistics*. Available from: www.cancerre searchuk.org/cancer-info/cancerstats/types/thyroid/incidence/#By [accessed 27 July 2014].

Cancer Research UK (2014j) *Liver Cancer September 14*. Available from: http://publications.can cerresearchuk.org/downloads/Product/CS_KF_LIVER.pdf [accessed 27 July 2014].

Cancer Research UK (2014k) *Brain, CNS and other Intracranial Tumours Incidence Statistics*. Available from: www.cancerresearchuk.org/cancer-info/cancerstats/types/brain/incidence/ [accessed 27 July 2014].

Cancer Research UK (2014l) *Brain, CNS and other Intracranial Tumours, Key Facts June 14*. Available from: http://publications.cancerresearchuk.org/downloads/Product/CS_KF_ BRAIN.pdf [accessed 27 July 2014].

Cancer Research UK (2014m) *Childhood Cancer, September 14*. Available from: http://pub lications.cancerresearchuk.org/downloads/Product/CS_KF_CHILDHOOD.pdf [accessed 27 July 2014].

Cancer Research UK (2014n) *Teenage and Young Adult Cancer, September 14*. Available from: http://publications.cancerresearchuk.org/downloads/Product/CS_KF_TYA.pdf [accessed 27 July 2014].

Cancer Research UK (2014o) *Our Policy on National Cancer Plans*. Available from: www.cancer researchuk.org/about-us/we-develop-policy/our-policy-on-nhs-cancer-services/our-policy-on-national-cancer-plans [accessed 27 July 2014].

Cancer Research UK (2014p) *The History of Cancer Surgery*. Available from: www.cancerresearchuk. org/cancer-info/cancerandresearch/all-about-cancer/what-is-cancer/treating-cancer/history-of-surgery/surgery3 [accessed 27 July 2014].

Cancer Research UK (2014q) *Cancer Survival Statistics*. Available from: www.cancerresearchuk. org/cancer-info/cancerstats/survival/ [accessed 27 July 2014].

Cancer Research UK (2014r) *Lifetime Risk of Developing Cancer*. Available from: www.cancer researchuk.org/cancer-info/cancerstats/cancerstats-explained/lifetime-risk-methodology [accessed 18 April 2014].

Cancer Research UK (2014s) *Cancer Incidence By Age*. Available from: www.cancerresearchuk. org/cancer-info/cancerstats/incidence/age/ [accessed 18 April 2014].

Cancer Research UK (2014t) *Melanoma Risks and Causes*. Available from: www.cancerre searchuk.org/cancer-help/type/melanoma/about/melanoma-risks-and-causes [accessed 18 April 2014].

Cancer Research UK (2014u) *Cervical Cancer Screening*. Available from: www.cancerresearchuk.org/ cancer-help/type/cervical-cancer/about/cervical-cancer-screening [accessed 21 April 2014].

Cancer Research UK (2014v) *About Bowel Cancer Screening*. Available from: www.cancer researchuk.org/cancer-help/type/bowel-cancer/about/screening/about-bowel-cancer-screening [accessed 21 April 2014].

Cancer Research UK (2014w) *Childhood Cancer Statistics*. Available from: www.cancerresearchuk. org/cancer-info/cancerstats/childhoodcancer/ [accessed 1 February 2014].

Cancer Research UK (2014x) *Childhood Cancer Incidence Statistics*. Available from: www.can cerresearchuk.org/cancer-info/cancerstats/childhoodcancer/incidence/#lymph (accessed 28 December 2014).

Cancer Research UK (2014y) *Long Term Side Effects of Radiotherapy*. Available from: www. cancerresearchuk.org/about-cancer/cancers-in-general/treatment/radiotherapy/follow-up/ long-term-side-effects-of-radiotherapy (accessed 10 September 2014).

Cancer Research UK, International Agency for Research on Cancer, World Health Organization (2014) *World Cancer Fact Sheet: World Cancer Burden 2012*. Available from: http://publications. cancerresearchuk.org/downloads/product/CS_REPORT_WORLD.pdf [accessed 27 July 2014].

Candy, B., Jones, L., Drake, R., Leurent, B. and King, M. (2011) 'Interventions for supporting informal caregivers of patients in the terminal phase of a disease', *Cochrane Database Syst Rev.* (6):CD007617. doi: 0.1002/14651858.CD007617.pub2.

Cannon S. (1989) 'Social research in stressful settings: difficulties for the sociologist studying the treatment of breast cancer', *Sociology of Health & Illness,* 11(1): 62–77.

Cantwell, B.M., Ramirez, A.J. (1997) 'Doctor–patient communication: a study of junior house officers', *Medical Education,* 31(1): 17–21.

Capodice, J.L. (2010) 'Acupuncture in the oncology setting: clinical trial update', *Current Treatment Options in Oncology,* 11(3–4): 87–94.

Carayol, M., Bernard, P., Boiché, J., Riou, F., Mercier, B., Cousson-Gélie, F., Romain, A.J., Delpierre, C. and Ninot, G. (2013) 'Psychological effect of exercise in women with breast cancer receiving adjuvant therapy: what is the optimal dose needed?', *Annals of Oncology,* 24(2): 291–300.

Cardy, P. (2006) *Worried Sick: The Emotional Impact of Cancer.* Macmillan Cancer Support.

Care Quality Commission (CQC) (2011) *Equality and Human Rights in the Essential Standards of Quality and Safety: Equality and Human Rights in Outcomes. Guidance for Compliance Inspectors and Registration Assessors.* London: Care Quality Commission. Available from www.cqc.org.uk/information-our-staff/equality-and-human-rights-guidance-our-inspectors.

Carel, H. (2008) *Illness: The Cry of the Flesh.* Acumen: Stocksfield.

Carers UK (2011) *Carers at a Distance: Bridging the Gap.* London: Carers UK.

Carers UK (2013a) *Older Carers in the UK.* [Online] Available from: www.carersuk.org/professionals/resources/research-library/item/491-older-.

Carers UK (2013b) *Find Support In Your Area.* Available from: www.carersuk.org/help-and-advice/finding-help-where-you-live [accessed 9 December 2013].

Carey, M., Lambert, S., Smits, R., Paul, C., Sanson-Fisher, R. and Clinton-McHarg, T. (2012) 'The unfulfilled promise: a systematic review of interventions to reduce the unmet supportive care needs of cancer patients', *Supportive Care in Cancer,* 20(2): 207–219.

Carlson, L.E., Clifford, S.K., Groff, S.L., Maciejewski, O. and Bultz, B. (2010a) 'Screening for depression in cancer care', in A.J. Mitchell and J.C. Coyne (eds), *Screening for Depression in Clinical Practice.* New York, NY: Oxford University Press, pp. 265–298.

Carlson, L.E., Groff, S.L., Maciejewski, O. and Bultz, B.D. (2010b) 'Screening for distress in lung and breast cancer outpatients: a randomized controlled trial', *Journal of Clinical Oncology,* 28(33): 4884–91.

Carlson, L.E., Speca, M., Hagen, N. and Taenzer, P. (2001) 'Computerized quality-of-life screening in a cancer pain clinic', *Journal of Palliative Care,* 17: 46–52.

Carlson, L.E., Speca, M., Patel, K.D. and Goodey, E. (2004) 'Mindfulness-based stress reduction in relation to quality of life, mood, symptoms of stress and levels of cortisol, dehydroepiandrosteronesulfate (DHEAS) and melatonin in breast and prostate cancer outpatients', *Psychoneuroendocrinology,* 29: 448–74.

Carlson, L.E., Waller, A. and Mitchell, A.J. (2012a) 'Screening for distress and unmet needs in patients with cancer: review and recommendations', *J Clin Oncol.,* 30(11): 1160–1177.

Carlson, L.E., Waller, A., Groff, S.L., Zhong, L. and Bultz, B.D (2012b) 'Online screening for distress, the 6th vital sign, in newly diagnosed oncology outpatients: randomised controlled trial of computerised vs personalised triage', *Br J Cancer,* 107(4): 617–625.

Carlson, R.W., Moench, S., Hurria, A., et al. (2008) 'NCCN task force report: Breast cancer in the older woman', *Journal National Comprehensive Cancer Network,* 6(sup.p 4): S1–S25.

Carney, C.P. and Jones, L.E. (2006) 'The influence of type and severity of mental illness on receipt of screening mammography', *Journal of General and Internal Medicine,* 21(10): 1097–104.

Carr, A. (2012) *Family Therapy: Concepts, Process and Practice.* London: Wiley.

Carroll, K.M., Libby, B., Sheehan, J. and Hyland, N. (2001) 'Motivational interviewing to enhance treatment initiation in substance abusers: an effectiveness study', *American Journal of Addictions,* 10(4): 335–39. doi:10.1111/j.1521-0391.2001.tb00523.x.

Carter, G., Lewin, T., Rashid, G., Adams, C. and Clover, K. (2008) 'Computerised assessment of quality of life in oncology patients and carers', *Psycho-oncology*, 17(1): 26–33.

Carter, P. and Chang, B.L. (2000) 'Sleep and depression in cancer caregivers', *Cancer Nursing*, 23(6): 410–14.

Cartwright-Alcarese, F. (1995) 'Addressing sexual dysfunction following radiation therapy for a gynecologic malignancy', *Oncology Nursing Forum*, 22: 1227–32.

Carver, C.S., Scheier, M.F. and Weintraub, J.K. (1989) 'Assessing coping strategies: a theoretically based approach', *Journal of Personality and Social Psychology*, 56: 267–83.

Cassidy, T. (2013) 'Benefit finding through caring: the cancer caregiver experience', *Psychology and Health*, 28(3): 250–66.

Cassileth, B.R, Vickers, A.J. and Magill, L.A. (2003) 'Music therapy for mood disturbance during hospitalization for autologous stem cell transplantation: a randomized controlled trial', *Cancer*, 98(12): 2723–9.

Cataldo, J.K., Jahan, T.M. and Pongquan, V.L. (2012) 'Lung cancer stigma, depression, and quality of life among ever and never smokers', *European Journal of Oncology Nursing*, 16(3): 264–9.

Cavalli-Bjorkman, N., Qvortrup, C., Sebjørnsen, S., Pfeiffer, P., Wentzel-Larsen, T., et al. (2012) 'Lower treatment intensity and poorer survival in metastatic colorectal cancer patients who live alone', *British Journal of Cancer*, 107(1): 89–94.

Cella, D.F., Tulsky, D.S., Gray, G., Sarafian, B., Linn, E., Bonomi, A., Silberman, M., Yellen, S.B., Winicour, P. and Brannon, J. (1993) 'The Functional Assessment of Cancer Therapy scale: development and validation of the general measure', *Journal of Clinical Oncology*, 11: 570–9.

Center to Advance Palliative Care (2011) *Growth of Palliative Care in US Hospitals 2012 Snapshot*. Available from: http://reportcard.capc.org/pdf/capc-growth-analysis-snapshot-2011.pdf [accessed 23 February 2015].

Centrewatch (2014) *Overview of Clinical Trials*. Available from: www.centerwatch.com/clinical-trials/overview.aspx [accessed 26 June 2014].

Centre for Policy on Ageing (2010) *CPA Briefings: A Review of Age Discrimination in Primary and Community Health Care, Mental Health Care and Social Services in the United Kingdom* [Online]. Available from: www.cpa.org.uk/policy/briefings/discrimination_in_health_and_social_care.pdf [Accessed 9 December 2013] .

Cesari, M., Colloca, G., Cerullo, F., Ferrini, A. and Testa, A.C. (2011) 'Onco-geriatric approach for the management of older patients with cancer', *Journal American Medical Directors Association*, 12(2): 153–9.

Chadwick, A., Street, C., McAndrew, S. and Deacon, M. (2012) Minding our own bodies: reviewing the literature regarding the perceptions of service users diagnosed with serious mental illness on barriers to accessing physical health care. *International Journal of Mental Health Nursing*, 21, 211–19.

Chamberlain, J. and Moss, S. (eds) (1996) *Evaluation of Cancer Screening*. London: Springer.

Chang, W.H. (2006) Cancers in infancy: percent distribution and incidence rates', *Acta Paediatrica Taiwanica*, 47 (6) :273–277.

Chaplin, J. and Mitchell, D. (2005) 'Spirituality in palliative care', in J. Lugton and R. McIntyre (eds), *Palliative Care: The Nursing Role*. London: Elservier, Churchill Livingstone. pp. 169–97.

Chapman, R.M. (1982) 'Effect of cytotoxic therapy on sexuality and gonadal function', *Seminars in Oncology*, 9: 84–94.

Charles, C. and DeMaio, S. (1993) 'Lay participation in health care decision making: a conceptual framework', *Journal of Health Politics, Policy and Law*, 18(4): 881–904.

Charles, C., Gafni, A. and Whelan, T. (1997) Shared decision-making in the medical encounter: what does it mean? (or it takes at least two to tango)', *Social Science & Medicine*, 44(5): 681–692.

Charlton, C.R., Dearing, K.S., Berry, J.A. and Johnson, M.J. (2008) 'Nurse practitioners' communication styles and their impact on patient outcomes: an integrated literature review', *Journal of the American Academy of Nurse Practitioners*, 20(7): 382–8.

Charman, C. and Hulbert-Williams, N.J. (2013) 'Which therapeutic techniques are used by psychologists working in cancer care: findings from a pilot study', *Psycho-oncology*, 22(111): 23.

Charmaz, K. (1983) 'Loss of self: a fundamental form of suffering in the chronically ill', *Sociology of Health & Illness,* 5(2): 168–195.

Charmaz, K. (1994) 'Identity dilemmas of chronically ill men', *Sociological Quarterly,* 35(2): 269–88.

Charmaz, K. (1995) 'The body, identity, and self: adapting to impairment', *Sociological Quarterly,* 36(4): 657–80.

Charmaz, K. (2002) 'Stories and silences: disclosures and self in chronic illness', *Qualitative Inquiry,* 893: 302–328.

Chattoo, S., Crawshaw, M. and Atkin, K. (2010) *The Experience of Cancer-Related Fertility Impairment Among People of South Asian and White Origin.* Final Report to Cancer Research UK (C8351/A9005) (unpublished). [Summaries associated with this project can be found at: www.york.ac.uk/healthsciences/research-information/conference-cancer-survivorship/].

Chaturvedi, A.K., Engels, E.A., Gilbert, E.S., Chen, B.E., Storm, H., Lynch, C.F., Hall, P., Langmark, F., Pukkala, E., Kaijser, M. Andersson, M., Fosså, S.D., Joensuu, H., Boice, J.D., Kleinerman, R.A. and Travis, L.B. (2007) 'Second cancers among 104,760 survivors of cervical cancer: evaluation of long-term risk', *Journal of the National Cancer Institute,* 99: 1634–43. doi:10.1093/jnci/djm201.

Chau, I., Norman, A.R., Cunngingham, D. et al. (2005) 'A randomised comparison between 6 months of bolus fluorouracil/leucovorin and 12 weeks of protracted venous infusion fluorouracil as adjuvant treatment in colorectal cancer', *Annals of Oncology,* 16: 549–57.

Chen, C.-H., Shun, C.-T., Huang, K.-H., Huang, C.-Y., Tsai, Y.-C., Yu, H.-J. and Pu, Y.-S. (2007) 'Stopping smoking might reduce tumour recurrence in nonmuscle-invasive bladder cancer', *British Journal of Urology International,* 100(2): 281–6. doi:10.1111/j.1464-410X.2007.06873.x.

Cheng, C., Hui, W. and Lam, S. (2004) 'Psychosocial factors and perceived severity of functional dyspeptic symptoms: a psychosocial interactionist model', *Psychosomatic Medicine,* 66: 85–91.

Chewning, B., Bylund, C.L., Shah, B., Arora, N.K., Gueguen, J.A. and Makoul, G. (2012) 'Patient preferences for shared decisions: a systematic review', *Patient Education and Counseling,* 86(1): 9–18. doi: 10.1016/j.pec.2011.02.004. Epub 2011 Apr 6.

Chiang, V.C, Keatinge, D. and Williams, A.K. (2001) 'Challenges of recruiting a vulnerable population in a grounded theory study', *Nursing and Health Sciences,* 3: 205–11.

Childs, P.J. and Bidmead, M (2012) 'Principles and practice of radiation treatment planning', in P. Symonds, C. Deehan, J.A. Mills and C. Meredith (eds), *Walter and Miller's Textbook of Radiotherapy,* 7th edn. London: Elsevier Churchill Livingstone. pp. 159–88.

Chinot, O.L., de La Motte Rouge. T., Moore, N. et al. (2011) 'AVAglio: phase 3 trial of bevacizumab plus temozolomide and radiotherapy in newly diagnosed glioblastoma multiforme', *Adv Ther.* 28(4): 334–40.

Cho, J., Smith, K., Choi, E.K., Kim, I.R., Chang, Y.J, Park, H.Y., Guallar, E. and Sim, Y. (2013) 'Public attitudes toward cancer and cancer patients: a national survey in Korea', *Psycho-oncology,* 22: 605–13.

Chochinov, H.M., Hack, T., Hassard, T., Kristjanson, L.J., McClement, S. and Harlos, M. (2005) 'Dignity therapy: a novel psychotherapeutic intervention for patients near the end of life', *Journal of Clinical Oncology,* 23(24): 5520–5.

Chochinov, H.M., Kristjanson, L. J., Breitbart, W., Mcclement, S., Hack, T. F., Hassard, T. and Harlos, M. (2011) 'Effect of dignity therapy on distress and end-of-life experience in terminally ill patients: a randomised controlled trial', *Lancet Oncol,* 12: 753–62.

Choi, W.S., Harris, K.J., Okuyemi, K. and Ahluwalia, J.S. (2003) 'Predictors of smoking initiation among college-bound high school students', *Annals of Behavioral Medicine,* 26(1): 69–74.

Chou, R., Croswell, J.M., Dana, T., Bougatsos, C., Blazina, I., Fu, R., Gleitsmann, K., Koenig, H.C., Lam, C., Maltz, A., Rugge, B. and Lin, K. (2011) 'Screening for prostate cancer: a review of the evidence for the US Preventative Services Task Force', *Annals of Internal Medicine,* 155(11): 762–71.

Chouliara, Z., Kearney, N., Stott, D., Milassiotis, A.and Miller, M. (2004a) 'Perceptions of older people with cancer of information, decision making and treatment: a systematic review of selected literature', *Annals of Oncology,* 15(11): 1596–602.

Chouliara, Z., Kearney, N., Worth, A. and Stott, D. (2004b) 'Challenges in conducting research with hospitalized older people with cancer: drawing from the experience of an ongoing interview-based project', *European Journal of Cancer Care,* 13: 409–15.

Chow, A.Y. (2010) 'Cell cycle control by oncogenes and tumour suppressors: driving the transformation of normal cells into cancerous cells', *Nature Education,* 3(9): 7.

Chow, E., Tsao, M.N. and Harth, T. (2004) 'Does psychosocial intervention improve survival in cancer? A meta-analysis', *Palliative Medicine,* 18(1): 25–31.

Christakis, N.A. and Fowler, J.H. (2007) 'The spread of obesity in a large social network over 32 years', *New England Journal of Medicine,* 357(4): 370–9.

Christakis, N.A. and Lamont, E.B. (2000) 'Extent and determinants of error in doctors' prognoses in terminally ill patients: prospective cohort study', *British Medical Journal,* 320: 469.

Chung-Hon, P. and Evans, W. (2006) 'Treatment of acute lymphoblastic leukaemia', *The New England Journal of Medicine,* 354: 166–178.

Ciarrochi, J., Fisher, D. and Lane, L. (2011) 'The link between value motives, value success, and well-being among people diagnosed with cancer', *Psycho-oncology,* 20(11): 1184–92.

Clark, D. (2007) 'From margins to centre: a review of the history of palliative care in cancer', *Lancet Oncology,* 8: 430–8.

Clark, M., Isaacks-Downton, G., Wells, N., Redlin-Frazier, S., Eck, C., Hepworth, J.T., et al. (2006) 'Use of preferred music to reduce emotional distress and symptom activity during radiation therapy', *Journal of Music Therapy,* 43(3): 247–65.

Clarke-Steffen, L. (1997) 'Reconstructing reality: family strategies for managing childhood cancer', *Journal of Pediatric Nursing,* 12(5): 278–287.

Clarke, S., Thomas, P. and James, K. (2013) 'Cognitive analytic therapy for personality disorder: randomised controlled trial', *British Journal of Psychiatry,* 202: 129–34.

Clavel, J., Goubin, A., Auclercm, M.F., Auvrignon, A., Waterkeyn, C., Patte, C., Baruchel, A., Leverger, G., Nelken, B., Philippe, N., Sommelet, D., Vilmer, E., Bellec, S., Perrillat-Menegaux, F. and Hémon, D. (2004) 'Incidence of childhood leukaemia and non-Hodgkin's lymphoma in France: National Registry of Childhood Leukaemia and Lymphoma, 1990–1999', *European Journal of Cancer Prevention,* 13 (2): 97–103.

Claxton-Oldfield, S. and Claxton-Oldfield, J. (2008) 'Keeping hospice palliative care volunteers on board: dealing with issues of volunteer attrition, stress, and retention', *Indian Journal of Palliative Care,* 14(1): 30–7.

Clift, S., Camic, P.M., Chapman, B., Clayton, G., Daykin, N., Eades, G., Parkinson, C., Secker, J., Stickley, T. and White, M. (2009) 'The state of arts and health in England', *Arts and Health: An International Journal for Research, Policy and Practice,* 1(1): 6–35.

Coates, A., Abraham, S. and Kaye, S.B. (1983) 'On the receiving end: patient perception of the side-effects of cancer', *European Journal of Cancer and Clinical Oncology,* 19(2): 203–8.

Cobb, M., Dowrick, C. and Lloyd-Williams, M. (2012a) 'Understanding spirituality: a synoptic view', *British Medical Journal Supportive & Palliative Care,* 2: 339–343.

Cobb, M., Puchalski, C. and Rumbold, B. (eds) (2012b) *Oxford Textbook of Spirituality in Healthcare.* Oxford: Oxford University Press.

Cocksedge, S. and May C. (2005) 'The Listening Loop: a model of choice about cues within primary care consultations', *Medical Education,* 39: 999–1005.

Coebergh, J.W.W., Janssen-Heijnen M.L.G. and Razenberg, P.P.A. (1998) 'Prevalence of co-morbidity in newly diagnosed patients with cancer: a population-based study', *Critical Reviews in Oncology/Hematology,* 27(2): 97–100.

Cogliano, V.J., Baan, R. and Straif, K., et al. (2011) 'Preventable exposures associated with human cancers', *Journal of the National Cancer Institute,* 103(24): 1827–39. doi:10.1093/jnci/djr483.

Cohen, D.J. and Crabtree, B.F. (2008) 'Evaluative criteria for qualitative research in health care: controversies and recommendations', *Annals of Family Medicine,* 6(4): 331–9.

Coiffier, B., Lepage, E., Briere, P.D. et al. (2002) 'CHOP chemotherapy plus rituximab compared with CHOP alone in elderly patients with diffuse large B-cell lymphoma', *The New England Journal of Medicine,* 346: 235–42.

Cole, M.P., Jones, C.T. and Todd, I.D. (1971) 'A new anti-oestrogenic agent in late breast cancer. An early clinical appraisal of ICI46474', *British Journal of Cancer,* 25(2): 270–5.

Coleman, M.P., Forman, D., Bryant, H., Butler, J., Rachet, B., Maringe, C., Nur, U., Tracey, E., Coory, M., Hatcher, J., McGahan, C.E., Turner, D., Marrett, L., Gjerstorff, M.L., Johannesen, T.B., Adolfsson, J., Lambe, M., Lawrence, G., Meechan, D., Morris, E.J., Middleton, R., Steward, J., Richards, M.A. (2011) 'Cancer survival in Australia, Canada, Denmark, Norway, Sweden, and the UK (1995–2007 (the International Cancer Benchmarking Partnership): and analysis of population based cancer registry data', *Lancet,* 377(9760): 127–138. Available from: www.thelancet.com/journals/lancet/article/PIIS0140-6736%2810%2962231-3/abstract [accessed 17 November 2014].

Collins, A.L., Love, A.W., Bloch, S., Street, A.F., Duchesne, G.M, Dunai, J. and Couper, J.W. (2011) 'Cognitive existential couple therapy for newly diagnosed prostate cancer patients and their partners: a descriptive pilot study', *Psycho-oncology,* 22(2): 465–9.

Collins, R.L., Taylor, S.E. and Skokan, L.A. (1990) 'A better world or a shattered vision? Changes in perspectives following victimization', *Social Cognition,* 8: 263–85.

Colon Cancer Laparoscopic or Open Resection Study Group, Buunen, M., Veldkamp, R., Hop, W.C.J., Kuhry, E., Jeekel, J., Haglind, E., Påhlman, L., Cuesta, M.A., Msika, S., Morino, M., Lacy, A. and Bonjer, H.J. (2009) 'Survival after laparoscopic surgery versus open surgery for colon cancer: long-term outcome of a randomised clinical trial', *Lancet Oncology.* 10: 44–52. doi:10.1016/S1470-2045(08)70310-3.

Colyer, H. (2003) 'The context of radiotherapy care', in S. Faithfull and M. Wells (eds), *Supportive Care in Radiotherapy.* London: Churchill Livingstone. pp. 1–16.

Committee on Medical Aspects of Radiation in the Environment (COMARE) (2005) *The Incidence of Childhood Cancer Around Nuclear Installations in Great Britain.* London: Department of Health. Available from: www.gov.uk/government/publications/comare-10th-report (accessed 28 December, 2014).

Compass, B.E., Stoll, M.F., Thomsen, A.H., Oppedisan, G., Epping-Jordan, J.E. and Krag, D.N. (1999) 'Adjustment to breast cancer: age-related differences in coping and emotional distress', *Breast Cancer Research & Treatment,* 54(3): 195–203.

Connell, C. (1998) *Something Understood-Art Therapy in Cancer Care.* Wrexham, UK: Wrexham Publications. pp. 8–9.

Conner, A., Allport, S., Dixon, J., Somerville, A.M. (2008) 'Patient perspective: what do palliative care patients think about their care', *International Journal Palliative Nursing,* 14(11): 546–52.

Conner, A. and Muir, M. (2007) 'Managing symptoms, what can nurses do? A principle based approach', in S. Kinghorn and S. Gaines (eds), *Palliative Nursing: Improving End of Life Care.* 2nd rev. edn. Oxford, UK: Bailliere Tindall, UK. Chapter 2.

Connolly, M., Perryman, J., McKenna, Y., Orford, J., Thomson, L., Shuttleworth, J., Cocksedge, S. (2010) 'SAGE & THYME: A model for training health and social care professionals in patient-focussed support', *Patient Education and Counseling,* 79: 87–93.

Conway, J. and Johnson, J. (2012) 'Radiation treatment planning: immobilization, localization and verification techniques', in P. Symonds, C. Deehan, J.A. Mills and C. Meredith (eds), *Walter and Miller's Textbook of Radiotherapy,* 7th edn. London: Elsevier Churchill Livingstone. pp. 145–58.

Cooke, L. (1997) 'Cancer and learning disability', *Journal of Intellectual Disability Research,* 41 (4): 312–316.

Cooke, L., Gemmill, G., Kravits, K. and Grant, M. (2009) 'Psychological issues of stem cell transplant', *Seminars in Oncology Nursing,* 25(2): 139–50.

Cooley, C.H. (1902) *Human Nature and the Social Order.* New York, NY: Scribner.

Cooper, M.L., Agocha, V.B. and Sheldon, M.S. (2000) 'A motivational perspective on risky behaviors: the role of personality and affect regulatory processes', *Journal of Personality,* 68(6): 1059–88. doi:10.1111/1467-6494.00126.

Coote, J. (1998) 'Getting Started-Introducing the art therapy service and the individual's first experiences', in M. Pratt and J.M. Wood (eds), *Art Therapy in Palliative Care: The Creative Response.* London: Routledge. pp. 53–64.

Copelan, E.A. (2006) 'Hematopoietic stem cell transplantation', *New England Journal of Medicine,* 354: 1813–26.

Cormac, I., Ferriter, M., Benning, R. and Saul, C. (2005) 'Physical health and health risk factors in a population of long-stay psychiatric patients', *Psychiatric Bulletin,* 29(1): 18–20.

Corner, J. (2008) 'Addressing the needs of cancer survivors: issues and challenges. Expert Review', *Pharmacoeconomics Outcomes Research*, 8(5): 443–51.

Corner, J., Wright, D., Hopkinson, J., Gunaratnam, Y., McDonald, J.W. and Foster, C. (2007) 'The research priorities of patients attending UK cancer treatment centres: findings from a modified nominal group study', *British Journal of Cancer,* 96(6): 875–81.

Corner, J., Yardley, J., Maher, E.J., Roffe, L., Young, T., Maslin-Prothero, S., Gwilliam, C., Haviland, J. and Lewith, G. (2009) 'Patterns of complementary and alternative medicine use among patients undergoing cancer treatment', *European Journal of Cancer Care,* 18: 271–279.

Corrao, G., Bagnardi, V., Zambon, A. and La Vecchia, C. (2004) 'A meta-analysis of alcohol consumption and the risk of 15 diseases', *Preventive Medicine*, 38(5): 613–9.

Costa, P.T., Jr, and McCrae, R.R. (1988) 'Recalled parent–child relations and adult personality', *Journal of Personality and Social Psychology,* 54(5): 853–63.

Coulter, A. (1997) 'Partnerships with patients: the pros and cons of shared clinical decision making', *Journal of Health Services Research and Policy,* 2: 112–21.

Coulter, A. and Ellins, J. (2006) *Patient-focused Interventions: A Review of the Evidence*. London: Picker Institute Europe, The Health Foundation.

Coupland, C.A., Chilvers, C.E. and Davey, G. (1999) 'Risk factors for testicular germ cell tumours by histological tumour type. United Kingdom Testicular Cancer Study Group', *British Journal of Cancer,* 80: 1859–63.

Coupland, V.H., Okello, C., Davies, E.A., Bray, F., Moller, H. (2010) 'The future burden of cancer in London compared with England', *Journal of Public Health,* 32(1): 83–9.

Couto, E., Boffetta, P., Lagiou, P. and Fervari, P. (2010) 'Mediterranean dietary patter and cancer risk in the EPIC cohort', *Journal of Cancer,* 104: 1493–1499.

Cox, A., Jenkins, V., Catt, S., Langridge, C., Fallowfield, L. (2006) 'Information needs and experiences: an audit of UK cancer patients', *European Journal Oncology Nursing,* 10(4): 263–72.

Cox, J., Holden, J. and Sagovsky, R. (1987) 'Detection of postnatal depression: development of 10-item Edinburgh Postnatal Depression Scale', *British Journal of Psychiatry,* 150: 782–6.

Cox, J.D., Stetz, J and Pajak, T.F. (1995) 'Toxicity Criteria of the Radiation Therapy Oncology Group (RTOG) and the European Organisation for Research and Treatment of Cancer (EORTC)', *International Journal of Radiation Oncology Biology Physics,* 31(5): 1341–6.

Craig, P., Dieppe, P., Macintyre, S., Michie, S., Nazareth, I. and Petticrew, M. (2008) 'Developing and evaluating complex interventions: the new Medical Research Council guidance', *BMJ,* 337.

Crosier, A. (2005) *Smoking and Health Inequalities*. London: ASH.

Culley, L., Hudson, N. and van Rooij, F. (eds) (2009) *Marginalized Reproduction: Ethnicity, Infertility and Reproductive Technologies*. London: Earthscan Books. Available from: www. earthscan.co.uk/Portals/0/pdfs/Marginalized_Reproduction_II.pdf.

Cutler, T. (2012) 'Haemopoietic stem cell transplant', in M. Brown and T.J. Cutler (eds), *Haematology Nursing*. Chichester: Wiley-Blackwell. pp. 287–299.

Dalgleish, A., Richards, M. and Sikora, K. (2004) 'Cancer 2025: prevention', *Expert Review of Anticancer Therapy,* 4(3s1): S19–23.

Dallos, R. and Draper, R. (2010) *An Introduction to Family Therapy: Systemic Theory and Practice*. London: Open University Press.

Dalton, K.A and Gosselin, T.K (2013) 'Xerostomia', in C.H. Yarbro, D. Wujcik and B.H. Gobel (eds), *Cancer Symptom Management*, 4th edn. Burlington, VT: Jones and Bartlett Learning. pp. 421–36.

Dannie, E. (2006) 'Fertility issues', in M. Grundy (ed.), *Nursing in Haematological Oncology*, 2nd edn. Edinburgh: Ballière Tindall. pp. 405–423.

Davey, M., Tubbs, C., Kissil, K. and Nino, A. (2011) '"We are survivors too": African–American youths' experiences of coping with parental breast cancer', *Psycho-oncology,* 20: 77–87.

David, C.L., Williamson, K. and Owen Tilsley, D.W. (2012) 'A small scale qualitative focus group to investigate the psychosocial support needs of teenage young adult cancer patients undergoing radiotherapy in Wales', *European Journal on Oncology Nursing,* 16: 375–9.

Davies, N.J. (2009) 'Cancer survivorship: living with or beyond cancer', *Cancer Nursing Practice,* 8(7): 29–34.

Davis, T.C., Williams, M.V., Marin, E., et al. (2002) 'Health literacy and cancer communication', *Ca: a Cancer Journal for Clinicians,* 52(3): 134–49.

Daykin, N. (2007) 'Context, culture and risk: towards an understanding of the impact of music in health care settings', in J. Edwards (ed.), *Music: Promoting Health and Creating Community in Healthcare Contexts.* Newcastle: Cambridge Scholars Publishing. pp. 83–104.

Daykin, N., Bunt, L. and McClean, S. (2006) 'Music and healing in cancer care: a survey of supportive care providers', *The Arts in Psychotherapy,* 33(5): 402–13.

Daykin, N., McClean, S. and Bunt, L. (2007a) 'Creativity, identity and healing: participants' accounts of music therapy in cancer care', *Health: An Interdisciplinary Journal for the Social Study of Health, Illness and Medicine,* 11(3): 349–70.

Daykin, N., Evans, D., Petsoulas, C. and Sayers, A. (2007b) 'Evaluating the impact of patient and public involvement initiatives on UK health services: a systematic review of the literature'. *Evidence and Policy: A Journal of Research Debate and Practice,* 3(1): 47–65.

De Hert, M., Correll, C.U., Bobes, J., Cetkovich-Bakmas, D.C., Asai, I., Detraux, J., Gautam, S., Möller, H-J.,Ndetei, D.M., Newcomer, J.W., Uwakwe, R. and Leucht, S. (2011) 'Physical illness in patients with severe mental disorders: prevalence, impact of medications and disparities in health care', *World Psychiatry,* 10: 52–77.

Del Piccolo L., Goss C. and Bergvik, S. (2006) 'Consensus finding on the appropriateness of provider responses to patient cues and concerns', *Patient Education and Counselling,* 60: 313–325.

De Martel, C., Ferlay J, Franceschi S, et al. (2012) 'Global burden of cancers attributable to infections in 2008: a review and synthetic analysis', *Lancet Oncology,* 13(6): 607–15. doi:10.1016/S1470-2045(12)70137-7.

De Rosa, A., Gomez, D., Hossaini, S., Duke, K., Fenwick, S.W., Brooks, A., Poston, G.J., Malik, H.Z. and Cameron, I.C. (2013) 'Stage IV colorectal cancer: outcomes following the liver-first approach', *Journal of Surgical Oncology,* 108: 444–9. doi:10.1002/jso.23429.

De Shazer, S. (1985) *Keys to Solution in Brief Therapy.* New York, NY: WW Norton & Co.

De Shazer, S. and Berg, I. K. (1997) '"What works?" Remarks on research aspects of solution-focused brief therapy', *Journal of Family Therapy,* 19(2): 121–4. doi:10.1111/1467-6427.00043.

de Valois, B., Young, T., Robinson, N., McCourt, C. and Maher, E. (2010) 'Using traditional acupuncture for breast cancer-related hot flashes and night sweats', *Journal of Alternative and Complementary Medicine,* 16 (10): 1047–1057.

De Valois, B.A., Young T.E. and Melsome, E. (2012) 'Assessing the feasibility of using acupuncture and moxibustion to improve quality of life for cancer survivors with upper body lymphoedema', *European Journal of Oncology Nursing,* 16(3): 301–9.

de Visser, R.O. and Smith, J.A. (2007) 'Alcohol consumption and masculine identity among young men', *Psychology & Health,* 22(5): 595–614.

Deacon, M. (2013a) 'Oncology in mental health practice', in E. Collins, M. Drake and M. Deacon (eds), *The Physical Care of People with Mental Health Problems. A Guide for Best Practice.* London: Sage Publications. pp. 81–95.

Deacon, M. (2013b) 'Legal and ethical issues', in E. Collins, M. Drake and and M. Deacon (eds), *The Physical Care of People with Mental Health Problems. A Guide for Best Practice.* London: Sage Publications. pp. 188–99.

Deadman, J.M., Leinster, S.J., Owens RG., Dewey ME. and Slade PD. (2001) 'Taking responsibility for cancer treatment', *Social Science & Medicine,* 53: 669–77.

Dearden, C. and Becker, S. (2004) *Young Carers in the UK: the 2004 Report.* London: The Children's Society.

Decker, C. (2006a) 'Social support of adolescent cancer survivors: a review of the literature', *Psycho-oncology,* 16: 1–11.

Decker, C.L. (2006b) 'Coping in adolescents with cancer', *Journal of Psychosocial Oncology,* 24(4): 123–40.

Dein, S. (2005) 'Attitudes towards cancer among elderly Bangladeshis in London: a qualitative study', *European Journal of Cancer Care,* 14: 149–50.

Del Piccolo, L., Goss, C. and Bergvik, S. (2006) 'Consensus finding on the appropriateness of provider responses to patient cues and concerns', *Patient Education and Counseling,* 60: 313–25.

DeMarinis, V., Barsky, A J., Antin, J.H. and Chang, G. (2009) 'Health psychology and distress after haematopoietic stem cell transplantation', *European Journal of Cancer Care*, 18: 57–63.

Demark-Wahnefried, W., Rimer, B.K. and Winer, E.P.(1997) 'Weight gain in women diagnosed with breast cancer', *Journal of the American Dietetic Association*, 97(5): 519–26.

Dementia UK (2013) *About Dementia.* Available from: www.dementiauk.org/information-support/about-dementia/#1 [accessed 9 December 2013].

Demetri, G., Dvan Oosterom, A.T., Garrett, C.R. et al. (2006) 'Efficacy and safety of sunitinib in patients with advanced gastrointestinal stromal tumour after failure of imatinib: a randomised controlled trial', *Lancet*, 368(9544): 1329–38.

DeMeyer, E.S. (2009) 'Emerging immunology of stem cell transplantation', *Seminars in Oncology Nursing*, 25(2): 100–4.

Demicco, E.G. (2013) 'Sarcoma diagnosis in the age of molecular pathology', *Advances in Anatomic Pathology*, 20(4): 264–74.

Denters, M.J., Deutekom, M., Essink-Bot, M.L., et al. (2013) 'FITfalse-positives in colorectal cancer screening experience psychological distress up to 6 weeks after colonoscopy', *Supportive Care in Cancer*, 21(10): 2809–15. doi:10.1007/s00520-013-1867-7.

Deorah, S., Lynch, C., Sibenaller, Z. and Ryken, T. (2006) 'Trends in brain cancer incidence and survival in the United States: Surveillance, Epidemiology, and End Results Program 1973 to 2001', *Neurosurgical Focus*, 20(4): E1.

Department for Constitutional Affairs (2005) *Mental Capacity Act 2005* (Chapter 9) London: The Stationery Office.

Department for Transport (2011) *National Travel Survey 2010.* Available from: www.gov.uk/government/publications/national-travel-survey-2010 [accessed 9 December 2013].

Department of Health (1992) *The Health of the Nation.* London: Department of Health.

Department of Health (1995) *A Policy Framework for Commissioning Cancer Services: A Report by the Expert Advisory Group on Cancer to the Chief Medical Officers of England and Wales.* London: Department of Health.

Department of Health (1999) *Saving Lives: Our Healthier Nation.* London: Department of Health.

Department of Health (2000) *The NHS Cancer Plan: a Plan for Investment, a Plan for Reform.* London: Department of Health. Available from: www.dh.gov.uk/cancer [accessed].

Department of Health (2001a) *Manual of Cancer Services Standards.* London: Department of Health.

Department of Health (2001b) *National Service Framework: Older People.* Available from: https://www.gov.uk/government/publications/quality-standards-for-care-services-for-older-people [accessed 9 December 2013].

Department of Health (2001c) *Valuing People: A New Strategy For Learning Disability For The 21st Century.* London: Department of Health.

Department of Health (2003) *Personality Disorder: No Longer A Diagnosis Of Exclusion. Policy Implementation Guidance for the Development of Services for People with Personality Disorder.* Leeds: Department of Health.

Department of Health (2004a) *National Service Framework for Children, Young People and Maternity Services.* London: Department of Health.

Department of Health (2004b) *The NHS Cancer Plan and the New NHS.* London: Department of Health.

Department of Health (2005a) Mental Capacity Act 2005.

Department of Health (2005b) *Research Governance Framework for Health And Social Care.* Available from: http://webarchive.nationalarchives.gov.uk/20130107105354/www.dh.gov.uk/prod_consum_dh/groups/dh_digitalassets/@dh/@en/documents/digitalasset/dh_4122427.pdf [accessed 17 November 2014].

Department of Health (2006) *From Values to Action: The Chief Nursing Officer's Review of Mental Health Nursing.* London: Department of Health.

Department of Health (2007a) *Cancer Reform Strategy.* London: Department of Health.

Department of Health (2007b) Mental Health Act 2007.

Department of Health (2007c) *Getting It Right for People with Cancer. Clinical Case for Change.* London: Department of Health.

Department of Health (2008a) *High Quality Care for all (Darzi Report).* London: Department of Health.

Department of Health (2008b) *Refocusing the Care Programme Approach. Policy and Positive Practice Guidance.* London: Department of Health.

Department of Health (2008c) *End of Life Care Strategy: Promoting High Quality Care for all Adults at the End of Life.* London: Department of Health.

Department of Health (2008d) *NHS Permission for Research and Development Involving NHS Patients,* 2nd edn. Available from: www.dh.gov.uk/prod_consum_dh/groups/dh_digital assets/@dh/@en/documents/digitalasset/dh_091186.pdf [accessed 13 April 2012].

Department of Health (2008e) *National Manual of Cancer Services.* London: Department of Health.

Department of Health (2009) *Healthier Lives, Brighter Futures: The Strategy for Children and Young People's Health.* London: Department for Children, Schools and Families.

Department of Health (2009a) *National Chemotherapy Advisory Board Report. Ensuring Quality and Safety of Chemotherapy Services.* London: HMSO.

Department of Health (2009b) *Improving the Health and Wellbeing of People with Learning Disabilities.* London: Department of Health.

Department of Health (2010a) *Liberating the NHS: An Information Revolution.* London: Department of Health.

Department of Health (2010b) *National Cancer Survivorship Initiative Vision.* Available from: www. ncsi.org.uk/wp-content/uploads/NCSI-Vision-Document.pdf [accessed 18 November 2014].

Department of Health (2010c) *Reducing Cancer Inequality: Evidence, Progress and Making It Happen.* London: Department of Health. Available from: www.dh.gov.uk/prod_consum_dh/groups/ dh_digitalassets/@dh/@en/@ps/documents/digitalasset/dh_114354.pdf.

Department of Health (2010d) *The NHS Constitution: The NHS Belongs To Us All.* Available from: www. dh.gov.uk/en/Publicationsandstatistics/Publications/PublicationsPolicyAndGuidance/ DH_113613.

Department of Health (2011a) *Improving Outcomes: A Strategy for Cancer.* www.gov.uk/government/uploads/system/uploads/attachment_data/file/213785/dh_123394.pdf [accessed 21 April 2014].

Department of Health (2011b) *No Health without Mental Health: A Cross-Government Mental Health Outcomes Strategy for People of All Ages.* London: Department of Health.

Department of Health (2011c) *Manual of National Cancer Standards.* London: HMSO.

Department of Health (2011d) *The NHS Outcomes Framework 2012–13.* Available from: www. dh.gov.uk/en/Publicationsandstatistics/Publications/PublicationsPolicyAndGuidance/ DH_131700 [accessed 18 November 2014].

Department of Health (2012a) *Cancer Patient Experience Survey 2011/12.* Available from: www.wp.dh.gov.uk/publications/files/2012/08/Cancer-Patient-Experience-Survey-National-Report-2011-12.pdf.

Department of Health (2012b) 'Employers urged to take 3 steps to improve mental health', Press release. 24 July 2012.

Department of Health (2012c) *Holistic Needs Assessment for People with Cancer: A Practical Guide for Healthcare Professionals.* Available from: http://ncat.nhs.uk/sites/default/files/work-docs/ HNA_practical%20guide_web.pdf.

Department of Health (2012d) *Cancer Services Coming of Age.* Available from: www.gov.uk/ government/publications/improving-older-peoples-access-to-cancer-treatment-services [accessed 9 December 2013].

Department of Health (2012e) *The Impact of Patient Age on Clinical Decision Making in Oncology.* Available from: www.gov.uk/government/publications/the-impact-of-patient-age-on-clinical-decision-making-in-oncology [accessed 9 December 2013].

Department of Health (2012f) *No Health without Mental Health: Implementation Framework.* London: Department of Health.

Department of Health (2012g) *Preventing Suicide in England. A Cross-Government Outcomes Strategy To Save Lives.* London: Department of Health.

Department of Health (2013) *NHS Constitution: The NHS Belongs to us All.* London: Department of Health. Available from: www.nhs.uk/choiceintheNHS/Rightsandpledges/NHSConstitution/Pages/Overview.aspx (accessed 3 November).

Department of Health and Social Services (1996) *Cancer Services. Investing for the Future (The Campbell Report).* DHSS Northern Ireland.

Department of Health Cancer Policy Team (2012) *Radiotherapy in England 2012.* Available from: www.gov.uk/government/uploads/system/uploads/attachment_data/file/213151/Radiotherapy-Services-in-England-2012.pdf [accessed 1 September 2014].

Department of Health, Department of Health Social Services and Public Safety, The Scottish Government and Welsh Government (2011) *Physical Activity Guidelines for Adults (19–64 Years).* Available from: www.gov.uk/government/uploads/system/uploads/attachment_data/file/213740/dh_128145.pdf [accessed 18 April 2014].

Department of Health, Social Services and Public Safety (DHSSPS) (2008a) *Regional Cancer Framework. A Cancer Control Programme for Northern Ireland.* Available from: www.dhsspsni.gov.uk/eeu_cancer_control_programme_eqia.pdf [accessed 18 November 2014].

Department of Health, Social Services and Public Safety (DHSSPS) (2008b) *Service Framework for Cancer Prevention, Treatment and Care.* Belfast: DHSSPS.

Department of Work and Pensions (2010) *Over 10 Million People to Live to 100.* Available from: www.gov.uk/government/news/over-ten-million-people-to-live-to-100 [accessed 9 December 2013].

Derogatis, L.P., Morrow GR, Fetting J, Penman D, Piasetsky S, Schmale AM, et al. (1983) 'The prevalence of psychiatric disorders among cancer patients', *Journal of the American Medical Association,* 249: 751–7.

Des Guetz, G., Nicolas, P., Perret, G.-Y., Morere, J.-F., Uzzan, B. (2010) 'Does delaying adjuvant chemotherapy after curative surgery for colorectal cancer impair survival? A meta-analysis', *European Journal of Cancer England,* 46: 1049–55. doi:10.1016/j.ejca.2010.01.020.

Detmar, S.B., Muller, M.J., Schornagel, J.H., Wever, L.D. and Aaronson, N.K. (2002) 'Health-related quality-of-life assessments and patient-physician communication: a randomized controlled trial', *Journal of the American Medical Association,* 288: 3027–34.

Devane, C. (2009) 'Cancer Survivorship: the entire journey', *Nursing Times,* 105(12): 2–15.

Dewalt, D.A., Berkman, N.D., Sheridan, S., et al. (2004) 'Literacy and health outcomes: a systematic review of the literature', *Journal of General Internal Medicine,* 19(12): 1228–39.

Dhami, K. (2011) *Lesbian and Bisexual Women and Breast Cancer: A Policy Briefing.* Available from: www.breastcancercare.org.uk/campaigning-volunteering/policy/breast-cancer-inequalities/lesbian-bisexual-women-breast-cancer [accessed 13 August 2012].

Dibble, S.L., Chapman, J., Mack, K.A. and Shih, A. (2000) 'Acupressure for nausea: results of a pilot study', *Oncology Nursing Forum,* 27(1): 41–7.

Dickson-Swift, V., James, E.L, Kippen, S. and Liamputtong, P. (2007) 'Doing sensitive research: what challenges do qualitative researchers face?', *Qualitative Research,* 7(3): 327–53.

Dickson-Swift, V., James, E.L, Kippen, S. and Liamputtong, P. (2008) 'Risk to researchers in qualitative research on sensitive topics: issues and strategies', *Qualitative Health Research,* 18(1): 133–44.

Dickson-Swift, V., James, E.L, Kippen, S. and Liamputtong, P. (2009) 'Researching sensitive topics: qualitative research as emotion work', *Qualitative Research,* 9(1): 61–79.

Dimbleby Cancer Care (2014) *Researching Care and Cure.* Available from: www.dimblebycancercare.org/research [accessed 22 June 2014].

Directive 2004/27/EC of The European Parliament and of the Council of 31 March 2004, amending Directive 2001/83/EC on the Community. Available from: http://ec.europa.eu/health/files/eudralex/vol-1/dir_2004_27/dir_2004_27_en.pdf (accessed 5 November 2014).

Disability Rights Commission (2006) *Equal Treatment: Closing the Gap – A Formal Investigation into Physical Health Inequalities Experienced by People with Learning Disabilities and/or Mental Health Problems.* London: Disability Rights Commission.

Dixon, L., Adler, D., Berlant, J., Dulit, R., Goldman, B., Hackman, D., Oslin, D., Siris, S., Sonis, M. and Valenstein, M. (2007) 'Psychiatrists and primary caring: what are our boundaries of responsibility?', *Psychiatric Services,* 58(5): 600–2.

Dixon-Woods, M., Young, B. and Heney, D. (2005) *Rethinking Experiences of Childhood Cancer: A Multidisciplinary Approach to Chronic Childhood Illness.* Maidenhead, UK: Open University Press.

Djuretic, T., Laing-Morton, T., Guy, M. and Gill, M. (1999) 'Concerted effort is needed to ensure these women use preventive services', *British Medical Journal,* 318: 536.

Dobbie, M. and Mellor, D. (2008) 'Chronic illness and its impact: considerations for psychologists', *Psychology, Health and Medicine,* 13(5): 583–90.

Dochez, C., Bogers, J.J., Verhelst, R., et al. (2014) 'HPV vaccines to prevent cervical cancer and genital warts: an update', *Vaccine,* 32(14): 1595–601. doi:10.1016/j.vaccine.2013.10.081.

Dockter, L. and Keene, S. (2009) 'Ageism in chemotherapy', *The Internet Journal of Law, Healthcare and Ethics,* 6(1).

Dodd, S., Williams, L.J., Jacka, F.N., Pasco, J.A., Bjerkeset, O. and Berk, M. (2009) 'Reliability of the Mood Disorder Questionnaire: comparison with the Structured Clinical Interview for the DSM-IV-TR in a population sample', *Australian and New Zealand Journal of Psychiatry,* 43(6): 526–30.

Doehring, C. (2006) *The Practice of Pastoral Care: A Postmodern Approach.* Louisville, KY: Westminster John Knox Press.

Doka, K. (ed.) (1989) *Disenfranchised Grief.* Lexington, MA: Lexington Books.

Dolbeault, S., Szporn A. and Holland, J.C. (1999) 'Psycho-oncology: where have we been? Where are we going?', *European Journal of Cancer,* 35(11): 1554–8.

Doll, R. (2004) 'Mortality in relation to smoking: 50 years' observations on male British doctors', *British Medical Journal,* 328(7455): 1519. doi:10.1136/bmj.38142.554479.AE.

Doll, R. and Hill, A.B. (1950) 'Smoking and carcinoma of the lung', *British Medical Journal,* 2(4682): 739–48.

Donovan, M. and Glackin M. (2012) 'The lived experience of patients receiving radiotherapy for head and neck cancer: a literature review', *International Journal of Palliative Nursing,* 18(9): 448–55.

Doobaree, I.J., Landis, S.H., Linklater, K.M., El-Hariry, I., Moller, H. and Tyczynski, J. (2009) 'Head and neck cancer in South East England between 1995–1999 and 2000–2004: an estimation of incidence and distribution by site, stage and histological type', *Oral Oncology,* 45: 809–14.

Dorrell, S. (2005) 'The pain of venous cannulation', *Journal of the Royal Society of Medicine,* 98(6): 292.

Dorros, S.M., Card, N.A., Segrin, C. and Badger T. (2010) 'Interdependence in women with breast cancer and their partners: an interindividual model of distress', *Journal of Consulting & Clinical Psychology,* 78(1): 121–5.

Douma, K.F., Aaronson, N.K., Vasen, H.F., et al. (2008) 'Psychosocial issues in genetic testing for familial adenomatous polyposis: a review of the literature', *Psychooncology,* 17(8):737–745.

Dow Meneses, K., McNees, P., Loerzel, V.W., Su, X., Zhang, Y. and Hassey, L.A. (2007) 'Transition from treatment to survivorship: effects of a psychoeducational intervention on quality of life in breast cancer survivors', *Oncology Nursing Forum,* 34(5): 1007–16.

Dowling, E.C., Klabunde, C., Patnick J., et al. International Cancer Screening Network (ICSN) (2010) 'Breast and cervical cancer screening programme implementation in 16 countries', *Journal of Medical Screening,* 17: 139–146.

Downing, Storey, L. Dempster, McCorry (2012) *Who Am I Now? Creating a New Normality. Living with the Consequences of Surviving Breast Cancer.* Submitted as part of research portfolio for Doctorate in Clinical Psychology. Unpublished.

Drake, M. (2013) 'The physical health needs of individuals with mental health problems –
    setting the scene', in E. Collins, M. Drake and M. Deacon (eds), *The Physical Care of People
    with Mental Health Problems. A Guide for Best Practice.* London: Sage Publications. pp. 1–15.

Druker, B.J., Guilhot, F., O'Brien, S.G. et al (2006) 'IRIS Investigators: Five-year follow-up of
    patients receiving imatinib for chronic myeloid leukemia', *New England Journal of Medicine,*
    355(23): 2408–2417.

Druss, B.G. (2007) 'Improving medical care for persons with serious mental illness: challenges
    and solutions', *Journal Clinical Psychiatry,* 68(Suppl. 4): 40–44.

Dryden, W. and Reeves, A. (2013) *Handbook of Individual Therapy,* 6th edn. London: Sage
    Publications.

DuBois, D. and DuBois, E.F. (1916) 'A formula to estimate the approximate surface area if
    height and weight be known', *Archives of Internal Medicine,* 17: 863–71.

Duesbury, T. (2005) 'Art therapy in the hospice: rewards and frustrations', in D. Waller and
    C. Sibbert (eds), *Art Therapy and Cancer Care.* Maidenhead, UK: Open University Press. pp.
    199–210.

Duff, M., Scheepers, M., Cooper, M., Hoghton, M. and Baddeley, P. (2001) '*Helicobacter pylori*:
    has the killer escaped from the institution? A possible cause of increased stomach cancer in a
    population with intellectual disability', *Journal of Intellectual Disability Research,* 45(3): 219–25.

Dundee, J., Chaly, R. and Fitzpatrick, K. (1988) 'Randomized comparison of the antiemetic
    effects of metoclopramide and electroacupuncture in cancer chemotherapy', *British Journal
    of Clinical Pharmacology,* 25(6): 678–9.

Dunn, J., Ng, S.K., Holland, J., Aitken, J., Youl, P., Baade, P.D. and Chambers, S.K. (2013)
    'Trajectories of psychological distress after colorectal cancer', *Psycho-oncology,* 22(8):
    1759–65.

Dunne, D.F.J., Yip, V.S., Jones, R.P., McChesney, E.A., Lythgoe, D.T., Psarelli, E.E., Jones, L.,
    Lacasia-Purroy, C., Malik, H.Z., Poston, G.J. and Fenwick, S.W. (2014) 'Enhanced recovery
    in the resection of colorectal liver metastases', *Journal of Surgical Oncology.* 110(2): 197–202.

Eastwood, P. (2011) *Statistics on Obesity, Physical Activity and Diet: England 2011.* London: NHS
    Information Centre for Health and Social Care.

Eckert, R.M (2001) 'Understanding anticipatory nausea', *Oncology Nursing Forum,* 28(10): 1553–58.

Edwards, A., Pang, N., Shiu, V. and Chan, C. (2010) 'The understanding of spirituality and the
    potential role of spiritual care in end-of-life and palliative care: a meta-study of qualitative
    research', *Palliative Medicine,* 24(8): 753–70.

Edwards, D. (2004) *Art Therapy.* London: Sage Publications.

Egan, B., Gage, H., Hood, J., Poole, K., McDowell, C., Maguire, G., Storey, L., et al. (2012)
    'Availability of complementary and alternative medicine for people with cancer in the
    British National Health Service: results of a national survey', *Complementary Therapies in
    Clinical Practice,* 18(2): 75–80. doi:10.1016/j.ctcp.2011.11.003.

Egan, G. (2009) *The Skilled Helper: A Problem-Management and Opportunity-Development Approach
    to Helping. Belmont.* CA: Wadsworth Publishing Company.

Egbert, N. and Parrott, R. (2001) 'Self-efficacy and rural women's performance of breast and
    cervical cancer detection practices', *Journal Health Communication,* 6(3): 219–33.

Eguchi, T., Kodera, Y., Nakanishi, H., Yokoyama, H., Ohashi, N., Ito, Y., Nakayama, G., Koike, M.,
    Fujiwara, M., Nakao, A. (2008) 'The effect of chemotherapy against micrometastases and
    isolated tumor cells in lymph nodes: an *in vivo* study', *Vivo Athens Greece,* 22: 707–12.

Eide, H., Quera, V., Graygaard, P. and Finsent, A. (2004) 'Physician patient dialogue surround-
    ing patient's expression of concerns: applying sequence analysisto RIAS', *Social Science &
    Medicine,* 59: 145–55.

Eilers, J., Berger, A.M. and Peterson, M.P. (1988) 'Development testing and application of the
    oral assessment guide', *Oncology Nursing Forum,* 15(3): 325–30.

Einhorn, L.H., Rapoport, B., Koeller, J., Grunberg, S.M., Feyer, P., Rittenberg, C., Aapro, M. (2005)
    'Antiemetic therapy for multiple-day chemotherapy and high-dose chemotherapy with stem
    cell transplant: review and consensus statement', *Supportive Care in Cancer,* 13: 112–16.

Eiser, C. and Upton, P. (2007) 'The cost of caring for a child with cancer: a questionnaire sur-
    vey', *Child: Care, Health and Development,* 33(4): 455–9.

Ekfors, H. and Petersson, K. (2004) 'A qualitative study of the experience during radiotherapy of Swedish patients suffering from lung cancer', *Oncology Nursing Forum*, 31(2): 329–34.

El Turabi, A., Abel, G.A., Roland, M. and Lyratzopoulos, G. (2013) 'Variation in reported experience of involvement in cancer treatment decision making: evidence from the National Cancer Patient Experience Survey', *British Journal of Cancer*, 109(3): 780–7. doi:10.1038/bjc.2013.316.

Elliott, J., Fallows, A., Staetsky, L., Smith, P.W.F, Foster, C.L, Maher, E.J. and Corner, J. (2011) 'The health and well-being of cancer survivors in the UK: findings from a population-based survey. *British Journal of Cancer*, 105: S11–S20.

Ellis, P.M, Butow, P.N, Tattersall, M.H.N, Dunn, S.M. and Houssami, N. (2001) 'Randomised clinical trials in oncology: understanding and attitudes predict willingness to participate', *Journal of Clinical Oncology*, 19(15): 3554–61.

Elwell, L., Grogan, S. and Coulson, N. (2011) 'Adolescents living with cancer: the role of computer- mediated support groups', *Journal of Health Psychology*, 16(2): 235–248.

Emilsson, S., Svensk, A.C., Tavelin, B. and Lindh, J. (2012) 'Support group participation during the post-operative radiotherapy period increases level of coping resources among women with breast cancer', *European Journal of Cancer Care*, 21(5): 591–8.

Endler, N.S. and Parker, J.D. (1990) 'Multidimensional assessment of coping: a critical evaluation', *Journal of Personality and Social Psychology*, 58(5): 844–54.

Engstrom, C.A., Strohl, R.A., Rose, L. et al. (1999) 'Sleep alterations in cancer patients', *Cancer Nursing*, 22: 143–148.

Entwistle, V.A., Carter, S.M., Trevena, L, et al. (2008) 'Communicating about screening', *British Medical Journal*. 337: a1591. doi:10.1136/bmj.a1591.

Entwistle, V.A., Firnigi D., Ryan M., Francis J. and Kinghorn, P. (2012) 'Which experiences of health care delivery matter to service users and why? A critical interpretive synthesis and conceptual map', *Journal of Health Service Research & Policy*, 17(2): 70–8.

EORTC Quality of Life Group (1995) *EORTC QLQ-C30 (version 3)*. Available from: http://groups.eortc.be/qol/eortc-qlq-c30 [accessed 12 October 2014].

EORTC (2014) *EORTC QLQ-C30*. Available from: http://groups.eortc.be/qol/eortc-qlq-c30 (accessed 5 November 2014).

Epping-Jordan, J.E., Compas, B.E., Osowiecki, D.M., Oppedisano, G., Gerhardt, C., Primo, K. and Krag, D.N. (1999) 'Psychological adjustment in breast cancer: processes of emotional distress', *Health Psychology*, 18(4): 315–26.

The Equality Act 2010. London: HMSO. Available from: www.legislation.gov.uk/ukpga/2010/15/contents [accessed 10 November 2014].

Equality and Human Rights Commission (2010) *Your Rights to Equality from Health and Social Care Services. Equality Act 2010 Guidance of your Rights, Volume 5 of 9*. Manchester: Equality and Human Rights Commission.

Erickson, J., Spurlock, L.K., Kramer, J.C. and Davis, M.A. (2013) 'Self-care strategies to relive fatigue in patients receiving radiation therapy', *Clinical Journal of Oncology Nursing*, 17(3): 319–24.

Ernst, E., Resch, K.-L., Mills S, et al. (1995) 'Complementary medicine: a definition', *British Journal of General Practice*, 45: 506.

Ernst, E. and Pittler, M.H. (2000) 'Efficacy of ginger for nausea and vomiting: a systematic review of the randomised clinical trials', *British Journal of Anaesthesia* 84(3): 367–371.

Espie, C.A., Fleming, L., Cassidy, J., Samuel, L., Taylor, L.M., White, C.A., Douglas, N.J., Engleman, H.M., Kelly, H. and Paul, J. (2008) 'Randomized controlled clinical effectiveness trial of cognitive behavior therapy compared with treatment as usual for persistent insomnia in patients with cancer', *Journal of Clinical Oncology*, 26(28): 4651–8.

European Oncology Nursing Society (EONS) (2010) *Extravasation Guidelines*. Brussels: European Oncology Nursing Society.

Evans, M., Shaw, A., Thompson, E.A. et al. (2007) 'Decisions to use complementary and alternative medicine (CAM) by male cancer patients: information-seeking roles and types of evidence used', *BMC Complementary and Alternative Medicine*, 7: 25.

Extermann, M., Aapro, M., Bernabei, R., Cohen, H.J., et al (2005) 'Use of comprehensive geriatric assessment in older cancer patients. Recommendations from the task force on CGA of the International Society of Geriatric Oncology (SIOG)', *Critical Reviews in Oncology & Hematology,* 55: 241–52.

Extermann, M. and Huria, A. (2007) 'Comprehensive geriatric assessment for older patients with cancer', *Journal of Clinical Oncology,* 25: 1824–31.

Extermann, M., Overcash, J., Lyman, G.H., Parr, J. and Balducci, L. (1998) 'Co-morbidity and functional status are independent in older cancer patients', *Journal of Clinical Oncology,* 16: 1582–7.

Ezzo, J.M., Richardson, M.A., Vickers, A., Allen, C., Dibble, S.L., Issell, B.F., Lao, L., Pearl, M., Ramirez, G., Roscoe, J.A., Shen, J., Shivnan, J.C., Streitberger, K., Treish, I. and Zhang, G. (2006) 'Acupuncture-point stimulation for chemotherapy-induced nausea or vomiting', *Cochrane Database of Systematic Reviews,* Issue 2. Art.No: CD002285. doi:10.1002/14651858. CD002285.pub2.

Ezzone, S.A. (2010) 'Principles and techniques of blood and marrow transplantation', in C.H. Yarbro, D. Wujcik and B.H. Holmes (eds), *Cancer Nursing: Principles and Practice,* 7th edn. Sudbury, MA: Jones and Bartlett. pp. 504–12.

Fagerlin, A., Zikmund-Fisher, B.J. and Ubel, P.A. (2011) 'Helping patients decide: ten steps to better risk communication', *Journal of the National Cancer Institute,* 103(19): 1436–43. doi:10.1093/jnci/djr318.

Faithfull, S. (2008) 'Radiotherapy' in J. Corner and C. Bailey (eds), *Cancer Nursing: Care in Context,* 2nd edn. Oxford, UK: Blackwell Publishing. pp. 317–59.

Faller, H., Bulzebruck, H., Drings, P. and Lang, H. (1999) 'Coping, distress, and survival among patients with lung cancer', *Archives in General Psychiatry,* 56: 756–62.

Fallowfield, L. (1993) 'Giving sad bad news', *Lancet,* 341: 476–78.

Fallowfield, L. and Jenkins V. et al. (2003) 'Enduring impact of communication skills training: 12 month follow up results of a randomised trial', *British Journal of Cancer,* 89: 1445–49.

Fallowfield, L., Ratcliffe, D., Jenkins, V., et al. (2001) 'Psychiatric morbidity and its recognition by doctors in patients with cancer', *British Journal of Cancer,* 84(8): 1011–15.

Farrell, C. (2013) *An Exploration of the Role of Oncology Specialist Nurses within Nurse-led Chemotherapy Clinics: A Two-stage Study Using Survey and Ethnographic Methods.* Unpublished thesis (PhD). University of Manchester.

Farrell, C., Heaven, C., Beaver, K. and Maguire, P. (2005) 'Identifying the concerns of women undergoing chemotherapy', *Patient Education and Counseling,* 56: 72–7.

Fearon, K.C.H., Llungquist,O., Von Meyenfeldt, M. et al. (2005) 'Enhanced recovery after surgery: a consensus review of clinical care for patients undergoing colonic resection', *Clinical Nutrition,* 24(3): 466–477.

Featherstone, H. and Whitham, L. (2010) *The Cost of Cancer.* London: Policy Exchange. Available from: www.policyexchange.org.uk/images/publications/thecostofcancer-feb10.pdf.

Featherstone, M. and Hepworth, M. (1991) 'The mask of ageing', in M. Featherstone, M. Hepworth and B.S. Turner (eds), *The Body: Social Process and Cultural Theory.* London: Sage Publications. pp. 371–389.

Federico, S., Brennan, R. and Dyer, M.A. (2011) 'Childhood cancer and developmental biology a crucial partnership', *Current Topics in Developmental Biology,* 94: 1–13.

Fedirko, V., Tramacere, I. and Bagnardi, V. et al. (2011) 'Alcohol drinking and colorectal cancer risk: an overall and dose-response meta-analysis of published studies', *Annals of Oncology,* 22(9): 1958–72. doi:10.1093/annonc/mdq653.

Fenlon, D. and Foster, C. (2009) *Self-Management Support: A Review of the Evidence.* Working document for the National Cancer Survivorship Initiative Self-Management Work Stream. London.

Fenlon, D., Frankland, J., Foster, C., Brooks, C., et al. (2012a) 'Living into old age with the consequences of breast cancer', *European Journal of Oncology Nursing,* 17(3): 311–316.

Fenlon, D., Richardson, A., Addington-Hall, J., Smith P., Corner, J., Winter, J. and Foster, C. (2012b) 'A cohort study of the recovery of health and wellbeing following colorectal cancer (CREW study): protocol paper', *BMC Health Services Research,* 12(90). doi:10.1186/1472-6963-12-90.

Fenton, L., Rigney, M. and Herbst, R.S. (2009) 'Clinical trial awareness, attitudes, and participation among patients with cancer and oncologists', *Community Oncology,* 6(5): 207–228.

Ferlay, J., Soerjomataram, I., Ervik, M., Dikshit, R., Eser, S., Mathers, C., Rebelo, M., Parkin, D.M., Forman, D. and Bray, F. (2013) *GLOBOCAN 2012 v1.0, Cancer Incidence and Mortality Worldwide: IARC CancerBase No. 11* [Internet]. Lyon, France: International Agency for Research on Cancer.

Fern, L.A. and Whelan, J. (2010) 'Recruitment of adolescents and young adults to cancer clinical trials- international comparisons, barriers and implications', *Seminars in Oncology*, 37 (2): 1–8.

Fern, L.A., Birch, R.J., Whelan, J., Cooke, M., Sutton, S., Neal, R.D., Gerrard, C., Hubbard, G., Smith, S., Lethaby, C., Dommett, R. and Gibson, F. (2013) 'Why can't we improve the timeliness of cancer diagnosis in children, teenagers and young adults?', *British Medical Journal*, 347.

Feros, D.L., Lane, L., Ciarrochi, J. and Blackledge, J.T. (2013) 'Acceptance and Commitment Therapy (ACT) for improving the lives of cancer patients: a preliminary study', *Psycho-oncology*, 22(2): 459–64. doi:10.1002/pon.2083.

Ferrell, B.R. and Coyle, N. (2006) *Textbook of Palliative Nursing*, 2nd edn. Toronto: Oxford University Press.

Ferrell, B.R., Ervin, K., Smith, S., Marek, T. and Melancon, C. (2002) 'Family perspectives of ovarian cancer', *Cancer Practice,* 10(6): 269–76.

Fesharakizadeh, M., Taheri, D., Dolatkhah, S. and Wexner, S.D. (2013) 'Postoperative ileus in colorectal surgery: is there any difference between laparoscopic and open surgery?', *Gastroenterology Reports,* 1: 138–43. doi:10.1093/gastro/got008.

Festinger, L. (1957) *A Theory of Cognitive Dissonance.* London: Tavistock Publications.

Field, A. (2013) *Discovering Statistics Using IBM SPSS Statistics*, 4th edn. London: Sage Publications.

Fields, M.M. (2013) 'Increased intracranial pressure' in C.H. Yarbro, D. Wujcik and B.H. Gobel (eds), *Cancer Symptom Management*, 4th edn, Burlington, VT: Jones and Bartlett Learning. pp. 439–55.

Fife, B.L., Kennedy, V.N. and Robinson, L. (1994) 'Gender and adjustment to cancer: clinical implications', *Journal of Psychosocial Oncology,* 12(1–2): 1–21.

Filshie, J., Bolton, T., Browne, D. et al (2005) 'Acupuncture and self acupuncture for long term treatment of vasomotor symptoms in cancer patients – audit and treatment algorithm', *Acupuncture in Medicine,* 23: 171–80.

Finset, A. (2011) 'Emotional cues and concerns in medical conulstations', *Patient Education & Counseling,* 82: 139–40.

Fish, J. (2009) *Cervical Screening in Lesbian and Bisexual Women: A Review of the Worldwide Literature using Systematic Methods.* Report commissioned by the NHS Cervical Screening Programme, Sheffield. HPRU Report ISBN: 978-1-85721-396-6.

Fish, J. (2010) '"It's a mixed up, muddled up, shook up world, except for Lola": transforming health and social care for trans people', *Diversity in Health & Care,* 7(2): 87–9. (Guest editorial).

Fish, J. (2012) *Supporting LGBT People with Cancer: A Practical Guide for Cancer and Other Health Professionals.* Leicester: De Montfort University.

Fishbein, M. and Ajzen, I. (1975) *Belief, Attitude, Intention and Behavior: An Introduction to Theory and Research.* Vermont: ARRB Group.

Fjorback, L. O., Arendt, M., Ørnbøl, E., Fink, P. and Walach, H. (2011) 'Mindfulness-based stress reduction and mindfulness-based cognitive therapy: a systematic review of randomized controlled trials', *Acta Psychiatrica Scandinavica*, 124(2): 102–19. Available from: http://dx.doi.org/10.1111/j.1600-0447.2011.01704.x.

Flaherty, K.T., Puzanov I, Kim KB et al. (2010) 'Inhibition of mutated, activated BRAF in metastatic melanoma', *The New England Journal of Medicine*, 363(9): 809–19.

Fleming, A. and Chi, S.C. (2012) 'Brain tumors in children', *Current Problems in Pediatric and Adolescent Health Care*, 42(4): 80–103.

Fletcher, I. (2006) *Patterns of Verbal Interaction Between Health Professionals and Cancer Patients.* Thesis (PhD). University of Manchester.

Flick, U. (2002) *An Introduction to Qualitative Research*, 2nd edn. London: Sage Publications.

Flynn, M. and Quinn, J. (2010) 'Merseyside and Cheshire Cancer Network, Cancer Awareness Measure (CAM)', UK Data Archive/Economic and Social Data Service. Available from:

www.esds.ac.uk/doc/6640%5Cmrdoc%5CUKDA%5CUKDA_Study_6640_Information. htm.

Flynn, S., Hulbert-Williams, N.J., Tytherleigh, M., Roberts, S., Wilkinson, H. and Taylor, E. (2013) *Living Life after Cancer Treatment: A Cancer Survivorship Support Group Evaluation.* Chester Research Online.

Folkman, S. and Lazarus, R.S. (1985) *The Ways of Coping Questionnaire.* Menlo Park, CA: Mindgarden.

Folkman, S., Lazarus, R.S., Dunkel-Schetter, C., DeLongis, A. and Gruen, R.J. (1986) 'Dynamics of a stressful encounter: cognitive appraisal, coping and encounter outcomes', *Journal of Personality and Social Psychology,* 50(5): 992–1003.

Forbat, L., Hubbard, G. and Kearney, N. (2009a) 'Patient and public involvement: models and muddles', *Journal of Clinical Nursing,* 18: 2547–2554.

Forbat, L., Hubbard, G. and Kearney, N. (2009b) *Better Cancer Care: A Systemic Approach to Practice.* Edinburgh: Dunedin Press.

Forbat, L., Place, M., Kelly, D., Hubbard, G., Boyd, K., Howie, K. and Leung, H. (2013) 'A cohort study reporting clinical risk factors and individual risk perceptions of prostate cancer: Implications for PSA testing', *British Journal of Urology International,* 111(3):389–95.

Forbat, L., White, I., Marshall-Lucette, S. and Kelly, D. (2011) 'Discussing the sexual consequences of treatment in radiotherapy and urology consultations with couples affected by prostate cancer', *British Journal of Urology International,* 109(1): 98–103.

Forbes, L.J. and Ramirez AJ. (2014) 'Communicating the benefits and harms of cancer screening', *Current Oncology Reports,* 16(5): 382. doi:10.1007/s11912-014-0382-4.

Ford, E.S., Merritt, R.K., Heath, G.W., Powell, K.E., Washburn, R.A., Kriska, A. and Haile, G. (1991) 'Physical activity behaviors in lower and higher socioeconomic status populations', *American Journal of Epidemiology,* 133(12): 1246–56.

Forest, F., Duband, S. and Peoc'h, M. (2011) 'The attitudes of patients to their own autopsy: a misconception', *Journal of Clinical Pathology,* 64(11): 1037.

Forsythe, A.R. (2010) 'Gender differences in incidence rates of childhood B- Precursor Acute Lymphoblastic Leukaemia', *Journal of Pediatric Oncology Nursing,* 27(3): 164–167.

Foster, C., Breckons, M., Cotterell, P., Barbosa, D., Calman, L., Corner, J., Fenlon, D., Foster, R., Grimmett, C., Richardson, A. and Smith, P.W. (2014) 'Cancer survivors' self-efficacy to self-manage in the year following primary treatment', *Journal of Cancer Survivorship,* DOI 10.1007/s11764-014-0384-0.

Foster, C. and Fenlon, D. (2011) 'Recovery and self-management support following primary cancer treatment', *British Journal of Cancer,* 105: S21–S28.

Foster, C., Roffe, L., Scott, I. and Cotterell, P. (2010) *Self-Management of Problems Experienced Following Primary Cancer Treatment: An Exploratory Study.* London: Macmillan Cancer Support.

Foster, C., Wright, D., Hill, H., Hopkinson, J. and Roffe, L. (2009) 'Psychosocial implications of living 5 years or more following a cancer diagnosis: a systematic review of the research evidence', *European Journal of Cancer Care,* 18: 223–47.

FOxTROT Collaborative Group (2012) 'Feasibility of preoperative chemotherapy for locally advanced, operable colon cancer: the pilot phase of a randomised controlled trial', *Lancet Oncology,* 13, 1152–60. doi:10.1016/S1470-2045(12)70348-0.

Fraenkel, L. and McGraw, S. (2007) 'Participation in medical decision making: the patients' perspective', *Medical Decision Making,* 27: 533–538.

Fransson, P. (2011) 'Fatigue in prostate cancer patients treated with external beam radiotherapy: a prospective 5-year long-term patient-reported evaluation', *Journal of Cancer Research and Therapeutics,* 6(4): 2678–86.

Freud, S. (1917) 'Mourning and melancholia', in J. Strachey (ed.), *The Standard Edition of the Complete Psychological Works of Sigmund Freud,* Vol. 14 (1957). London: Hogarth Press.

Frick, E., Tyroller, M., Panzer, M. (2007) 'Anxiety, depression and quality of life of cancer patients undergoing radiation therapy: a cross sectional study in a community hospital outpatient centre', *European Journal of Cancer Care,* 16: 130–6.

Fridriksdottir, N., Saevarsdottir, T., Halfdanardottir, S.I., et al. (2011) 'Family members of cancer patients: needs, quality of life and symptoms of anxiety and depression', *Acta Oncologica*, 50(2): 252–8.

Frisch, M., Smith, E. et al. (2003) 'Cancer in a population-based cohort of men and women in registered homosexual partnerships', *American Journal of Epidemiology* 157: 966–972.

Frisch, M., Smith, E., Grulich, A. and Johansen, C. (2003) 'Cancer in a population-based cohort of men and women in registered homosexual partnerships', *American Journal of Epidemiology*, 157: 966–972.

Fröjd, C., Lampic, C., Larsson, G., Birgegård, G. and von Essen, L. (2007) 'Patient attitudes, behaviours, and other factors considered by doctors when estimating cancer patients' anxiety and desire for information', *Scand J Caring Sci.*, 21(4): 523–529.

Fröman, N. (2014) 'Marie and Pierre Curie and the discovery of polonium and radium', Nobelprize.org. Available from: www.nobelprize.org/nobel_prizes/themes/physics/curie [accessed 23 July 2014].

Fundamental Rights Agency (FRA) (2013) *Inequalities and Multiple Discrimination in Access to and Quality of Healthcare*. Vienna: Fundamental Rights Agency. Available from: http://fra.europa.eu/en/publication/2013/inequalities-discrimination-healthcare [accessed 9 December 2013].

Furukawa, T.A., Anraku, K. and Hiroe, T., et al. (1999) 'A polydiagnostic study of depressive disorders according to DSM-IV and 23 classical diagnostic systems', *Psychiatry and Clinical Neurosciences*, 53(3): 387.

Gabriel, J. (2007) *The Biology of Cancer*. London: Whurr.

Gabrielsson, A. (2011) *Strong Experiences with Music*. Oxford: Oxford University Press.

Galfin JM, Watkins ER, Harlow T. (2011) 'A brief guided self-help intervention for psychological distress in palliative care patients: a randomised controlled trial', *Palliative Medicine*, 26(3): 197–205.

Galiatsatos, P. and Foulkes., W.D. (2006) 'Familial adenomatous polyposis', *American Journal of Gastroenterology*, 101(2): 385–98.

Galimberti, V., Cole, B.F., Zurrida, S., Viale, G., Luini, A., Veronesi, P., Baratella, P., Chifu, C., Sargenti, M., Intra, M., Gentilini, O., Mastropasqua, M.G., Mazzarol, G., Massarut, S., Garbay, J.-R., Zgajnar, J., Galatius, H., Recalcati, A., Littlejohn, D., Bamert, M., Colleoni, M., Price, K.N., Regan, M.M., Goldhirsch, A., Coates, A.S., Gelber, R.D., Veronesi, U., International Breast Cancer Study Group Trial 23-01 Investigators (2013) 'Axillary dissection versus no axillary dissection in patients with sentinel-node micrometastases (IBCSG 23-01): a phase 3 randomised controlled trial', *Lancet Oncology*. 14: 297–305. doi:10.1016/S1470-2045(13)70035-4.

Ganai, S. (2014) 'Disclosure of surgeon experience', *World Journal of Surgery*. 38 (7): 1622–1625.

Gandubert, C., Carrière I., Escot, C., et al. (2009) 'Onset and relapse of psychiatric disorders following early breast cancer: a case–control study', *Psycho-oncology*, 18: 1029–37.

Garber, J. and Offit K. (2005) 'Hereditary cancer predisposition syndromes', *Journal of Clinical Oncology*, 23(2): 276–92.

Gates, M., Lackey N (1998) 'Youngsters caring for adults with cancer', *Image–The Journal of Nursing Scholarship*, 30(1): 11–15.

Gelling, L. (1999) 'Role of research ethics committee', *Nurse Education Today*, 19: 564–569.

Gelling, L. (2010) 'Gaining access to the research site', in K. Gerrish and A. Lacey (eds), *The Research Process in Nursing*. Chichester: Wiley-Blackwell. pp. 114–126.

General Medical Council (2007) *Consent: Patients and Doctors Making Decisions Together: A Draft for Consultation*. London: General Medical Council.

Geyer, C.E., Forster, J., Lindquist, D., et al. (2006) 'Lapatinib plus Capecitabine for HER2-Positive Advanced Breast Cancer', *The New England Journal of Medicine*, 355(26): 2733–43.

Gibbard, I. and Hanley, T. (2008) 'A five-year evaluation of the effectiveness of person centred counselling in routine clinical practice in primary care', *Counselling and Psychotherapy Research*, 8(4): 215–22.

Gielissen, M.F.M., Verhagen, C.A.H.H.V.M. and Bleijenberg, G. (2007) 'Cognitive behaviour therapy for fatigued cancer survivors: long-term follow-up', *British Journal of Cancer*, 97: 612–18.

Gigerenzer, G., Gaissmaier, W., Kurz-Milcke, E. et al. (2007) 'Helping doctors and patients make sense of health statistics', *Psychological Science in the Public Interest,* 8: 53–96.

Gil, F., Grassi, L., Travado L, et al. Southern European Psycho-oncology Study Group (2005) 'Use of distress and depression thermometers to measure psychosocial morbidity among Southern European cancer patients', *Supportive Care in Cancer,* 13: 600–6.

Gilbert, K.R. (2001) *The Emotional Nature of Qualitative Research.* Boca Raton, FL: CRC Press LLC.

Gilham, C., Peto, J., Simpson, J., Roman, E., Eden, T., Greaves, M., Alexander, F. (2005) 'Day care in infancy and risk of childhood acute lymphoblastic leukaemia: findings from UK case-control study', *British Medical Journal,* 330: 1294–300.

Gill, P.S., Kai, J., Bhopal, R.S. and Wild, S. (2004) 'Black and Minority Ethnic Groups', in A. Stevens, J. Raftery, J. Mant and S. Simpson (eds), *Health Care Needs Assessment: The Epidemiology Based Needs Assessment Reviews (Series 3).* Oxford: Radcliffe.

Gilroy, A. (2007) *Art Therapy, Research and Evidence-based Practice.* Sage Publications.

Gingerich, W.J. and Peterson, L.T. (2013) 'Effectiveness of solution-focused brief therapy: a systematic qualitative review of controlled outcome studies', *Research in Social Work Practice,* 23(3): 266–83.

Girgis, A., Lambert SD. (2009) 'Caregivers of cancer survivors: the state of the field', *Cancer Forum,* 33: 167–71.

Glaser, B.G. and Strauss, A.L. (1965) *Awareness of Dying.* New York, NY: Aldine Publishing Company.

Glover, D. and Harmer, V. (2014) 'Radiotherapy-induced skin reactions: assessment and management', *British Journal of Nursing,* 23(4): 28–35.

Glover, G., Webb, M. and Evison, F. (2010) *Improving Access to Psychological Therapies: A Review of the Progress Made by Sites in the First Roll-out Year.* Available from: www.iapt.nhs.uk/wp-content/uploads/iapt-year-onesites-data-review-final-report.pdf.

Glynne-Jones, R., Counsell, N., Quirke, P., Mortensen, N., Maraveyas, A., Meadows, H.M., Ledermann, J., Sebag-Montefiore, D. (2014) 'Chronicle: results of a randomised phase III trial in locally advanced rectal cancer after neoadjuvant chemoradiation randomising postoperative adjuvant capecitabine plus oxaliplatin (Xelox) versus control', *Annals of Oncology,* 25(7): 1356–1362.

Gobbi, P.G., Bergonzi, M., Comelli, M., Villano, L., Pozzoli, D., Vanoli, A., Dionigi, P. (2013) 'The prognostic role of time to diagnosis and presenting symptoms in patients with pancreatic cancer', *Cancer Epidemiology,* 37: 186–90. doi:10.1016/j.canep.2012.12.002.

Gomella, L.G. (2007) 'Contemporary use of hormonal therapy in prostate cancer: managing complications and addressing quality-of-life issues', *BJU Int,* 99 (Suppl. 1): 25–9

Gomes, B., Calanzani, N., Gysels, M., Hall, S. and Higginson, I. (2013) 'Heterogeneity and changes in preferences for dying at home: a systematic review', *BMC Palliative Care* 12: 7.

Goodman, M. (1996) 'Menopausal symptoms', in S.L. Groenwald, M.H. Frogge, M. Goodman and C.H. Yarbro (eds), *Cancer Symptom Management.* Sudbury, MA: Jones and Bartlett. pp. 571–595.

Goodwin, J.S., Hunt, W.C., Key, C.R. and Samet, J.M. (1987) 'The effect of marital status on stage, treatment, and survival of cancer patients' *Journal of the American Medical Association,* 258(21): 3125–30.

Gosney, M.A. (2005) 'Clinical assessment of elderly people with cancer', *Lancet Oncology,* 6(10): 790–7.

Goss, R.E. and Klass, D. (2005) *Dead but not Lost: Grief Narratives in Religious Traditions.* Walnut Creek, C.A. Alta Mira.

Gott, M. and Hinchcliffe, S (2003) 'How important is sex in later life? The views of older people', *Social Science & Medicine,* 56(8): 1617–28.

Gould, B.E. and Dyer, R.M. (2011) *Pathophysiology for the Health Professions,* 4th edn. Maryland Heights, MO: Elsevier.

Grassi, L., Rossi, E., Caruso, R., Nanni, M.G., Pedrazzi, S., Sofritti, S. and Sabato, S. (2011) 'Educational intervention in cancer outpatient clinics on routine screening for emotional distress: an observational study', *Psycho-oncology,* 20(6): 669–74.

Gratwohl, A., Baldomero, H., Aljurf, M. et al., for the Worldwide Network of Blood and Marrow Transplantation (2010) 'Hematopoietic stem cell transplantation: a global perspective', *Journal of the American Medical Association*, 303(16): 1617–24.

Graves, K.D., Arnold, S.M., Love, C.L., Kirsh, K.L., Moore, P.G. and Passik, S.D. (2007) 'Distress screening in a multidisciplinary lung cancer clinic: prevalence and predictors of clinically significant distress', *Lung Cancer*, 55: 215–24.

Gray, R. (2012) 'Physical health and mental illness: a silent scandal', *International Journal of Mental Health Nursing*, 21: 191–2.

Grazin, N. (2007) 'Long-term conditions: help patients to help themselves', *Health Services Journal*, 117: 28–9.

Grbich, C., Parker, D. and Maddocks, I. (2001) 'The emotions and coping strategies of caregivers of family members with a terminal cancer', *Journal of Palliative Care*, 17(1): 30–6.

Greaves, M.F., Maia, A.T., Wiemels, J.L. and Ford, A.M. (2003) 'Leukemia in twins: lessons in natural history', *Blood*, 102: 2321–33.

Greaves, M.F. and Wiemels, J. (2003) 'Origins of chromosome translocations in childhood leukaemia', *Nature Reviews: Cancer*, 3: 639–49.

Greco, L.A., Lambert, W. and Baer, R.A. (2008) 'Psychological inflexibility in childhood and adolescence: development and evaluation of the avoidance and fusion questionnaire for youth', *Psychological Assessment*, 20(2): 93–102.

Green, B.L., Marshall, H.C., Collinson, F., Quirke, P., Guillou, P., Jayne, D.G., Brown, J.M. (2013) 'Long-term follow-up of the Medical Research Council CLASICC trial of conventional versus laparoscopically assisted resection in colorectal cancer', *British Journal of Surgery*, 100: 75–82. doi:10.1002/bjs.8945.

Greenberg, G., Ganshorn, K. and Danilkewich, A. (2001) 'Solution-focused therapy: counseling model for busy family physicians', *Canadian Family Physician*, 47(11): 2289–95.

Greer, S. (2008) 'CBT for emotional distress of people with cancer: some personal observations. *Psycho-oncology*, 17(2): 170–3.

Greimel, E., Kristensen, G.B., van der Burg, M.E.L., Coronado, P., Rustin, G., del Rio, A.S., Reed, N.S., Nordal, R.R., Coens, C., Vergote, I., European Organization for Research and Treatment of Cancer – Gynaecological Cancer Group and NCIC Clinical Trials Group (2013) 'Quality of life of advanced ovarian cancer patients in the randomized phase III study comparing primary debulking surgery versus neo-adjuvant chemotherapy', *Gynecologic Oncology*, 131: 437–44. doi:10.1016/j.ygyno.2013.08.014.

Grinyer, A. and Thomas C. (2001) 'Young adults with cancer: the effect of the illness on parent and families', *International Journal of Palliative Nursing*, 7: 162–70.

Grocke, D. and Wigram, T. (2007) *Receptive Methods in Music Therapy: Techniques and Clinical Applications for Music Therapy Clinicians, Educators and Students*. London: Jessica Kingsley.

Grube, B. and Wells, M. (2010) 'New technologies, new skills, better knowledge', Guest Editorial European Oncology Nursing Society Newsletter, Theme: Radiotherapy Care. Available from: www.cancernurse.eu/documents/newsletter/2010summer/EONSNewsletter 2010summerfullpdf.pdf [accessed 12 October 2014].

Grunberg, S.M., Deuson, R.R., Mavros, P., Geling, O., Hansen, M., Cruciani, G., Daniele, B., De Pouvourville, G., Rubenstein, E.R. and Daugaard, G. (2004) 'Incidence of chemotherapy-induced nausea and emesis after modern antiemetics', *Cancer*, 100(10): 2261–8.

Grunfeld, E., Zitzelsberger, L., Coristine, M., Whelan, T.J., Aspelund, F. and Evans, W.K. (2005) 'Job stress and job satisfaction of cancer care workers', *Psycho-oncology*, 14: 61–9.

Güleser, G.N., Taşci, S. and Kaplan, B. (2012) 'The experience of symptoms and information needs of cancer patients undergoing radiotherapy', *Journal of Cancer Education*, 27: 46–53.

Guo, Z., Tang, H.Y., Li, H., Tan, S.K., Feng, K.H., Huang, Y.C., Bu, Q. and Jiang, W. (2013) 'The benefits of psychosocial interventions for cancer patients undergoing radiotherapy', *Health and Quality of Life Outcomes*, 11: 121. Available from: www.hqlo.com/content/11/1/121 [accessed 7 November 2014].

Gupta, V. and Woodman C. (2010) 'Managing stress in the palliative care team', *Paediatric Nursing*, 22: 10: 14–18.

Gurney, J.G., Smith, M.A., Ross. J., A. (2012) *Cancer Among Infants*. National Cancer Institute. Available from: www.cancer.gov/search/results.

Haase, J.E. and Rostad, M. (1994) 'Experiences of completing cancer therapy: child and parent perspectives', *Journal of Pediatric Oncology Nursing*, 13(3): 160–161.

Hagedoorn, M., Buunk, B., Kuijer, R., Wobbes, T. and Sanderman, T. (2000) 'Couples dealing with cancer: role and gender differences regarding psychological distress and quality of life', *Psycho-oncology*, 9: 232–42.

Hagerty, R.G., Butow, P.N., Ellis, P.M. et al. (2005) 'Communicating with realism and hope: incurable cancer patients' views on the disclosure of prognosis', *Journal Clinical Oncology*, 23: 1278–88.

Hagger-Johnson, G., Taibjee R., Semlyen J., Fitchie, I., Fish, J. Meads, C. and Varney, J. (2013) 'Sexual orientation identity in relation to smoking history and alcohol use at age 18/19: cross-sectional associations from the Longitudinal Study of Young People in England (LSYPE)', *British Medical Journal Open*, 3: e002810.

Hagopian, R., Lafta, R., Hassan, J. (2010) 'Trends in childhood leukaemia in Basra, Iraq. 1993–2007', *American Journal of Public Health*, 100(6): 1081–1087

Haines, M. and Spear, S.F. (1996) 'Changing the perception of the norm: a strategy to decrease binge drinking among college students', *Journal of American College Health*, 45(3): 134–40.

Halcón, L.L., Chlan, L.L., Kreitzer, M.J. and Leonard, B.J. (2003) 'Complementary therapies and healing practices: faculty/student beliefs and attitudes and the implications for nursing education', *Journal of Professional Nursing*, 19: 387–97.

Hall, D., Meador, K. and Koenig, H. (2008) 'Measuring religiousness in health research: review and critique', *Journal of Religion and Health*, 47: 134–163.

Hallam, R.S. (2013) *Individual Case Formulation*. Oxford: Academic Press.

Hamilton, W. (2007) *Cancer Diagnosis in Primary Care*. Edinburgh, UK: Churchill Livingstone.

Hamilton, W. (2009) 'The CAPER studies: five case-control studies aimed at identifying and quantifying the risk of cancer in symptomatic primary care patients.' *British Journal of Cancer*, 101(S2): S80–6.

Hamilton, W., Peters, J., Bankhead, C. and Sharp, D. (2009) 'Risk of ovarian cancer in women with symptoms in primary care: population based case control study', *British Medical Journal*, 339: 2998.

Hammer, K., Mogensen, O. and Hall, E.O.C. (2009) 'Hope as experienced in women newly diagnosed with gynaecological cancer', *European Journal of Oncology Nursing*, 13(4): 274–9.

Hanahan, D. and Weinberg, R.A. (2000) 'The hallmarks of cancer', *Cell*, 100(1): 57–70.

Hanahan, D. and Weinberg, R.A. (2011) 'Hallmarks of cancer: the next generation', *Cell*, 144: 646–74.

Hanley, B. (2005) *Research as Empowerment? Report of a Series of Seminars Organised by the Toronto Group*. Joseph Rowntree Foundation. Available from: www.jrf.org.uk/bookshop/eBooks/1859353185.pdf [accessed 16 January 2012].

Hanna, L., Taggart, L. and Cousins, W. (2011) 'Cancer prevention and health promotion for people with intellectual disabilities: an exploratory study of staff knowledge', *Journal of Intellectual Disability Research*, 55(3): 281–91.

Hanoch, Y., Wood S. and Rice T. (2007) 'Bounded rationality, emotions and older adult decision making: not so fast and yet so frugal', *Human Development*, 50: 333–58.

Hanser, S.B., Bauer-Wu, S., Kublcek, L., Healey, M., Manola, J. Hernandez, M. and Bunnell, C. (2006) 'Effects of a music therapy intervention on quality of life and distress in women with metastatic breast cancer', *Journal of the Society for Integrative Oncology*, 4(3): 116–24.

Hanson, E.J. (1994) 'An exploration of the taken-for-granted world of the cancer nurse in relation to stress and the person with cancer', *Journal of Advanced Nursing*, 19: 12–20.

Harakeh, Z., Scholte, R.H., de Vries, H. and Engels, R.C. (2006) 'Association between personality and adolescent smoking', *Addictive Behaviors*, 31(2): 232–45.

Harcourt, D. and Frith, H. (2008) 'Women's experiences of an altered appearance during chemotherapy', *Journal of Health Psychology,* 13(5): 597–606.

Harding, C., Harris, A. and Chadwick, D. (2009) 'Auricular acupuncture: a novel treatment for vasomotor symptoms associated with luteinizing-hormone releasing hormone agonist treatment for prostate cancer', *British Journal of Urology International,* 103(2): 186–90.

Harding, R. and Higginson I.J. (2003) 'What is the best way to help caregivers in cancer and palliative care? A systematic review of interventions and their effectiveness', *Palliative Medicine,* 17: 63–74.

Hardy, S. and Thomas, B. (2012) 'Mental and physical health comorbidity: political imperatives and practice implications', *International Journal of Mental Health Nursing,* 21: 289–98.

Harris, E.C. and Barraclough, B. (1998) 'Excess mortality of mental disorder', *British Journal of Psychiatry,* 173: 11–53.

Harris, J., Hay, J., Kuniyuki, A., Asgan, M., Press, N. and Bowen, D. (2010) 'Using a family system approach to investigate cancer risk communication with melanoma families', *Psychooncology,* 19: 1102–11.

Harris, J. and Huntington, A. (2001) 'Emotions as analytic tools: qualitative research, feelings and psychotherapeutic insight', in K. Gilbert (ed.), *The Emotional Nature of Qualitative Research.* Boca Raton, FL: CRC Press LLC. pp. 129–45.

Harris, R., Probst, H., Beardmore, C., James, S., Dumbleton, C., Bolderston, A., Faithfull, S., Wells. M. and Southgate, E. (2012) 'Radiotherapy skin care: a survey of practice in the UK', *Radiography,* 18: 21–7.

Harrison, J., Maquire, P., Ibbotson, T., Macleod, R. and Hopwood, P. (1994) 'Concerns, confiding and psychiatric disorder in newly diagnosed cancer patients: a descriptive study', *Psycho-oncology,* 3: 173–9.

Harrison, J.A., Mullen, P.D. and Green, L.W. (1992) 'A meta-analysis of studies of the Health Belief Model with adults', *Health Education Research,* 7(1): 107–16. doi:10.1093/her/7.1.107.

Harrison, J.D., Young, J.M., Price, M.A., Butow, P.N. and Solomon, M.J. (2009) 'What are the unmet supportive care needs of people with cancer? A systematic review', *Supportive Care in Cancer,* 17(8): 1117–28.

Harvie, M., Hooper, L. and Howell, A. H. (2003) 'Central obesity and breast cancer risk: a systematic review', *Obesity Reviews,* 4(3): 157–73.

Haveman, M., Heller, T., Lee, L., Maaskant, M., Shooshtari, S. and Strydom, A. (2009) *Report on the State of Science on Health Risks and Ageing in People with Intellectual Disabilities.* University of Dortmund, IASSID Special Interest Research Group on Ageing and Intellectual Disabilities/ Faculty Rehabilitation Sciences.

Haviland, J., Owen, J.R., Dewar, J., Agrawal, R., Barrett, J., Barrett-Lee, P., Dobbs, H.J., Hopwood, P., Lawton, P., Magee, B., Mills, J., Simmons, S., Syndenham, M., Venables, K., Bliss, J. and Yarnold, J. (2013) 'The UK Standardisation of Breast Radiotherapy (START) trials of radiotherapy hypofractionation for treatment of early breast cancer: 10-year follow-up of two randomised controlled trials', *The Lancet Oncology,* 14(11): 1086–94.

Hayes, S.C. (ed) (1989) *Rule-Governed Behavior.* New York, NY: Plenum Publishing Corporation.

Hayes, S.C. (2002) 'Acceptance, mindfulness, and science', *Clinical Psychology Science and Practice,* 9(1): 101–6.

Hayes, S.C., Barnes-Holmes, D. and Roche, B. (2001) *Relational Frame Theory: A Post-Skinnerian Account of Human Language and Cognition.* New York: Plenum Publishers.

Hayes, S.C. and Gifford, E. (1997) 'The trouble with language: experiential avoidance, rules, and the nature of verbal events', *Psychological Science,* 8(3): 170.

Hayes, S.C., Luoma, J.B., Bond, F.W., Masuda, A. and Lillis, J. (2006) 'Acceptance and Commitment Therapy: model, processes and outcomes', *Behaviour Research and Therapy,* 44(1): 1–25.

Hayes, S.C., Strosahl, K.D. and Wilson, K.G. (2011) *Acceptance and Commitment Therapy: The Process and Practice of Mindful Change,* 2nd edn. New York, NY: Guilford Press.

Health and Care Professions Council (HCPC) (2013) *Standards of Proficiency: Radiographers.* HCPC. Available from: www.hpc-uk.org/assets/documents/10000dbdstandards_of_proficiency_radiographers.pdf [accessed 3 November 2014].

Health and Social Care Information Centre (2012) *National Head and Neck Cancer Audit 2011.* Available from: www.ic.nhs.uk/canceraudits [accessed]

Health Professionals Council (2008) *Standards of Conduct, Performance and Ethics,* 2nd edn. Available from: www.hpc-uk.org/publications/index.asp?id=38 [accessed 18 November 2014].

Health Protection Agency (2011) *Risk of Solid Cancer following Radiation Exposure. Estimates in the UK Population.* Report of the Independent Advisory Group of Ionising Radiation. Available from: www.gov.uk/government/uploads/system/uploads/attachment_data/file/334311/RCE-19_for_website_v2.pdf [accessed 6 November 2014].

Health Quality Ontario (2010) 'Robotic-assisted minimally invasive surgery for gynecologic and urologic oncology: an evidence-based analysis', *Ontario Health Technology Assessment Series,* 10: 1–118.

Heath, J.A. and Ross, J.A. (2010) 'Epidemiology of cancer in childhood', in W. Carroll, and J.L. Finlay (eds), *Cancer in Children and Adolescents.* New York, NY: Jones and Bartlett. pp. 3–34.

Heaven, C.M., Clegg, J. and Maguire P. (2006) 'Transfer of communication skills training from workshop to workplace: the impact of clinical supervision', *Patient Education and Counseling,* 60: 313–25.

Heaven, C.M. and Maguire, P. (1993) *Assessing Patients with Cancer: The Content, Skills And Process Of Assessment.* Cancer Research UK.

Heaven, C.M. and Maguire, P. (1997) 'Disclosure and identification of hospice patients' concerns', *Palliative Medicine,* 11: 283–90.

Heaven, C.M., Maguire P. and Green C. (2003) 'A patient-centred approach to defining and assessing interviewing competency', *Epidemiologia e Psichiatria Sociale,* 12: 86–91.

Hedrick, T.L., Sawyer, R.G., Hennessy, S.A., Turrentine, F.E. and Friel, C.M. (2014) 'Can we define surgical site infection accurately in colorectal surgery?', *Surgical Infections,* 15(4): 372–376.

Hegarty, P., Kayes, O., Freeman, A., Christopher, N., Ralph, D. and Minhas, S. (2006) 'A prospective study of 100 cases of penile cancer managed according to European Association of Urology guidelines', *British Journal of Urology International,* 98: 526–31.

Hellwig, J (2011) 'Sex after cancer: many women want medical help', *Nursing for Women's Health,* 15(2): 103–8.

Helms, R,. O'Hea, E.L. and Corso, M. (2008) 'Body image issues in women with breast cancer', *Psychology, Health & Medicine,* 13(3): 313–25.

Hemminki, K. and Mutanen, P. (2001) 'Parental cancer as a risk factor for nine common childhood malignancies', *British Journal of Cancer,* 84(7): 990–3.

Henderson, S. (2003) 'Power imbalance between nurses and patients: a potential inhibitor of partnership care', *Journal of Clniical Nursing,* 12(4): 501–8.

Henoch, I. and Danielson, E. (2009) 'Existential concerns among patients with cancer and interventions to meet them: an integrative literature review', *Psycho-oncology,* 18(3): 225–36.

Heritage J., Robinson, J., Elliot, M., Beckett, M. and Wilkes, M. (2007) 'Reducing patients' unmet concerns in primary care: the difference one word can make', *Journal of General Internal Medicine,* 22(10): 1429–33.

Her Majesty's Government (2011) *House of Commons Committee of Public Accounts: Delivering the Cancer Reform Strategy.* London: The Stationery Office.

Herschbach, P., Berg, P., Dankert, A., Duran, G., Engst-Hastreiter, U., Waadt, S., Keller, M., Ukat, R. and Henrich, G. (2005) 'Fear of progression in chronic diseases: psychometric properties of the Fear of Progression Questionnaire', *Journal of Psychosomatic Research,* 58(6): 505–11.

Hesketh, P.J. (2008) 'Chemotherapy-Induced nausea and vomiting', *The New England Journal of Medicine,* 358(23): 2482–94.

Hesketh, R. (2013) *Introduction to Cancer Biology.* Cambridge: Cambridge University Press.

Heslop, P., Blair, P., Fleming, P., Hoghton, M., Marriott, A. and Russ, L. (2013) *Confidential Inquiry into Premature Deaths of People with Learning Disabilities (CIPOLD).* Bristol. Available from: www.bris.ac.uk/cipold/reports/index.html [accessed 17 November 2014].

Hewitson, P., Glasziou, P., Watson, E., Towler, B. and Irwig, L. (2008) 'Cochrane Systematic Review of colorectal cancer screening using the fecal occult blood test (hemoccult): an update', *American Journal of Gastroenterology,* 103(6): 1541–9.

Hewitt, M., Greenfield S and Stovall E (eds), (2005) *From Cancer Patient to Cancer Survivor: Lost in Transition.* Washington, DC: National Academies Press.

Hewitt, M., Rowland, J.H. and Yancik, R. (2003) 'Cancer survivors in the United States: age, health and disability', *Journals of Gerontology Series A,* 58(1): 82–91.

Heyn, L., Ruland C.M. and Finset, A. (2012) 'Effects of an interactive tailored patient assessment tool on eliciting and responding to cancer patients' cues and concerns in clinical consultations with physicians and nurses', *Patient Education & Counseling,* 86: 158–65.

Heywood, K. (2003) 'Introducing Art Therapy into the Christie Hospital Manchester UK 2001–2002', *Complementary Therapies in Nursing and Midwifery,* 9: 125–32.

Hickok, J.T., Roscoe, J.A., Morrow, G.R., King, D.K., Atkins, J.N. and Fitch, T.R. (2003) 'Nausea and emesis remain significant problems of chemotherapy despite prophylaxis with 5-hydroxytriptamine-3 antiemetics', *Cancer,* 97(11): 2880–86.

Hickok, J.T., Roscoe, J.A., Morrow, G.R., Mustian, K., Okunieff, P., Bole, C.W. (2005) 'Frequency, severity, clinical course and correlates of fatigue in 372 patients during 5 weeks of radiotherapy for cancer', *Cancer,* 104(8): 1772–8.

Higgins, M.J. and Baselga, J. (2011) 'Targeted therapies for breast cancer', *Journal of Clinical Investigation,* 121(10): 3797–803.

Hilarius, D.L., Kloeg, P.H., Gundy, C.M. and Aaronson, N.K. (2008) 'Use of health-related quality-of-life assessments in daily clinical oncology nursing practice: a community hospital-based intervention study', *Cancer,* 113(3): 628–37.

Hill, S. (2003) *PROCEED: Responding to the Needs of People with Cancer from Minority Ethnic Communities.* Cancer Research UK (CERP Portal).

Hilliard, R.E. (2003) 'The effects of music therapy on the quality and length of life of people diagnosed with terminal cancer', *Journal of Music Therapy,* 40(2): 113–37.

Hilton, S. and Hunt, K. (2010) 'Coverage of Jade Goody's cervical cancer in UK newspapers: a missed opportunity for health promotion?', *Bio Med Central Public Health,* 10: 368.

Hinchliff, S., Gott, M. and Galena, E. (2005) '"I daresay I might find it embarrassing": general practitioners' perspectives on discussing sexual health issues with lesbian and gay patients', *Health and Social Care in the Community,* 13: 345–53.

Hinsley, R. and Hughes, R. (2007) '"The reflections you get": an exploration of body image and cachexia', *International Journal of Palliative Nursing,* 13(2): 84–9.

Hinton, J. (1994) 'Can home care maintain an acceptable quality of life for patients with terminal cancer and their relatives?', *Palliative Medicine,* 8: 183–96.

Hippisley-Cox, J., Vinogradova, Y., Coupland, C. and Parker, C. (2007) 'Risk of malignancy in patients with schizophrenia or bipolar disorder. Nested case-control study', *Archives of General Pyschiatry,* 64(12): 1368–76.

Hirschfeld, R., Williams, J., Spitzer, R., Calabrese, J., Flynn, L., Keck, P., et al. (2000) 'Development and validation of screening instrument for bipolar spectrum disorder: the mood disorder questionnaire', *American Journal of Psychiatry,* 157: 1873–5.

Hjort Jakobsen, D., Rud, K., Kehlet, H. and Egerod, I. (2014) 'Standardising fast-track surgical nursing care in Denmark', *British Journal of Nursing,* 23: 471–6.

Hobfoll, S.E. (1989) 'Conservation of resources: a new attempt at conceptualizing stress', *American Psychologist,* 44(3): 513–24.

Hochberg, J., Waxman, I.M., Kelly, K.M., Morris, E. and Cairo, M.S. (2009) 'Adolescent non-Hodgkin lymphoma and Hodgkin lymphoma: state of the science', *British Journal of Haematology,* 144(1): 24–40.

Hochschild, A.R. (1983) *The Managed Heart.* Berkeley, CA: University of California Press.

Hodges, L.J. and Humphris, G.M. (2009) 'Fear of recurrence and psychological distress in head and neck cancer patients and their carers', *Psycho-oncology* 18: 841–8.

Hodges, L.J., Humphris, G.M. and Macfarlane, G. (2005) 'A meta-analytic investigation of the relationship between the psychological distress of cancer patients and their carers', *Social Science & Medicine,* 60: 1–12.

Hodgkinson, K., Butow, P., Hobbs, K.M., Hunt, G.E., Lo, S.K. and Wain, G. (2007) 'Assessing unmet supportive care needs in partners of cancer survivors: the development and evaluation of the cancer survivors' partners unmet needs measure (CaSPUN)', *Psycho-oncology,* 16: 805–13.

Hodgson, R., Wildgust, H.J. and Bushe, C.J. (2010) 'Cancer and schizophrenia: is there a paradox?', *Journal of Psychopharmacology,* 24(11): 51–60.

Hodkinson, S., Bunt, L. and Daykin, N. (2014) 'Music therapy in children's hospices: an evaluative survey of provision', *The Arts in Psychotherapy,* 41(5): 570–576.

Hoey, L.M., Ieropoli, S.C., White, V.M. and Jefford, M. (2008) 'Systematic review of peer-support programs for people with cancer', *Patient Education and Counseling,* 70: 315–37.

Hoffbrand, A.V. and Moss, P.A.H. (2011) *Essential Haematology,* 6th edn. Chichester, UK: Wiley-Blackwell.

Hoffman, C.J., Ersser, S.J., Hopkinson, J.B., Nicholls, P.G., Harrington, J.E. and Thomas, P.W. (2012) 'Effectiveness of mindfulness-based stress reduction in mood, breast- and endocrine-related quality of life, and well-being in stage 0 to III breast cancer: a randomized, controlled trial', *Journal of Clinical Oncology,* 30 (12): 1335–42.

Hofmann, S. and Asmundson, G. (2008) 'Acceptance and mindfulness-based therapy: new wave or old hat?', *Clinical Psychology Review,* 28(1): 1–16.

Hofmann, W., Friese, M. and Wiers, R.W. (2008) 'Impulsive versus reflective influences on health behavior: a theoretical framework and empirical review', *Health Psychology Review,* 2(2): 111–37. doi:10.1080/17437190802617668.

Hogg, J. and Tuffrey-Wijne, I. (2008) 'Cancer and intellectual disabilities: a review of some key contextual issues', *Journal of Applied Research in Intellectual Disabilities,* 21(6): 509–18.

Holland, J.C., Breitbart, W., Dudley, M.M., Fulcher, C., Greiner, C.B., Hoofring, L. et al. (2010) 'Distress management: clinical practice guidelines in oncology', *Journal of the National Comprenhensive Cancer Network,* 8: 448–85.

Holland, J.C., Bultz, B.D. and National Comprehensive Cancer Network (NCCN) (2007) 'The NCCN guideline for distress management: a case for making distress the sixth vital sign', *Journal of the National Comprenhensive Cancer Network,* 5(1): 3–7.

Holland, J.C. and Gooen-Piels, J. (2000) 'Principles of psycho-oncology', in J.C. Holland and E. Frei (eds), *Psychological Care of the Cancer Patient.* New York, NY: Oxford University Press.

Holland, J.M., Neimeyer, R.A., Boelen, P.A. and Prigerson, H.G. (2009) 'The underlying structure of grief: a taxometric investigation of prolonged and normal reactions to loss', *Journal of Psychopathology and Behavioural and Assessment,* 31(3): 190–201.

Hollingworth, W., Harris, S., Metcalfe, C., Mancero, S., Biddle, L., Campbell, R. and Brennan, J. (2012) 'Evaluating the effect of using a distress thermometer and problem list to monitor psychosocial concerns among patients receiving treatment for cancer: preliminary results of a randomised controlled trial', *Psycho-oncology,* 21(S2).

Hollins, S., Attard, M.T., von Fraunhofer, N., McGuigan, S. and Sedgwick, P. (1998) 'Mortality in people with learning disability: risks, causes, and death certification findings in London', *Developmental Medicine & Child Neurology,* 40(1): 50–6.

Hollins, S. and Downer, J. (2000) *Keeping Healthy 'Down Below'.* London: Royal College of Psychiatrists.

Hollins, S. and Perez, W. (2000) *Looking after My Breasts.* London: Gaskell/St George's Hospital Medical School.

Hollins, S. and Wilson, J. (2004) *Looking after My Balls.* London: Gaskell/St George's Hospital Medical School.

Holloway, I. and Todres, L. (2010a) 'Ethnography', in K. Gerrish and A. Lacey (eds), *The Research Process in Nursing.* Chichester: Wiley-Blackwell. pp. 165–76.

Holloway, I. and Todres, L. (2010b) 'Grounded theory', in K. Gerrish and A. Lacey (eds), *The Research Process in Nursing.* Chichester, UK: Wiley-Blackwell. pp. 153–164.

Holloway, I. and Wheeler, S. (2010) *Qualitative Research in Nursing and Healthcare,* 3rd edn. Chichester, UK: Wiley-Blackwell.

Hollstein, M., Sidransky, D., Vogelstein, B. and Harris, C.C. (1991) 'p53 mutations in human cancers,' *Science,* 253: 49–53.

Holmes, T.S. and Rahe, R.H. (1967) 'The Social Readjustment Rating Scale', *Journal of Psychosomatic Research,* 11: 213–18.

Home Office (2010) *Equality Act 2010: Guidance*. Available from: www.gov.uk/equality-act-2010-guidance [accessed 9 December 2013].

Hopkinson, J.B. and Corner, J.L. (2006) 'Helping patients with advanced cancer live with concerns about eating: a challenge for palliative care professionals', *Journal of Pain and Symptom Management*, 31(4): 293–305.

Hopwood, P. (1994) 'The assessment of body image in cancer patients', *European Journal of Cancer*, 29(2): 276–81.

Hordern, A. and Street, A. (2007) 'Communicating about patient sexuality and intimacy after cancer: mismatched expectations and unmet needs', *Medical Journal of Australia*, 186: 224–7.

Horne, B., Gilleece, M., Jackson, G., Snowden, J.A., Liebersbach, S., Velikova, G. and Wright, P. (2013) 'Psychosocial supportive care services for haematopoietic stem cell transplant patients: a service evaluation of three UK transplant centres', *European Journal of Cancer Care*, 23(3): 349–362.

Horne, D. and Watson, M. (2011) 'Cognitive-behavioural therapies in cancer care', in M. Watson and D. Kissane (eds), *Handbook of Psychotherapy in Cancer Care*. Oxford: Wiley-Blackwell Publishers.

Horne, G., Seymour, J. and Payne, S. (2012) 'Maintaining integrity in the face of death: a grounded theory to explain the perspectives of people affected by lung cancer about the expression of wishes for end of life care', *International Journal of Nursing Studies*, 49(6): 718–26.

Hoskin, P. (2006) (ed.) *Radiotherapy in Practice: External Beam Therapy*. Oxford: Oxford University Press.

House of Lords (2000) *House of Lords Select Committee on Science and Technology Report on Complementary and Alternative Medicine (HL Paper 123 2000)*.

Houtzager, B., Grootenhuis, M., Caron, H. and Last, B. (2004) 'Quality of life and psychological adaptation in siblings of paediatric cancer patients, 2 years after diagnosis', *Psycho-oncology*, 13: 499–511.

Howard, L.M., Barley, E.A., Davies, E., Rigg, A., Lempp, H., Rose, D., Taylor, D. and Thornicroft, G. (2010) 'Cancer diagnosis in people with severe mental illness: practical and ethical issues. *Lancet Oncology*, 11: 797–804.

Howell, D., Currie, S. and Mayo, S., et al. (2009) *A Pan-Canadian Clinical Practice Guideline: Psychosocial and Supportive Care of Adults with Cancer. Part I—Psychosocial Health Care Needs Assessment and Screening for Distress*. Toronto: Canadian Association of Psychosocial Oncology, p. 4.

Høybye, M.T., Johansen, C. and Tjørnjhøj-Thomsen, T. (2005) 'Online interaction. effects of storytelling in an Internet breast cancer support group', *Psycho-oncology*, 14: 211–20.

Huang, Z., Hankinson, S.E., Colditz, G.A., et al. (1997) 'Dual effects of weight and weight gain on breast cancer risk', *Journal of the American Medical Association*, 278(17): 1407–11.

Hubbard, G., Backett-Milburn, K. and Kemmer, D. (2001) 'Working with emotion: issues for the researcher in fieldwork and teamwork', *International Journal of Social Research Methodology*, 4(2): 119–37.

Hubbard, G. and Forbat, L. (2012) 'Cancer as biographical disruption: constructions of living with cancer', *Supportive Care in Cancer*, 20(9): 2033–40.

Hubbard, G., Illingworth, N., Rowa-Dewar, N., Forbat, E. and Kearney, N. (2010) 'Treatment decision making in cancer care: the role of the carer,' *Journal of Clinical Nursing*, 19: 2023–31.

Hubbard, G., Kidd, L., Donaghy, E., McDonald, C. and Kearney, N. (2007) 'A review about involving people affected by cancer in research, policy and planning and practice', *Patient Education and Counseling*, 65: 21–33.

Hubbard G. Knighting K. Rowa-Dewar, N Forbat, L. Illingworth, Wilson, Kearney, N. (2007) *People's Experience of Cancer within the First Year Following Diagnosis*. Stirling: University of Stirling.

Hubbard, G., Menzies, S., Flynn, P., Adams, S., Haseen, F., Thomas, I., Scanlon, K., Reed, L. and Forbat, L. (2013) 'Relational mechanisms and psychological outcomes in couples affected by breast cancer: a systematic narrative review of the literature. *British Medical Journal: Supportive and Palliative Care*, 3(3): 309–317.

Hudes G., Carducci, M., Tomczak, P., et al. (2007) 'Temsirolimus, interferon alfa, or both for advanced renal-cell carcinoma', *New England Journal of Medicine*, 356(22): 2271–81.

Hudson, P.A. (2005) 'Critical review of supportive interventions for family caregivers of patients with palliative-stage cancer', *Journal Psychosocial Oncology*, 22(4): 77–92.

Hughes, J.G., Goldbart, J., Fairhurst, E. and Knowles, K. (2007) 'Exploring acupuncturists' perceptions of treating patients with rheumatoid arthritis', *Complementary Therapies in Medicine*, 15: 101–8.

Hughes, J.G. (2009) '"When I first started going I was going in on my knees, but I came out and I was skipping": exploring rheumatoid arthritis patients' perceptions of receiving treatment with acupuncture', *Complementary Therapies in Medicine*, 17: 269–73.

Hulbert-Williams, N.J., Flynn, S., Heaton-Brown, L. and Scanlon, K. (unpublished data) 'Interventions to help improve well-being in breast cancer survivors at the end of active treatment: a systematic review of the literature'.

Hulbert, N.J. and Morrison, V.L. (2006) 'A preliminary study into stress in palliative care: optimism, self-efficacy and social support', *Psychology, Health & Medicine*, 11(2): 246–54.

Hulbert-Williams, N.J., Neal, R.D., Morrison, V., Hood, K. and Wilkinson, C. (2012a) 'Anxiety, depression and quality of life after cancer diagnosis: what psychosocial variables predict how patients adjust?', *Psycho-oncology*, 21(8): 857–67.

Hulbert-Williams, N.J., Hulbert-Williams, S.L., Morrison, V., Neal, R.D. and Wilkinson, C. (2012b) 'The Mini-Mental Adjustment to Cancer Scale: re-analysis of its psychometric properties in a sample of 160 mixed cancer patients', *Psycho-oncology*, 21(7): 792–7.

Hulbert-Williams, N.J., Armes, J., Brown, J., Calman, L., Hubbard, G., Levandowski, J., Nelson, A. and Wright, P. (2012c) 'Developing a nationally collaborative framework for psychosocial oncology research: a review of the UK NCRI Psychosocial Oncology Clinical Studies Group', *Asia–Pacific Journal of Clinical Oncology*, 8(Suppl. S3): 234.

Hulbert-Williams, N.J., Morrison, V., Neal, R.D. and Wilkinson, C. (2013) 'Investigating the cognitive precursors of emotional response to cancer stress: re-testing Lazarus's Transactional Model', *British Journal of Health Psychology*, 18(1): 97–112.

Hulbert-Williams, N.J., Storey, L. and Wilson, K. (2014) 'Psychological interventions for patients with cancer: psychological flexibility and the potential utility of Acceptance and Commitment Therapy', *European Journal of Cancer Care*, online first access.

Hulbert-Williams, N.J. and Owen, R. (2015) 'ACT: Acceptance and Commitment Therapy for cancer patients', in J.C. Holland, W.S. Breitbart, P.B., Jacobsen, et al. (eds), *Psycho-oncology*, 3rd edn. New York, NY: Oxford University Press.

Hummel, S. and Chilcott, J. (2013) *Option Appraisal: Screening for Prostate Cancer – Model Update*. Report to the UK National Screening Committee. March 2013 version 1.0. University of Sheffield School of Health and Related Research (ScHARR).

Hurria , A. and Balducci, L. (2009) *Geriatric Oncology: Treatment, Assessment and Management*. New York: Springer Science and Business Media.

Hunter, M.S., Coventry, S., Hamed, H., Fentiman, I. and Grunfeld, E.A. (2008) 'Evaluation of a group cognitive behavioural intervention for women suffering from menopausal symptoms following breast cancer treatment', *Psycho-oncology*, 18(5): 560–3.

Huynh, T., Alderson, M. and Thompson, M. (2008) 'Emotional labour underlying caring: an evolutionary concept analysis', *Journal of Advanced Nursing*, 64(2): 195–208.

ICH GCP (n.d.) *Good Clinical Practice*. Available from: http://ichgcp.net/ [accessed 5 November 2014].

Idowu, O.E. and Idowu, M.A. (2008) 'Environmental causes of childhood brain tumours', *Journal of African Health Sciences*, 8(1): 1–4.

Illingworth, N., Forbat, L., Hubbard, G. and Kearney, N. (2010) 'The importance of relationships in the experience of cancer: a re-working of the policy ideal of whole-systems working', *European Journal of Oncology Nursing*, 14(1): 23–8.

Inagaki, T., Yasukawa, R., Okazaki, S., Yasuda, H., Kawamukai, T., Utani, E., Hayashida, M., Mizuno, S., Miyaoka, T., Shinno, H. and Horiguchi, J. (2006) 'Factors disturbing treatment for cancer in patients with schizophrenia', *Psychiatry and Clinical Neurosciences*, 60: 327–31.

Incrocci, L. and Jensen, P.T. (2013) 'Pelvic radiotherapy and sexual function in men and women', *Journal of Sexual Medicine Special Issue: Cancer Survivorship and Sexual Health*, 10: 53–64.

Independent UK Panel on Breast Cancer Screening (2012) 'The benefits and harms of breast-cancer screening: an independent review', *Lancet*, 380(9855): 1778–86.

Ingleton, C. and Davies, S. (2004) 'Research and scholarship in palliative care nursing', in S. Payne, J. Seymour and C. Ingleton (eds), *Palliative Care Nursing: Principles & Evidence for Practice*. Maidenhead, UK: Open University Press. pp. 677–96.

Institute for Women's Health (2014) *United Kingdom Collaborative Trial of Ovarian Cancer Screening*. Available from: www.instituteforwomenshealth.ucl.ac.uk/womens-cancer/gcrc/ukctocs [accessed 21 April 2014].

Institute of Medicine (IOM) (2007) *Cancer Care for the Whole Patient: Meeting Psychosocial Health Needs*. Washington, DC: National Academy Press. p. 430.

International Agency for Research on Cancer (IARC) (1988) *IARC Monographs on the Evaluation of Carcinogenic Risks to Humans. Volume 44 Alcohol Drinking*.

International Agency for Research on Cancer (IARC) (2008) *World Cancer Report 2008*. Geneva: World Health Organization Press.

International Agency for Research on Cancer (IARC) (2014) *World Cancer Report 2014*. Geneva: World Health Organization Press.

International Agency for Research on Cancer (IARC) Working Group on the Evaluation of Carcinogenic Risk to Humans (2009) *Personal Habits and Indoor Combustions (Volume 100)*. Geneva: International Agency for Research on Cancer.

International Society of Lymphology (2003) 'The diagnosis and treatment of peripheral lymphedema: a consensus document of the international society of lymphedema', *Lymphology*, 36: 84–91.

Ionising Radiation (Medical Exposure) Regulations 2000 (SI 2000 No 1059). London: HMSO. Available from: www.opsi.gov.uk/si/si2000/20001059.htm [accessed 11 September 2014].

Ionising Radiation (Medical Exposure) (Amendment) Regulations (2006) (SI 2006/2523) London: HMSO. Available from: www.opsi.gov.uk/si/si2006/20062523.htm [accessed 11 September 2014].

Ionising Radiation (Medical Exposure) (Amendment) Regulations (2011) (SI 2011/1567). London: HMSO. Available from: www.legislation.gov.uk/uksi/2011/1567/contents/made [accessed 11 September 2014].

Ipsos MORI for Cancerbacup (2006) *Cancer – A Public Priority? Attitudes Towards Cancer Treatment in Britain*. London: Cancerbacup.

Iqbal, G., Gumber, A., Johnson, M.R.D., Szczepura, A., Wilson, S. and Dunn, J.A. (2009) 'Improving ethnicity data collection for health statistics in the UK,' *Diversity in Health & Care*, 6(4): 267–85.

Iqbal, G., Gumber, A., Szczepura, A., Johnson, M.R.D., Wilson, S. and Dunn, J.A. (2008) *Improving Ethnic Data Collection for Statistics of Cancer Incidence, Management, Mortality and Survival in the UK*. Report for Cancer Research UK. Coventry: Warwick Medical School Clinical Trials Unit. Available from: http://www2.warwick.ac.uk/fac/med/research/csri/ethnicityhealth/research/crc.pdf.

Iredale, R., Brain, K., Williams, B., France, E. and Gray, J. (2006) 'The experiences of men with breast cancer in the United Kingdom. *European Journal of Cancer*, 42: 334–41.

Ireland, M. and Pakenham, K. (2010) 'The nature of youth care tasks in families experiencing chronic illness/disability: development of the Youth Activities of Caregiving Scale (YACS)', *Psychology and Health*, 25(6): 713–31.

Ito, T., Shimizu, K., Ichida, Y. et al (2011) 'Usefulness of pharmacist-assisted screening and psychiatric referral program for outpatients with cancer undergoing chemotherapy', *Psycho-oncology*, 20: 647–54.

Iveson, C. (2002) 'Solution-focused brief therapy', *Advances in Psychiatric Treatment*, 8: 149–56.

Jack, B.A., O'Brien, M.R., Kirton, J.A., Marley, K., Whelan, A., Baldry, C.R. and Groves, K.E. (2013) 'Enhancing communication with distressed patients, families and colleagues: the value of the Simple Skills Secrets model of communication for the nursing and healthcare workforce', *Nurse Education Today*, 33(12): 1550–6.

Jack, R.H., Davies, E.A. Møller, H. (2011) 'Lung cancer incidence and survival in different ethnic groups in South East England', *British Journal of Cancer*, 105(7): 1049–53.

Jacobs, T. (1990) 'There is no age time: early adolescence and its consequences', in S. Dowling (ed.), *Early Adolescence and its Consequences: Its Significance for Clinical Work*. Madison, CT: International Universities Press.

Jacobsen, N.S. and Truax, P. (1991) 'Clinical significance: a statistical approach to defining meaningful change in psychotherapy research', *Journal of Consulting and Clinical Psychology*, 59(1): 12–19.

Jacobsen, P.B. and Ransom, S. (2007) 'Implementation of NCCN distress management guidelines by member institutions', *Journal of the National Comprehensive Cancer Network*, 5: 99–103.

James, A., Daley, C.M. and Greiner, M. (2011) '"Cutting" on cancer: attitudes about cancer spread and surgery among primary care patients in the USA', *Social Science and Medicine*, 73(11): 1669–1673.

James, K., Keegan-Wells, D., Hinds, P., Kelly, K., Bond, D., Hall, B., Mahan, R., Moore, I., Roll, L. and Speckhart, B. (2002) 'The care of my child with cancer: parents' perceptions of caregiving demands', *Journal of Pediatric Oncology Nursing*, 19: 218.

Jamrozik, K. (2005) 'Estimate of deaths attributable to passive smoking among UK adults: database analysis. *British Medical Journal*, 330(7495): 812.

Janaki, M.G., Kadam, A.R., Mukesh, S., Nirmala, S., Ponni, A., Ramesh B.S. and Rajeev, A.G. (2010) 'Magnitude of fatigue in cancer patients receiving radiotherapy and its short term effects on quality of life', *Journal of Cancer Research and Therapeutics*, 6(1): 22–6.

Jancar, J. (1990) 'Cancer and mental handicap: a further study', *British Journal of Psychiatry*, 156: 531–3.

Jansen, J., van Weert, J., deGroot, J., van Dulmen, S., Heeren, T. and Bensing, J. (2010) 'Emotional and informational patient cues: the impact of nurses' responses on recall', *Patient Education and Counseling*, 79(2): 218–24.

Janssen, A.L. and Macleod, R.D. (2010) 'What can people approaching death teach us about how to care', *Patient Education and Counseling*, 8: 251–6.

Jarvis, A. (2003) 'Transforming the patient experience in radiation therapy', *Radiology Management*, 25(6): 34–6.

Jefford, M., Karahalios, E., Pollard, A., Baravelli, C., Carey, M., Franklin, J., Aranda, S. and Schofield, P. (2008) 'Survivorship issues following treatment completion: results from focus groups with Australian cancer survivors and health professionals', *Journal of Cancer Survivorship*, 2(1): 20–32.

Jenkinson, C., Coulter, A. and Bruser, S. (2002) 'The Picker Patient Experience Questionnaire: development and validation using data from in-patient surveys in five countries', *International Journal for Quality in Health Care*, 14(5): 353–8.

Jim, H.S.L., Syrjala, K.L. and Rizzo, D. (2012) 'Supportive care of hematopoietic cell transplant patients', *Biology of Blood and Marrow Transplantation*, 18: S12–S16.

Johnson, B. and Clarke, J.M. (2003) 'Collecting sensitive data: the impact on researchers', *Qualitative Health Research*, 13(3): 421–434.

Johnson, M.R.D. (2008) 'Making difference count: ethnic monitoring in health (and social care)', *Radical Statistics*, 96: 38–45.

Johnson, M.R.D. (2012) 'Making diversity count: equality and diversity monitoring', *Diversity & Equality in Health & Care*, 9(4): 291–6.

Johnson, M.R.D. (2012a) 'Communication in cross-cultural cancer care', *Nursing Times*, 10 August. Available from: www.nursingtimes.net/nursing-practice/clinical-zones/cancer/communication-in-cross-cultural-cancer-care/5048153.article?blocktitle=This-Week's-Practice&contentID=4386

Johnson, N. (2009) 'The role of self and emotion within qualitative sensitive research: a reflective account', *ENQUIRE*, 4: 23–50.

Johnston, W. T., Lightfoot, T.J. and Simpson, J. (2010) 'Childhood cancer survival rates: a report from the United Kingdom Childhood Cancer Study', *Cancer Epidemiology*, 34(6): 659–666.

Joint Committee on Human Rights (2007) *The Human Rights of Older People in Healthcare.* Available from: www.publications.parliament.uk/pa/jt200607/jtselect/jtrights/156/156i.pdf [accessed 9 December 2013].

Jones, A., Tuffrey-Wijne, I., Bernal, J., Butler, G. and Hollins, S. (2007) 'Meeting the cancer information needs of people with learning disabilities: experiences of paid carers', *British Journal of Learning Disabilities,* 35(1): 12–18.

Jones, F.M.E., Fellows, J.L., Horne, DJ. (2011) 'Coping with cancer: a brief report on stress and coping strategies in medical students dealing with cancer patients', *Psycho-oncology,* 20: 219–23.

Jones, G. (2000) 'An art therapy group in palliative care', *Nursing Times,* (10): 42–43.

Jones, G.D.D. and Symonds, P. (2012) 'Molecular, cellular and tissue effects of radiotherapy', in P. Symonds, C. Deehan, J.A. Mills and C. Meredith (eds), *Walter and Miller's Textbook of Radiotherapy,* 7th edn. London: Elsevier Churchill Livingstone. pp. 279–92.

Jones, J.M., Cheng, T., Jackman, M., Walton, T., Haines, S., Rodin, G. and Catton, P. (2011) 'Getting back on track: evaluation of a brief group psychoeducation intervention for women completing primary treatment for breast cancer', *Psycho-oncology,* 22(1): 117–24.

Jones, L.E. and Doebbeling CC. (2007) 'Suboptimal depression screening following cancer diagnosis', *General Hospital Psychiatry,* 29: 547–54.

Jones, P., Blunda, M., Biegel, G., Carlson, L.E., Biel, M. and Wiener, L. (2013) 'Can mindfulness-based interventions help adolescents with cancer?', *Psycho-oncology,* 22(9): 1–6.

Jones, R.P., Vauthey, J.-N., Adam, R., Rees, M., Berry, D., Jackson, R., Grimes, N., Fenwick, S.W., Poston, G.J. and Malik, H.Z. (2012) 'Effect of specialist decision-making on treatment strategies for colorectal liver metastases', *British Journal of Surgery,* 99, 1263–9.

Jones, S., Howard, L. and Thornicroft, G. (2008) 'Diagnostic overshadowing: worse physical health care for people with mental illness', *Acta Psychiatrica Scandinavica,* 118(3): 169–71.

Joseph, F., Woodward, A. and Reynolds, J. (2011) *The Continuum Companion to Existentialism.* London: Continuum.

Joseph Rowntree Foundation (2012) *Monitoring Poverty and Social Exclusion 2012.* Available from: www.jrf.org.uk/publications/monitoring-poverty-2012?gclid=CIji_b72p7sCFW_Mt AodSgYAUg [accessed 9 December 2013].

Joyce, M. (2013) 'Dyspnoea', in C.H. Yarbro, D. Wujcik and B.H. Gobel (eds), *Cancer Symptom Management,* 4th edn. Burlington, VT: Jones and Bartlett Learning. pp. 317–29.

Junejo, M.A., Mason, J.M., Sheen, A.J., Bryan, A., Moore, J., Foster, P., Atkinson, D., Parker, M.J. and Siriwardena, A.K. (2014) 'Cardiopulmonary exercise testing for preoperative risk assessment before pancreaticoduodenectomy for cancer', *Annals of Surgical Oncology,* 21(6): 1929–1936.

Jung, C.G. (1978) *Man and his Symbols.* London: Picador.

Juslin, P.N. and Sloboda, J.A. (eds) (2010) *Handbook of Music and Emotion: Theory, Research, Applications.* Oxford: Oxford University Press.

Kaatsch, P., Spinx, C., Schulze-Rath, R., Schmieda, S. and Blettner, M. (2008) 'Leukaemia in young children living in the vicinity of German nuclear power plants', *International Journal of Cancer,* 15: 721–726.

Kabat-Zinn, J. (1990) *Full Catastrophe Living.* London: Delta.

Kabat-Zinn, J. (1994) *Wherever You Go, There You Are.* New York, NY: Hyperion.

Kabat-Zinn, J. (2003) 'Mindfulness-based interventions in context: past, present, and future', *Clinical Psychology: Science and Practice,* 10(2): 144–56.

Kabat-Zinn, J. (2013) *Full Catastrophe Living. Using the Wisdom of Your Body and Mind to Face Stress, Pain, and Illness.* London: Bantam.

Kai, J., Beavan, J. and Faull, C. (2011) 'Challenges of mediated communication, disclosure and autonomy in cross-cultural cancer care', *British Journal of Cancer,* 105(7): 918–24.

Karasek, R.A. (1979) 'Job demands, job decision latitude, and mental strain: implications for job redesign', *Administrative Science Quarterly,* 24(2): 285–308.

Karbani, G., Lim, J.N.W., Hewison, J., Atkin, K., Horgan, K., Lansdown, M. and Chu, C.E. (2011) 'Culture, attitude and knowledge about breast cancer and preventive measures: a qualitative study of South Asian breast cancer patients in the UK', *Asian Pacific Journal of Cancer Prevention,* 12(6): 1619–26.

Karnilowicz, W. (2011) 'Identity and psychological ownership in chronic illness and disease state', *European Journal of Cancer,* 20(2): 276–82.

Kay, M.A., Glorioso, J.C., Naldini, L. (2001) 'Viral vectors for gene therapy: the art of turning infectious agents into vehicles of therapeutics', *Nature Medicine,* 7: 33–40.

Kearney, N., Miller, M., Paul, J., Smith, K. and Rice, A.M. (2003) 'Oncology health care professionals attitudes to cancer: a professional concern', *Annals of Oncology,* 14: 57–61.

Kedge, E.M. (2009) 'A systematic review to investigate the effectiveness and acceptability of interventions for moist desquamation in radiotherapy patients', *Radiotherapy,* 15(3): 247–57.

Keely (2000) 'Classification of lymphodoema', in R. Twycross, K. Jenns and J. Todd (eds), *Lymphoedema.* Abingdon: Radcliffe Medical Press Ltd. pp.22–43.

Keen, A. and Lennan, E. (2011) *Women's Cancers.* Oxford: Wiley.

Keeney, S., McKenna, H., Fleming, P. and McIlfatrick, S. (2010) 'Attitudes to cancer and cancer prevention: what do people aged 35–54 years think?' *European Journal of Cancer Care,* 19: 769–77.

Kehlet, H. and Wilmore, D.W. (2008) 'Evidence-based surgical care and the evolution of fast-track surgery', *Annals of Surgery,* 248: 189–98.

Kelly, D. (2004) 'Male sexuality and prostate cancer in theory and practice', *Nursing Clinics of North America,* 39: 341–57.

Kelly, D. (2013) 'Developing age appropriate psychosexual support for adolescent cancer survivors: a discussion paper', *Journal of Sexual Medicine,* 10(S1): 133–8.

Kelly, D. and Gibson F. (eds) (2008) *Cancer Care for Adolescents and Young Adults.* Oxford: Blackwell-Wiley.

Kelly, D., Pearce, S and Mullhall, A (2004) '"Being in the same boat": ethnographic insights into an adolescent cancer unit', *International Journal of Nursing Studies,* 41: 847–57.

Kelly, D., White, I., Marshall-Lucette, S. and Forbat, L. (2010) *The Private Side of Prostate Cancer: A Study of the Impact on Couples.* Final report to Macmillan Cancer Support. London.

Kelly, R.S., Patnick, J., Kitchener, H.C., Moss, S.M. on behalf of the NHSCSP HPV Special Interest Group (2011) 'HPV testing as a triage for borderline or mild dyskaryosis on cervical cytology: results from the Sentinel Sites study', *British Journal of Cancer,* 105(7): 983–8.

Kendall, M., Boyd, K., Sheikh, A., Murray, S.A, Brown, D., Mallinson, I., Kearney, N. and Worth, A. (2007) 'Key challenges and ways forward in researching the "good death": qualitative in-depth interview and focus group study', *British Medical Journal,* 334(7592): 521–6.

Kennard, B.D., Smith, S.M., Olvera, R., et al. (2004) 'Nonadherence in adolescent oncology patients: preliminary data on psychological risk factors and relationships to outcome', *Journal of Clinical Psychology in Medical Settings,* 11: 30–9.

Kennedy, A., Reeves, D., Bower, P., Lee, V., Middleton, E., Richardson, G., Gardner, C., Gately, C. and Rogers, A. (2007) 'The effectiveness and cost effectiveness of a national lay-led self care support programme for patients with long-term conditions: a pragmatic randomised controlled trial', *Journal of Epidemiology and Community Health,* 61(3): 254–61.

Kennedy, F., Hicks, B. and Yarker, J. (2013) 'Work stress and cancer researchers: an exploration of the challenges, experiences and training needs of UK cancer researchers', *European Journal of Cancer Care,* 23(4): 462–71.

Kerr, I.B. and Ryle, A. (2006) 'Cognitive analytic therapy', in S. Bloch (ed.), *An Introduction to the Psychotherapies,* 4th edn. Oxford: Oxford University Press. pp. 267–86.

Key, J., Hodgson, S., Omar, R.Z., et al. (2006) 'Meta-analysis of studies of alcohol and breast cancer with consideration of the methodological issues', *Cancer Causes Control,* 17(6): 759–70.

Kidd, J. and Finlayson, M. (2006) 'Navigating uncharted water: research ethics and emotional engagement in human inquiry', *Journal of Psychiatric and Mental Health Nursing,* 13: 423–28.

Kim, C., McGlynn, K.A., McCorkle, R., Li, Y., Erickson, R.L., Ma, S., Niebuhr, D.W., Zhang, G., Zhang, Y., Bai, Y., Dai, L., Graubard, B.I., Zheng, T., Aschebrook-Kilfoy, B., Barry, K.H. and Zhang, Y. (2012) 'Sexual functioning among testicular cancer survivors: a case-control study in the US', *Journal of Psychosomatic Research,* 73(1): 68–73.

Kim, S.S., Kaplowitz, S. and Johnston, M.V. (2004) 'The effect of patient empathy on patient satisfaction and compliance', *Evaluation and the Health Professions,* 27(3): 237–51.

Kim, Y., Carver, C.S., Rocha-Lima, C. and Shaffer, K.M. (2013) 'Depressive symptoms among caregivers of colorectal cancer patients during the first year since diagnosis: a longitudinal investigation', *Psycho-Oncology,* 22 (2): 362–367.

King, C.R. (1997) 'Nonpharmacological management of chemotherapy-induced nausea and vomiting', *Oncology Nursing Forum,* 24(7): 41–8.

King, M., Marston, L. and Bower, P. (2013) 'Comparison of non-directive counselling and cognitive behaviour therapy for patients presenting in general practice with an ICD-10 depressive episode: a randomized control trial', *Psychological Medicine,* online first access.

King, R.J.B. and Robins, M.W. (2006) *Cancer Biology,* 3rd edn. London: Pearson Education.

Kings Fund (2013) *Experience-Based Co-Design Toolkit.* Available from: www.kingsfund.org.uk/projects/ebcd [accessed 9 December 2013].

Kirchheiner, K., Czajka, A., Ponocny-Seliger, E., Lütgendorf-Caucig, C., Schmid, M.P., Komarek, E., Pötter R. and Dörr, W. (2013) 'Physical and psychosocial support requirements of 1,500 patients starting radiotherapy', *Strhlentherapie und Onkologie,* 189(5): 424–9.

Kisely, S., Sadek, J., MacKenzie, A., Lawrence, D. and Campbell, L.A. (2008) 'Excess cancer mortality in psychiatric patients', *The Canadian Journal of Psychiatry,* 53(11): 753–60.

Kissane, D. and Bloch, S. (2002) *Family Focused Grief Therapy: A Model of Family-Centred Care during Palliative Care and Bereavement.* Maidenhead, UK: Open University Press.

Kitzinger, J. (2006) 'Focus groups', in C. Pope and N. Mays (eds), *Qualitative Research In Health Care,* 3rd edn. Malden, MA: Blackwell Publishing Ltd.

Klass, D., Silverman, P.R. and Nickman, S.L. (1996) *Continuing Bonds: New Understandings of Grief.* Washington, DC: Taylor and Francis.

Klein, R., Dean, A. and Bogdonoff, M. (1967) 'The impact of illness upon the spouse', *Journal of Chronic Diseases,* 20: 241–8.

Klein, S., Tracy D., Kitchener, H.C. and Walker, L.G. (1999) 'The effects of the participation of patients with cancer in teaching communication skills to medical undergraduates: a randomised study with follow-up after 2 years', *European Journal of Cancer,* 36(2): 1448–56.

Klinkhammer-Schalke, M., Koller, M., Steinger, B., Ehret, C., Ernst, B., Wyatt, J.C., Hofstädter, F., Lorenz, W. and Regensburg QoL Study Group. (2012) 'Direct improvement of quality of life using a tailored quality of life diagnosis and therapy pathway: randomised trial in 200 women with breast cancer', *British Journal of Cancer,* 106(5): 826–38.

Kluin, P. and Schuuring, E. (2011) 'Molecular cytogenetics of lymphoma: where do we stand in 2010?', *Histopathology,* 58: 128–44.

Knols, R., Aaronson, N.K., Uebelhart, D., Fransen, J. and Aufdemkampe, G. (2005) 'Physical exercise in cancer patients during and after medical treatment: a systematic review of randomized and controlled clinical trials', *Journal of Clinical Oncology,* 23(16): 3830–42.

Koehler, K. (2010) 'Helping families help bereaved children', in C.A. Corr and D.E. Balk (eds) *Children's Encounters with Death, Bereavement and Coping.* New York: Springer. pp. 311–336.

Koen, M.P., Van Eeden, C. and Wissing, M.P. (2011) 'The prevalence of resilience in a group of professional nurses. *Health South Africa Gesondheid,* 16(1): 1–11.

Koenig, H.G., King, D.E. and Carson, V.B. (2012) *Handbook of Religion and Health.* Oxford: Oxford University Press.

Koffman, J., Morgan, M., Edmonds, P., Speck, P. and Higginson, I.J. (2008) '"I know he controls cancer": the meanings of religion among Black Caribbean and White British patients with advanced cancer', *Social Science Medicine,* 67(5): 780–9.

Koh, Y.-X., Chok, A.-Y., Zheng, H.-L., Tan, C.-S., Goh, B.K.P. (2014) 'Systematic review and meta-analysis comparing the surgical outcomes of invasive intraductal papillary mucinous neoplasms and conventional pancreatic ductal adenocarcinoma', *Annals of Surgical Oncology,* 21(8): 2782–2800.

Kohara, I. and Inoue, T. (2010) 'Searching for a way to live to the end: decision making process in patients considering participation in cancer phase I clinical trials. *Oncology Nursing Forum,* 37(2): 124–32.

Korfage, I.J., Fuhrel-Forbis, A., Ubel, P.A., et al. (2013) 'Informed choice about breast cancer prevention: randomized controlled trial of an online decision aid intervention', *Breast Cancer Research,* 15(5): R74.

Kotkamp-Mothes, N., Slawinsky, D., Hindermann, S. and Strauss, B. (2005) 'Coping and psychological wellbeing in families of elderly cancer patients', *Critical Reviews in Oncology-Hematology,* 55: 213–29.

Kovács, M., Kovács, E. and Hegedűs, K. (2010) 'Is emotional dissonance more prevalent in oncology care? Emotion work, burnout and coping', *Psycho-oncology,* 19: 855–62.

Kovar, H. and Izraeli, S. (2012) 'The biology of cancer in children', in M.C.G. Stevens, C.N. Hubert and A. Biondi (eds), *Cancer in Children: Clinical Management,* 6th edn. Oxford University Press: Oxford. pp. 14–35.

Kulkarni, K.P. and Marwaha, R.K.M., (2011) 'Childhood acute lymphoblastic leukemia: need of a national population based registry', *Indian Pediatrics,* 48(10): 841.

Kozachik, S.L., Given, C.W., Given, B.A., et al. (2001) 'Improving depressive symptoms among cargivers of patients with cancer: results of a randomised clinical trial', *Oncology Nursing Forum,* 28: 1149–57.

Kralik, D., Koch, T., Price, K. and Howard N. (2004) 'Chronic illness self-management: taking action to create order', *Journal of Clinical Nursing,* 13(2): 259–267.

Kravdal, O. (2001) 'The impact of marital status on cancer survival', *Social Science & Medicine,* 52(3): 357–68.

Kristeller, J.L., Sheets, V., Johnson, T. and Frank, B. (2011) 'Understanding religious and spiritual influences on adjustment to cancer: individual patterns and differences', *Journal of Behavioral Medicine,* 34(6): 550–61.

Kristjanson, L.J., Chalmers, K.I. and Woodgate, R. (2004) 'Information and support needs of adolescent children of women with breastcancer', *Oncology Nursing Forum,* 31: 111–9.

Kristjanson, L.J. and Coyle N. (2010) 'Qualitative research', in G. Hanks et al., (eds), *Oxford Textbook of Palliative Medicine,* 4th edn. Oxford: Oxford University Press.

Kroenke, K., Spitzer RL, Williams JBW. (2003) 'The Patient Health Questionnaire-2: validity of a two-item screener', *Medical Care,* 41: 1284–92.

Kua, J. (2005) 'The prevalence of psychological and psychiatric sequelae of cancer in the elderly: how much do we know?', *Annals Academic Medicine Singapore,* 34(3): 250–6.

Kuchinski, A.M., Reading, M. and Lash, A.A. (2009) 'Treatment related fatigue and exercise in patients with cancer: a systematic review', *Medsurg Nursing,* 18(3): 174–80.

Kuijer, R.G., Ybema, J.F., Buunk, B.P., Maiella De Jong, G., Thijs-Boer, F. and Sanderman, R. (2000) 'Active engagement, protective buffering, and overprotection: three ways of giving support by intimate partners of patients with cancer', *Journal of Social and Clinical Psychology,* 19(2): 256–275.

Kumar, A., Puri, R., Gadgil, P.V. and Jatoi, I. (2012) 'Sentinel lymph node biopsy in primary breast cancer: window to management of the axilla', *World Journal of Surgery,* 36: 1453–59.

Kupka, R.W., Altshuler, L.L., Nolen, W.A., Suppes, T., Luckenbaugh, D.A., Leverich, G.S., Frye, M.A., Keck Jr, P.E., McElroy, S.L., Grunze, H. and Post, R.M. (2007) 'Three times more days depressed than manic or hypomanic in both bipolar I and bipolar II disorder', *Bipolar Disorder,* 9(5): 531–5.

Kuthning, M. and Hundt, F. (2013) 'Aspects of vulnerable patients and informed consent in clinical trials german medical science', *German Medical Science E-Journal,* 11: Doc03. doi:10.3205/000171.

Kwan, M.L., Kushi, L.H., Weltzien, E., Tam, E.K., Castillo, A., Sweeney, C. and Caan, B.J. (2010) 'Alcohol consumption and breast cancer recurrence and survival among women with early-stage breast cancer: the life after cancer epidemiology study', *Journal of Clinical Oncology,* 28(29): 4410–16.

La Cour, P. and Hvidt, N.C. (2010) 'Research on meaning-making and health in secular society: secular, spiritual and religious existential orientations', *Social Science & Medicine,* 71(7): 1292–9.

Laaksonen, M., Rahkonen, O., Karvonen, S. and Lahelma, E. (2005) 'Socioeconomic status and smoking analysing inequalities with multiple indicators', *The European Journal of Public Health,* 15(3): 262–9.

Lab Tests Online UK (2014) Available from: www.labtestsonline.org.uk/ [accessed 5 January 2014].

Labay, L.E. and Walco, G.A. (2004) 'Brief report: empathy and psychological adjustment in siblings of children with cancer', *Journal of Pediatric Psychology*, 29(4): 309–314.

Lacey Jr, J.V., Mink, P.J., Lubin, J.H., Sherman, M.E., Troisi, R., Hartge, P., Schatzkin, A. and Schairer, C. (2002) 'Menopausal hormone replacement therapy and risk of ovarian cancer', *Journal of the American Medical Association*, 288(3): 334–41. Erratum in *Journal of the American Medical Association*, 288(20): 2544.

Lai, D.T., Cahill, K., Qin, Y. and Tang, J. L. (2010) 'Motivational interviewing for smoking cessation', *Cochrane Database System Review*. doi: 10.1002/14651858.CD006936.pub2

Lalla, R.V., Sonis, S.T. and Peterson, D.E. (2008) 'Management of oral mucositis in patients who have cancer', *Dental Clinics of North America*, 52(1): 61–77.

Lalor, J.G., Begley, C.M. and Devane, D. (2006) 'Exploring painful experiences: impact of emotional narratives on members of a qualitative research team', *Journal of Advanced Nursing*, 56(6): 607–16.

Lam, W.T., Shing, Y.T., Bonanno, G.A., Mancini, A.D. and Fielding, R. (2010) 'Distress trajectories at the first year diagnosis of breast cancer in relation to six years survivorship', *Psycho-oncology*, 21(1): 90–9.

Lamb, M.A. (1995) 'Effects of cancer on the sexuality and fertility of women', *Seminars in Oncology Nursing*, 11(2): 120–7.

Lambert, S.D., Jones, B., Girgis, A. and Lecathelinais, C. (2012) 'Distressed partners and caregivers do not recover easily: adjustment trajectories among partners and caregivers of cancer survivors', *Annals of Behavioural Medicine*, 44(2): 225–35.

Lambert, V.A. and Lambert CE. (2008) 'Nurses' workplace stressors and coping strategies', *Indian Journal of Palliative Nursing*, 14(1): 38–44.

Land, S.R. (2012) 'Methodologic barriers to addressing critical questions about tobacco and cancer prognosis', *Journal of Clinical Oncology*, 30(17): 2030–2.

Lang, B.H.-H., Lo, C.-Y., Chan, W.-F., Lam, K.-Y., Wan, K.-Y. (2007) 'Prognostic factors in papillary and follicular thyroid carcinoma: their implications for cancer staging', *Annals of Surgical Oncology*, 14: 730–8.

Langewitz, W., Heydrich, L., Nübling, M., Szirt, L., Weber, H. and Grossman, P. (2010) 'Swiss Cancer League communication skills training programme for oncology nurses: an evaluation', *Adv Nurs.*, 66 (10): 2266–2277.

Langston, B., Armes, J., Levy, A., Tidey, E. and Ream, E. (2013) 'The prevalence and severity of fatigue in men with prostate cancer: a systematic review of the literature', *Supportive Care in Cancer*, 21(6): 1761–71.

Lanzkowsky, P. (2011) *Manual of Pediatric Hematology and Oncology*, 5th edn. London: Elsevier.

Larsen-Disney, P. (2007) *Fertility Preservation for Cancer*. Sussex Cancer Network.

Laubmeier, K.K., Zakowski, S.G. and Bair, J.P. (2004) 'The role of spirituality in the psychological adjustment to cancer: a test of the transactional model of stress and coping', *International Journal of Behavioral Medicine*, 11(1): 48–55.

Lavelle, K., Todd, C., Moran, A., Howell, A., Bundred, N. and Campbell, M. (2007) 'Non-standard management of breast cancer increases with age in the UK: a population based cohort of women > or =65 years', *British Journal of Cancer*, 96: 1197–203.

Lawenda, B.D., Gagne, H.M., Gierga, D.P., Niemierko, A., Wong, W.M., Tarbell, N.J., Chen, G.T., Hochberg, F.H. and Loeffler, J.S. (2004) 'Permanent alopecia after cranial irradiation: dose–response relationship', *International Journal of Radiation Oncology Biology Physics*, 60(3): 879–87.

Lawrence, D. and Kisely, S. (2010) 'Inequalities in healthcare provision for people with severe mental illness', *Journal of Psychopharmacology*, 24(11): Suppl. 4, 61–68.

Laz, C. (2003) 'Age embodied', *Journal of Aging Studies*, 17(4): 503–19.

Lazare, A. (1979) 'Unresolved Grief', in A. Lazare, *Outpatient Psychiatry: Diagnosis and Treatment*. Baltimore, MD: Williams and Wilkins.

Lazarus, R.S. (1993) 'From psychological stress to the emotions: a history of changing outlooks', *Annual Review of Psychology*, 44: 22–39.

Lazarus, R.S. (1999) *Stress and Emotion. A New Synthesis*. London: Free Association Books.

Lazarus, R.S. (2006) 'Emotions and interpersonal relationships: towards a person-centred conceptualization of emotions and coping', *Journal of Personality,* 74(1): 9–46. doi:10.1111/j.1467-6494.2005.00368.x.

Lazarus, R.S. and Folkman, S. (1984) *Stress, Appraisal and Coping.* New York, NY: Springer.

Le Blanc, M. and Tangen, C. (2012) 'Choosing phase II endpoints and designs: evaluating the possibilities', *Clinical Cancer Research,* 18(8): 2130–2.

Le Blanc, P.M, Bakker A.B, Peeters M.C.W, van Heesch N.C.A. and Schaufeli W.B. (2001) 'Emotional job demands and burnout among oncology care providers', *Anxiety, Stress & Coping,* 14: 243–63.

Lee, C., Dominik, R., Levin, C., Barry, M., Cosenza, C., O'Connor, A. and Mulley, A. (2010) 'Development of instruments to measure quality of breast cancer treatment decisions', *Health Expectations,* 33(3): 258–272.

Lee, L., Li, C., Landry, T., Latimer, E., Carli, F., Fried, G., Feldman, L.S. (2014) 'A systematic review of economic evaluations of enhanced recovery pathways for colorectal surgery', Ann. Surgo., 259(4): 670–676.

Lee, M.S., Kun-Hyung, K., Byung-Cheul, S., Sun-Mi, C. and Ernst, E. (2009) 'Acupuncture for treating hot flushes in men with prostate cancer: a systematic review', *Supportive Care in Cancer,* 17(7): 763–70.

Lees, J. and Chan, A. (2011) 'Polypharmacy in elderly patients with cancer: clinical implications and management', *Lancet Oncology* 12(13): 1249–57.

Lees, N. and Lloyd-Williams, M. (1999) 'Assessing depression in palliative care patients using the visual analogue scale: a pilot study', *European Journal of Cancer Care,* 8(4): 220–3.

Leijte, J., Kirrander, P., Antonini, N., Windahl, T. and Horenblas, S. (2008) 'Recurrence patterns of squamous cell carcinoma of the penis: recommendations for follow-up based on a two-centre analysis of 700 patients', *European Urology,* 54: 161–9.

Lennan, E. (2011) 'Chemotherapy as a treatment for breast cancer', in V. Harmer (ed.), *Breast Cancer Nursing Care and Management.* London: Wiley-Blackwell. pp. 149–172.

Lent, RW (2007) 'Restoring emotional well-being: a theoretical model', in M. Feuerstein (ed.), *Handbook of Cancer Survivorship.* New York, NY: Springer. pp. 231–248.

Leonard, K. (2010) 'Late effects of radiotherapy', European Oncology Nursing Society Newsletter, Theme: Radiotherapy Care. Available from: www.cancernurse.eu/documents/newsletter/2010summer/EONSNewsletter2010summerfullpdf.pdf [accessed 12 October 2014].

Lethborg, C., Aranda, S. and Kissane, D. (2008) 'Meaning in adjustment to cancer: a model of care', *Palliative & Supportive Care,* 6: 61–70.

Lethborg, C., Schofield, P. and Kissane, D. (2012) 'The advanced cancer patient experience of undertaking meaning and purpose (MaP) therapy', *Palliative & Supportive Care,* 10(3): 177–88.

Leucht, S., Burkard, T., Henderson, J., Maj, M. and Sartorius, N. (2007) 'Physical illness and schizophrenia: a review of the literature', *Acta Psychiatrica Scandinavica,* 116: 317–33.

Lev, E.L., Paul, D. and Owen, S.V. (1999) 'Age, self-efficacy, and change in patients' adjustment to cancer', *Cancer Practice,* 7(4): 170–6.

Lev, E.L., Daley, K.M., Conner, N.E., Reith, M., Fernandez, C. and Owen, S.V. (2001) 'An intervention to increase quality of life and self-care self-efficacy and decrease symptoms in breast cancer patients', *Scholarly Inquiry for Nursing Practice,* 15(3): 277–94.

Leventhal, H., Diefenbach, M. and Leventhal, E. (1992) 'Illness cognition: using common sense to understand treatment adherence and effect cognitive interactions', *Cognitive Therapy & Research,* 16(2): 143–63.

Leventhal, H., Meyer, D. and Nerenz, D. (1980) 'The common sense model of illness danger', in S. Rachman (ed.), *Medical Psychology.* Vol. 2. New York. NY: Pergamon.

Levy-Lahad, E. and Friedman, E. (2007) 'Cancer risks among BRCA1 and BRCA2 mutation carriers', *British Journal of Cancer,* 96(1): 11–15.

Lewis, C.S. (1961) *A Grief Observed.* London: Faber and Faber.

Lewis, F.M. (2006) 'The effects of cancer survivorship on families and caregivers', *American Journal of Nursing,* 106(3): 20–5.

Lewis, M. (2007) *Medicine and Care of the Dying: A Modern History*. New York, NY: Oxford University Press.

Liechty, T. and Yarnal, C.M. (2010) 'Older women's body image: a lifecourse perspective', *Ageing & Society,* 30: 1197–218.

Lim, J., Bogossian, F. and Ahern, K. (2010) 'Stress and coping in Australian nurses: a systematic review', *International Nursing Review,* 57: 22–31.

Li-Min, W., Chi-Chun, C., Haase, J.E. and Chung-Hey, C. (2009) 'Coping experiences of adolescents with cancer: a qualitative study', *Journal of Advanced Nursing,* 65(11): 2358–66.

Linabery, A.M. and Ross, J.A. (2008) 'Trends in childhood cancer incidence in the United States (1992–2004)', *Cancer,* 112(2): 416–432.

Lindemann, E. (1944) 'Symptomatology and management of acute grief', *American Journal of Psychiatry,* 101(22): 141–8.

LINKS website, www.nhs.uk/NHSEngland/links/Pages/links-make-it-happen.aspx [accessed 16 January 2012].

Little, M., Paul, K., Jordens C.F.C. and Sayers E. (2002) 'Survivorship and discourses of identity', *Psycho-oncology,* 11: 170–8.

Little, P., Everitt H., Williamson I., Warner G., Moore M., Gould C., Ferrier K. and Payne, S. (2001) 'Observational study of the effect of patient centredness and positive approach on outcomes of general practice consultations', *British Medical Journal,* 323(7318): 908–11.

Littlewood, J. (1992) *Aspects of Grief: Bereavement in Adult Life*. London: Tavistock/Routledge.

Ljungman, P., Bregni, M., Brune, M. et al, for the European Group for Blood and Marrow Transplantation (2010) 'Allogeneic and autologous transplantation for haematological diseases, solid tumours and immune disorders: current practice in Europe in 2009', *Bone Marrow Transplantation,* 45: 219–34.

Ljungqvist, O. (2014) 'ERAS–enhanced recovery after surgery: moving evidence-based perioperative care to practice', *Journal of Parenteral and Enteral Nutrition,* doi:10.1177/0148607114523451.

Loeb, S., van den Heuvel, S., Zhu, X., Bangma, C.H., Schroder, F.H. and Roobol, M.J. (2012) 'Infectious complications and hospital admissions after prostate biopsy in a European randomized trial', *European Urology,* 61(6): 1110–14.

Lombardo, P., Vaucher, P., Haftgoli, N., Burnand, B., Favrat, B., Verdon, F., Bischoff, T. and Herzig, L. (2011) 'The "help" question doesn't help when screening for major depression: external validation of the three-question screening test for primary care patients managed for physical complaints', *BMC Medicine,* 9: 114.

Long, K. and Marsland, A. (2011) 'Family adjustment to childhood cancer: a systematic review', *Clinical Child and Family Psychology Review,* 14: 57–88.

Longmore, R.J. and Worrell, M. (2007) 'Do we need to challenge thoughts in cognitive behavior therapy?', *Clinical Psychology Review,* 27(2): 173–87.

Lopez, K.A. and Willis, D.G. (2004) 'Descriptive versus interpretive phenomenology: their contributions to nursing knowledge', *Qualitative Health Research,* 14(5): 726–35.

Lord, K., Mitchell, A.J., Ibrahim, K., Kumar, S., Rudd, N. and Symonds, P. (2012) 'The beliefs and knowledge of patients newly diagnosed with cancer in a UK ethnically diverse population', *Clinical Oncology,* 24(1): 4–12.

Lorig, K. (2002) 'Partnerships between expert patient and physician', *Lancet,* 359: 814–15.

Lorig, K. and Holman H (2003) 'Self-management education: history, definition, outcomes and mechanisms', *Annals of Behavioural Medicine,* 26(1): 1–7.

Lorig, K., Ritter, P., Steward, A.L., Sobel, D.S., William Brown, B., Bandura, A., Gonzalez, V., Laurent, D. and Holman, H. (2001) 'Chronic disease self-management program: 2-year health status and health care utilization outcomes', *Medical Care,* 39(11): 1217–23.

Lubbock, T. (2012) *Until Further Notice, I Am Alive*. London: Granta.

Luckett, T., Butow, P.N. and King, M.T. (2009) 'Improving patient outcomes through the routine use of patient-reported data in cancer clinics: future directions', *Psycho-oncology,* 18: 1129–38.

Luckett, T., Butow, P.N., King, M.T., Oguchi, M., Heading, G., Hackl, N.A., Rankin, N., Price, M.A. (2010) 'A review and recommendations for optimal outcome measures of anxiety, depression and general distress in studies evaluating psychosocial interventions for English-speaking adults with heterogeneous cancer diagnoses', *Supportive Care in Cancer,* 18(10): 1241–62.

Luszczynska, A., Sarkar, Y. and Knoll, N. (2007) 'Received social support, self-efficacy, and finding benefits in disease as predictors of physical functioning and adherence to antiretroviral therapy', *Patient Education and Counseling*, 66(1): 37–42.

Luzzatto, P. (2005) 'Musing with death in group art therapy with cancer patients', in D. Waller and C. Sibbert (eds), *Art Therapy and Cancer Care*. Maidenhead, UK: Open University Press. pp. 163–172.

Luzzatto, P. and Gabriel, B. (1998) 'Art psychotherapy', in J.C. Holland, W.S. Breitbart, P.B., Jacobsen, et al. (eds), *Psycho-oncology*. Oxford: Oxford University Press. p. 750.

Luzzatto, P. and Gabriel, B. (2000) 'The creative journey, a model for short-term group art therapy with posttreatment cancer patients', *Art Therapy: Journal of The American Art Therapy Association*, 17: 265–9.

Lykken, D.T. (1968) 'Statistical significance in psychological research', *Psychological Bulletin*, 70(3): 151–9.

Lymphoedema Framework (2006) *Best Practice for the Management of Lymphoedema*. London: MEP Ltd.

Lynch, H.T., Lynch, P.M., Lanspa, S.J., et al. (2009) 'Review of the Lynch syndrome: history, molecular genetics, screening, differential diagnosis, and medicolegal ramifications', *Clinical Genetics*, 76(1): 1–18.

Lynn, J., Adamson, D.M. (2003) *Living Well at the End of Life: Adapting Health Care to Serious Chronic Illness in Old Age*. Washington, DC: Rand Health.

Lyratzopoulos, G., Abel, G.A., Barbiere, J.M., Brown, C.H., Rous, B.A., Greenberg, D.C. (2012) 'Variation in advanced stage at diagnosis of lung and female breast cancer in an English region 2006–2009', *British Journal of Cancer*, 106: 1068–75.

Lyseng-Williamson, K.A. (2013) 'Erlotinib: a guide to its use in first-line treatment of non-small-cell lung cancer with epidermal growth factor-activating mutations', *Molecular Diagnosis and Therapy*, 17(1): 57–62.

Ma, R. W.-L. and Chapman, K. (2009) 'A systematic review of the effect of diet in prostate cancer prevention and treatment', Journal of Human Nutrition and Dietetics, 22: 187–199.

Ma, Y., Yang, Y., Wang, F., Zhang, P., Shi, C., Zou, Y. and Qin, H. (2013) 'Obesity and risk of colorectal cancer: a systematic review of prospective studies', *PLoS One*, 8(1): e53916.

MacBride, S.K., Wells, M.E., Hornsby, C., Sharp, L., Finnila, K. and Downie, L. (2008) 'A case study to evaluate a new soft silicone dressing, Mepilex Lite, for patients with radiation skin reactions', *Cancer Nursing*, 31: E8–14.

MacCubbin, H.I., MacCubbin, M.A., Thompson, A.I. and Thompson, E.A. (1998) 'Resilience in ethnic families: a conceptual model for predicting family adjustment and adaptation', in H.I. MacCubbin, E.A. Thompson, A.I. Thompson and J.E. Fromer (eds), *Resiliency in Native American and Immigrant Families*. London: Sage Publications. pp. 107–250.

Macdonald, A. (2008) *Solution-Focused Therapy*. London: Sage Publications.

MacDonald, R.A.R., Hargreaves, D.J. and Miell, D. (2002) *Musical Identities*. Oxford: Oxford University Press.

MacDonald, R.A.R., Kreutz, G. and Mitchell, L. (2012) *Music, Health and Wellbeing*. Oxford: Oxford University Press.

Mack, T.M., Cozen, W. and Shibata, D.K. (1995) 'Concordance for Hodgkin's disease in identical twins suggesting genetic susceptibility to the young-adult form of the disease', *New England Journal of Medicine*, 332: 413–8.

MacKellar, M. (2010) *When it Rains: A Memoir*. Sydney: Random House.

Mackenbach, J.P., Kunst, A.E., Cavelaars, A.E., Groenhof, F., Geurts, J.J. and EU Working Group on Socioeconomic Inequalities in Health (1997) 'Socioeconomic inequalities in morbidity and mortality in Western Europe', *Lancet*, 349: 1655–9.

Macmillan Cancer Support (n.d.) *'Top Tips' series*. Available from: www.macmillan.org.uk/Aboutus/Healthprofessionals/Primary_care_cancer_leads/Resources.aspx [accessed August 2012].

Macmillan Cancer Support (n.d) *Living with after Cancer*. Available from: www.macmillan.org.uk/Cancerinformation/Livingwithandaftercancer/Livingwithandaftercancer.aspx [accessed 17 February 2015].

Macmillan Cancer Support (2007) *Living With or Beyond Cancer.* London: Macmillan Cancer Support.

Macmillan Cancer Support (2009) *Life after Treatment.* London: Macmillan Cancer Support.

Macmillan Cancer Support (2011a) *More than a Million – Understanding the UK's Carers of People with Cancer.* A report by Ipsos MORI for Macmillan Cancer Support. London: Macmillan Cancer Support.

Macmillan Cancer Support (2011b) *Psychological and Emotional Support Provided by Macmillan Professionals: An Evidence Review.* Available from: www.macmillan.org.uk/servicesimpact.

Macmillan Cancer Support (2012a) *Chewing and Swallowing Problems.* Available from: www.macmillan.org.uk/Cancerinformation/Livingwithandaftercancer/Eatingwell/Eatingproblems/Swallowingproblems.aspx [accessed 31 October 2014].

Macmillan Cancer Support (2012b) *Holistic Needs and Care Planning.* Available from: www.macmillan.org.uk/Aboutus/Healthandsocialcareprofessionals/Newsandupdates/MacVoice/MacVoiceWinter2012/Holisticneedsassessmentandcareplanning.aspx [accessed 1 August 2014].

Macmillan Cancer Support (2012c) *Improving the Quality of Cancer Care in Primary Care.* 2nd edn. London: Macmillan Cancer Support. Available from: www.macmillan.org.uk/Aboutus/Healthprofessionals/Primary_care_cancer_leads/Resources.aspx.

Macmillan Cancer Support (2013a) *Cancer Patient Experience Survey: Insight Report and League Table 2012–13.* London: Macmillan Cancer Support.

Macmillan Cancer Support (2013b) *Cancer's Hidden Price Tag – Revealing the Costs Behind the Illness.* London: Macmillan Cancer Support.

Macmillan Cancer Support (2013c) *Cured But At What Cost?* London: Macmillan Cancer Support.

Macmillan Cancer Support (2013d) *Throwing Light on the Consequences of Cancer and its Treatment.* Available from: www.macmillan.org.uk/Documents/AboutUs/Research/Researchandevaluationreports/Throwinglightontheconsequencesofcanceranditstreatment.pdf [accessed 12 October 2014].

Macmillan Cancer Support (2014) *The Older People's Project pilot sites.* Available from: www.macmillan.org.uk/Aboutus/Healthandsocialcareprofessionals/Macmillansprogrammesandservices/Improvingservicesforolderpeople/Pilots/PilotSites.aspx, [accessed 1 August 2014].

Maddams, J., Utley, M. and Møller, H. (2012) 'Projections of cancer prevalence in the United Kingdom 2010–2040', *British Journal of Cancer,* 107(7): 1195–202.

Maguire, P. (1999) 'Improving communication with cancer patients: a millennium review', *European Journal of Cancer,* 35(10): 1415–22.

Maguire, P. (2000) 'Psychological Aspects', in M. Dixon (ed.), *ABC of Breast Diseases.* London: British Medical Journal Books. pp. 150–153.

Maguire, P., Booth K et al. (1996) 'Helping health professionals involved in cancer care acquire key interviewing skills: the impact of workshops', *European Journal of Cancer,* 3A(90): 1486–9.

Maguire, P. and Faulkner, A. (1988) 'Communication with cancer patients: handling bad news and difficult questions', *British Medical Journal,* 297(6653): 907–9.

Maguire P. (2002) 'Improving the recognition of concerns and affective disorders in cancer patients', *Ann Oncol.,* 13 (Suppl 4):177–181.

Maher, E.J. and Makin, W. (2007) 'Life after cancer treatment – a spectrum of chronic survivorship conditions', *Clinical Oncology,* 19: 743–5.

Malapelle, U., Carlomagno, C., de Luca, C., Bellevicine, C. and Troncone, G. (2014) 'KRAS testing in metastatic colorectal carcinoma: challenges, controversies, breakthroughs and beyond,' *Journal of Clinical Pathology,* 67(1): 1–9.

Malone, A. and Price, J. (2012) 'The significant effects of childhood cancer on siblings', *Cancer Nursing Practice,* 11(4): 20–31.

Malpas, J.E. and Solomon, R.C. (1998) *Death and Philosophy.* London: Routledge.

Mandelblatt, J.S., Sheppard, V.B., Hurria, A., Kimmick, G., Isaacs, C., et al (2010) 'Breast cancer adjuvant chemotherapy decisions in older women: the role of patient preference and interactions with physicians', *Journal of Clinical Oncology,* 28(19): 3146–53.

Mann, L. and Ford, A. (2011) 'Distress thermometers in radiotherapy: a holistic assessment tool', *Imaging & Therapy Practice,* 1 April: 8.

Manne, S. and Badr, H. (2008) 'Intimacy and relationship processes in couples' psychosocial adaptation to cancer', *Cancer*, 112(Suppl. 11): 2541–55.

Mannix, K.A., Blackburn, I.M., Garland, A., Gracie, J., Moorey, S., Reid, B., Standart, S. and Scott, J. (2006) 'Effectiveness of brief training in cognitive behavioural therapy techniques for palliative care practitioners', *Palliative Medicine*, 20: 579–84.

Mansi, J.L., Smith, I.E., Walsh, G., et al (1989) 'Primary medical therapy for operable breast cancer', *European Journal of Cancer & Clinical Oncology*, 25(11): 1623–27.

Marcell, A.V., Ford, C.A., Pleck, J.H. and Sonenstein, F.L. (2007) 'Masculine beliefs, parental communication, and male adolescents' health care use', *Pediatrics*, 119(4): e966–e975.

Marieb, E.N. and Hoehn, K. (2013) *Human Anatomy and Physiology*, 9th edn. Boston, MA: Pearson Education.

Marmot, M. (2010) *Fair Society Healthy Lives. The Strategic Review of Health Inequalities in England Post-2010 (The Marmot Review)*. Available from: www.instituteofhealthequity.org/projects/fair-society-healthy-lives-the-marmot-review [accessed 6 November].

Marris, P. (1974) *Loss and Change*. London: Routledge.

Martelli, M., Ferreri, A. J. M., Agostinelli, C. (2013) 'Diffuse large B-cell lymphoma'. *Critical reviews in oncology/hematology*, 87(2): 146–72.

Martínez-Iñigo, D., Totterdell, P., Alcover, C.M. and Holman, D. (2007) 'Emotional labour and emotional exhaustion: interpersonal and intrapersonal mechanisms', *Work & Stress*, 21(1): 30–47.

Martini, F.H., Nath, J.N. and Bartholomew, E.F. (2012) *Fundamentals of Anatomy and Physiology*. San Francisco, CA: Pearson.

Maskarinec, G., Murphy, S., Shumay, D.M. and Kakai, H. (2001) 'Dietary changes among cancer survivors', *European Journal of Cancer Care*, 10: 12–20.

Maslach, C. (1982) *Burnout: The Cost of Caring*. Englewood Cliffs,NJ: Spectrum.

Maslow, A.H. (1970) *Motivation and Personality*. New York, NY: Harper & Row.

Mathew, J. and Perez, E.A. (2011) 'Trastuzumab emtansine in human epidermal growth factor receptor 2-positive breast cancer: a review', *Current Opinion in Oncology*, 23(6): 594–600.

Mathieson, C.M. (1999) 'Interviewing the ill and the healthy: paradigm or process?', in M. Murray and K. Chamberlain (eds), *Qualitative Health Psychology: Theories and Methods*. London: Sage Publications. pp. 117–133.

Maunder, E.Z. (2006) 'Emotion work in the palliative nursing care of children and young people', *International Journal of Palliative Nursing*, 12(1): 27–33.

Maunsell, E., Brisson, J., Deschenes, L. and Frasure-Smith, N. (1996) 'Randomized trial of a psychologic distress screening program after breast cancer: effects on quality of life', *Journal of Clinical Oncology*, 14: 2747–55.

May, C., Montori, V.M. and Mair, F.S. (2009) 'We need minimally disruptive medicine', *British Medical Journal*, 339: 485–7.

Mayne, M. (2006) *The Enduring Melody*. London: Darton, Longman & Todd.

McCance, K.L. and Huether, S.E. (2010) *Pathophysiology: The Biological Basis for Disease in Adults and Children*, 6th edn. London: Elsevier.

McCaughan, E. and Parahoo, K. (2000) 'Attitudes to cancer of medical and surgical nurses in a district general hospital', *European Journal of Oncology Nursing*, 4(3): 162–70.

McCaul, K.D., Sandgren, A.K., King, B., O'Donnell, S., Branstetter, A. and Foreman, G. (1999) 'Coping and adjustment to breast cancer', *Psycho-oncology*, 8(3): 230–6.

McClain, C.S., Rosenfeld, B, Breitbart, W. (2003) 'Effect of spiritual well-being on end-of-life despair in terminally-ill cancer patients'. *Lancet*, 361(9369): 1603.

McClean, S., Bunt, L. and Daykin, N. (2012) 'The healing and spiritual properties of music therapy at a cancer care centre', *Journal of Alternative and Complementary Medicine*, 18(4): 402–7.

McCloskey, S. and Taggart L. (2010) 'How much compassion have I left? An exploration of occupational stress among children's palliative care nurses', *International Journal of Palliative Nursing*, 16(5): 233–40.

McConnell, T.H. and Hull, K.L. (2011) *Human Form, Human Function*. Philadelphia, PA: Wolters Kluwer/Lippincott Williams & Wilkins.

McCorkle, R., Ercolano, E., Lazenby, M., Schulman-Green, D., Schilling, L.S., Lorig, K. and Wagner, E.H. (2011) 'Self-management: enabling and empowering patients living with cancer as a chronic illness', *CA: A Cancer Journal for Clinicians*, 61: 50–62.

McCubbin, H. I., McCubbin, M.A., Thompson, A.I. and Thompson, E.A. (1998) 'Resiliency in ethnic families: a conceptual model for predicting family adjustment and adaptation', *Resiliency in Native American and Immigrant Families*, 2: 3–48.

McCutcheon, T. (2013) 'The ileus and oddities after colorectal surgery', *Gastroenterology Nursing*, 36: 368–75, quiz 376–77. doi:10.1097/SGA.0b013e3182a71fdf.

McGrath, P. (2003) 'Spiritual pain: a comparison of findings from survivors and hospice patients', *American Journal of Hospice and Palliative Care*, 20(1): 23–33.

McGrath, P. and Phillips, E. (2008) '"It is very hard": treatment for childhood lymphoma from the parents' perspective', *Issues in Comprehensive Pediatric Nursing*, 31: 37–54.

McGuinness, B. and Finucane, N. (2011) 'Evaluating a creative arts bereavement support intervention: innovation and rigour', *Bereavement Care*, 30(1): 37–42.

McHugh, R.K., Hearon, B.A. and Otto, M.W. (2010) 'Cognitive-behavioral therapy for substance use disorders', *The Psychiatric Clinics of North America*, 33(3): 511.

McIlfatrick, S., Sullivan, K. and McKenna, H. (2006) 'Exploring the ethical issues of the research interview in the cancer context', *European Journal of Oncology Nursing*, 10(1): 39–47.

McKay, J.R., Franklin, T.R., Patapis, N. and Lynch, K.G. (2006) 'Conceptual, methodological, and analytical issues in the study of relapse', *Clinical Psychology Review*, 26(2): 109–27.

McLachlan, SA, Allenby A, Matthews J, Wirth A, Kissane D, Bishop M. et al. (2001) 'Randomized trial of coordinated psychosocial interventions based on patient self-assessments versus standard care to improve the psychosocial functioning of patients with cancer', *Journal of Clinical Oncology*, 19: 4117–25.

McNeely, M.L., Campbell, K.L., Rowe, B.H., Klassen, T.P., Mackey, J.R. and Courneya, K.S. (2006) 'Effects of exercise on breast cancer patients and survivors: a systematic review and meta-analysis', *Canadian Medical Association Journal*, 175(1): 34–41.

McNeilly, P. and, Gilmore F. (2009) 'Interdisciplinary working', in J. Price and P. McNeilly (eds), *Palliative Care for Children and Families: An Interdisciplinary Approach*. Basingstoke, UK: Palgrave Macmillan. pp. 18–37.

McQueen, A.C.H. (2004) 'Emotional intelligence in nursing work', *Journal of Advanced Nursing*, 47(1): 101–8.

McSherry, R., Pearce, P., Grimwood, K. and McSherry, W. (2012) 'The pivotal role of nurse managers, leaders and educators in enabling excellence in nursing care', *Journal of Nursing Management*, 20(1): 7–19.

McSherry, W. and Ross, L. (2010) *Spiritual Assessment in Healthcare Practice*. Keswick, UK: M&K Publishing.

Mead, G.H. (1934) *Mind, Self, and Society*. Chicago, IL: University of Chicago Press.

Medscape (2013) *Hypoalbuminemia*. Available from: http://emedicine.medscape.com/article/166724-overview [accessed 9 December 2013].

Meehl, P.E. (1967) 'Theory-testing in psychology and physics: a methodological paradox', *Philosophy of Science*, 34(2): 103–15.

Meehl, P.E. (1978) 'Theoretical risks and tabular asterisks: Sir Karl, Sir Ronald, and the slow progress of soft psychology', *Journal of Consulting and Clinical Psychology*, 46: 806–34.

Megdal, S.P., Kroenke, C.H., Laden, F., et al. (2005) 'Nightwork and breast cancer risk: a systematic review and meta-analysis', *European Journal of Cancer*, 41(13): 2023–32.

Mehrebian, A. (1971) *Silent Messages*. Belmont, CA: Wandsworth.

Mehta, A., Cohen, R., Chan, L. (2009) 'Palliative care: a need for a family systems approach', *Palliative and Supportive Care*, 7: 235–43.

Meijer, A., Roseman, M., Milette, K., et al. (2011) 'Depression screening and patient outcomes in cancer: a systematic review', *PLOS One*, 6(11): e27181.

Meiklejohn, J.A., Heesch, K.C., Janda, M. and Hayes, S.C. (2013) 'How people construct their experience of living with secondary lymphoedema in the context of their everyday lives in Australia', *Supportive Care in Cancer*, 21(2): 459–66.

Mellon, S., Northouse, L. and Weiss, L. (2006) 'A population-based study of the quality of life of cancer survivors and their family caregivers', *Cancer Nursing*, 29(2): 120–131.

Mencap (2004) *Treat Me Right: Better Healthcare for People with a Learning Disability*. London: Mencap.

Mencap (2007) *Death by Indifference*. London: Mencap.

Mencap (2012) *Death by Indifference: 74 Deaths and Counting*. London: Mencap.

Merseyside and Cheshire Cancer Network (MCCN) (2009) *Early Detection and Prevention of Cancer, Social Marketing Insight*. pp. 1–58. Available from: www.mccn.nhs.uk/userfiles/documents/SocialMarketingInsight.pdf [accessed 18 November 2014]

Merseyside and Cheshire Cancer Network (MCCN)/Cancer Research UK (2009) *Malignant Melanoma over 50s Campaign*. Available from: www.cancerresearchuk.org/prod_consump/groups/cr_common/@nre/@hea/documents/generalcontent/cr_045568.pdf.

Merseyside and Cheshire Cancer Research Network (2013) *Annual Progess Report 1 April 2012 31 March 2013*. Warrington: MCCRN.

Michael, J. (2008) *Healthcare for All: Report of the Independent Inquiry into Access to Healthcare for People with Learning Disabilities*. London: Aldrick Press.

Mick, J., Hughes, M. and Cohen, M. (2003) 'Sexuality and cancer: how oncology nurses can address it BETTER', *Oncology Nursing Forum*, 30: 152–3.

Middleton, J. and Lennan, E. (2011) 'Effectively managing chemotherapy induced nausea and vomiting', *British Journal of Nursing*, 22(17): S7–S15.

Miller, M. and Kearney, N. (2004) 'Chemotherapy-related nausea and vomiting: past reflections, present practice and future management', *European Journal of Cancer Care*, 13: 71–81.

Miller, W.R. and Rollnick, S. (2002) *Motivational Interviewing*, 2nd edn. New York, NY: Guilford Press.

Mills, E.J., Seely, D., Rachlis, B., Griffiths, L., Wilson, K., Ellis, P. and Wright, J.R. (2006) 'Barriers to participation in clinical trials of cancer: a meta-analysis and systematic review of patient-reported factors', *Lancet Oncology*, 7(2): 141–8.

Mills, J.A., Porter, H. and Gill, D. (2012) 'Radiotherapy beam production', in P. Symonds, C. Deehan, J.A. Mills and C. Meredith (eds), *Walter and Miller's Textbook of Radiotherapy*, 7th edn. London: Elsevier Churchill Livingstone. pp. 121–44.

Mills, M.E, Murray, L.J., Johnston, B.T., Cardwell, C., Donnelly, M. (2009) 'Does a patient-held quality-of-life diary benefit patients with inoperable lung cancer?'. *Journal of Clinical Oncology*, 27(1): 70–7.

Mind (2013) *We Still Need to Talk: A Report on Access to Talking Therapies*. Available from: www.mind.org.uk/media/494424/we-still-need-to-talk_report.pdf [accessed 9 December 2013].

Minuchin, S. (1968) *Families of the Slums*. New York, NY: Basic Books.

Mitchell, A.J. (2007) 'Pooled results from 38 analyses of the accuracy of distress thermometer and other ultrashort methods of detecting cancer-related mood disorders', *Journal of Clinical Oncology*, 25: 4670–81.

Mitchell, A.J. (2010) 'Short screening tools for cancer-related distress: a review and diagnostic validity meta-analysis', *Journal of the National Comprehensive Cancer Network*, 8(4): 487–94.

Mitchell, A.J. (2012) *Rapid Screening for Depression and Emotional Distress in Routine Cancer Care: Local Implementation and Meta-analysis*. Thesis (MD). University of Leicester.

Mitchell, A.J., Kaar, S., Coggan, C. and Herdman, J. (2008) 'Acceptability of common screening methods used to detect distress and related mood disorders-preferences of cancer specialists and non-specialists', *Psycho-oncology*, 17(3): 226–36.

Mitchell, A.J. and Kakkadasam, V. (2011) 'Ability of nurses to identify depression in primary care, secondary care and nursing homes: a meta-analysis of routine clinical accuracy', *International Journal of Nursing Studies*, 48(3): 359–68.

Mitchell, A.J. and Malladi, S. (2010) 'Screening and case finding tools for the detection of dementia. Part I: evidence-based meta-analysis of multidomain tests', *Am J Geriatr Psychiatry*, 18(9): 759–782.

Mitchell, A.J., Vaze, A. and Rao, S. (2009) 'Clinical diagnosis of depression in primary care: a meta-analysis', *Lancet*, 374(9690): 609–19.

Mitchell, A.J., Hussain, N., Grainger, L. and Symonds, P (2010a) 'Identification of patient-reported distress by clinical nurse specialists in routine oncology practice: a multicentre UK study', *Psycho-oncology,* 20(10): 1076-1083.

Mitchell, A.J., Meader, N. and Symonds, P. (2010b) 'Diagnostic validity of the Hospital Anxiety and Depression Scale (HADS) in cancer and palliative settings: a meta-analysis', *J Affect Disord.,* 126(3): 335–348.

Mitchell, A.J., Chan, M., Bhatti, H., Halton, M., Grassi, L., Johansen, C. and Meader, N. (2011a) 'Prevalence of depression, anxiety, and adjustment disorder in oncological, haematological, and palliative-care settings: a meta-analysis of 94 interview-based studies', *Lancet Oncol.,* 12(2): 160–174.

Mitchell, A.J., Vahabzadeh, A. and Magruder, K. (2011b) 'Screening for distress and depression in cancer settings: 10 lessons from 40 years of primary-care research', *Psychooncology.* 20(6): 572–584.

Mitchell, A.J., Meader, N., Davies, E., Clover, K., Carter, G.L., Loscalzo, M.J., Linden, W., Grassi, L., Johansen, C., Carlson, L.E. and Zabora, J. (2012a) 'Meta-analysis of screening and case finding tools for depression in cancer: evidence based recommendations for clinical practice on behalf of the Depression in Cancer Care consensus group', *J Affect Disord.,* 140 (2): 149–160.

Mitchell, A.J., Lord, K., Slattery, J., Grainger, L. and Symonds, P. (2012b) 'How feasible is implementation of distress screening by cancer clinicians in routine clinical care?', *Cancer,* 118(24): 6260–6269.

Mitchell, D. and Lozano, R.G. (2012) 'Understanding patient psychosocial issues: my perspective', *Radiation Therapist,* 21(1): 96–99.

Mitchell, G. (2013) 'The rationale for fractionation in radiotherapy', *Clinical Journal of Oncology Nursing,* 17(4): 412–17.

Mitchell, S. (2013) 'Cancer related fatigue', in C.H. Yarbro, D. Wujcik and B.H. Gobel (eds), *Cancer Symptom Management,* 4th edn. Burlington, VT: Jones and Bartlett Learning. pp. 27–43.

Moffatt, C.J., Franks, P.J., Doherty, D.C. et al. (2003) 'Lymphoedema: an underestimated health problem', *Quarterly Journal of Medicine,* 96: 731–8.

Mohty, B. and Mohty, M. (2011) 'Long-term complications and side effects after allogeneic hematopoietic stem cell transplantation: an update', *Blood Cancer Journal,* 1(4): e16, doi. org/10.1038/bcj.2011.14.

Molassiotis, A. and Borjeson, S. (2006) 'Nausea and vomiting', in N. Kearney and A. Richardson (eds), *Nursing Patients with Cancer: Principles and Practice.* Edinburgh: Elsevier Churchill Livingstone. pp. 415–437.

Molassiotis, A., Helin, A.M., Dabbour, R. and Hummerston, S. (2006) 'The effects of P6 pressure in the prophylaxis of chemotherapy-related nausea and vomiting in breast cancer patients', *Complementary Therapies in Medicine,* 15(1): 3–12.

Molassiotis, A. and Jacobs, C. (2012) 'An evaluation of the current state of cancer-related palliative and supportive care research in the UK', *Palliative Care & Medicine,* 2(4): 112–19.

Molassiotis, A. and Rogers, M. (2012) 'Symptom experience and regaining normality in the first year following a diagnosis of head and neck cancer: a qualitative longitudinal study', *Palliative & Supportive Care,* 10(3): 197–204.

Moller, H.J. (2000) 'Rating depressed patients: observer- vs self-assessment', *European Psychiatry,* 15: 160–72.

Moller, H.J., Linklater, K.M. and Robinson, D. (2009) 'A visual summary of the Eurocare 4 results', *British Journal of Cancer,* 101(S2): S110–14.

Mols, F., Lemmens, V., Bosscha, K., van den Broek, W., Thong, M.S.Y. (2014) 'Living with the physical and mental consequences of an ostomy: a study among 1–10-year rectal cancer survivors from the population-based PROFILES registry', *Psycho-oncology,* 23(9): 998–1004.

Montazeri, A. (2008) 'Health-related quality of life in breast cancer patients: a bibliographic review of the literature from 1974 to 2007', *Journal of Experimental and Clinical Cancer Research,* 27: 32. doi:10.1186/1756-9966-27-32.

Montazeri, A. (2009) 'Quality of life data as prognostic indicators of survival in cancer patients: an overview of the literature from 1982 to 2008', *Health and Quality of Life Outcomes*, 23(7): 102–123.

Moorcraft, S.Y., Smyth, E.C. and Cunningham, D. (2014) 'Adjuvant or neoadjuvant therapy for operable esophagogastric cancer?', *Gastric Cancer*, 18(1): 1–10.

Moore, P.M., Rivera Mercado, S., GrezArtigues, M. and Lawrie, T.A. (2013) 'Communication skills training for healthcare professionals working with people who have cancer', *Cochrane Database of Systematic Reviews*, Issue 3. Art. No.: CD003751.

Moore, S.C., Gierach, G.L., Schatzkin, A. and Matthews, C.R. (2010) 'Physical activity, sedentary behaviours, and the prevention of endometrial cancer', *British Journal of Cancer*, 103(7): 933–8.

Moorey, S., Cort, E., Kapari, M., Monroe, B., Hansford, P., Mannix, K., Henderson, M., Fisher, L. and Hotopf, M. (2009) 'A cluster randomized controlled trial of cognitive behaviour therapy for common mental disorders in patients with advanced cancer', *Psychological Medicine*, 39(5): 713–23.

Moorey, S., Greer, S., Bliss, J. and Law, M. (1998) 'A comparison of adjuvant psychological therapy and supportive counselling in patients with cancer', *Psycho-oncology*, 7(3): 218–28.

Moos, R.H. and Schaefer, A. (1984) 'The crisis of physical illness: an overview and conceptual approach', in R.H. Moos (ed.), *Coping with Physical Illness: New Perspectives*. Vol 2. New York, NY: Plenum.

Morasso, G., Costantini, M., Baracco, G., Borreani, C. and Capelli, M. (1996) 'Assessing psychological distress in cancer patients: validation of a self-administered questionnaire', *Oncology*, 53(4): 295–302.

Morgan, M., Ten Haken, R., and Lawrence, T (2011) 'Radiation oncology', in V.T. DeVita, T.S. Lawrence and S.A. Rosenberg (eds), *Cancer: Principles and Practice of Oncology*, 9th edn. London: Wolters Kluwer/Lippincott Williams and Wilkins. pp. 289–311.

Morris, J., Perez, D. and McNoe, B. (1998) 'The use of quality of life data in clinical practice', *Quality of Life Research*, 7: 85–91.

Morse, J.M. and Johnson, J.L. (1991) 'Towards a theory of illness. The illness constellation model', in J.M. Morse and J.L. Johnson (eds), *The Illness Experience: Dimensions of Suffering*. Newbury Park, CA: Sage Publications.

Morse, L. (2013) 'Skin and nail bed changes', in C.H. Yarbro, D. Wujcik and B.H. Gobel (eds), *Cancer Symptom Management*, 4th edn. Burlington, VT: Jones and Bartlett Learning. pp. 587–616.

Moser, K., Sellars, S., Wheaton, M., et al. (2011) 'Extending the age range for breastscreening in England: pilot study to assess the feasibility and acceptability of randomization', *Journal of Medical Screening*, 18(2): 96–102.

Mosher, C.E. and Danoff-Burg, S. (2007) 'Death and anxiety related stigma', *Death Studies*, 31: 885–907.

Moss, S.M., Campbell, C., Melia, J., et al. (2011) 'Performance measures in three rounds of the English bowel cancer screening pilot', *Gut*, 61(1): 101–7.

Mota, F. (2003) 'Microinvasive squamous carcinoma of the cervix: treatment modalities,' *Acta Obstetrica et Gynecologica Scandinavica*, 82: 505–9.

Motzer, R.J., Hutson, T.E., Tomczak, P., et al. (2009) 'Overall survival and updated results for sunitinib compared with interferon alfa in patients with metastatic renal cell carcinoma', *Journal of Clinical Oncology*, 27(22): 3584–90.

Moyes, L.H., McCaffer, C.J., Carter, R.C., Fullarton, G.M., Mackay, C.K. and Forshaw, M.J. (2013) 'Cardiopulmonary exercise testing as a predictor of complications in oesophagogastric cancer surgery', *Annals of the Royal College of Surgeons of England*, 95: 125–130.

Mulley, A., Trimble C. and Elwyn G. (2012) *Patients' Preferences Matter: Stop the Silent Misdiagnosis*. London: The King's Fund.

Munzenberger, N., Fortaainer, C., Macquart-Maoulin, G., Faucher, C., Novakovitch, G., Maraninchi, D., Moatti, J.P. and Blaise, D. (1999) 'Psychological aspects of haematopoietic stem cell donation for allogeneic transplantation: how family donors cope with this experience', *Psycho-oncology*, 8: 55–63.

Murphy, M.F.G., Bithell, J.F., Stiller, C.A., Kendall, G.M. and O'Neill, K.A. (2013) 'Childhood and adult cancers: contrasts and commonalities', *Maturitas*, 76: 95–8.

Murphy, R., Straebler, S., Cooper, Z. and Fairburn, C. G. (2010) 'Cognitive behavioral therapy for eating disorders', *Psychiatric Clinics of North America*, 33(3): 611–27.

Murray, S.A., Kendall, M., Boyd, K.and Sheikh, A. (2005) 'Illness trajectories and palliative care', *British Medical Journal*, 330: 100.

Mustafa, M., Carson-Stevens, A., Gillespie, D. and Edwards, A.G.K. (2013) 'Psychological interventions for women with metastatic breast cancer (review)', *Cochrane Database of Systematic Reviews*, Issue 6.

Mustafa, O., Mustafa, S., Hakan, S.B., Erkan, C., Mehmet, A., Burhan, S., Arzu, K., Zekiye, T. and Yeliz, S. (2004) '"Do not tell": what factors affect relatives' attitudes to honest disclosure of diagnosis to cancer patients?', *Supportive Care in Cancer*, 12(7): 497–502.

Myint, A.S. (2013) 'Contact radiotherapy for elderly patients with early low rectal cancers', *British Journal of Hospital Medicine*, 74: 391–6.

Nagel, T. (2010) *Secular Philosophy and the Religious Temperament: Essays 2002–2008*. New York, NY: Oxford University Press.

Nainis, N., Paice, J.A., Ratner, J., Wirth, J.H., Lai, J. and Shott, S. (2006) 'Relieving symptoms in cancer: innovative use of art therapy', *Journal of Pain Symptom Management*, 31(2): 162–9.

Nanton, V., Osborne, D. and Dale, J. (2010) 'Maintaining control over illness: a model of partner activity in prostate cancer', *European Journal of Cancer Care*, 19(3): 329–39.

National Alliance for Caregiving (2009) *Caregiving in the USA*. Available from: www.caregiving.org/data/Caregiving_in_the_USA_2009_full_report.pdf.

National Audit Office (2010) *Delivering the Cancer Reform Strategy*. London: National Audit Office.

National Cancer Action Team (2007) *Holistic Common Assessment of Supportive and Palliative Care Needs for Adults with Cancer: Assessment Guidance*. London: National Cancer Action Team.

National Cancer Action Team (2013) *Holistic Needs Assessment for People with Cancer. A Practical Guide for Health Care Professionals*. London: National Cancer Action Team.

National Cancer Action Team/National Cancer Equality Initiative (2011) *WECAN: Reducing Inequalities In Commissioning Cancer Services – Principles and Practical Guidance For Good Equality Working*. London: National Cancer Action Team. Available from: www.ncat.nhs.uk/sites/default/files/work-docs/FINAL%20PRINCIPLES%20%26%20GUIDANCE%20DOC.pdf

National Cancer Equality Initiative (NCEI) (2010) *Reducing Cancer Inequality: Evidence, Progress and Making it Happen*. London: Department of Health/National Cancer Action Team (Gateway ref 13852).

National Cancer Institute (NCI) (1998) *Eating Hints for Cancer Patients*: NIH Publication no 98-2079. Bethesda, MD :National Institutes of Health.

National Cancer Institute (NCI) (2000) *PDQ Supportive Care Summary for Patients: Nutrition*. Cancernet. Available from: http://cancernet.nci.nih.gov [accessed 16 October 2009].

National Cancer Institute (NCI) (2010) *Common Toxicity Criteria*. National Cancer Institute NIH Publication No. 09–5410.

National Cancer Intelligence Network (NCIN) (2009) *Cancer Incidence and Survival By Major Ethnic Group, England 2002–2006*. London: National Cancer Inequality Network for National Cancer Action Team. Available from: www.ncin.org.uk/view.aspx?rid=75or http://library.ncin.org.uk/docs/090625-NCIN-Incidence_and_Survival_by_Ethnic_Group-Report.pdf

National Cancer Intelligence Network (NCIN) (2010a) *Routes to Diagnosis: NCIN Data Briefing*. Available from: www.ncin.org.uk/publications/data_briefings/routes_to_diagnosis.aspx [accessed 18 November 2014].

National Cancer Intelligence Network (NCIN) (2010b) *Evidence to March 2010 on Cancer Inequalities in England*. Available from: www.ncin.org.uk/publications/reports/ [accessed 9 December 2013].

National Cancer Intelligence Network (NCIN) (2011a) *Major Surgical Resections, England 2004–06*. Available from: www.ncin.org.uk/publications/reports/ [accessed 9 December 2013].

National Cancer Intelligence Network (NCIN) (2011b) *The Second All Breast Cancer Report.* Available from: www.ncin.org.uk/publications/reports/ [accessed 9 December 2013].

National Cancer Intelligence Network (NCIN) (2012) *Cancer Patient Experience Survey 2011/2012.* London: Department of Health. Available from: www.ncin.org.uk/cancer_information_tools/cancer_patient_experience [accessed 5 November 2014].

National Cancer Intelligence Network (2012b) *Routes to Diagnosis. 2006–2008.* NCIN. Information supplement available from: www.ncin.org.uk/publications/routes_to_diagnosis.aspx

National Cancer Patient Experience Survey (NCPES) (2010) *National Cancer Patient Experience Survey Programme – 2010: National Survey Report.* Available from: www.dh.gov.uk/en/publicationsand statistics/./DH_122516

National Cancer Patient Experience Survey (NCPES) (2013) *National Cancer Patient Experience Survey 2012–13.* Leeds: NHS England.

National Cancer Peer Review–National Cancer Action Team (2010) *Manual for Cancer Services 2008. Psychological Support Measures.* London: Department of Health. Available from: www.dh.gov.uk [accessed 31 March 2011].

National Cancer Peer Review-National Cancer Action Team (2013) *Manual for Cancer Services: Radiotherapy Measures Version 5.0.* National Cancer Action Team.

National Cancer Research Institute (NCRI) (2013) *Cancer Research Spend in the UK 2002–2011: An Overview of the Research Funded by NCRI Partners.* London: National Cancer Research Institute.

National Cancer Survivorship Initiative (2012) www.ncsi.org.uk [accessed 21 March 2012].

National Cancer Survivorship Initiative (NCSI) (2013) *Living With and Beyond Cancer: Taking Action to Improve Outcomes.* London, Department of Health, Macmillan Cancer Support & NHS Improvement.

National Center for Biotechnology Information (NCBI) (2013) NCBI Pubmed Database. Available from: www.ncbi.nlm.nih.gov/pubmed [accessed 9 December 2013].

National Centre for Complementary and Alternative Medicine (NCCAM) (2002) *What is CAM?* Available from: www.nccam.nih.gov/sites/nccam.nih.gov/files/D347.

National Chemotherapy Advisory Group (2009) *Chemotherapy Services in England: Ensuring Quality and Safety.* London: NCAG.

National Comprehensive Cancer Network (NCCN) (2004) 'Prostate cancer: NCCN clinical: practice guidelines in oncology', *J Natl Compr Canc Network.* 2(3): 224–248.

National Comprehensive Cancer Network (NCCN) (2008) *Distress Management. NCCN Clinical Practice Guidelines in Oncology.* National Comprehensive Cancer Network. Available from: www.nccn.org/professionals/physician_gls/PDF/distress.pdf.

National Comprehensive Cancer Network (NCCN) (2010) *NCNN Clinical Practice Guidelines in Oncology.* Available from: www.nccn.org/professionals/physician_gls/pdf/antiemesis.pdf

National Confidential Enquiry into Patient Outcome and Death (2006) *The Coroner's autopsy – do we deserve better?* Available from: www.ncepod.org.uk/2006Report/Downloads/ncepod_2006_report.pdf [accessed 3 January 2014].

National Confidential Inquiry into Patient Outcome and Death (2008) *Systemic Anticancer Therapy: For Better for Worse.* London: National Confidential Inquiry into Patient Outcome and Death.

National End of Life Care Intelligence Network (2012) *What Do We Know Now That We Didn't Know a Year Ago? New Intelligence On End Of Life Care in England.* Available from: www.endoflifecare-intelligence.org.uk/resources/publications/what_we_know_now [accessed 23 January 2015].

National Health Service (NHS) (2011) *Draft Spiritual Support and Bereavement Care Quality Markers and Measures for End of Life Care.* London: Department of Health.

National Health Service (NHS) Cancer Screening Programmes (2005) *Breast Cancer Grading: Nottingham Criteria.* London: Department of Health. Available from: www.cancerscreening.nhs.uk/breastscreen/publications/nhsbsp58-poster.pdf [accessed 3 November 2014].

National Health Service Choices website from: www.nhs.uk/Conditions/Malignant-melanoma/Pages/Symptoms.aspx and www.nhs.uk/conditions/malignant-melanoma/pages/realstorypage.aspx [accessed August 2012].

National Health Service England (2013) *NHS Standard Contract for Stereotactic Radiosurgery and Stereotactic Radiotherapy*. Available from: www.england.nhs.uk/wp-content/uploads/2013/06/d05-stere-radiosurg-stere-radiother.pdf [accessed 1 August 2014].

National Health Service Health Research Authority (2013) *Defining Research*. London: Health Research Authority.

National Health Service (NHS) England (2014) 'One chance to get it right: improving people's experience of care in the last few days and hours of life', *Leadership Alliance for the Care of Dying People*. NHS England. Available from: www.england.nhs.uk/ourwork/qual-clin-lead/lac/ [accessed 6 January 2015].

National Health Service Health Research Authority (2014) *Proportionate Review: Frequently Asked Questions, v3.0*. Available from: www.hra.nhs.uk/resources/applying-to-recs/nhs-rec-proportionate-review-service/

National Health Service London [on behalf of the Strategic AHP leads group (SAHPLE)] (2012) *Allied Health Professions Cancer Care Toolkit: A Guide for Health Care Commissioners*. London: National Health Service.

National Health Service Quality Improvement Scotland (2010) *Skin Care of Patients Receiving Radiotherapy*. Edinburgh: NHS Quality Improvement Scotland.

National Health Service Southwest. (2010) *Achieving Age Equality in Health and Social Care: NHS Practice Guide*. Available from: http://age-equality.southwest.nhs.uk/downloads/guides/age-equality-nhs-practice-guide-ALL-chapters.pdf [accessed 9 December 2013].

National Institute for Clinical Excellence (NICE) (2003) *Improving Outcomes for Haematological Cancers – The Research Evidence*. London: NICE.

National Institute for Clinical Excellence (NICE) (2004a) *Improving Outcomes in Head and Neck Cancers*. Available from: www.nice.org.uk/nicemedia/live/10897/28851/28851.pdf.

National Institute for Clinical Excellence (NICE) (2004b) *Guidance on Cancer Services. Improving Supportive and Palliative Care for Adults with Cancer: The Manual*. London: NICE.

National Institute for Clinical Excellence (NICE) (2004c) *Improving Supportive and Palliative Care for Adults with Cancer: The Manual*. Available from: www.nice.org.uk/nicemedia/pdf/csgsp-manual.pdf.

National Institute for Clinical Excellence (NICE) (2004d) *Guidance on Cancer Services: Improving Supportive and Palliative Care for Adults with Cancer*. London: NICE.

National Institute for Clinical Excellence (NICE) (2004e) *Improving Outcomes in Supportive and Palliative Care*. London: NICE.

National Institute for Clinical Excellence (NICE) (2005a) *Improving Outcomes in Children and Young People with Cancer*. London: HMSO.

National Institute for Health and Clinical Excellence (NICE) (2005b) *Referral Guidelines for Suspected Cancer*. London: NICE. www.nice.org.uk/CG027NICEguideline [accessed 18 November 2014].

National Institute for Health and Clinical Excellence (NICE) (2008) *Prostate Cancer: Diagnosis and Treatment*. London: NICE.

National Institute for Health and Clinical Excellence (NICE) (2009a) *Advanced Breast Cancer: Diagnosis and Treatment. NICE Clinical Guideline*. London: National Collaborating Centre.

National Institute for Health and Clinical Excellence (NICE) (2009b) *NICE Guidelines [CG90]: Depression in Adults: the Treatment and Management of Depression in Adults*. Available from: www.nice.org.uk/guidance/CG90/chapter/introduction [accessed 7 September 2014].

National Institute for Health and Clinical Excellence (NICE) (2011) *Guideline 122. Ovarian Cancer: The Recognition and Initial Management of Ovarian Cancer*. London: NICE. http://guidance.nice.org.uk/CG122.

National Institute for Health and Clinical Excellence (NICE) (2012a) *Quality Standard for Lung Cancer*. London: NICE.

National Institute for Health and Clinical Excellence (NICE) (2012b) *Quality Standard for Colorectal Cancer*. Available from: http://publications.nice.org.uk/quality-standard-for-colorectal-cancer-qs20.

National Institute for Health and Clinical Excellence (NICE) (2012c) *CG151 Neutropenic Sepsis: Full Guidelines*. London: NICE.

National Institute for Health and Care Excellence (NICE) (2013a) *Quality Standard for Patient Experience in Adult NHS Services*. Available from: http://publications.nice.org.uk/quality-standard-for-patient-experience-in-adult-nhs-services-qs15 [accessed 18 November 2014].

National Institute for Health and Care Excellence (NICE) (2013b) *Familial Breast Cancer: Classification and Care of People at Risk of Familial Breast Cancer and Management of Breast Cancer and Related Risks in People with a Family History of Breast Cancer. [CG164]*. London: NICE.

National Institute for Health and Care Excellence (NICE) (n.d.) http://guidance.nice.org.uk/Topic/Cancer

National Institute for Health Research (NIHR) (2010) *Research in the NHS: HR Good Practice Resource Pack, Version 1*. Available from: www.nihr.ac.uk/files/Research%20Passport%20Current/Instructions%20for%20Completing%20the%20Research%20Passport%20Form%20_V1.1.pdf [accessed 24 April 2012].

National Institute for Health Research (NIHR) (2013) *UK Clinical Trials Gateway (UKCTG)*. Available from: www.ukctg.nihr.ac.uk/default.aspx [accessed 9 December 2013].

National Office of the NHS Screening Programme (2014a) *NHS Cancer Screening Programme*. Available from: www.cancerscreening.nhs.uk/cervical/about-cervical-screening.html [accessed 21 April 2014].

National Office of the NHS Screening Programme (2014b) *NHS Cervical Screening Programme*. Available from: www.cancerscreening.nhs.uk/cervical/statistics.html [accessed 21 April 2014].

National Office of the NHS Screening Programme (2014c) *NHS Breast Screening Programme*. Available from: www.cancerscreening.nhs.uk/breastscreen/index.html [accessed 21 April 2014].

National Office of the NHS Screening Programme (2014d) *Breast Screening Programme, England 2010-11*. Available from: www.cancerscreening.nhs.uk/breastscreen/breast-statistics-bulletin-2010-11.pdf [accessed 13 November 2014].

National Office of the NHS Screening Programme (2014e) *NHS Bowel Scope Screening*. Available from: www.cancerscreening.nhs.uk/bowel/bowel-scope-screening.html [accessed 21 April 2014].

National Office of the NHS Screening Programme (2014f) *Prostate Cancer Risk Management Programme*. Available from: www.cancerscreening.nhs.uk/prostate/index.html [accessed 21 April 2014].

National Office of the NHS Screening Programme (2014g) *Informed Choice About Cancer Screening*. Available from: www.informedchoiceaboutcancerscreening.org/ [accessed 21 April 2014].

National Quality Forum (2006) *A National Framework and Preferred Practice for Palliative and Hospice Care Quality*. Washington, DC: National Quality Forum.

Navari, R.M. (2013) 'A review of the prevention of nausea and vomiting induced by chemotherapy', *European Oncology and Haematology*, 9(1): 51–5.

Navarro, V. (2009) 'What we mean by social determinants of health', *International Journal of Health Services*, 39 (3): 423–441.

Naylor, W. and Mallett, J. (2001) 'Management of acute radiotherapy induced skin reactions: a literature review,' *European Journal of Oncology Nursing*, 5(4): 221–33.

Neal, R.D. (2009) 'Do diagnostic delays in cancer matter?', *British Journal of Cancer* 101(S2): S9–12.

Neary, P., Makin, G.B., White, T.J., White, E., Hartley, J., MacDonald, A., Lee, P.W.R. and Monson, J.R.T. (2003) 'Transanal endoscopic microsurgery: a viable operative alternative in selected patients with rectal lesions', *Annals of Surgical Oncology*, 10: 1106–11.

Needham, C. (2003) *Citizen-Consumers: New Labour's Marketplace Democracy*. London: Catalyst.

Neimeyer, R.A. (2001) (ed.) *Meaning Reconstruction and the Experience of Loss*. Washington, DC: American Psychological Association Press.

Nekolaichuk, C.L., Cumming, C., Turner, J., Yushchyshyn, A. and Sela, R. (2011) 'Referral patterns and psychosocial distress in cancer patients accessing a psycho-oncology counseling service', *Psycho-oncology*, 20: 326–32.

Nelson, E. and While, D. (2002) 'Children's adjustment during the first year of a parent's cancer diagnosis', *Journal of Psychosocial Oncology*, 20: 15–36.

Nelson, H.D., Fu, R., Goddard, K., et al. (2013) *Risk Assessment, Genetic Counseling, and Genetic Testing for BRCA-Related Cancer: Systematic Review to Update the U.S. Preventive Services Task Force Recommendation*. Rockville, MD: Agency for Healthcare Research and Quality (US).

Nelson, R.L., Gladman, E. and Barbateskovic, M. (2014) 'Antimicrobial prophylaxis for colorectal surgery', *Cochrane Database of Systematic Reviews*, Issue 5, CD001181. doi:10.1002/14651858. CD001181.pub4.

Neuss, M.N., Desch, C.E., McNiff, K.K., Eisenberg, P.D., Gesme, D.H., Jacobson, J.O., Jahanzeb, M., Padberg, J.J., Rainey, J.M., Guo, J.J. and Simone, J.V. (2005) 'A process for measuring the quality of cancer care: the Quality Oncology Practice Initiative', *Journal of Clinical Oncology*, 23(25): 6233–9.

Newell, S.A., Sanson-Fisher, R.W. and Savolainen, N.J. (2002) 'Systematic review of psychological therapies for cancer patients: overview and recommendations for future research', *Journal of the National Cancer Institute*, 94(8): 558–84.

Nguyen, T.N., Nilsson, S., Hellström, A-L. and Bengston, A. (2010) 'Music therapy to reduce pain and anxiety in children with cancer undergoing lumbar puncture: a randomized clinical trial', *Journal of Pediatric Oncology Nursing*, 27(3): 146–55.

NHS Confederation (2010) *Feeling Better? Improving Patient Experience in Hospital*. London: The NHS Confederation. Available from: www.nhsconfed.org/Publications/Documents/ Feeling_better_Improving_patient_experience_in_hospital_Report.pdf (Guideline Ref ID NHSC2010).

Nho, J.H. (2013) 'Effect of PLISSIT model sexual health enhancement program for women with gynecologic cancer and their husbands', *Journal of the Korean Academy of Nursing*, 43(5): 681–9.

Nicholls, W., Hulbert-Williams, N.J. and Bramwell, R. (2014) 'The role of relationship attachment in psychological adjustment to cancer in patients and caregivers: a systematic review of the literature', *Psycho-Oncology*, 23(10): 1083–1095.

Nijman, J.L., Sixma, H., van Triest, B., Keus, R.B. and Denricks, M. (2011) 'The quality of radiation care: the results of focus group interviews and concept mapping to explore the patient's perspective', *Radiotherapy and Oncology*, 102: 154–60.

Nivison-Smith, I., Hawkins, P. and Ma, D.D.F. (2000) *Outcomes of 124 Allogeneic Transplants Involving Matched Related Non-Sibling Donors – A Comparative Study from the Australasian Bone Marrow Transplant Recipient Registry*. Poster presentation at IBMTR/ABMTR Participants' meeting, Anaheim, CA, March.

Nix, T.W. and Barnette, J.J. (1998) 'The data analysis dilemma: ban or abandon. A review of null hypothesis significance testing', *Research in the Schools*, 5(2): 3–14.

Noble-Adams, R. (1999) 'Radiation-induced reactions 2: development of a measurement tool', *British Journal of Nursing*, 8(18): 1208–11.

Nofech-Mozes, S., Vella, E.T., Dhesy-Thind, S., Hagerty, K.L., Mangu, P.B., Temin, S. and Hanna, W.M. (2012) 'Systematic review of hormone receptor testing in breast cancer', *Applied Immunohistochemistry and Molecular Morphology*, 20(3): 214–63.

Nogier, P.M.T. (1981) *Handbook on Auricular Therapy*. Moulins-les-Metz, France: Maisonneuve.

Nolan, S. (2012) *Spiritual Care at the End Of Life: The Chaplain as a 'Hopeful Presence'*. London: Jessica Kingsley.

Norberg, A.L. and Steneby S. (2009) 'Experiences of parents of children surviving brain tumour: a happy ending and a rough beginning', *European Journal of Cancer Care*, 18: 371–380.

Nord, C., Mykletun, A., Thorsen, L., Bjoro, T. and Fossa, S.D. (2005) 'Self-reported health and use of health care services in long term cancer survivors', *International Journal of Cancer*, 114(2): 307–16.

Norman, P., Bennett, P., Smith, C. and Murphy, S. (1997) 'Health locus of control and leisure-time exercise', *Personality and Individual Differences*, 23(5): 769–74.

Northouse, L.L., Katapodi, M., Song, L., et al. (2010) 'Interventions with family care-givers of cancer patients', *Ca: A Cancer Journal for Clinicians*, 60: 317–39.

Northouse, L.L, Rosset, T., Phillips, L., Mood, D., Schafenacker, A. and Kershaw, T. (2006) 'Research with families facing cancer: the challenges of accrual and retention', *Research in Nursing & Health,* 29: 199–211.

Nottingham City and County PCT (2011) *In The Pink: Providing Excellent Care for LGBT People.* Available from: http://btckstorage.blob.core.windows.net/site2702/In%20the%20pink.pdf [accessed 18 November 2014].

Nursing and Midwifery Council (2010) *The Code: Standards of Conduct, Performance and Ethics for Nurses and Midwives.* Available from: www.nmc-uk.org

O'Connell, K.A. and Skevington, S.M. (2010) 'Spiritual, religious, and personal beliefs are important and distinctive to assessing quality of life in health: a comparison of theoretical models', *British Journal of Health Psychology,* 15(Pt 4): 729–48.

O'Kelly, J. and Koffman, J. (2007) 'Multidisiplinary perspectives of music therapy in adult palliative care', *Palliative Medicine,* 21(3): 235–241.

O'Regan, P., Wills, T. and O'Leary, A. (2010) 'Complementary therapies: a challenge for nursing practice', *Nursing Standard,* 24(21): 35–40.

O'Shaughnessy, J., Miles, D., Vukelja, S., Moiseyenko, V., Ayoub, J.P., Cervantes, G., et al. (2002) 'Superior survival with capecitabine plus docetaxel combination therapy in anthracycline-pretreated patients with advanced breast cancer: phase III trial results', *J Clin Oncol.,* 20(12): 2812–2823.

Oakley, C., Lennan, E., Roe, H., Craven, O., Harrold, K. and Vidall, C. (2010) 'Safe practice and nursing care of patients receiving oral anti-cancer medicines: a position statement from UKONS', *Ecancermedicalscience,* 4: 177.

Office for National Statistics (2006) *General Health.* UK Government.

Office for National Statistics (2011) *Interim Life Tables, England and Wales 1980–82 to 2008–10.* Available from: www.ons.gov.uk/ons/search/index.html?newquery=United+Kingdom+Health+Statistics&newoffset=1150&pageSize=50&sortBy=&sortDirection=DESCENDING&applyFilters=true [accessed 9 December 2013].

Office for National Statistics (2012) *General Lifestyle Survey 2010.* Available from: www.ons.gov.uk/ons/rel/ghs/general-lifestyle-survey/2010/index.html [accessed 9 December 2013].

Office for National Statistics (2013a) *Deaths Registered in England and Wales (Series DR) 2012.* London: Office for National Statistics.

Office for National Statistics (2013b) *Health Expectancies at Birth and Age 65 in the United Kingdom.* Available from: www.ons.gov.uk/ons/rel/disability-and-health-measurement/health-expectancies-at-birth-and-age-65-in-the-united-kingdom/index.html [accessed 9 December 2013].

Office for National Statistics (2013c) *Statistical Bulletin, Deaths Registered in England and Wales (Series DR) 2012.* Available from: www.ons.gov.uk/ons/dcp171778_331565.pdf [accessed 22 October 2013].

Oguchi, M., Jansen, J., Butow, P., Colagiuri, B., Divine, R. and Dhillon, H. (2011) 'Measuring the impact of nurse cue-response behaviour on cancer patients' emotional cues', *Patient Education and Counseling,* 82: 163–8.

Oken, M.M., Hocking, W.G., Kvale, P.A. et al. (2011) 'Screening by chest radiograph and lungcancer mortality: the Prostate, Lung, Colorectal, and Ovarian (PLCO) randomized trial', *Journal of the American Medical Association,* 306(17): 1865–73.

Oluwasola, O.A., Fawole, O.I., Otegbayo, A.J., Ogun, G.O., Adebamowo, C.A. and Bamigboye, A.E. (2009) 'The autopsy: knowledge, attitude and perceptions of doctors and relatives of the deceased', *Archives of Pathology and Laboratory Medicine,* 133: 78–82.

Örtqvist, D. and Wincent, J. (2010) 'Role stress, exhaustion, and satisfaction: a cross-lagged structural equation modelling approach supporting Hobfoll's loss spirals', *Journal of Applied Social Psychology,* 40(6): 1357–84.

Osborn, D.P.J., Levy, G., Nazareth, I., Peterson, I., Islam, A. and King, M.B. (2007) 'Relative risk of cardiovascular and cancer mortality in people with severe mental illness from the United Kingdom's general: practice research database', *Archives of General Psychiatry.* 64: 242–9.

Osborn, R.L., Demoncada, A.C. and Feuerstein, M. (2006) 'Psychosocial interventions for depression, anxiety, and quality of life in cancer survivors: meta-analyses', *International Journal of Psychiatry in Medicine*, 36(1): 13–34.

Ostafin, B. and Marlatt, G. (2008) 'Surfing the urge: experiential acceptance moderates the relation between automatic alcohol motivation and hazardous drinking', *Journal of Social and Clinical Psychology*, 27(4): 404–18.

Oxford Dictionaries (2014) *Stress*. Available from: www.oxforddictionaries.com/definition/english/stress?q=stress [accessed 8 March 2014].

Packman, W., Weber, S., Wallace, J. and Bugescu, N. (2010) 'Psychological effects of hematopoietic SCT on pediatric patients, siblings and parents: a review', *Bone Marrow Transplantation*, 45: 1134–46.

Palazzoli, M., Boscolo, L., Cecchin, G. and Prata, G.l (1978) *Paradox and Counterparadox*. New York, NY: Jason Aronson.

Parekh, N., Chandran, U. and Bandera, E.V. (2012) 'Obesity in cancer survival', *Annual Review of Nutrition*, 32(1): 311–42.

Pargament, K.I. (2007) *Spiritually Integrated Psychotherapy: Understanding and Addressing the Sacred*. New York, NY: Guilford Press.

Park, T.G., Jeong, J.H. and Kim, S.W. (2006) 'Current status of polymeric gene delivery systems', *Advance Drug Delivery Reviews*, 58: 467–86.

Parkes, C.M. (1970) 'The first year of bereavement: a longitudinal study of the reaction of London widows to the death of their husbands', *Psychiatry*, 33: 444–467.

Parkes, C.M. (1975) *Bereavement: Studies of Grief in Adult Life*. London: Pelican Books.

Parkes, C.M. and Prigerson, H.G. (2010) *Bereavement: Studies of Grief in Adult Life*, 4th edn. London: Routledge.

Parkes, C.M. and Weiss, R.S.(1983) *Recovery from Bereavement*. New York: Basic Books.

Parkin, D.M. (2006) 'The global health burden of infection-associated cancers in the year 2002', *International Journal of Cancer*, 118(12): 3030–44.

Parkin, D.M. (2011) 'Cancers attributable to occupational exposures in the UK in 2010', *British Journal of Cancer*, 105(S2): S70–2.

Parkin, D.M. and Boyd, L. (2011) 'Cancers attributable to overweight and obesity in the UK in 2010', *British Journal of Cancer*, 105(Suppl. 2): S34–7. doi:10.1038/bjc.2011.481.

Parkin, D.M., Mesher, D. and Sasieni, P. (2010) 'Cancers attributable to solar (ultraviolet) radiation exposure in the UK in 2010', *British Journal of Cancer*, 105(Suppl. 2): S66–9. doi:10.1038/bjc.2011.486.

Parkin, M., Boyd, L. and Walker, L.C. (2010) 'The fraction of cancer attributable to lifestyle and environmental factors in the UK in 2010', *British Journal of Cancer*, 105(Supp. 2): S77–81.

Parle, M., Jones, B. and Maguire, P. (1996) 'Maladaptive coping and affective disorders among cancer patients', *Psychological Medicine*, 26, 735–44.

Parle, M., Maguire P. and Heaven C. (1997) 'The development of a training model to improve health professionals' skills, self efficacy and outcome expectancy when communicating with cancer patients', *Social Science & Medicine*, 44: 231–40.

Parliamentary and Health Service Ombudsman (2009) *Six Lives: The Provision of Public Services to People with Learning Disabilities*. London: The Stationery Office.

Partridge, A.H., Gelbar, S., Peppercorn, J., et al. (2004) 'Web-based survey of fertility issues in young women with breast cancer', *Journal of Clinical Oncology*, 22(20): 4174–83.

Passweg, J.R., Baldomero, H., Gratwohl, A., Bregni, M., Cesaro, S., Dreger, P., De Witte, T., Farge-Bancel, D., Gaspar, B., Marsh, J., Mohty, M., Peters, C., Tichelli, A., Velardi, A., Ruiz de Elvira, C., Falkenburg, F., Sureda, A., Madrigal, A. and for the European Group for Blood and Marrow Transplantation (EBMT) (2012a) 'The EBMT activity survey: 1990–2010', *Bone Marrow Transplantation*, 47: 906–23.

Passweg, J.R., Halter, J., Bucher, C., Gerull, S., Heim, D., Rovo, A., Buser, A., Stern, M. and Tichelli, A. (2012b) 'Hematopoietic stem cell transplantation: a review and recommendations for follow-up care for the general practitioner', *Swiss Medical Weekly*, 142: w13696.

Patenaude, A.F. and Kupst, M.J. (2005) 'Psychosocial functioning in pediatric cancer', *Journal of Pediatric Psychology*, 30(1): 9–27.

Paterson, C. and Britten, N. (2003) 'Acupuncture for people with chronic illnesses: combining qualitative and quantitative outcome assessment', *The Journal of Alternative and Complementary Medicine*, 9(5): 671–81.

Paterson, C., Thomas, K., Manasse, A., Cooke, H. and Peace, G. (2007) 'Measure yourself concerns and wellbeing (MYCaW): an individualised questionnaire for evaluating outcome in cancer support care that includes complementary therapies', *Complement Ther Med*, 15: 38–45.

Pathology Harmony (2012) *Tumour Marker Requesting: Guidance for Non-Specialists*. Available from: www.pathologyharmony.co.uk/harmony-bookmark-v7.pdf [accessed 5 January 2014].

Patja, K., Eero, P. and Iivanainen, M. (2001) 'Cancer incidence among people with intellectual disability', *Journal of Intellectual Disability Research*, 45(4): 300–307.

Patja, K., Mölsä, P. and Iivanainen, M. (2001) 'Cause-specific mortality of people with intellectual disability in a population-based, 35-year follow-up study', *Journal of Intellectual Disability Research*, 45(1): 30–40.

Patja, K., Pukkala, E., Sund, R., Iivanainen, M. and Kaski, M. (2006) 'Cancer incidence of persons with Down syndrome in Finland: a population-based study', *International Journal of Cancer*, 118(7): 1769–72.

Patrick, D.L., Ferketich S.L., Frame P.S., Harris J.J., Hendricks C.B., et al. (2003) 'National Institutes of Health State-of-the-Science Conference Statement: Symptom Management in Cancer: Pain, Depression, and Fatigue, July 15–17, 2002', *Journal of the National Cancer Institute*, 95: 1110–7.

Patterson, J.M., Holm, K.E. and Gurney, J.G. (2004) 'The impact of childhood cancer on the family: a qualitative analysis of strains, resources, and coping behaviors', *Psycho-oncology*, 13: 390–407.

Pavlicevic, M. (ed.) (2005) *Music Therapy in Children's Hospices: Jessie's Fund in Action*. London: Jessica Kingsley.

Pavlicevic, M. and Ansdell, G. (eds) (2004) *Community Music Therapy*. London: Jessica Kingsley.

Pavlidis, N. and Fizazi, K. (2009) 'Carcinoma of unknown primary (CUP)', *Critical Reviews in Oncology/Hematology*, 69(3): 271–8.

Payne, S.A. and Seymour J.E. (2004) 'Overview', in S. Payne, J. Seymour and C. Ingleton (eds), *Palliative Care Nursing: Principles and Evidence for Practice*. Maidenhead, UK: Open University Press. pp. 15–38.

Payne, S.A., Seymour, J.E., Chapman, A. and Holloway, M. (2008) 'Older Chinese people's views on food: implications for supportive cancer care', *Ethnicity & Health*, 13(5): 497–514.

Pearce, C.L., Chung, K., Pike, M.C., Wu, A.H. (2009) 'Increased ovarian cancer risk associated with menopausal estrogen therapy is reduced by adding a progestin', *Cancer*, 115(3): 531–9.

Pearce, S. (2008) 'The impact of adolescent cancer in healthcare professionals', in D. Kelly and F. Gibson (eds), *Cancer Care for Adolescents and Young Adults*. Oxford: Blackwell-Wiley. pp. 59–77.

Pearson, V. (1998) 'Only one quarter of women with learning disabilities in Exeter have cervical screening', *British Medical Journal*, 316: 1979.

Pekmezi, D.W. and Demark-Wahnefried, W. (2011) 'Updated evidence in support of diet and exercise interventions in cancer survivors', *Acta Oncologica*, 50(2): 167–78.

Pendley, J.S., Dahlquist, L.M. and Dreyer, Z. (1997) 'Body image and psychosocial adjustment in adolescent cancer survivors', *Journal of Pediatric Psychology*, 22(1): 29–43.

Peng, Z. (2005) 'Current status of Gendicine® in China: recombinant humanAd-p53 agent for treatment of cancers', *Human Gene Therapy*, 16: 1016–27.

Penson, R.T., Daniels, K.J. and Lynch Jr, T.J. (2004) 'Too old to care?', *Oncologist*, 9(3): 343–52.

Penson, R.T., Gu, F., Harris, S., Thiel, M., Lawton, N., Fuller, A. and Lynch, T. (2007) 'Hope', *Oncologist*, 12(9): 1105–13.

Perkins, H.W. (2007) 'Misperceptions of peer drinking norms in Canada: another look at the "reign of error" and its consequences among college students', *Addictive Behaviors*, 32(11): 2645–56.

Peto, R. (2011) 'The fraction of cancer attributable to lifestyle and environmental factors in the UK in 2010', *British Journal of Cancer*, 105(Suppl. 2): S1. doi:10.1038/bjc.2011.473.

Picardi, A. (2009) 'Rating scales in bipolardisorder', *Current Opinion in Psychiatry,* 22(1): 42–9.

Piccart-Gebhart et al (2005) 'Trastuzumab after Adjuvant Chemotherapy in HER2–Positive Breast Cancer', *New England Journal of Medicine,* 353: 1659–72.

Pickett, M., Brennan, A.W, Greenberg, H.S, Licht, L. and Worrell, J.C. (1994) 'Use of debriefing techniques to prevent compassion fatigue in research teams', *Nursing Research,* 43(4): 250–2.

Pike, M.C., Pearce, C.L. and Wu, A.H. (2004) 'Prevention of cancers of the breast, endometrium and ovary', *Oncogene,* 23(38): 6379–91.

Piper, B.F., Dibble, S.L., Dodd, M.J., Weiss, M.C., Slaughter, R.E. and Paul, S.M. (1998) 'The revised Piper Fatigue Scale: psychometric evaluation in women with breast cancer', *Oncology Nurse Forum,* 25(4): 677–84.

Pirl, W., Muriel, A., Hwang, V., Kornblith, A., Greer, J. and Donelan, K. (2007) 'Screening for psychosocial distress: a national survey of oncologists', *Journal of Supportive Oncology,* 5(1): 499–504.

Pitcairn, A. (2008) 'Life after treatment, or chemotherapy saves the lost boy', in D. Kelly and F. Gibson (eds), *Cancer Care for Adolescents and Young Adults.* Oxford: Blackwell-Wiley. pp. 163–6.

Pitceathly, C., Tolosa, I., Kerr, I.B. and Grassi, L. (2011) 'Cognitive analytic therapy in psycho-oncology', in M. Watson and D. Kissane (eds), *Handbook of Psychotherapy in Cancer Care.* Oxford, UK: Wiley-Blackwell Publishers.

Pivot, P. Gligorov, J., Muller, V., Barreett-Lee, P., Verma, S., Knoop, A., Curigliano, G., Semiglazov, V., Lopez-Vivano, G., Jenkins, V., Scotto, N., Osbourne, S. and Fallowfield, L. (2013) 'Preference for subcutaneous or intravenous administration of trastuzumab in patients with HER2-positive early breast cancer (PrefHer): an open-label randomised study', *Lancet Oncology,* 14(10): 962–70.

Poirier, P. (2011) 'The impact of fatigue on role functioning during radiation therapy', *Oncology Nursing Forum,* 38(4): 457–65.

Polit, D.F. and Beck C.T. (2004) *Nursing Research: Principles and Methods,* 7th edn. Philadelphia, PA: Lippincott Williams & Wilkins.

Politi, M.C., Clark, M.A., Ombao, H., et al. (2011) 'Communicating uncertainty can lead to less decision satisfaction: a necessary cost of involving patients in shared decision making?', *Health Expectations,* 14(1): 84–91.

Politi, M.C., Han, P.K. and Col, N.F. (2007) 'Communicating the uncertainty of harms and benefits of medical interventions', *Medical Decision Making,* 27(5): 681–95.

Poon, P.C.M. (2012) 'The information needs, perceptions of communication and decision-making process of cancer patients receiving palliative chemotherapy', *Journal of Pain Management,* 5(1): 93–105.

Pope, C. and Mays, N. (2006) 'Qualitative methods in health research', in C. Pope and N. Mays (eds), *Qualitative Research in Health Care,* 3rd edn. Malden, MA: Blackwell Publishing.

Pope, C., Ziebland, S. and Mays, N. (2000) 'Analysing qualitative data', *British Medical Journal,* 320(7227): 114–16.

Pope, C., Ziebland, S. and Mays, N. (2006) 'Analysing qualitative data', in C. Pope and N. Mays (eds), *Qualitative Research in Health Care,* 3rd edn. Malden, MA: Blackwell Publishing.

Porcu, E., Ciotti, P.M. and Venturoli, S. (2013) *Handbook of Human Oocyte Preservation.* Cambridge: Cambridge University Press.

Porth, C.M. (2011) *Essentials of Pathophysiology,* 3rd edn. Philadelphia, PA: Wolters Kluwer/ Lippincott Williams & Wilkins.

Portnoy, D.B., Han, P.K., Ferrer, R.A., et al. (2013) Physicians' attitudes about communicating and managing scientific uncertainty differ by perceived ambiguity aversion of their patients', *Health Expectations,* 16(4): 362–72.

Potter, P., Deshields, T., Divanbeigi, J., Berger, J., Cipriano, D., Norris, L. and Olsen, S. (2010) 'Compassion fatigue and burnout: prevalence amongst oncology nurses', *Clinical Journal of Oncology Nursing,* 14(5): 56–62.

Power, E., Miles, A., von Wagner, C., et al. (2009) 'Uptake of colorectal cancer screening: system, provider and individual factors and strategies to improve participation', *Future Oncology,* 5(9): 1371–88.

Power, S. and Condon, C. (2008) 'Chemotherapy induced alopecia: a phenomenological study', *Cancer Nursing Practice*, 7(7): 44–7.

Poylin, V., Curran, T., Lee, E. and Nagle, D. (2014) 'Laparoscopic colectomy decreases the time to administration of chemotherapy compared with open colectomy', *Annals of Surgical Oncology*, 21(11): 3587–3591.

Prager K. (1995) *The Psychology of Intimacy*. New York, NY: Guilford Press.

PREDICT (2008) *Increasing the Participation of the Elderly in Clinical Trials: Work Package 1. Literature Review*. Available from: www.predicteu.org/Reports/PREDICT_WP1_Report.pdf [accessed 9 December 2013].

PREDICT (2013) *Increasing the PaRticipation of the ElDerly in Clinical Trials*. Available from: www.predicteu.org/index.html [accessed 9 December 2013].

Primrose, J.N., Perera, R., Gray, A., Rose, P., Fuller, A., Corkhill, A., George, S., Mant, D. and FACS Trial Investigators (2014) 'Effect of 3 to 5 years of scheduled CEA and CT follow-up to detect recurrence of colorectal cancer: the FACS randomized clinical trial', *Journal of the American Medical Association*, 311: 263–70. doi:10.1001/jama.2013.285718.

Princess Royal Radiotherapy Review Team (2011) *Managing Radiotherapy Induced Skin Reactions, A Toolkit for Healthcare Professionals*. St James's Institute of Oncology. Available from: www.ycn.nhs.uk/html/downloads/ltht-managingradiotherapyinducedskinreactions-oct2011.pdf [accessed 29 August 2014].

Prochaska, J.O. and di Clemente, C.C. (1984) *The Transtheoretical Approach: Crossing Traditional Boundaries of Therapy*. Homewood, IL: Brooks.

Prostate Cancer UK (2012) *Prostate Cancer – A Guide for Newly Diagnosed Men*. Available from http://prostatecanceruk.org [accessed 4 January 2014].

Pruitt, R.H. and Privette A.B. (2001) 'Planning strategies for the avoidance of pitfalls in intervention research', *Journal of Advanced Nursing*, 35(4): 514–20.

Public Health England (2010) Th*e Tobacco Advertising and Promotion (Display) (England) Regulations (2010, Statutory Instrument No.445*. Available from: www.legislation.gov.uk/uksi/2010/445/made [accessed 7 June 2014].

Puchalski, C., Ferrell, B., Virani, R., Otis-Green, S., Baird, P., Bull, J., Chochinov, H., Handzo, G., Nelson-Becker, H., Prince-Paul, M., Pugliese, K. and Sulmasy, D. (2009) 'Improving the quality of spiritual care as a dimension of palliative care: the report of the Consensus Conference', *Journal of Palliative Medicine*, 12(10): 885–904.

Puig, A., Lee, S.M., Goodwin, L. and Sherrard, P.A.D. (2006) 'The efficacy of creative arts therapies to enhance emotional expression, spirituality and psychological well-being of newly diagnosed stage I and stage II breast cancer patients', *The Arts in Psychotherapy*, 33 (3): 218–228.

Pulgar, A., Garrido, S., Alcala, A. and Reyes del Passo, G.A. (2012) 'Psychological predictors of immune response following bone marrow transplantation', *Behavioural Medicine*, 38(1): 12–18.

Pulte, D. and Brenner, H. (2010) 'Changes in survival in head and neck cancers in the late 20th and early 21st century: a period analysis', *Oncologist*, 15: 994–1001.

Purandare, L. (1997) 'Attitudes to cancer may create a barrier to communication between the patient and caregiver', *European Journal of Cancer Care*, 6: 92–99.

Quality Health (2013a) *National Cancer Patient Experience Survey National Report*. Available from: www.quality-health.co.uk/resources/surveys/national-cancer-experience-survey/2013-national-cancer-patient-experience-survey-reports [accessed 9 December 2013].

Quality Health (2013b) *Radiotherapy Patient Experience Survey 2013 National Report*. NHS England.

Queenan, J.A., Feldman-Stewart, D., Brundage, M. and Groome, P.A. (2010) 'Social support and quality of life of prostate cancer patients after radiotherapy treatment', *European Journal of Cancer Care*, 19: 251–9.

Quinn, B. and and Kelly, D. (2000) 'Sperm banking and fertility concerns: enhancing the support available to men with cancer', *European Journal of Oncology Nursing*, 4: 55–8.

Quinn, B. and Stephens, M. (2006) 'Bone marrow transplantation' in N. Kearney and A. Richardson (eds), *Nursing Patients with Cancer: Principles and Practice*. Edinburgh: Elsevier Churchill Livingstone. pp. 329–351.

Quinn, G., Koskan, A., Wells, K.J., Gonzales, L.E., Meade, C.D., Christie, L. and Jacobsen, P. (2012) 'Cancer patients' fears related to clinical trial participation: a qualitative study', *Journal of Cancer Education,* 27: 257–62.

Quinten, C., Coens, C., Mauer, M., Comte, S., Sprangers, M.A.G., Cleeland, C., Osoba, D., Bjordal, K. and Bottomley, A. (2009) 'Baseline quality of life as a prognostic indicator of survival: a meta-analysis of individual patient data from EORTC clincial trials', *Lancet Oncology,* 10(9): 865–71.

Radecki, S.E., Kane, R.L., Solomon, D.H., Mendenhall, R.C. and Beck, J.C. (1988) 'Do physicians spend less time with older patients?', *Journal of the American Geriatric Society,* 36(8): 713–8.

Radloff, L.S. (1977) 'The CESD Scale: a self report scale for research in the general population', *Applied Psychological Measurement,* 1: 385–401.

Raffle, A.E., Alden, B., Quinn, M., Babb, P. and Brett, M. (2003) 'Outcomes of screening to prevent cancer: analysis of cumulative incidence of cervical abnormality and modelling of cases and deaths prevented', *British Medical Journal,* 326: 901–6.

Raffle, A.E. and Gray, J.A.M. (2007) *Screening: Evidence and Practice.* Oxford: Oxford University Press.

Rager, K.B. (2005) 'Compassion stress and the qualitative researcher', *Qualitative Health Research,* 15(3): 423–30.

Rajaraman, P., Simpson, J., Neta, G., Berrington de Gonzalez, A., Ansell, P., Linet, M.S., Ron, E. and Roman, E. (2011) 'Early life exposure to diagnostic radiation and ultrasound scans and risk of childhood cancer: case-control study', *British Medical Journal:* 342: 472–7.

Ramirez, A.J, Graham, J., Richards, M.A., Cull, A. and Gregory, W.M. (1996) 'Mental health of hospital consultants: the effects of stress and satisfaction at work', *Lancet,* 347: 724–8.

Rand, K.L., Cripe, L.D., Monahan, P.O., Tong, Y., Schmidt, S. and Rawl, S.M. (2012) 'Illness appraisal, religious coping, and psychological responses in men with advanced cancer', *Supportive Care in Cancer,* 20(8): 1719–28.

Rasmussen, D.M. and Elverdam, B. (2007) 'Cancer survivors' experience of time: time disruption and time appropriation', *Journal of Advanced Nursing,* 57(6): 614–22.

Ratchet, B., Maringe, C., Nur, U., Quaresma, M., Shah, A., Woods, L., et al (2009) 'Population-based cancer survival trends in England and Wales up to 2007: an assessment of the NHS cancer plan for England', *Lancet Oncology,* 10: 351–69.

Ream, E., Finnegan-John, J., Foster, R., et al. (2013) *I'm Just in the Shadow to Keep an Eye: an Investigation to Understand the Need for Support in Family Members of People Having Chemotherapy.* Macmillan Cancer Care.

Regan-Smith, M., Hirschmann, K., Lobst, W. and Battersby, M. (2006) 'Teaching residents chronic disease management using the Flinders model', *Journal of Cancer Education,* 21(2): 60–2.

Regnard, C., Reynolds, J., Watson, B., Matthews, D., Gibson, L., and Clarke, C. (2007) 'Understanding distress in people with severe communication difficulties: developing and assessing the Disability Distress Assessment Tool (DisDAT)', *Journal of Intellectual Disability Research,* 51(4): 277–92.

Relf, M., Machin, L. and Archer, N. (2008) *Guidance For Bereavement Needs Assessment in Palliative Care.* London: Help the Hospices.

Renehan, A.G., Tyson, M., Egger, M., Heller, R.F. and Zwahlen, M. (2008) 'Body-mass index and incidence of cancer: a systematic review and meta-analysis of prospective observational studies', *Lancet,* 371(9612): 569–78.

Renner, B., Spivak, Y., Kwon, S. and Schwarzer, R. (2007) 'Does age make a difference? Predicting physical activity of South Koreans', *Psychology and Aging,* 22(3): 482–93.

Repetto, L. (2003) 'Greater risks of chemotherapy toxicity in elderly patients with cancer', *Journal of Supportive Oncology,* 1(S2): 18–24.

Reynolds, F. and Lim, K.H. (2007) 'Contribution of visual art-making to the subjective well-being of women living with cancer: a qualitative study', *The Arts in Psychotherapy,* 34(1): 1–10.

Ribbens McCarthy, J. and Edwards, R. (2011) *Key concepts in Family Studies.* London: Sage Publications.

Richards, M.A. (2009) 'The National Awareness and Early Diagnosis Initiative in England: assembling the evidence', *British Journal of Cancer,* 101(S2): S1–4.

Richards, M.A. and Hiom, S. (eds) (2009) 'Diagnosing cancer earlier: evidence for a National Awareness and Early Detection Initiative', *British Journal of Cancer,* 101(Suppl. 2): ??.

Richardson, A., Tebbit, P., Brown, V. and Sitzia, J. on behalf of the Cancer Action Team (2007) *Holistic Common Assessment of Supportive and Palliative Care Needs for Adults with Cancer. Report to the Cancer Action Team.* London: King's College London.

Richardson, B.E. and Lehmann, R. (2010) 'Mechanisms guiding primordial germ cell migration: strategies from different organisms', *Nature Reviews Molecular Cell Biology,* 11: 37–49.

Richardson, C. and Atkinson, J. (2006) 'Blood and marrow transplantation', in M. Grundy (ed.), *Nursing in Haematological Oncology,* 2nd edn. Edinburgh: Ballière Tindall.

Ridner, S.H., Bonner, C.M., Deng, J. and Sinclair, V.G. (2012) 'Voices from the shadows: living with lymphedema', *Cancer Nursing,* 35(1): E18–26.

Riely, G.J., Pao, W., Pham, D. et al. (2006) 'Clinical course of patients with non-small cell lung cancer and epidermal growth factor receptor exon 19 and exon 21 mutations treated with gefitinib or erlotinib', *Clinical Cancer Research,* 12(3): 839–44.

Ring, A. (2010) 'The influences of age and co-morbidities on treatment decisions for patients with HER2-positive early breast cancer', *Critical Reviews in Oncology and Hematology,* 76(2): 127–32.

Ring, A., Harder, H., Langridge, C., Ballinger, R.S. and Fallowfield, L.J. (2013) 'Adjuvant Chemotherapy in Elderly Women with breast cancer (AChEW): an observational study identifying MDT perceptions and barriers to decision making', *Annals of Oncology,* 24(5): 1211–9.

Rischer, J., Scherwath, A., Zander, A.R., Koch, U. and Schulz-Kindermann, F. (2009) 'Sleep disturbances and emotional distress in the acute course of hematopoietic stem cell transplantation', *Bone Marrow Transplantation,* 44(2): 121–8.

Ritchie J. and Spencer L. (1994) 'Qualitative data analysis for applied policy research', in A. Bryman and R.G. Burgess (eds), *Analyzing Qualitative Data.* London: Routledge. pp. 173–94.

Ritchie, J., Spencer, L. and O'Connor, W. (2003) 'Carrying out qualitative analysis', in J. Ritchie and J. Lewis (eds), *Qualitative Research Practice.* London: Sage Publications. pp. 219–62.

Ritter, J. and Bielack, S. (2010) 'Osteosarcoma', *Annals of Oncology,* 21(Suppl. 7): 320–5.

Robb, K., Stubbings, S., Ramirez, A., Macleod, U., Austoker, J., Waller, J., Hiom, S., Wardle, J. (2009) 'Public awareness of cancer in Britain: a population based survey of adults', *British Journal of Cancer,* 101(S2): S18–23.

Robb, S.L, Clair, A.A., Watanabe, M., Monahan, P.O., Azzouz, F., Stouffer, J.W., Ebberts, A., Darsie, E., Whitmer, C., Walker, J., Nelson, K., Hanson-Abromeit, D., Lane, D. and Hannan, A. (2008) 'Randomised controlled trial of the active music engagement (AME) intervention on children with cancer', *Psycho-oncology,* 17(7): 699–708.

Robert, G., Cornwell, J., Brearley, S., Foot, C., Goodrich, J., Joule, N., Levenson, R., Maben, J., Murrells, T., Tsianakas, V. and Waite, D. (2011) *What Matters to Patients? Developing the Evidence Base for Measuring and Improving Patient Experience. Project Report for the Department of Health and NHS Institute for Innovation & Improvement.* London: Kings Fund. Available from: www.institute.nhs.uk/images/Patient_Experience/Final%20Project%20Report%20pdf%20doc%20january%202012.pdf [accessed 18 November 2014]

Roberts, G. and Holmes, J. (1998) *Healing Stories: Narrative in Psychiatry and Psychotherapy.* Oxford: Oxford University Press.

Roberts, I.S.D., Benamore, R.E., Benbow, E.W., Lee, S.H., Harris, J.N., Jackson, A., Mallett, S., Patankar, T., Peebles, C., Roobottom, C. and Traill, Z.C. (2012) 'Post-mortem imaging as an alternative to autopsy in the diagnosis of adult deaths: a validation study', *Lancet,* 379: 136–42.

Roberts, M. (2012) 'Fewer premature births after smoking ban in Scotland', *BBC News Health.* Available from: www.bbc.co.uk/news/health-17262897 [accessed 22 July 2012].

Robinson, K.A, Dennison, C.R, Wayman, D.M., Pronovost, P.J. and Needham, D.M. (2007) 'Systematic review identifies number of strategies important for retaining study participants', *Journal of Clinical Epidemiology,* 60: 757–65.

Robson, D. and Gray, R. (2007) 'Serious mental illness and physical health problems: a discussion paper', *International Journal of Nursing Studies*, 44: 457–66.

Rock, C.L. and Demark-Wahnefried, W. (2002) 'Nutrition and survival after the diagnosis of breast cancer: a review of the evidence', *Journal of Clinical Oncology*, 20(15): 3302–16.

Rodriguez, K.L., Bayliss, N., Alexander, S.C. et al. (2010) 'How oncologists and their patients with advanced cancer communicate about health-related quality of life', *Psycho-oncology*, 19(5): 490–9.

Roe, H. (2011) 'Chemotherapy-induced alopecia: advice and support for hair loss', *British Journal of Nursing (Oncology Suppl.)*, 20(10): S4–11.

Roellig, C., Theide, C., Gramatzky, M. et al (2010) 'A novel prognostic model in elderly patients with acute myeloid leukaemia. Results of 909 patients entered into the prospective AML 96 trial', *Blood*, 116: 971–8.

Rolland, J.S. (1994) *Families, Illness and Disability: An Integrative Treatment Model*. New York, NY: Basic Books.

Rolland, J.S. (1999) 'Parental illness and disability: a family systems framework', *Journal of Family Therapy*, 21: 242–66.

Roscoe, J.A., Morrow, G., Bushunow, P., Tian, L. and Matteson, S. (2002) 'Acustimulation wristbands for the relief of chemotherapy-induced nausea', *Alternative Therapies in Health and Medicine*, 8(4): 56–63.

Rose, H. and Cohen, K. (2010) 'The experiences of young carers: a meta-synthesis of qualitative findings', *Journal of Youth Studies*, 13(4): 473–87.

Rose, M., Owens, S. and Hastings, D. (2012) 'Therapy with unsealed radionuclides', in P. Symonds, C. Deehan, J.A. Mills and C. Meredith (eds), *Walter and Miller's Textbook of Radiotherapy*, 7th edn. London: Elsevier Churchill Livingstone. pp. 113–20.

Rose, P. (2011) 'The experience of receiving radiation therapy', *The Australian Journal of Cancer Nursing*, 12(1): 10–15.

Rosenblatt, P.C. (1983) *Bitter, Bitter Tears: Nineteenth Century Diaries and Twentieth Century Grief Theories*. Minneapolis, MN: University of Minnesota Press.

Rosenblatt, P.C., Walsh, R. and Jackson, D.A. (1976) *Grief and Mourning in Cross-cultural Perspective*. New Haven, CT: Human Relations Area File.

Rosenbloom, S.K., Victorson, D.E., Hahn, E.A., Peterman, A.H. and Cella, D. (2007) 'Assessment is not enough: a randomized controlled trial of the effects of HRQL assessment on quality of life and satisfaction in oncology clinical practice', *Psycho-oncology*, 16: 1069–79.

Rosenstock, I.M. (1974) 'The Health Belief Model and preventive health behavior', *Health Education & Behavior*, 2: 364–86.

Rossi-Ferrario, S., Zotti, A.M., Massara, G. and Nuvolone, G. (2003) 'A comparative assessment of psychological and psychosocial characteristics of cancer patients and their caregivers', *Psycho-oncology*, 12: 1–7.

Rost, A.D., Wilson, K.G., Buchanan, E., Hildebrandt, M.J. and Mutch, D. (2012) 'Improving psychological adjustment among late-stage ovarian cancer patients: examining the role of avoidance in treatment', *Cognitive & Behavioural Practice*, 19: 508–17.

Roth, A.J., Kornblith, A.B., Batel-Copel, L., et al. (1998) 'Rapid screening for psychologic distress in men with prostate carcinoma: a pilot study', *Cancer*, 82: 1904–08.

Roth, A.J. and Modi, R. (2003) 'Psychiatric issues in older cancer patients', *Critical Reviews in Oncology and Hematology*, 48(2): 185–97.

Rotter, J.B. (1966) 'Generalized expectancies for internal versus external control of reinforcement', *Psychological Monographs: General and Applied*, 80(1): 1–28.

Rouillon, F., Gasquet, I., Garay, R.P. and Lancrenon, S. (2011) 'Screening for bipolar disorder in patients consulting general practitioners in France', *Journal of Affective Disorders*, 130(3): 492–5.

Roulson, J., Benbow, E.W. and Hasleton, P.S. (2005) 'Discrepancies between clinical and autopsy diagnosis and the value of post mortem histology: a meta-analysis and review', *Histopathology*, 47: 551–9.

Rowa-Dewar, N., Ager, W., Kearney, N. and Seaman, P. (2007) *Glasgow Public Involvement in Cancer*. Glasgow Centre for Population Health & Cancer Care Research Centre.

Rowland, J.H. (1989) 'Developmental stage and adaptation: child and adolescent model', in J.C. Hollandand and J.H. Rowland (eds), *Handbook of Psyhooncology*. London: OUP. pp. 519–543.

Roxby, P. (2012) 'Smoking ban's impact five years on', *BBC News Health*. Available from: www.bbc.co.uk/news/health-18628811 [accessed 22 July 2012].

Roy, R., Chun, J. and Powell, S.N. (2011) 'BRCA1 and BRCA2: different roles in a common pathway of genome protection', *Nature Reviews Cancer*, 12: 68–78.

Royal College of General Practitioners (1993) 'Barthel Activities of Daily Living (ADL) Index', *Occasional Paper Royal College General Practitioners*, 59: 24.

Royal College of General Practitioners (2011) *Management of Depression in Older People: Why This is Important in Primary Care*. Available from: www.rcgp.org.uk/gp-training-and-exams/~/media/Files/GP-training-and-exams/Management-of-Depression-factsheet.ashx [accessed 9 December 2013].

Royal College of Nursing (2012) *Patient Focus*. Available from: www.rcn.org.uk/development/practice/clinical_governance/patient_focus [accessed 18 November 2014].

Royal College of Pathologists (2009) *The Retention and Storage of Pathological Records and Specimens*, 4th edn. Available from: www.rcpath.org/Resources/RCPath/Migrated%20Resources/Documents/G/g031retentionstorageaugust09.pdf [accessed 31 July 2012].

Royal College of Physicians, Royal College of Radiologists, Royal College of Obstetricians and Gynaecologists (2007) *The Effects of Cancer Treatment on Reproductive Functions*. London: Royal College of Physicians.

The Royal College of Radiologists (2006) *Radiotherapy Dose-fractionation*. London: Royal College of Radiologists.

The Royal College of Radiologists (2008) *The Timely Delivery of Radical Radiotherapy, Standards and Guidelines for the Management of Unscheduled Treatment Interruptions*, 3rd edn. Board of Faculty of Clinical Radiologists, The Royal College of Radiologists. Available from: www.rcr.ac.uk/docs/oncology/pdf/BFCO(08)6_Interruptions.pdf [accessed 11 September 2014].

Royal College of Surgeons (2012) Access All Ages: Assessing the Impact of Age on Access to Surgical Treatment. Available from: www.rcseng.ac.uk/publications/docs/access-all-ages [accessed 9 December 2013].

Rubin, G., McPhail, S. and Elliott, K. (2011) *National Audit of Cancer Diagnosis in Primary Care*. London: Royal College of General Practitioners, National Cancer Intelligence Network, National Cancer Action Team, Department of Health. Gateway approval 16345.

Rubino, C., Perry, S.J., Milam, A.C. and Spitzmueller, C. (2012) 'Demand–Control–Person: Integrating the Demand–Control and Conservation of Resources Models to Test an Expanded Stressor–Strain Model', *Journal of Occupational Health Psychology*, 17 (4): 456–472.

Rudinger, E. (ed.) (1982) *Living with Stress*. London: Consumer Association.

Rushton, L., Hutchings, S.J., Fortunato, L., et al. (2012) 'Occupational cancer burden in Great Britain', *British Journal of Cancer*, 107(S1): S3–7.

Russ, T.C., Stamatakis, E., Hamer, M., Starr, J.M., Kivimäki, M. and Batty, G.D. (2012) 'Association between psychological distress and mortality: individual participant pooled analysis of 10 prospective cohort studies', *British Medical Journal*. doi:10.1136/bmj.e4933.

Russell, M., Raheja, V. and Jaiyesimi, R. (2013) 'Human papillomavirus vaccination in adolescence', *Perspectives in Public Health*, 133(6): 320–4.

Ruud, E. (1998) *Music Therapy: Improvisation, Communication and Culture*. Gilsum, NH: Barcelona Publishers.

Ryan, H., Schofield, P. and Butow, P. (2005) 'How to recognise and manage psychological distress in cancer patients', *European Journal of Cancer Care*, 14: 7–15.

Ryan, J.L., Bole, C., Hickok, J.T., Figueroa-Moseley, C., Colman, L., Khanna, R.C., Pentland, A.P. and Morrow, G.R. (2007) 'Post-treatment skin reactions reported by cancer patients differ by race, not by treatment or expectations', *British Journal of Cancer*, 97: 14–21.

Ryle, A. (1991) *Cognitive-Analytic Therapy: Active Participation in Change*. Chichester, UK: Wiley.

Ryle, A. and Kerr, I.B. (2002) *Introducing Cognitive Analytic Therapy*. Chichester, UK: Wiley.

Saegrov, S. and Halding, A.G. (2004) 'What is it like living with the diagnosis of cancer?' *European Journal of Cancer Care*, 13: 145–53.

Sage, N., Sowden M., Chorlton E., Edeleanu, A. (2008) *CBT for Chronic Illness and Palliative Care*. Hoboken, NJ: John Wiley and Sons Ltd.

Saleh, M., Barlow-Stewart, K., Meiser, B., Tucker, K., Eisenbruch, M. and Kirk, J. (2012) 'Knoweldge, attitudes and beliefs of Arabic–Australians concerning cancer', *Psycho-oncology*, 21: 195–202.

Saltz, L.B., Douillard, J.Y., Pirotta, N., Alakl, M., Gruia, G., Awad, L., et al. (2001) 'Irinotecan plus fluorouracil/leucovorin for metastatic colorectal cancer: a new survival standard', *Oncologist*, 6(1): 81–91.

Sanson-Fisher, R., Girgis, A., Boyes, A., Bonevski, B., Burton, L. and Cook P. (2000) 'The unmet supportive care needs of patients with cancer. Supportive Care Review Group', *Cancer*, 88(1): 226–237.

Sarna, L. (1998) 'Effectiveness of structured nursing assessment of symptom distress in advanced lung cancer', *Oncology Nursing Forum*, 25(6): 1041–8.

Sasco, A., Secretan, M.B. and Straif, K. (2004) 'Tobacco smoking and cancer: a brief review of the epidemiological evidence', *Lung Cancer*, 45: S3–9.

Sasieni, P. and Castanon, A. (2012) *Audit of Invasive Cervical Cancer: National Report 2007–2011*. Sheffield: NHS Cancer Screening Programmes.

Sasieni, P., Adams, J. and Cuzick, J. (2003) 'Benefits of cervical screening at different ages: evidence from the UK audit of screening histories', *British Journal of Cancer*, 89(1): 88–93.

Sasieni, P.D., Shelton, J., Ormiston-Smith, N., et al. (2011) 'What is the lifetime risk of developing cancer? The effect of adjusting for multiple primaries', *British Journal of Cancer*, 105(3): 460–5.

Satgé, D. and Vekemans, M. (2011) 'Down syndrome patients are less likely to develop some (but not all) malignant solid tumours', *Clinical Genetics*, 78(1): 35–7.

Satin, J.R., Linden, W. and Phillips MJ. (2009) 'Depression as a predictor of disease progression and mortality in cancer patients: a meta-analysis', *Cancer*, 115(22): 5349–61.

Sauer-Heilborn, A., Kadidlo, D. and McCullough, J. (2004) 'Patient care during infusion of hematopoietic progenitor cells', *Transfusion*, 44(6): 907–16.

Saunders, C.M. (1978) *The Management of Terminal Malignant Disease*. London: Edward Arnold.

Sawada, N.O., de Paula, J.M., Sonobe, H.M., Zago, M.M.F., Guerrero, G.P. and Nicolussi, A.C. (2012) 'Depression, fatigue, and health-related quality of life in head and neck cancer patients: a prospective pilot study', *Supportive Care in Cancer*, 20(11): 2705–11.

Scanlon, K. (2004) *An Investigation into Breast Cancer Related Knowledge, Beliefs and Attitudes Among Women from Minority Ethnic Groups Living in London and Sheffield: A Qualitative Study*. Breast Cancer Care UK (see CERP portal resources).

Schalock, R., Borthwick-Duffy, S., Bradley, V., Buntinx, W., Coulter, D., Craig, E., Gomez, S., Lachapelle, Y., Luckasson, R., Reeve, A., Shogren, K., Snell, M., Spreat, S., Tasse, M., Thompson, J., VerdugoAlonso, M., Wehmeyer, M. and Yeager, M. (2010) *Intellectual Disability: Definition, Classification, and System of Supports*, 11th edn. Washington, DC: American Association on Intellectual and Developmental Disabilities.

Schaverien, J. (2000) 'The triangular relationship and the aesthetic countertransference in analytical art psychotherapy', in A. Gilroy and G. McNeilly (eds), *The Changing Shape of Art Therapy*. London: Jessica Kingsley. pp. 55–84.

Schernhammer, E., Haidinger, G., Waldhor, T. Vargos, R. and Vutuc, C. (2010) 'A study of trends in beliefs and attitudes toward cancer', *Journal of Cancer Education*, 25(2): 211–16.

Schiffman, M., Castle, P.E., Jeronimo, J., et al. (2007) 'Human papillomavirus and cervical cancer', *Lancet*, 370(9590): 890–907.

Schiffman, M. and Wacholder, S. (2012) 'Success of HPV vaccination is now a matter of coverage', *Lancet*, 13(1): 10–12.

Schilling, C. (1993) *The Body and Social Theory*. London: Sage.

Schneider, S., Moyer, A., Knapp-Oliver, S., Sohl, S., Cannella, D. and Targhetta, V. (2010) 'Pre-intervention distress moderates the efficacy of psychosocial treatment for cancer patients: a meta-analysis', *Journal of Behavioural Medicine*, 33: 1–14.

Schnoll, R.A., Harlow, L.L., Stolbach, L.L. and Brandt, U. (1998) 'A structural model of the relationships among stage of disease, age, coping, and psychological adjustment in women with breast cancer', *Psycho-oncology*, 7(2): 69–77.

Schofield, P.E., Butow, P.N., Tompson, J.F., Tattersall, M.H., Beeney, L.J. and Dunn, S.M. (2003) 'Psychological responses of patients receiving a diagnosis of cancer', *Annals of Oncology*, 14: 48–56.

Scholz, U., Schüz, B., Ziegelmann, J.P., Lippke, S. and Schwarzer, R. (2008) 'Beyond behavioural intentions: planning mediates between intentions and physical activity', *British Journal of Health Psychology*, 13(3): 479–94.

Schröder, F.H., Hugosson, J., Roobol, M.J. et al. (2009) 'Screening and prostate-cancer mortality in a randomized European study', *The New England Journal of Medicine*, 360(13): 1320–8.

Schroevers, M. and Brandsma R. (2010) 'Is learning mindfulness associated with improved affect after mindfulness-based cognitive therapy?', *British Journal of Health Psychology*, 101: 95–107.

Schut, H. and Stroebe, M. (2010) 'Effects of support, counselling and therapy before and after loss: can we really help bereaved people?' *Psychologica Belgica*, 50(1&2): 89–102.

Schwarzer, R. (1992) *Self-Efficacy in the Adoption and Maintenance of Health Behaviors: Theoretical Approaches and a New Model*. Washington, DC: Hemisphere Publishing Corp.

Schwarzer, R. and Fuchs, R. (1996) 'Self-efficacy and health behaviours', in M. Conner and P. Norman (eds), *Predicting Health Behaviour: Research and Practice with Social Cognition Models*. Buckingham: Open University Press. pp. 163–96.

Schwarzer, R. and Luszczynska, A. (2008) 'How to overcome health-compromising behaviors: the health action process approach', *European Psychologist*, 13(2): 141–51.

Scott-Findlay, S. and Chalmers, K. (2001) 'Rural families perspectives on having a child with cancer', *Journal of Pediatric Nursing*, 205–207.

Scotté, F., Tourani, J.M., Banu, E., Peyromaure, M., Levy, E., Marsan, S., Magherini, E., Fabre-Guillevin, E., Andrieu, J.M. and Oudard, S. (2005) 'Multicenter study of a frozen glove to prevent docetaxel-induced onycholysis and cutaneous toxicity of the hand', *Journal of Clinical Oncology*, 23(19): 4424.

Scottish Executive (2001) *Cancer in Scotland: Action for Change*. Edinburgh: Scottish Executive.

Scottish Government (2008a) *Better Health, Better Care*. Edinburgh: Scottish Government.

Scottish Government (2008b) *Better Cancer Care, An Action Plan*. Edinburgh: Scottish Government.

Scottish Health Council (n.d.). Available from: www.scottishhealthcouncil.org/home.aspx [accessed 16 January 2012].

Scully, C., Epstein, J. and Sonis, S. (2003) 'Oral mucositis: a challenging complication of radiotherapy, chemotherapy, and radiochemotherapy: part 1 pathogenesis and prophylaxis of mucositis', *Head Neck*, 25(12): 1057–70.

Seddon, D., Timoney, M., Freeman, M. (2010) *National Primary Care Audit of Cancer Diagnoses: Findings of Linked Observations from Participating Practices in Merseyside and Cheshire, March 2010*. Available from: www.mccn.nhs.uk/fileuploads/File/NPCAudit%20write%20up%20-%20FULL%20FINAL%2014%20April%2010.pdf [accessed 18 November 2014].

Seitz, H.K., Pelucchi, C., Bagnardi, V. and La Vecchia, C. (2012) 'Epidemiology and pathophysiology of alcohol and breast cancer: update 2012', *Alcohol and Alcoholism*, 47(3): 204–12.

Selye, H. (1953) 'The General Adaptation Syndrome in its relationship to neurology, psychology and psychopathology', in A. Weider (ed.), *Contributions toward Medical Psychology: Theory and Psychodiagnostic Methods*. Vol. 1. New York, NY: Ronald Press Company. pp. 234–274.

Serra, R. and de Franciscis, S. (2014) 'The importance of extended thromboprophylaxis in patients undergoing major surgery for cancer', *Thrombosis Research*, 133: 965–6. doi:10.1016/j.thromres.2014.02.016.

Shah, A. and Coleman, M.P. (2007) 'Increasing incidence of of Leukaemias: a controversy re-examined', *British Journal of Cancer*, 77: 1009–1012.

Shaw, C. (1999) 'A framework for the study of coping, illness behaviour and outcomes', *Journal of Advanced Nursing,* 29(5): 1246–55.

Sheehan, D. and Draucker, C. (2011) 'Interaction patterns between parents with advanced cancer and their adolescent children', *Psycho-oncology,* 20(10): 1108–15.

Sheehan, D.V., Lecrubier, Y., Sheehan, K.H., Amorim, P., Janavs, J., Weiller, E., Hergueta, T., Baker, R. and Dunbar, G.C. (1998) 'The Mini-International Neuropsychiatric Interview (M.I.N.I.): the development and validation of a structured diagnostic psychiatric interview for DSM-IV and ICD-10', *Journal of Clinical Psychiatry,* 59(Suppl. 20): 22–33. [The complete M.I.N.I version 5.0.0 follows on pp. 34–57].

Shelburne, N. and Bevans, M. (2009) 'Non-myeloablative allogeneic hematopoietic stem cell transplantation', *Seminars in Oncology Nursing,* 25(2): 120–8.

Shennan, C., Payne. S. and Fenlon, D. (2011) 'What is the evidence for the use of mindfulness-based interventions in cancer care? A review', *Psycho-oncology,* 20: 681–97.

Shepherd, F.A., Rodrigues, P.J., Ciuleanu, T., et al. (2005) 'Erlotinib in previously treated non-small-cell lung cancer', *New England Journal of Medicine,* 353(2): 123–132.

Shewale, S. and Parekh, S. (2013) 'In concert with pediatric clinical trials', *Clinical Practice,* 10(2): 167–75.

Shim, E.J., Mehnert, A., Koyama, A., Cho, S.J., Inui, H., Paik, N.S. et al. (2006) 'Health-related quality of life in breast cancer: a cross-cultural survey of German, Japanese, and South Korean patients', *Breast Cancer Research and Treatment,* 99: 341–50.

Shimizu, K., Ishibashi, Y., Umezawa, S., et al (2010) 'Feasibility and usefulness of the "distress screening program in ambulatory care" in clinical oncology practice', *Psycho-oncology,* 19: 718–25.

Shin, D.W., Cho, J., Roter, D.L, Kim, S.Y., Sohn, S.K., Yoon, M.S., Kim, Y.W., Cho, B. and Park, J.H. (2013) 'Preferences for and experiences of family involvement in cancer treatment decision-making: patient-caregiver dyads study', *Psycho-oncology,* 22(11): 2624–31.

Shippee, N., Shah, N., May, C.R., Mair, F.S. and Montori, V.M. (2012) 'Cumulative complexity: a functional, patient-centred model of patient complexity can improve research and practice', *Journal of Clinical Epidemiology,* 65(10): 1041–51.

Shontz, F.C. (1975) *The Psychological Aspects of Physical Illness & Disability.* New York, NY: Macmillan.

Siegel, K., Raveis, V.H. and Karus, D. (2000) 'Correlates of self-esteem among children facing the death of a parent to cancer', in L. Baider, C.L. Cooper and A. Kaplan De-Nour (eds), *Cancer and the Family.* Chichester, UK: Wiley. pp. 223–37.

Sigurdson, A. and Jones, I. (2003) 'Second cancers after radiotherapy: any evidence for radiation induced genomic instability?' *Oncogene,* 22: 7018–27.

Silverman, J., Kurtz, S. and Draper, J. (2008) *Skills for Communicating with Patients,* 2nd edn. Oxford: Radcliffe Publishing.

Silverman, P.R., Nickman, S. and Worden, J.W. (1992) 'Detachment revisited', *American Journal of Orthopsychiatry,* 62(4): 494–593.

Silverstone, L. (1997) *Art Therapy – the Person-Centred Way: Art and Development Of The Person.* London: Jessica Kingsley.

Simillis, C., Li, T., Vaughan, J., Becker, L.A., Davidson, B.R. and Gurusamy, K.S. (2014) 'Methods to decrease blood loss during liver resection: a network meta-analysis', *Cochrane Database of Systematic Reviews,* Issue 4, CD010683. doi:10.1002/14651858.CD010683.pub2.

Singh, J.A., Sloan, J.A., Atherton, P.J., Smith, T., Hack, T.F., et al (2010) 'Preferred roles in treatment decision making among patients with cancer: a pooled analysis of studies using the Control Preferences Scale', *American Journal of Managed Care,* 16(9): 688–96.

Sjovall, K., Strombeck, G., Lofgren, A., Bendahl P.O. and Gunnars, B. (2010) 'Adjuvant radiotherapy of women with breast cancer – information, support and side effects', *European Journal of Oncology Nursing,* 14: 147–53.

Skaali, T., Fossa, S.D., Bremmes, R., Dahl, O., Haaland, C.F., Hauge, E.R., Klepp, O.N., Oldenburg, J., Wist, E. and Dahl, A.A. (2009) 'Fear of recurrence in long term testicular cancer survivors', *Psycho-oncology,* 18: 580–8.

Skarstein, J., Aass, N., Fossa, S.D., et al. (2000) 'Anxiety and depression in cancer patients: relation between the Hospital Anxiety and Depression Scale and the European Organization for Research and Treatment of Cancer Core Quality of Life Questionnaire', *Journal of Psychosomatic Research*, 49: 27–34.

Slade, T. and Andrews, G. (2001) 'DSM-IV and ICD-10 generalized anxiety disorder: discrepant diagnoses and associated disability', *Social Psychiatry and Psychiatric Epidemiology*, 36(1): 45–51.

Sleeper, R.B. (2009) 'Geriatric primer – common geriatric syndromes and special problems', *Consultant Pharmacist*, 24(6): 447–62.

Smallwood, C. (2005) *The Role of Complementary and Alternative Medicine in the NHS*. Kings's Fund.

Smedslund, G. and Ringdal, G.I. (2004) 'Meta-analysis of the effects of psychosocial interventions on survival time in cancer patients', *Journal of Psychosomatic Research*. 57(2): 123–31; discussion 133–5.

Smith, A., Juraskova, I., Butow P., Miguel C., Lopez A., Chang S., Brown R. and Bernhard, J. (2011) 'Sharing vs caring: the relative impact of sharing decisions versus managing emotions on patient outcomes', *Patient Education and Counseling*, 82: 233–9.

Smith, J.A. (2004) 'Reflecting on the development of interpretative phenomenological analysis and its contribution to qualitative research in psychology', *Qualitative Research in Psychology*, 1: 39–54.

Smith, J.A. (2011) 'Evaluating the contribution of interpretative phenomenological analysis', *Health Psychology Review*, 5(1): 9–27.

Smith, J.A., Flowers, P. and Larkin, M. (2009) *Interpretative Phenomenological Analysis: Theory, Method & Research*. London: Sage Publications.

Smith, J.E., Richardson, J., Hoffman, C. and Pilkington, K. (2005) 'Mindfulness-based stress reduction as supportive therapy in cancer care: systematic review', *Journal of Advanced Nursing*, 52(3): 315–27.

So, W.K. and Chui, Y.Y. (2007) 'Women's experience of internal radiation treatment for uterine cervical cancer', *Journal of Advanced Nursing*, 60(2): 154–61.

Sobin, L., Gospodarowicz, M. and Wittekind, C. (eds) (2010) *TNM Classification of Malignant Tumours*, 7th edn. UICC International Union Against Cancer. London: Wiley-Blackwell.

Social Care Institute for Excellence (2011) *Research Briefing 39: Preventing Loneliness and Social Isolation: Interventions and Outcomes*. Available from: www.scie.org.uk/publications/briefings/files/briefing39.pdf [accessed 9 December 2013].

Socie, G., Salooja, N., Cohen, A., Rovelii, A., Carreras, E., Locasciulli, A., Korthof, E., Weis, J., Levy, V. and Tichelli, A. (2003) 'Nonmalignant late effects after allogeneic stem cell transplantation', *Blood*, 101(9): 3373–85.

Society of Radiographers (2011a) *Summary of Interventions for Acute Radiotherapy-Induced Skin Reactions in Cancer Patients: A Clinical Guideline Recommended for Use by The Society and; College of Radiographers*. Available from: www.sor.org/learning/document-library/summary-interventions-acute-radiotherapy-induced-skin-reactions-cancer-patients-clinical-guideline [accessed 29 August 2014].

Society of Radiographers (2011b) *A UK Survey of Radiotherapy Skin Care by SCoR*. Available from: www.sor.org/learning/document-library/uk-survey-radiotherapy-skin-care-scor [accessed 11 September 2014].

Society of Radiographers (2013) *A Guide to Modern Radiotherapy*. Available from: www.sor.org/learning/document-library/guide-modern-radiotherapy [accessed 4 November 2014].

Sohn, P.M. and Loveland Cook, C.A. (2002) 'Nurse practitioner knowledge of complementary and alternative health care: foundation for practice', *Journal of Advanced Nursing*, 39(1): 9–16.

Söllner, W., DeVries, A., Steixner, E., Lukas, P., Sprinzl, G., Rumpold, G. and Maislinger, S. (2001) 'How successful are oncologists in identifying patient distress, perceived social support, and need for psychosocial counselling?' *British Journal of Cancer*, 84(2): 179–85.

Solsona, E., Algabab, F., Horenblasc, S., Pizzocarod, G. and Windahle, T. (2004) 'EAU guidelines on penile cancer', *European Urology*, 46: 1–8.

Søndenaa, K., Quirke, P., Hohenberger, W., Sugihara, K., Kobayashi, H., Kessler, H., Brown, G., Tudyka, V., D'Hoore, A., Kennedy, R.H., West, N.P., Kim, S.H., Heald, R., Storli, K.E.,

Nesbakken, A. and Moran, B. (2014) 'The rationale behind complete mesocolic excision (CME) and a central vascular ligation for colon cancer in open and laparoscopic surgery : proceedings of a consensus conference', *International Journal of Colorectal Disease,* 29: 419–28. doi:10.1007/s00384-013-1818-2.

Soriano, A., Castells, A., Ayuso, C., Ayuso, J.R., de Caralt, M.T., Ginès, M.A., Real, M.I., Gilabert, R., Quintó, L., Trilla, A., Feu, F., Montanyà, X., Fernández-Cruz, L. and Navarro, S. (2004) 'Preoperative staging and tumor resectability assessment of pancreatic cancer: prospective study comparing endoscopic ultrasonography, helical computed tomography, magnetic resonance imaging, and angiography', *American Journal of Gastroenterology,* 99: 492–501.

Spira, M. and Kenemore E. (2000) 'Adolescent daughters of mothers with breast cancer: impact and implications', *Clinical Social Work Journal,* 28: 183–95.

Spitzer, R.L., Williams, J.B., Gibbon, M. and First, M.B. (1992) 'The structured clinical interview for DSM-III-R (SCID). I: History, rationale, and description', *Archives of General Psychiatry,* 49(8): 624–9.

Spitzer, R.L., Kroenke, K., Williams, J.B., et al. (1999) 'Validation and utility of a self-report version of the PRIME-MD: the PHQ primary care study', *Journal of the American Medical Association,* 282: 1737–1744.

Staden, H. (1998) 'Alertness to the needs of others: a study of the emotional labour of caring', *Journal of Advanced Nursing,* 27: 147–56.

Stajduhar,K.I., Thorne, S.E., McGuinness, L. and and Kim-Sing, C. (2010) 'Patient perceptions of helpful communication in the context of advanced cancer', *Journal of Clinical Nursing,* 19: 2039–2047.

Stang, A., Trocchi, P., Ruschke, K., Schmidt-Pokrzywniak, A, Holzhausen, H-J., Loning, T., Buchmann, J., Thomssen, C., Lantzsch, T., Hauptmann, S., Bocker, W. and Kluttig, A. (2011) 'Factors influencing the agreement in histopathological assessments of breast biopsies among pathologists', *Histopathology,* 59: 939–49.

Stanton, A.L., Danoff-Burg, S., Cameron, C., Bishop, M., Collins, C.A., Kirk, S.B., Sworwski, L.A. and Twillman, R. (2000) 'Emotional expressive coping predicts psychological and physical adjustment to breast cancer', *Journal of Consulting and Clinical Psychology,* 68(5): 875–82.

Stanworth, R. (2004) *Recognizing Spiritual Needs in People Who Are Dying.* Oxford: Oxford University Press.

Stayt, L.C. (2009) 'Death, empathy and self-preservation: the emotional labour of caring for families of the critically ill in adult intensive care', *Journal of Clinical Nursing,* 18: 1267–75.

Stebbins, W.G., Garibyan, L. and Sober, A.J. (2010) 'Sentinel lymph node biopsy and melanoma: 2010 update: Part I,' *Journal of the American Academy of Dermatology,* 62(5): 723–34.

Stefanek, M., McDonald, P. and Hess, S. (2005) 'Religion, spirituality and cancer: current status and methodological challenges', *Psycho-oncology,* 14(6): 450–63.

Steginga, S.K., Occhipinti, S., Dunn, J., Gardiner, RA., Heathcote, P. and Yaxley, J. (2001) 'The supportive care needs of men with prostate cancer', *Psycho-oncology,* 10(1): 66–75.

Steliarova-Foucher, E., Stiller, C., Kaatsch, P., Berrino, F. and Coebergh, J. (2005) 'Trends in childhood cancer incidence in Europe 1970–1999', *Lancet,* 365(9477): 2088.

Stenberg, U., Ruland, C.M. and Miaskowski, C. (2010) 'Review of the literature on the effects of caring for a patient with cancer', *Psycho-oncology,* 19: 1013–25.

Stickel, F., Schuppan, D., Hahn, E.G. and Seitz, H.K. (2002) 'Cocarcinogenic effects of alcohol in hepatocarcinogenesis', *Gut,* 51(1): 132–9.

Stiller, C.A. (2007) *Childhood Cancer in Britain: Incidence, Survival, Mortality.* Oxford: Oxford University Press.

Stiller, C.A. (2009) *Incidence of Childhood Leukaemia: Factsheet.* Environmental and Health Information System, World Health Organization.

Stiller, C.A. (2010) *National Registry of Childhood Tumours: Progress Report 2010.* Childhood Cancer Research Group. Available from: www.ncin.org.uk/view.aspx?rid=492 [accessed 8 August 2012].

Stiller, C.A. and Shah, A. (2012) 'The epidemiology of cancer in children and adolescents', in M.C.G. Stevens, C.N. Hubert and A. Biondi (eds), *Cancer in Children: Clinical Management*, 6th edn. Oxford: Oxford University Press. pp. 1–13.

Stiller, C.A., Kroll, M.E. and Pritchard-Jones, K. (2012) 'Population survival from childhood cancer in Britain during 1978-2005 by eras of entry into clinical trials', *Annals of Oncology*, 9: 2464–2469.

Stilos, K. Doyle, C. and Daines, P. (2008) 'Addressing the sexual health needs of patients with gynecologic cancers', *Clinical Journal of Oncology Nursing*, 12(3): 457–63.

Street, A. F., Couper, J. W., Love, A. W., Bloch, S., Kissane, D. W., and Street, B.C. (2010) 'Psychosocial adaptation in female partners of men with prostate cancer', *European Journal of Cancer Care*, 19: 234–242.

Street, C. (2013) 'Promoting physical well-being', in E. Collins, M. Drake and and M. Deacon (eds), *The Physical Care of People with Mental Health Problems: A Guide for Best Practice*. London: Sage. pp. 158–170.

Stroebe, M.S. and Schut, H. (1999) 'The dual process model of coping with bereavement: rationale and description', *Death Studies*, 23: 197–224.

Strong, V., Waters, R., Hibberd, C., Murray, G., Wall, L., Walker, J., McHugh, G., Walker, A. and Sharpe, M. (2008) 'Management of depression for people with cancer (SMaRT oncology 1): a randomised trial', *Lancet*, 372(9632): 40–8.

Stubbings, S., Robb, K., Waller, J., Ramirez, A., Austoker, J., Macleod, U., Hiom, S. and Wardle, J. (2009) 'Development of a measurement tool to assess public awareness of cancer', *British Journal Cancer,* 101(Suppl. 2): S13–17.

Studer, G., Graetz, K. and Glanzmann, C. (2008) 'Outcome in recurrent head neck cancer treated with salvage-IMRT', *Radiation Oncology,* 3: 43–50.

Stussi, G. and Tsakiris, D.A. (2012) 'Late effects on haemostasis after haematopoietic stem cell transplantation', *Hämostaseologie*, 32: 63–6.

Sullivan, S.G., Hussain, R., Slack-Smith, L.M. and Bittles, A.H. (2003) 'Breast cancer and the uptake of mammography screening services by women with intellectual disabilities', *Preventative Medicine*, 37: 507–12.

Sulmasy, D.P. (2006) *The Rebirth of the Clinic: An Introduction to Spirituality in Health Care*. Washington, DC: Georgetown University Press.

Summerton, N. (1999) *Diagnosing Cancer in Primary Care*. Abingdon, UK: Radcliffe Medical Press.

Sun, C.-L., Francisco, L., Baker, K., Weisdorf, D.J., Forman, S.J. and Bhatia, S. (2011) 'Adverse psychological outcomes in long-term survivors of hematopoietic cell transplantation: a report from the Bone Marrow Transplant Survivor Study (BMTSS)', *Blood*, 118(17): 4723–31.

Sutton, S. (2004) 'Determinants of health-related behaviours: theoretical and methodological issues', in S. Sutton, A. Baum, and M. Johnston (eds), *The Sage Handbook of Health Psychology*. London: Sage Publications. pp. 94–126.

Svavarsdottir, E. (2005) 'Caring for a child with cancer: a longitudinal perspective', *Journal of Advanced Nursing*, 50(2): 153–61.

Svirbeley, J. (2009) *Series on Medical Algorythms*. Houston, TX: Springer.

Swash, B., Hulbert-Williams, N.J. and Bramwell, R. (2014) 'Unmet psychosocial needs in haematological cancer: a systematic review', *Supportive Care in Cancer*, 22(4): 1131–41.

Symonds, P. and Deehan, C. (2012) 'Brachytherapy', in P. Symonds, C. Deehan, J.A. Mills and C. Meredith (eds), *Walter and Miller's Textbook of Radiotherapy*, 7th edn. London: Elsevier Churchill Livingstone. pp. 189–200.

Symonds, P. and Meredith, C. (2012) 'Principles of management of patients with cancer', in P. Symonds, C. Deehan, J.A. Mills and C. Meredith (eds), *Walter and Miller's Textbook of Radiotherapy*, 7th edn. London: Elsevier Churchill Livingstone. pp. 293–300.

Szarewski, A., Cadman L, Mesher D et al. (2011) 'HPV self-sampling as an alternative in non-attenders for cervical screening: a randomised controlled trial', *British Journal of Cancer*. doi:10.1038/bjc.2011.48.

Taenzer, P., Bultz, B.D., Carlson, L.E., Speca, M., DeGagne, T., Olson, K., et al. (2000) 'Impact of computerized quality of life screening on physician behaviour and patient satisfaction in lung cancer outpatients', *Psycho-oncology,* 9: 203–13.

Tafalla, M., Sanchez-Moreno, J., Diez, T. and Vieta, E. (2009) 'Screening for bipolar disorder in a Spanish sample of outpatients with current major depressive episode', *Journal of Affective Disorders,* 114(2009): 299–304.

Tammemagi, C.M., Neslund-Dudas, C., Simoff, M. and Kvale, P. (2004) 'Smoking and lung cancer survival: the role of comorbidity and treatment,' *CHEST Journal,* 125(1): 27–37.

Tang, H., Greenwood, G.L., Cowling, D.W., Lloyd, J.C., Roeseler, A.G. and Bal, D.G. (2004) 'Cigarette smoking among lesbians, gays, and bisexuals: how serious a problem?', *Cancer Causes and Control,* 15(8): 797–803.

Tantamango-Bartley, Y., Jaceldo-Siegl, K., Fan, J. and Fraser, G. (2013) 'Vegetarian diets and the incidence of cancer in a low-risk population', *Cancer Epidemiology Biomarkers & Prevention,* 22(2): 286–94.

Tariman, J.D., Berry, D.L., Cochrane, B., Doorenbos, A. and Schepp, K. (2010) 'Preferred and actual participation roles during health care decision making in persons with cancer: a systematic review', *Annals of Oncology,* 21: 1145–51.

Taylor, A. and Gosney, M.A. (2011) 'Sexuality in older age: essential considerations for healthcare professionals', *Age and Ageing,* 40(5): 538–43.

Taylor, C., Richardson, A. and Cowley, S. (2011) 'Surviving cancer treatment: an investigation of the experience of fear about, and monitoring for, recurrence in patients following treatment for colorectal cancer', *European Journal of Oncology Nursing,* 15(3): 243–9.

Taylor, G.W., Jayne, D.G., Brown, S.R., Thorpe, H., Brown, J.M., Dewberry, S.C., Parker, M.C. and Guillou, P.J. (2010) 'Adhesions and incisional hernias following laparoscopic versus open surgery for colorectal cancer in the CLASICC trial', *British Journal of Surgery,* 97: 70–78.

Taylor, R.E. (2006) 'Principles of paediatric radiation oncology', in P. Hoskin (ed.), *Radiotherapy in Practice: External Beam Therapy.* Oxford: Oxford University Press. pp. 405–38.

Taylor, R.E and Powell, M.E.B. (2006) 'Uterus', in P. Hoskin (ed.), *Radiotherapy in Practice: External Beam Therapy.* Oxford: Oxford University Press. pp. 235–52.

Taylor, S., Harley, C., Campbell, L.J., Bingham, L., Podmore, E.J., Newsham, A.C., Selby, P.J., Brown, J.M. and Velikova, G. (2011) 'Discussion of emotional and social impact of cancer during outpatient oncology consultations', *Psycho-oncology,* 20(3): 242–51.

Taylor, S.E. (2008) *Health Psychology,* 7th edn. New York, NY: McGraw-Hill Higher Education.

Teasdale, J.D.S. (1995) 'How does cognitive therapy prevent depressive relapse and why should attentional control (mindfulness) training help?', *Behaviour Research and Therapy,* 33(1).

Temel, J.S., Greer, J.A., Muzikansky, A., Gallagher, E.R., Admane, S., Jackson, V.A., Dahlin, C.M., Blinderman, C.D., Jacobsen, J., Pirl, W.F., Billings, J.A. and Lynch, T.J. (2010) 'Early Palliative care for patients with secondary non small cell lung cancer', *New England Journal of Medicine,* 363: 733–42.

Temming, P. and Jenney, M.E.M. (2011) 'The neuro-developmental sequelae of childhood leukaemia and its treatment', *Archives of Disease in Childhood,* 95: 936–940.

Terracini, B. (2009) 'Epidemiology of childhood cancer', *Environmental Health,* Suppl. 1(58): 1–3.

Terzioglu, F., Şimsek, S., Karaca, K., Sariince, N., Altunsoy, P. and Salman, M.C. (2013) 'Multimodal interventions (chewing gum, early oral hydration and early mobilisation) on the intestinal motility following abdominal gynaecologic surgery', *Journal of Clinical Nursing,* 22: 1917–25.

Thain, C. (2006) 'Ethical issues', in M. Grundy (ed.) *Nursing in Haematological Oncology,* 2nd edn. Edinburgh: Ballière Tindall.

The Princess Royal Trust for Carers (2011) *Always on Call, Always Concerned.* Available from: www.carers.org/sites/default/files/always_on_call_always_concerned.pdf [accessed 9 December 2013].

The, A-M. (2002) *Palliative Care and Communication: Experiences in the Clinic.* Buckingham, UK: Open University Press.

Thewes, B., Butow, P., Stuart-Harris, R., et al, (2009) 'Does routine psychological screening of newly diagnosed rural cancer patients lead to better patient outcomes? Results of a pilot study', *Australian Journal of Rural Health*, 17: 298–304.

Thewes, B., Butow, P., Zachariae, R., Christensen, S., Simard, S. and Goaty, C. (2011) 'Fear of cancer recurrence: a systematic literature review of self-report measures', *Psycho-oncology*. doi:10.1002/pon.2070.

Thomas, C., Morris, S. and Harman, J. (2002) 'Companions through cancer: the care given by informal carers in cancer contexts', *Social Science & Medicine*, 54: 529–44.

Thomas, G. (1998) 'What lies within us: individuals in a Marie Curie Hospice', in M. Pratt and M.J. Wood (eds), *Art Therapy in Palliative Care: The Creative Response*. Oxford: Routledge. pp. 64–75.

Thombs, B.D., Coyne, J.C. and Cuijpers, P. et al. (2011) 'Rethinking recommendations for screening for depression in primary care', *Canadian Medical Association Journal*, 184(4): 413–18.

Thompson, A.G.H. (2007) 'The meaning of patient involvement and participation in health-care consultations: a taxonomy', *Social Science & Medicine*, 64: 1297–1310.

Thompson, A. and Chambers, E. (2011) 'Ethical issues in qualitative mental health research', in D. Harper and A.R. Thompson (eds), *Qualitative Research Methods in Mental Health and Psychotherapy: A Guide for Students and Practitioners*. London: Wiley-Blackwell. pp. 23–38.

Thompson, A. and Russo, K. (2012) 'Ethical dilemmas for clinical psychologists in conducting qualitative research', *Qualitative Research in Psychology*, 9: 32–46.

Thorne, B. (2012) *Counselling and Spiritual Accompaniment*. Chichester, UK: Wiley-Blackwell.

Thorne, S.E., Bultz, B.D., Baile, W.F. and SCRN Communication Team (2005) 'Is there a cost to poor communication in cancer care? A critical review of the literature', *Psycho-oncology*, 14: 875–84.

Thornicroft, G. (2011) 'Physical health disparities and mental illness: the scandal of premature mortality', *British Journal of Psychiatry*, 199: 441–2.

Tillich, P. (1980) *The Courage To Be*. New Haven, CT: Yale University Press.

Tipton, J. (2013) 'Nausea and vomiting', in C.H. Yarbro, D. Wujcik and B.H. Gobel (eds), *Cancer Symptom Management*, 4th edn. Burlington, VT: Jones and Bartlett Learning. pp. 213–240.

Tjasink, M. (2010) 'Art psychotherapy in medical oncology: a search for meaning', *International Journal of Art Therapy*, 15(2): 75–83.

Todres, L. and Holloway, I. (2010) 'Phenomenological research', in K. Gerrish and A. Lacey (eds), *The Research Process in Nursing*. Chichester, UK: Wiley-Blackwell. pp. 177–87.

Torrance, A.D.W., Almond, L.M., Fry, J., Wadley, M.S. and Lyburn, I.D. (2013) 'Has integrated 18F FDG PET/CT improved staging, reduced early recurrence or increased survival in oesophageal cancer?', *Surgeon-Journal of The Royal Colleges of Surgeons of Edinburgh and Ireland*, 13(1): 19–33.

Townsend, N., Wickramasinghe, K., Bhatnagar, P., Smolina, K., Nichols, M., Leal, J., Luengo-Fernandez, R. and Rayner, M. (2012) *Coronary Heart Disease Statistics 2012 Edition*. London: British Heart Foundation.

Tracey, A. (2011) 'Perpetual loss and pervasive grief', *Cruse Bereavement Care*, 30(3): 17–24.

Tramacere, I., Negri, E., Bagnardi, V., Garavello, W., Rota, M., Scotti, L., et al. (2010) 'A meta-analysis of alcohol drinking and oral and pharyngeal cancers. Part 1: overall results and dose-risk relation', *Oral Oncology*, 46(7): 497–503.

Trask, P.C., Paterson, A., Riba, M., Brines, B., Griffith, K., Parker, P., Weick, J., Steele, P., Kyro, K. and Ferrara, J. (2002) 'Assessment of psychological distress in prospective bone marrow transplant patients', *Bone Marrow Transplantation*, 29: 917–25.

Travis, K. (2009) 'Psychosocial oncology research faces uncertain future in UK', *Journal of the National Cancer Institute*, 101(11): 777–9.

Trepanier, A., Ahrens, M., McKinnon, W. et al. (2004) 'Genetic cancer risk assessment and counseling: recommendations of the National Society of Genetic Counselors', *Journal of Genetic Counselling*, 13(2): 83–114.

Trigg, M.E., Harland, N., Sather, H.N., Reaman, G.H., Tubergen, D.G., Steinherz, P.G., Gaynon, P.S., Fatih, M. and Hammond, D. (2008) 'Ten-year survival of children with acute lymphoblastic leukaemia: a report from the Childhood Oncology Group', *Journal of Clinical Oncology*, 49(6): 1142–1154.

Tsang, M. and Guy, R.H. (2010) 'Effect of aqueous cream BP on human stratum corneum in vivo', *British Journal of Dermatology*, 163(5): 954–8.

Tsitsikas, D.A., Brothwell, M., Chin Aleong, J-A. and Lister, A.T. (2011) 'The attitudes of relatives to autopsy: a misconception', *Journal of Clinical Pathology*, 64: 412–14.

Tuah, N.A., Amiel, C., Qureshi, S., Car, J., Kaur, B. and Majeed, A. (2012) 'Transtheoretical model for dietary and physical exercise modification in weight loss management for overweight and obese adults', The Cochrane Library, 8: 1–73.

Tuffrey-Wijne, I. (2010) *Living with Learning Disabilities, Dying With Cancer: Thirteen Personal Stories*. London: Jessica Kingsley.

Tuffrey-Wijne, I. (2013) 'A new model for breaking bad news to people with intellectual disabilities', *Palliative Medicine*, 27(1): 5–12.

Tuffrey-Wijne, I., Giatras, N., Butler, G. and Cresswell, A. (2012) 'People with intellectual disabilities who are affected by a relative or friend with cancer: a qualitative study exploring experiences and support needs', *European Journal of Oncology Nursing*, 16(5): 512–519.

Tuffrey-Wijne, I., Giatras, N., Goulding, L., Abraham, E., Fenwick, L., Edwards, C. and Hollins, S. (2013) 'Identifying the factors affecting the implementation of strategies to promote a safer environment for patients with learning disabilities in NHS hospitals: a mixed-methods study', *Health Services & Delivery Research*, 1(13). doi: 10.3310/hsdr01130.

Tuffrey-Wijne, I. and McEnhill, L. (2008) 'Communication difficulties and intellectual disability in end-of-life care', *International Journal of Palliative Nursing*, 14(4): 192–7.

Turati, F., Garavello, W., Tramacere, I., Pelucchi, C., Galeone, C., Bagnardi, V., et al. (2012) 'A meta-analysis of alcohol drinking and oral and pharyngeal cancers: results from subgroup analyses', *Alcohol and Alcoholism*, 48(1): 107–18.

Turner, B.S. (1991) 'Missing bodies: towards a sociology of embodiment', *Sociology of Health and Illness*, 13(2): 265–73.

Turner, D., Adams, E. and Boulton, M., et al. (2011) 'Partners and close family members of long-term cancer survivors: health status, psychosocial well-being and unmet supportive care needs', *Psycho-oncology*, 22(1): 12–19.

Turner, M., Payne S. and O'Brien T. (2011) 'Mandatory communication skills training for cancer and palliative care staff: does one size fit all', *European Journal of Oncology Nursing*, 15: 398–403.

Turner, N.J., Haward, R.A., Mulley, G.P. and Selby, P.J. (1999) 'Cancer in old age: is it inadequately investigated and treated?', *British Medical Journal*, 1999: 319.

Tuttle, R.M., Tala, H., Lebouef, R., Ghossein, R., Gonen, M., Brokhin, M., et al (2010) 'Estimating risk of recurrence in differentiated thyroid cancer after total thyroidectomy and radioactive iodine remnant ablation: using response to therapy variables to modify the initial risk estimates predicted by the new American Thyroid Association staging system', *Thyroid*, 20: 1341–9.

Tveit, K.M., Guren, T., Gilmelius, B. et al. (2012) 'Phase III trial of cetuximab with continuous or intermitant fluorouracil, leocovorin and oxaliplatin (Nordic FLOX) verus FLOX alone in first line treatment of metastatic colorectal cancer: the NORDIC-VII study', *Journal of Clinical Oncology*, 30: 1755–62.

Twigg, J (2000) 'Carework as a form of body work', *Aging and Society*, 20: 389–411.

Twycross, R. (1995) *Introducing Palliative Care*. Oxford, UK: Radcliffe Medical.

Uitterhoeve, R.J., Bensing, J., Dilven, E., Donders, R., deMulder, P. and van Achterberg, T. (2009) 'Nurse-patient communication in cancer care: does responding to patient's cues predict patient satisfaction with communication', *Psycho-oncology*, 18(10): 1060–8.

Uitterhoeve, R.J., Vernooy, M., Litjens, M., Potting, K., Bensing, J., De Mulder, P. and van Achterberg, T. (2004) 'Psychosocial interventions for patients with advanced cancer – a systematic review of the literature', *British Journal of Cancer*, 91: 1050–62.

UK National Screening Committee (2010) *The UK NSC Policy on Prostate Cancer Screening/Psa Testing in Men over the age of 50*. Policy database. Available from www.screening.nhs.uk/prostatecancer [accessed 1 January 2014].

UK National Screening Committee (2014). Available from: www.screening.nhs.uk/ [accessed 6 January 2015].

UK National Statistics (2013) *Older People*. Available from: www.statistics.gov.uk/hub/population/ageing/older-people [accessed 8 January 2013].

UK Oncology Nursing Society (UKONS) (2013a) *UKONS Reports and Resources*. Available at: http://ukons.org/index.php/reports/P12 (accessed 22 January 2015).

UK Oncology Nursing Society (UKONS) (2013b) *UKONS: Acute Oncology Prevention and Management Guidelines: Chemotherapy-Induced Nausea and Vomiting (CINV)*. Available from: ukons.org/contentimages/Treatment-protocol-A5-v7.pdf [accessed 26 February 2015].

UK Stem Cell Strategic Forum (2010) *The Future of Unrelated Donor Stem Cell Transplantation in the UK Part 1: Findings and Recommendations*. Watford: NHS Blood and Transplant.

US Department for Health and Human Services (2009) *National Cancer Institute's Common Terminology Criteria for Adverse Events (CTCAE) Version 4.0*. Published: May 28, 2009 (v4.03: June 14, 2010).

Vachon, M.L.S. (2010) 'Oncology staff stress and related interventions', in J.C. Holland, W.S. Breitbart, P.B. Jacobsen, M.S. Lederberg, M.J. Loscalzo and R.S. McCorkle (eds), *Psychooncology*, 2nd edn. New York, NY: Oxford University Press.

Vadaparampil, S.T., Miree, C.A., Wilson, C., et al. (2006–2007) 'Psychosocial and behavioral impact of genetic counseling and testing', *Breast Dis.*,27: 97-108.

Vallurupalli, M., Lauderdale, K., Balboni, M.J., et al (2012) 'The role of spirituality and religious coping in the quality of life of patients with advanced cancer receiving palliative radiation therapy', *Journal of Supportive Oncology*, 10: 81–7.

Van Cutsem, E., Köhne, C.H., Hitre, E. et al. (2009) 'Cetuximab and chemotherapy as initial treatment for metastatic colorectal cancer', *The New England Journal of Medicine*, 360(14): 1408–17.

van de Poll-Franse, L.V., Mols, F., Vingerhoets, A.J., Voogd, A.C., Roumen, R.M. and Coebergh, J.W. (2006) 'Increased health care utilisation among 10-year breast cancer survivors', *Supportive Care in Cancer*, 14(5): 436–43.

Van Oers, J.A., Bongers, I.M., Van de Goor, L.A. and Garretsen, H.F. (1999) 'Alcohol consumption, alcohol-related problems, problem drinking, and socioeconomic status', *Alcohol and Alcoholism*, 34(1): 78–88.

Van Putte, C., Regan, J. and Russo, A. (2014) *Seeley's Anatomy and Physiology*, 10th edn. New York, NY: McGraw-Hill International.

Van Ryn, M., Sanders, S., Kahn, K., van Houtven, C., Griffin, J., Martin, M., Atienza, A., Phelan, S., Finstad, D. and Rowland J. (2011) 'Objective burden, resources and other stressors among informal cancer caregivers: a hidden quality issue?', *Psycho-oncology*, 20: 44–52.

van Scheppingen, C., Schroevers, M.J., Pool, G., Smink, A., Mul, V. E., Coyne, J. C. and Sanderman, R. (2014) 'Is implementing screening for distress an efficient means to recruit patients to a psychological intervention trial?', *Psycho-Oncology*, 23: 516–523.

van Scheppingen, C., Schroevers, M.J., Smink, A., et al. (2011) 'Does screening for distress efficiently uncover meetable unmet needs in cancer patients?' *Psycho-oncology*, 20(6): 655–63.

van Uden-Kraan, C.F., Drossaert, C.H.C., Taal, E., Seydel, E.R. and van de Laar, M.A.F.J. (2009) 'Participation in online patient support groups endorses patients' empowerment', *Patient Education and Counseling*, 74: 61–9.

Vanderwerker, L.C., Laff, R.E., Kadan-Lottick, N.S., McColl, S. and Prigerson, H.G. (2005) 'Psychiatric disorders and mental health service use among caregivers of advanced cancer patients', *Journal of Clinical Oncology*, 23: 6899–907.

Vandyk, A.D. and Baker, C. (2012) 'Qualitative descriptive study exploring schizophrenia and the everyday effect of medication-induced weight gain', *International Journal of Mental Health Nursing*, 21: 349–57.

Velikova, G., Booth, L., Smith, A.B., Brown, P.M., Lynch, P., Brown, J.M., et al. (2004) 'Measuring quality of life in routine oncology practice improves communication and patient well-being: a randomized controlled trial', *Journal of Clinical Oncology*, 22: 714–24.

Velikova, G., Keding, A., Harley, C., Cocks, K., Booth, L., Smith, A.B., Wright, P., Selby, P.J. and Brown, J.M. (2010) 'Patients report improvements in continuity of care when quality of life assessments are used routinely in oncology practice: secondary outcomes of a randomised controlled trial', *European Journal of Cancer*, 46(13): 2381–8.

Venables, K. (2006) 'Basic physics', in P. Hoskin (ed.), *Radiotherapy in Practice: External Beam Therapy*. Oxford: Oxford University Press. pp. 7–26.

Verschuur, A., Van Tinkren, H., Graf, H., Bergeron, C., Sandstedt, B. and de Kraker, J. (2012) 'Treatment of pulmonary metastases in children with stage IV nephroblastoma with risk-based use of pulmonary radiation', *Journal of Clinical Oncology*, 30(28): 3533–3539.

Vidall, C., Dielenseger, P., Farrell, C., Lennan, E., Muxagata, P., Fernández-Ortega, P. and Paradies, K. (2011) 'Evidence-based management of chemotherapy-induced nausea and vomiting: a position statement from a European cancer nursing forum', *Ecancermedicalscience*, 5: 211.

Virshup, D.M. and McCance, K., L. (2010) 'Biology of cancer', in K.L. McCance, S.E. Huether (eds), *Pathophysiology: the Biologic Basis for Disease in Adult and Children*, 6th edn. Elsevier: London. pp. 333–74.

Visser, A., Huizinga, G.A., van der Graaf, W.T., Hoekstra, H.J. and Hoekstra-Weebers, J.E. (2004) 'The impact of parental cancer on children and the family: a review of the literature', *Cancer Treatment Reviews*, 30: 683–94.

Vodermaier, A. and Linden, W. (2008) 'Emotional distress screening in Canadian cancer care: a survey of utilization, tool choices and practice patterns'. *Oncology Exchange*, 7(4): 37–9.

Vodermaier, A., Linden, W. and Siu, C. (2009) 'Screening for emotional distress in cancer patients: a systematic review of assessment instruments', *Journal of the National Cancer Institute*, 101(21): 1464–88.

Vogel, B.A., Bengal, J. and Helmes, A.W. (2008) 'Information and decision making: patients' needs and experiences in the course of breast cancer treatment', *Patient Education and Counseling*, 71(1): 70–85.

Voigtmann, K., Kollner, V., Einsle., Franziska., Alheit, H., Joraschky, P., Herrmann, T. (2010) 'Emotional state of patients in radiotherapy and how they deal with their disorder', *Strahlentherapie und Onkologie*, 186(4): 229–35.

von Essen, L., Larsson, G., Oberg, K. and Sjoden, P.O. (2002) '"Satisfaction with care": associations with health-related quality of life and psychosocial function among Swedish patients with endocrine gastrointestinal tumours', *European Journal of Cancer*, 11: 91–9.

Von Korff, M., Gruman, J., Schaefer, J., Curry, S.J. and Wagner, E.H. (1997) 'Collaborative management of chronic illness', *Annals of Internal Medicine*, 127: 1097–102.

Wagener, P. (2009) *The History of Oncology*. Houston, TX: Springer.

Wald, N. and Nicolaides-Bouman, A. (1991) *UK Smoking Statistics 1991*. Maidenhead, UK: Open University Press.

Waldrop, D.P. (2007) 'Caregiver grief in terminal illness and bereavement: a mixed-methods study', *Health & Social Work*, 52(3): 197–206.

Waller, D. (1991) *A History of Art Therapists 1940–82*. London: Routledge.

Waller, J., Macedo, A., von Wagner, C., et al. (2012) 'Communication about colorectal cancer screening in Britain: public preferences for an expert recommendation', *British Journal of Cancer*, 107(12): 1938–43.

Waller, J., Robb, K., Stubbings, S., Ramirez, A., Macleod, U., Austoker, J., Hioms, S., Wardle, J. (2009) 'Awareness of cancer symptoms and anticipated help seeking among ethnic minority groups in England', *British Journal of Cancer*, 101(S2): S24–30.

Wallston, K.A. (1992) 'Hocus-pocus, the focus isn't strictly on locus: Rotter's social learning theory modified for health', *Cognitive Therapy and Research*, 16(2): 183–99.

Wallston, K.A., StrudlerWallston, B. and DeVellis, R. (1978) 'Development of the multidimensional health locus of control (MHLC) scales', *Health Education & Behavior*, 6(1): 160–70.

Walter, T. (2010) *Grief and Culture. Best of Bereavement Care 2009/2010*. London: CRUSE.

Ward, S., Viergutz, G., Tormey, D., DeMuln, J. and Paillen, A. (1992) 'Patients' reactions to completion of adjuvant breast cancer therapy', *Nursing Research*, 42(6): 362–6.

Warren, G.W., Kasza, K.A., Reid, M.E., Cummings, K.M. and Marshall, J.R. (2012) 'Smoking at diagnosis and survival in cancer patients', *International Journal of Cancer*, 132(2): 401–410.

Watson, E., Sugden, E.M. and Rose, P. (2010) 'Views of primary care physicians and oncologists on cancer follow-up initiatives in primary care: an online survey', *Journal of Cancer Survivorship*, 4, 159–66.

Watson, M., Dos Santos, M., Greer, S., Baruch, J. and Bliss, J. (1994) 'The Mini-MAC: further development of the Mental Adjustment to Cancer Scale', *Journal of Psychosocial Oncology*, 12(3): 33–46.

Watson, M., Greer, S., Young, J., Inayat, Q., Burgess, C. and Robertson, B. (1988) 'Development of a questionnaire measure of adjustment to cancer: the MAC scale', *Psychological Medicine*, 18: 203–9.

Weaver, K., Rowland, J., Alfano, C. and McNeel, T. (2010) 'Parental cancer and the family', *Cancer*, 116: 4395–401.

Wei, S., Said-Al-Naief, N. and Hameed, O. (2009) 'Estrogen and progesterone receptor expression is not always specific for mammary and gynecologic carcinomas: a tissue microarray and pooled literature review study', *Applied Immunohistochemistry and Molecular Morphology*, 17(5): 393–402.

Weiner, L.S., Steffen-Smith, E., Battles, H.B., Wayne, A., Love, C.P. and Fry, T. (2007) 'Sibling stem cell donor experiences at a single institution', *Psycho-oncology*, 17(3): 304–7.

Weinstein, N.D. (1982) 'Unrealistic optimism about susceptibility to health problems, *Journal of Behavioral Medicine*, 5(4): 441–60.

Weinstein, N.D. (1987) 'Unrealistic optimism about susceptibility to health problems: conclusions from a community-wide sample', *Journal of Behavioral Medicine*, 10(5): 481–500.

Weir, H.K., Kreiger, N. and Marrett, L.D. (1998) 'Age at puberty and risk of testicular germ cell cancer (Ontario, Canada)', *Cancer Causes and Control*, 9: 253–8.

Welch, A.S., Wadworth, M.E. and Compas, B.E. (1996) 'Adjustment of children and adolescents to parental cancer: parents' and children's perspectives', *Cancer*, 77: 1409–18.

Weller, D.P. and Campbell, C. (2009) 'Uptake in cancer screening programmes: a priority in cancer control', *British Journal of Cancer*, 101(Suppl. 2): S55–9. doi:10.1038/sj.bjc.6605391.

Weller, D.P., Patnick, J., McIntosh, H.M. and Dietrich, A.J. (2009) 'Uptake in cancer screening programmes', *Lancet Oncology*, 10(7): 693–9.

Wells, D.J. (2004) 'Gene therapy progress and prospects: electroporation and other physical methods', *Gene Therapy*, 11: 1363–9.

Wells, M. (1998) 'The hidden experience of radiotherapy to the head and neck: a qualitative study of patients after completion of treatment', *Journal Advanced Nursing*, 28: 840–8.

Wells, M. (2003) 'The treatment trajectory', in S. Faithfull and M. Wells (eds), *Supportive Care in Radiotherapy*. Edinburgh: Churchill Livingstone. pp. 39–59.

Wells, M. and MacBride, S. (2003) 'Radiation skin reactions', in S. Faithfull and M. Wells (eds), *Supportive Care in Radiotherapy*. Edinburgh: Churchill Livingstone. pp. 135–59.

Wells, M., Macmillan, M., Raab, G., MacBride, S., Bell, N., MacKinnon, K., MacDougall, H., Samuel, L. and Munro, A. (2004) 'Does aqueous or sucralfatecream affect the severity of erythematous radiation reactions? A randomised control trial', *Radiotherapy and Oncology*, 73(2): 153–62.

Welsh Government (2012) *Together for Health-Cancer Delivery Plan: A Delivery Plan up to 2016 for NHS Wales and its Partners*. Welsh Government.

Wengström, V.Y., Häggmark, C., Strander, H. and Forsberg, C. (1999) 'Effects of a theory based nursing intervention on breast cancer patients receiving radiation therapy: a randomized controlled study', *Acta Oncologica*, 38(6): 763–770.

Wenzlaff, R.M. and Wegner, D.M. (2000) 'Thought suppression', *Annual Review of Psychology*, 51(1): 59–91.

West, M.A., Lythgoe, D., Barben, C.P., Noble, L., Kemp, G.J., Jack, S. and Grocott, M.P.W. (2014) 'Cardiopulmonary exercise variables are associated with postoperative morbidity after major colonic surgery: a prospective blinded observational study', *British Journal of Anaesthesia*, 112: 665–71.

Westbrook, D., Kennerley, H. and Kirk, J. (2011) *An Introduction to Cognitive Behaviour Therapy: Skills and Applications*, 2nd edn. London: Sage Publications.

White, A.K., Thomson, C.S., Forman, D. and Meryn, S. (2009) 'Men's health and the excess burden of cancer in men', *European Urology Supplements*, 9: 467–70.

White, D. (2006) 'The hidden costs of caring: what managers need to know', *Health Care Manager,* 25(4): 341–7.

White, I., Faithfull, S. and Allan, H. (2013) 'The re-construction of women's sexual lives after pelvic radiotherapy: a critique of social constructionist and biomedical perspectives on the study of female sexuality after cancer treatment', *Social Science & Medicine,* 76: 188–96.

White, M. and Epston, D. (1990) *Narrative Means to Therapeutic Ends.* New York, NY: WW Norton & Co.

Whitehead, M. (1987) *The Health Divide*, London: Health Education Council.

Whooley, M.A., Avins, A.L., Miranda, J et al. (1997) 'Case-finding instruments for depression. Two questions are as good as many', *Journal of General Internal Medicine,* 12: 439–45.

Wigram, T. (2004) *Improvisation.* London: Jessica Kingsley.

Wigram, T., Pedersen, I.N. and Bonde, L.O. (eds) (2002) *A Comprehensive Guide to Music Therapy.* London: Jessica Kingsley.

Wilkins, J. (2000) 'Pioneering spirit: cervical screening for women with learning disabilities', *Learning Disability Practice,* 3(1): 4–8.

Wilkinson, R. and Pickett, K. (2010) *The Spirit Level: Why Equality is Better for Everyone* Harmondsworth: Penguin.

Wilkinson, S., Aldridge, J., Salmon, I., Cain, E. and Wilson, B. (1999) 'An evaluation of aromatherapy massage in palliative care', *Palliat Med.,*13(5): 409–417.

Wilkinson S., Barnes K. and Storey L. (2008) 'Massage for symptom relief in patients with cancer: systematic review', *Journal of Advanced Nursing,* 63(5): 430–439

Wilkinson, S., Perry, R., Blanchard, K. (2008) 'Effectiveness of a 3-day communication skills-course in changing nurses communication skills with cancer/palliative care patients: a randomised control trial', *Palliative Medicine,* 22: 365–75.

Wilkinson, S.M. (1991) 'Factors which influence how nurses communicate with cancer patients', *Journal of Advanced Nursing,* 16: 677–88.

Williams, A.F., Franks, P.J. and Moffat, C.J. (2005) 'Lymphoedema: estimating the size of the problem', *Palliative Medicine,* 19: 300–13.

Williams, C. and Johnson, M.R.D. (2010) *Race and Ethnicity in a Welfare Society.* New York, NY: Open University Press/McGraw Hill. Available from: www.mcgraw-hill.co.uk/html/0335225314.html

Williams, L., McCarthy, M.C., Eyles D, Drew S. (2013) 'Parenting a child with cancer: perceptions of adolescents and parents of adolescents and younger children following completion of childhood cancer treatment', *Journal of Family Studies,* 19(1): 80–9.

Williams, S. and Dale, J. (2006) 'The effectiveness of treatment for depression/depressive symptoms in adults with cancer: a systematic review', *British Journal of Cancer,* 94: 372–90.

Williamson, J.M.L., Jones, I.H. and Hockey, D.B. (2011) 'How does the media profile of cancer compare with prevalence?', *Annals of the Royal College of Surgeons England,* 93: 9–12.

Wilson, J.M.G. and Jungner G. (1968) *Principles and Practice of Screening for Disease.* Public Health Paper Number 34. Geneva: World Health Organization.

Wilson, K.G. and DuFrene, T. (2009) *Mindfulness for Two: An Acceptance and Commitment Therapy Approach to Mindfulness in Psychotherapy.* Oakland, CA: New Harbinger Press.

Wingard, J.R. (2002) 'The conundrum of chronic graft-versus-host disease'. *Bone Marrow Transplantation,* 12: 3–16.

Wingard, J.R., Majhil, N.S., Brazauskas, R. et al (2011) 'Long-term survival and late deaths after allogeneic hematopoietic stem cell transplantation', *Journal of Clinical Oncology,* 29: 2230–9.

Winzelberg, A.J., Classen, C., Alpers, G.W., Roberts, H., Koopman, C., Adams, R.E., Ernst, H., Dev, P. and Barr Taylor, C. (2003) 'Evaluation of an internet support group for women with primary breast cancer', *Cancer,* 97(5): 1164–73.

Witek-Janusek, L., Albuquerque, K., Chroniak, K.R., Chroniak, C., Durazo-Arvizu, R. and Mathews H.L. (2008) 'Effect of mindfulness based stress reduction on immune function, quality of life and coping in women newly diagnosed with early stage breast cancer', Brain Behavior, and Immunity, 22(6): 969–81.

Withey, S., Pracy, P. and Whys-Evans, P. (2000) 'Lymphodoema of the head and neck', in R. Twycross, K. Jenns and J. Todd (eds), Lymphoedema. Abingdon: Radcliffe Medical Press Ltd.

Wittchen, H.U., Robins, L.N., Cottler, L.B., Sartorius, N., Burke, J.D. and Regier, D. (1991) 'Cross-cultural feasibility, reliability and sources of variance of the Composite International Diagnostic Interview (CIDI). The multicentre WHO/ADAMHA field trials', British Journal of Psychiatry, 159: 645–53, 658.

Wolin, K., Yan, Y., Colditz, G.A. and Lee, I.M. (2009) 'Physical activity and colon cancer prevention: a meta-analysis', British Journal of Cancer, 100(4): 611–6.

Wood, M.J.M. (2005) 'Shoreline: the realities of working in cancer and palliative care', in D. Waller and C. Sibbert (eds), Art Therapy and Cancer Care. Madenhead, UK: Open University Press. pp. 82–102.

Wood, M.J.M., Low, J., Molassiotis A. and Tookman, A. (2013) 'Art therapy's contribution to the psychological care of adults with cancer: a survey of art therapists and service users in the UK', International Journal of Art Therapy-Inscape, 18(2): 42–53.

Wood, M.J.M., Molassiottis, A. and Payne, S. (2011) 'What research evidence is there for the use of art therapy in the management of symptoms in adults with cancer? A systematic review', Psycho-oncology, 20: 135–45.

Woodgate, R. (2006) 'Life is never the same: childhood cancer narratives', European Journal of Cancer Care, 15: 8–18.

Woodgate, R. and Degner, L. (2003) 'A substantive theory of keeping the spirit alive: the spirit within children with cancer and their families', Journal of Pediatric Oncology Nursing, 20(3): 103–119.

Woodgate, R.L. and Degner, L.F. (2004) 'Cancer symptom transition periods of children and families', Journal of Advanced Nursing, 46(4): 358–368.

Worden, J.W. (1991) Grief Counselling and Grief Therapy: A Handbook for the Mental Health Practitioner. 2nd edn. London: Springer.

Worden, J.W. (1996) Children and Grief: When a Parent Dies. New York, NY: Guilford Press.

Worden, J.W. (2008) Grief Counselling and Grief Therapy. A Handbook for the Mental Health Practitioner. 4th edn. London: Springer.

World Cancer Research Fund and the American Institute for Cancer Research. (2007) Food, Nutrition, Physical Activity, and the Prevention of Cancer: A Global Perspective. Washington, DC: American Institute for Cancer Research. Available from: www.wcrf.org/cancer_research/cup/

World Health Organization (WHO) (1948) Manual of the International Classification of Diseases, Injuries and Causes of Death, 6th edn. Geneva: World Health Organization.

World Health Organization (WHO) (1995) World Health Report. Geneva: World Health Organization.

World Health Organization (1999) WHOQOL Annotated Bibliography of the WHO Quality of Life Assessment Instrument – WHOQOL. Geneva: World Health Organization.

World Health Organization (WHO) (2001) The World Health Organization Report 2001 – Mental Health: New Understanding New Hope. Geneva: World Health Organization.

World Health Organization (WHO) (2002) National Cancer Control Programmes: Policies and Mangerial Guidelines, 2nd edn. Geneva: WHO.

World Health Organization (WHO) (2003) Framework Convention on Tobacco Control World Health Organization 2003. Available from: http://whqlibdoc.who.int/publications/2003/9241591013.pdf [accessed 18 April 2014].

World Health Organization (WHO) (2009) Cancer Mortality Database. Available from: www.who.int/whosis/mort/download/en/index.html [accessed on 15 February 2012].

World Health Organization (WHO) (2011). Factsheet Number 339. Tobacco. Available from: www.who.int/mediacentre/factsheets/fs339/en/ [accessed 18 April 2014].

World Health Organization (WHO) (2013a) WHO Definition of Palliative Care. Available from: www.who.int/cancer/palliative/definition/en/ [accessed March 2013].

World Health Organization (WHO) (2013b) *Health Status Statistics: Mortality*. Available from: www.who.int/healthinfo/statistics/indhale/en/ (accessed 10 November 2014].

World Literacy Foundation (2012) *The Economic and Social Cost of Illiteracy: A Snapshot of Illiteracy and its Causes in the UK and a Global Context*. Available from: www.worldliteracy-foundation.org/interim-report.html [accessed 18 November 2014].

Worster, B. and Holmes, S. (2009) 'A phenomenological study of the postoperative experiences of patients undergoing surgery for colorectal cancer', *European Journal of Oncology Nursing*, 13(5): 315–322.

Wright, J.R., Whelan, T.J., Schiff, S., Dubois, S., Crooks, D., Haines, P.T., de Rosa, D., Robers, R.S., Gafni, A., Pritchard, K. and Levine, M.N. (2004) 'Why cancer patients enter randomized clinical trials: exploring the factors that influence their decision', *Journal of Clinical Oncology*, 22(21): 4321–8.

Wright, M. and Leahey M. (2005) *Nurses and Families. A Guide to Family Assessment and Interventions*. 4th edn. Philadelphia, PA: FA Davis.

Wu, Y., Zhang, D. and Kang, S. (2013) 'Physical activity and risk of breast cancer: a meta-analysis of prospective studies. *Breast Cancer Research*, 137(3): 869–82.

Wujcik, D. (2013) 'Mucositis', in C.H. Yarbro, D. Wujcik and B.H. Gobel eds *Cancer Symptom Management*, 4th edn. Burlington, VT: Jones and Bartlett Learning. pp. 403–420.

Wyatt, D. and Talbot P. (2013) 'What knowledge and attitudes do paid carers of people with a learning disability have about cancer?', *European Journal of Cancer Care*, 22(3): 300–7.

Wyatt, G., Sikorskii, A., Rahbar, M.H., Victorson, D. and Adams, L. (2010) 'Intervention fidelity: aspects of complementary and alternative medicine research', *Cancer Nursing*, 33(5): 331–42.

Yalom, I.D. (2011) *Staring at the Sun*. London: Piatkus.

Yalom, I.D. and Lesczc, M. (2005) *The Theory and Practice of Group Psychotherapy*. New York, NY: Basic Books.

Yang, C.P., Hung, I.J., Jaing, T.H. and Chang, W.H. (2006) Cancers in infancy: percent distribution and incidence rates', *Acta Paediatrica Taiwanica*, 47 (6) :273–277.

Yarbro, C., Wujcik, D. and Gobel, B.H., et al (eds) (2011) *Cancer Nursing Principles and Practice*. London: Jones and Bartlett.

Yarbro, C.H., Wujcik, D. and Holmes Gobel, B. (eds) (2013) *Cancer Symptom Management*, 4th edn. Burlington, VT: Jones and Bartlett Learning.

Yardley, L. and Marks, D.F. (2004) 'Introduction to research methods in clinical and health psychology', in D. Marks and L. Yardley (eds), *Research Methods for Clinical & Health Psychology*. London: Sage Publications. pp. 1–20.

Yellen, S.B., Cella, D.F., Webster, K., Blendowski, C. and Kaplan, E. (1997) 'Measuring fatigue and other anemia-related symptoms with the Functional Assessment of Cancer Therapy (FACT) measurement system', *Journal of Pain and Symptom Management*, 13: 63–74.

Yi, J.C. and Syrjala, K.L. (2009) 'Sexuality after hematopoietic stem cell transplantation', *Cancer Journal*, 15(1): 57–64.

Yi, S.G., Wray, N.P., Jones, S.L., Bass, B.L., Nishioka, J., Brann, S., Ashton, C.M. (2013) 'Surgeon-specific performance reports in general surgery: an observational study of initial implementation and adoption', *Journal of the American College of Surgeons*, 217: 636–647.

Yoshida, T., Kakimoto, K., Takezawa, K., Arai, Y., Ono, Y., Meguro, N., Kinouchi, T., Nishimura, K. and Usami, M. (2009) 'Surveillance following orchiectomy for stage I testicular seminoma: long-term outcome', *International Journal of Urology*, 16: 756–9.

You, E., Song, H., Cho, J. and Lee, J. (2014) 'Reduction in the incidence of hospital-acquired *Clostridium difficile* infection through infection control interventions other than the restriction of antimicrobial use', *International Journal of Infectious Diseases*, 22: 9–10.

Young, A., Crowe, M, Lennan, E., Roe, H., Sharp, S., Vidall, C. and White, T. (2009) 'Delivery of chemotherapy at planned dose and on time', *Cancer Nursing Practice*, 8(5): 16–19.

Young, B., Dixon-Woods, M., Findlay, M. and Heney, D. (2002) 'Parenting in a crisis: conceptualising mothers of children with cancer', *Social Science & Medicine*, 55: 1835–47.

Young, A.N., Master, V.A., Paner, G.P., Wang, M.D. and Amin, M.B. (2008) 'Renal epithelial neoplasms: diagnostic applications of gene expression profiling', *Advances in Anatomic Pathology*, 15(1): 28–38.

Zaider, T. and Kissane, D.W. (2010) 'Psychosocial interventions for couples and families coping with cancer', in J. Holland, W.S. Breitbart, P.B. Jacobsen, M.S. Lederberg, M.J. Loscalzo and R. McCorkle, *Psycho-Oncology*, 2nd edn. Oxford: Oxford University Press. pp. 483–90.

Zapf, D. (2002) 'Emotion work and psychological well-being: a review of the literature and some conceptual considerations', *Human Resource Management,* Review, 12: 237–68.

Zaritsky, E. and Dibble, S.L. (2010) 'Risk factors for reproductive and breast cancers among older lesbians', *Journal of Women's Health*, 19 (1): 125–131.

Zealley, A.K. and Aitken, R.C.B. (1969) 'Measurement of mood', *Proceedings of the Royal Society of Medicine*, 62: 993–6.

Zhu, Z., Zhang, J., Liu, Y., Chen, M., Guo, P. and Li, K. (2014) 'Efficacy and toxicity of external-beam radiation therapy for localised prostate cancer: a network meta-analysis', *British Journal of Cancer*, 110(10): 2396–2404.

Zigmond, A.S. and Snaith, R.P. (1983) 'The Hospital Anxiety and Depression Scale', *Acta Psychiatrica Scandinavica*, 67: 361–70.

Zimmerman, C., Del Piccolo, L., Mazzi, M.A. (2003) 'Patient cues and medical interviewing in general practice. Example of the application of sequence analysis', *Epidemiolgia Epsichitria Sociale,* 12(2): 115–24.

Zimmerman, C., Del Piccalo, L., Finset, A. (2007) 'Cues and concerns by patients in medical consultations: a literature review', *Psychological Bulletin*, 133: 438–63.

Zinzani, P.L. Gandolfi, L. and Stefoni, V., et al. (2010) 'Yttrium-90 ibritumomab tiuxetan as a single agent in patients with pretreated B-cell lymphoma: evaluation of the long-term outcome', *Clinical Lymphoma Myeloma Leukemia*, 10(4): 258–61.

Zitella, L.J. (2013) 'Infection', in C.H. Yarbro, D. Wujcik and B.H. Gobel (eds), *Cancer Symptom Management,* 4th edn. Burlington, VT: Jones and Bartlett Learning.

Zollman, C. and Vickers, A. (1999) 'What is complementary medicine?', *British Medical Journal,* 319: 693–6.

AUTHOR INDEX

SUBJECT INDEX